Medicine and Surgery of South American Camelids

Medicine and Surgery of South American Camelids

Llama
Alpaca
Vicuña
Guanaco

MURRAY E. FOWLER, DVM

IOWA STATE UNIVERSITY PRESS / AMES

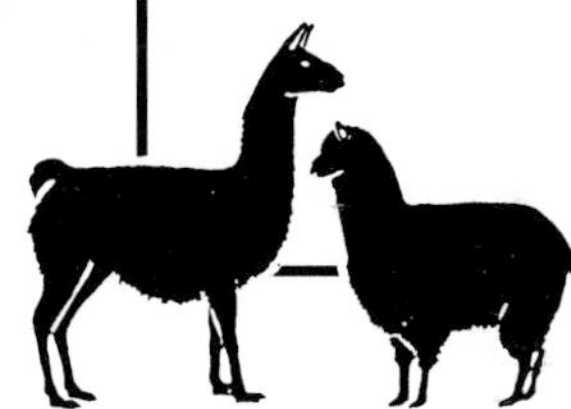

Grateful acknowledgment is given
for the special assistance of Audrey C. Fowler

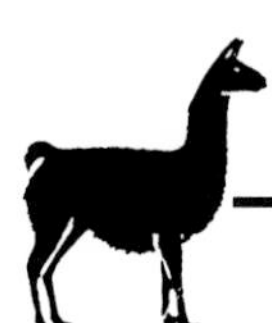

Murray E. Fowler is professor of veterinary medicine, School of Veterinary Medicine, University of California, Davis.

♾ Printed on acid-free paper in the United States of America

First edition, 1989
Second printing, 1991
Third printing, 1993

Library of Congress Cataloging-in-Publication Data
Fowler, Murray E.
Medicine and surgery of South American camelids: llama, alpaca, vicuña, guanaco/Murray E. Fowler.—1st ed.
p. cm.
Includes index.
ISBN 0-8138-0393-4
1. Lama (Genus)—Diseases. 2. Vicuña—Diseases. 3. Llama—Surgery. 4. Vicuña—Surgery. I. Title.
SF997.5.L35F68 1989
636.2′96—dc19 89–1870
CIP

Contents

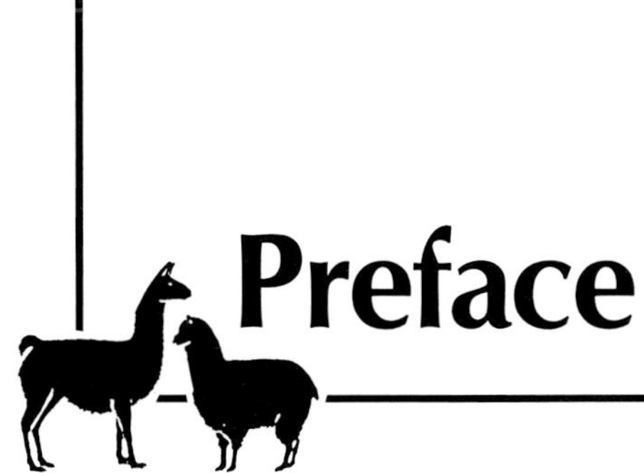

Preface

TWENTY years ago a book on South American camelid (SAC) medicine would have been of little interest for veterinarians except for the few who dealt with zoo populations. Today, the llama and alpaca industry is burgeoning in the United States and Canada, and interest has been expressed in Australia, New Zealand, England, and western Europe. Why the sudden popularity of these species? Even those close to the industry cannot explain it. Llamas and alpacas have been domesticated for over 6000 years and have been a vital factor of Andean society and economy for centuries.

Today, in North America, the large- or mixed-animal practitioner is being called upon to set up parasite control and vaccination programs and/or to treat llamas for colic. Most practitioners have little or no knowledge of camelids. There is essentially no literature dealing with them—at best a few papers in journals. Veterinary schools do not teach the specialized anatomy of these unique creatures.

The author has answered from two to five telephone calls daily in the past few years from practitioners inquiring about llama problems. This book is designed to begin to meet that need. It is written for the veterinarian faced with the interesting but challenging case of a sick llama or alpaca, or who must deal with preventive medical problems and infertility, or who is asked to conduct soundness examinations. Veterinarians are often required to advise a client in every aspect of animal management, including routine care and making wise choices for breeding stock or animals desired for packing or fiber production, since many llama owners lack farm or animal-raising experience.

The author is a clinician, and the orientation of the book is directed toward clinical medicine and surgery, but biologic and anatomic information is included. The llama and its cousins are like no other animal with which the veterinarian is familiar. The term "llama" includes all SACs unless otherwise specifically mentioned. Llamas may share some diseases with cattle and sheep and react to colic as would a horse, but camelid anatomy is unique; surgery techniques must differ. If understanding of these facts is lacking, diagnosis and subsequent therapy may fail.

Available world literature dealing with SACs has been used to augment the scope of the author's experience. Over 1000 references have been perused. Both North and South American camelid diseases have been discussed in order that this book may be comprehensive and usable throughout the world. As to why such books have not been published in South America, the value of the individual animal there is too little to warrant the time, energy, and expense required to deal with a single animal. Herd medicine is practiced, and the published literature of herd management has provided insight into individual camelid medicine.

The emphasis of this book is SAC medicine; however, some comparative medicine of Old World camels has been included.

Camelid medicine is in its infancy. There are many gaps in the world literature. No one person has the background to write the definitive text on camelids. This text may serve as a steppingstone for others who will enlarge on topics as more investigational work is completed and reported. The author makes no pretense of being a specialist in camelid medicine but hopes the experiences reported and summaries of world literature included may help move camelid medicine forward.

Each chapter has been reviewed by others with experience and expertise in the topic. Omissions may be the result of a lack of experience or available literature; however, errors or improper evaluations and conclusions based on the literature are the responsibility of the author.

The bringing together of this information has been an exciting task. Many have contributed. Llama owners have provided case material for obtaining experience and investigation. Colleagues have shared frustrations, philosophies, case material, ideas, and encouragement. I give special thanks to friend and colleague Dr. La Rue Johnson. Many individuals have contributed funds for research, which must continue for years to come. Many pleasant hours have been spent in close association with llamas and owners of llamas.

MURRAY E. FOWLER

Medicine and Surgery of South American Camelids

1 General Biology and Evolution

THE DOMESTICATED CAMELIDS of the world have had a significant impact on Old and New World cultures. Camels and South American camelids (SACs) went through a period of decline in the latter part of the nineteenth and early twentieth centuries. Governments neglected them as important components of the life of indigenous people and tried to replace them with other domestic animals. Only in the last few decades have these animals been recognized as a valuable resource and efforts made to research their unique physiology and adaptation to hostile environments.

TAXONOMY

Linnaeus placed the llama, alpaca, and Old World camels in a single genus, *Camelus,* in 1758. Other taxonomists proposed separate genus status for SACs in the early nineteenth century, but none of this work was accepted by the International Commission on Zoological Nomenclature. The genus name *Auchenia* was proposed by Illiger for SACs in 1811 and is frequently seen in print even today in the South American literature. However, *Auchenia* had been applied earlier to a genus of insects and thus was not a valid name for any other animal. In 1827, Lesson published an acceptable paper classifying the New World camelidae in the genus *Lama.* In 1924, Miller assigned the vicuña to a separate genus, *Vicugna* (5, 6).

The systematic classification of Old World camels has never been controversial. The one-humped camel (dromedary) is named *Camelus dromedarius* (Fig. 1.1) and the two-humped camel (Bactrian) *Camelus bactrianus* (Fig. 1.2). The classification of SACs has been more controversial. One system classifies the guanaco, llama, and alpaca within the genus *Lama* and vicuña as a single species in the genus *Vicugna.* Another system classifies all SACs within the genus *Lama.* Others classify the llama and alpaca as subspecies of *L. guanicoe guanicoe.*

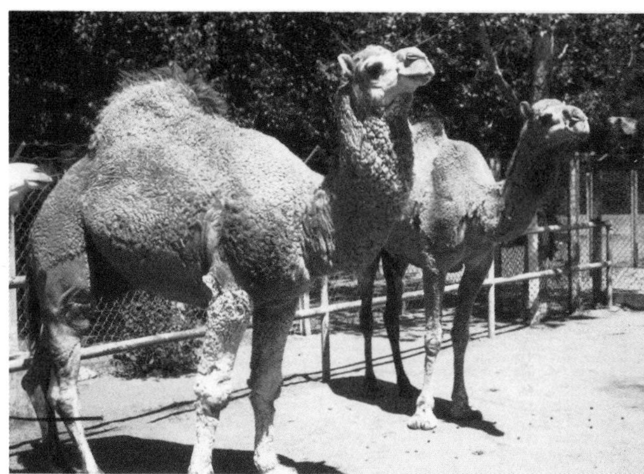

1.1 Dromedary camel.

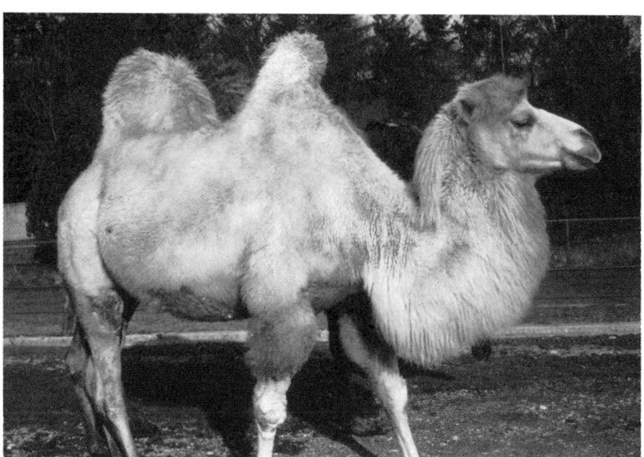

1.2 Bactrian camel.

Collectively, SACs are known as lamoids, although the term "auquenidae" is often found in older South American literature. Both camels and SACs are included in the term camelid.

The family Camelidae was previously designated as an infraorder, Tylopoda, under the suborder Ruminantia (12), but the most authoritative and current classification gives Tylopoda suborder status (10, 13, 14). This book will follow the classification for camelids as listed in Table 1.1.

Table 1.1. Camelid classification

Class—Mammalia
  Order—Artiodactyla
    Suborder—Tylopoda
      Family—Camelidae
        Genus—*Camelus,* Old World camelids
          Species
          C. dromedarius, dromedary camel
          C. bactrianus, Bactrian camel
        Genus—*Lama,* South American camelids
          Species
          L. glama, llama
          L. pacos, alpaca
          L. guanicoe, guanaco
        Genus—*Vicugna,* South American camelid
          Species
          V. vicugna or *L. vicugna,* vicuña
    Suborder—Ruminantia, deer, cattle, antelope, sheep, goat, gazelle

Alpacas and llamas exist only as domestic species. Guanacos and vicuñas are wild species. It is generally accepted that the alpaca shares some characteristics with the vicuña, e.g., incisor teeth with an open pulp cavity and continuous eruption into adulthood.

GENERAL BIOLOGY

All camelids have 37 pairs of chromosomes. All SACs have produced fertile crosses with one another (2, 7). Dromedary and Bactrian camels also produce fertile crosses (5). Despite size differences, the anatomy of all species of camelids is similar. The camels completed Pleistocene evolution in a semidesert environment and developed sophisticated adaptations for dealing with heat and dehydration (see Chap. 9). The SACs became adapted to the high altitudes of the Andes.

Camelids have a complex, three-compartmented stomach. Gastric digestion is similar to, but not analogous with, ruminant digestion. The two suborders separated from each other 30–40 million years ago when primordial species were simple stomached. Both groups utilized fibrous forage and developed similar foregut fermentation systems by parallel evolution (see Chap. 13). Camelids regurgitate and rechew ingested forage, as do ruminants, but are more efficient than ruminants in extracting protein and energy from poor-quality forages (see Chap. 2).

The SACs are communal dung pile users, while the camels defecate wherever they may be. Feces are pelleted in both groups and used for fuel by people who share their habitat. Camelids have a unique reproductive cycle (see Chap. 17).

The guanaco (Fig. 1.3) has the broadest distribution, both historically and currently, of the four SACs. Four geographic subspecies of guanaco have been described (7), ranging from sea level in Tierra del Fuego at the southernmost tip of South America to 4600 m in the Andes. The northernmost populations exist at latitude 8° south in Peru (2, 7). Guanacos live in both migratory and sedentary groups (2). They may be tamed and handled similarly to llamas; the Incas utilized them as pack animals (7). All guanaco subspecies share uniform coloration, with a dark brown upper body, neck, and limbs; whitish fiber on the underside of the neck and belly; and a grayish to black face.

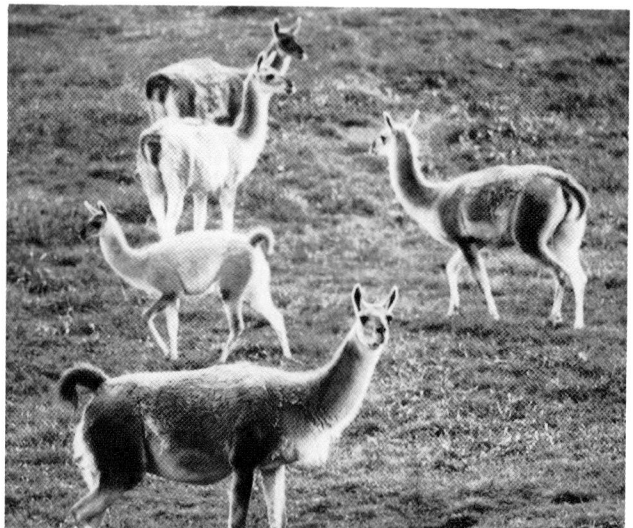

1.3 Guanaco.

Vicuña distribution is limited to the puna (Quechua for highland) life zone of the Andes (elevation 4200–4800 m) (2, 7). The vicuña (Fig. 1.4) is the smallest of the SACs and has the finest fiber coat. It has a cinnamon-colored coat, white underparts, a pale cinnamon face, and a bib of long, white hair on the chest. The vicuña was considered the property of the Inca kings, and only royalty was allowed to wear garments made from the fiber. There are two geographic subspecies of vicuña (2, 7).

The two breeds of alpaca, huacaya (Fig. 1.5) and suri (Fig. 1.6), are separated on the basis of fiber coat characteristics; 90% in Peru are of the huacaya breed (6), which is the only breed that has been exported to other countries. Huacaya fiber is shorter than that of the suri breed and is crimped and spongy, giving it the appearance of corriedale sheep wool (6). The coat of suri alpacas consists of long, straight fibers with no crimp. Alpaca coloration varies from white to black with in-

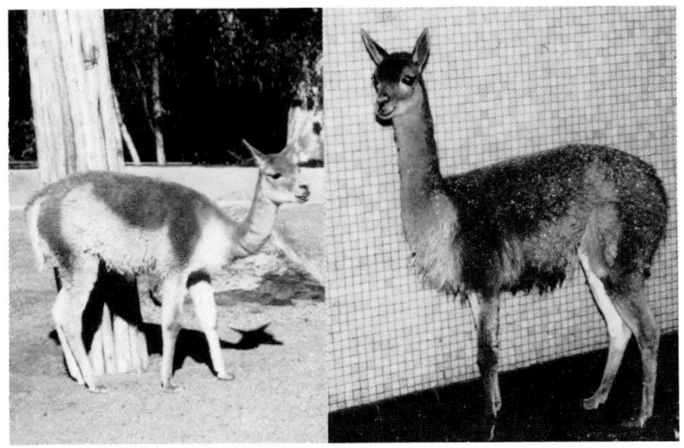

1.4 Vicuña.

termediate shades and combinations. The alpaca is the primary SAC fiber producer of the Andean highland.

The llama is the largest of the SACs; however, among individuals there is marked variation in size, overlapping sizes of other species (Fig. 1.7). The llama has been a beast of burden since its domestication. Two breeds are recognized in Peru: the more woolly varieties are called "ch'aku" in Quechua (Fig. 1.8) and those with less fiber on the neck and body are called "q'ara" (woolless) (Fig. 1.9). White llamas were killed as sacrificial offerings in the Inca culture.

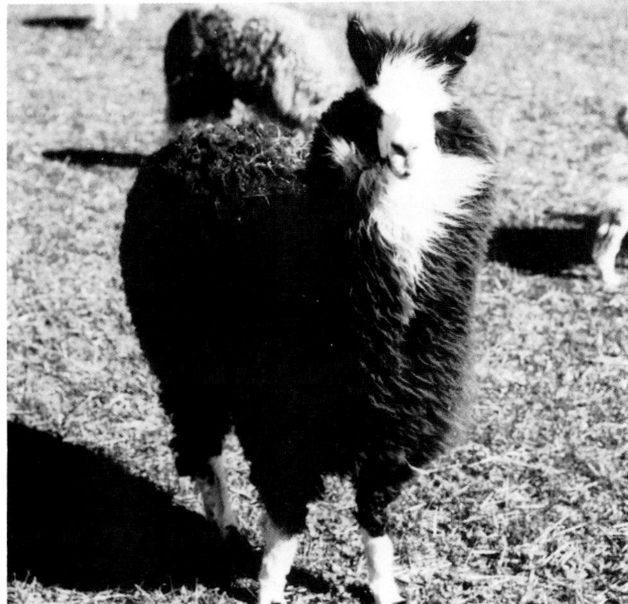

1.5 Huacaya alpaca.

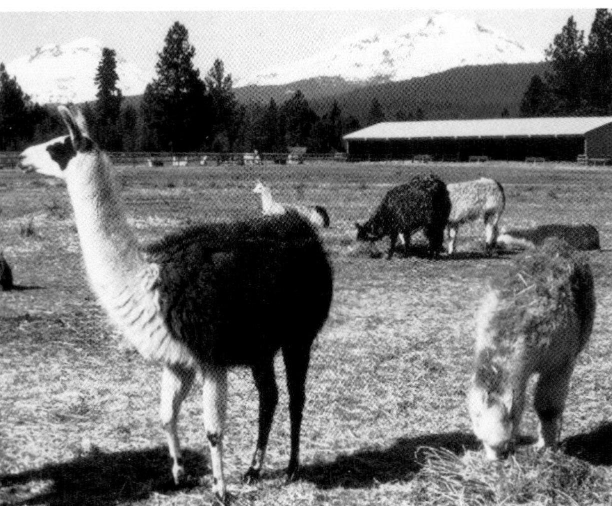

1.7 Llama.

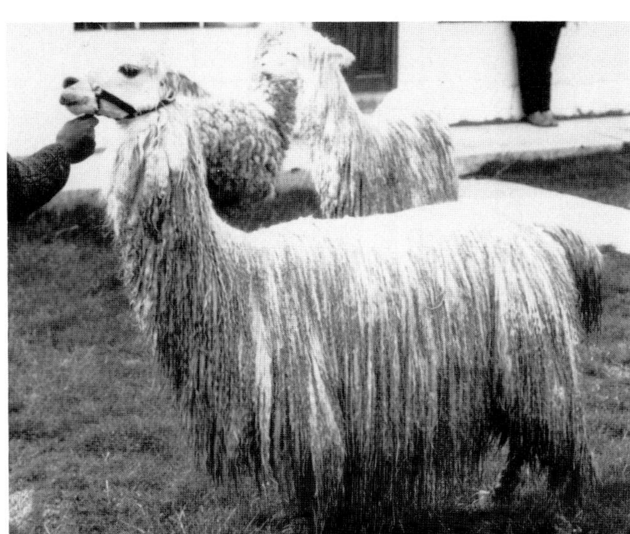

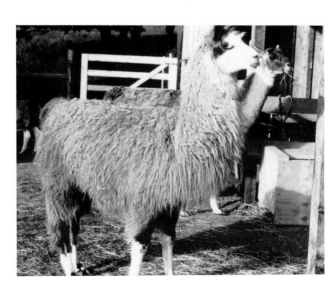

1.6 Suri alpaca.

1.8 Woolly-necked llama.

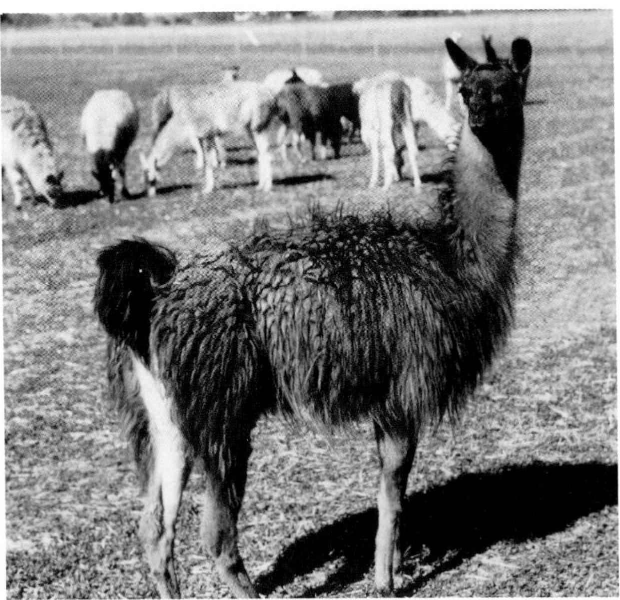

1.9 Relatively woolless-necked llama.

Both alpacas and llamas are slaughtered for meat in Andean countries. Lack of refrigeration necessitates immediate consumption, or the meat may be sun dried for storage. Dried meat is called "charqui," from which the North American word "jerky" originated for a similar product.

EVOLUTION
Camelid

Camelid evolution began in North America 40–50 million years ago in the early Eocene epoch. Geologic and paleantologic time scales are estimates and subject to revision. Figure 1.10 provides a diagram of the relationships of the various artiodactylid families since the Eocene epoch. Webb (14) published a definitive work on the evolution of Pleistocene camelids. He suggested three major tribes, separated as early as the Eocene epoch. This family tree (Fig. 1.11) is sketchy, with insufficient fossil records to trace lines accurately (postulates indicated by broken lines) (4, 14). Two tribes, Camelopini (*Camelops*) and Camelini (*Camelus*), evolved in North America only west of the Mississippi River. The tribe Lamini (*Lama*) was also found in Florida (4, 13).

The Pleistocene epoch was characterized by a series of periods of extreme cold and glaciation in northern North America and Europe (11). The last glacial retreat occurred about 10,000 years ago, marking the beginning of the recent epoch. It was during the Pleistocene epoch that the lamoids and camels flourished (8, 9). Many genera in the family Camelidae became extinct, for unknown reasons, before the recent epoch.

Epoch	Approximate beginning of Epoch, millions of years before	Suina	Tylopoda	Ruminantia: Traguloidea	Ruminantia: Cervoidea	Ruminantia: Bovoidea
Recent	0.01					
Pleistocene	3					
Pliocene	13					
Miocene	25	Suidae, Tayassuidae, Hippopotamidae	Camelidae	Tragulidae	Cervidae, Giraffidae	Antilocapridae, Bovidae
Oligocene	37					
Eocene	55					

*Adapted from Romer, Simpson

1.10 Suggested evolution of recent artiodactylids. Adapted from Romer 1966; Simpson 1980.

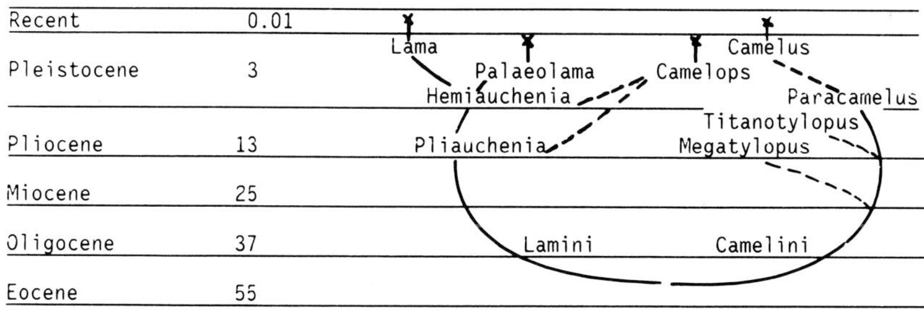

1.11 Suggested phylogeny of camelids. Adapted from Webb 1974; Harrison 1979.

Camel

Asia and Alaska are now separated by the 90-km (56-mile)-wide Bering Strait. However, during the height of one of the early Pleistocene glaciation periods, the sea level was lowered sufficiently to expose a wide land bridge (1). Plant and animal species moved back and forth across this bridge; the camel line of Camelidae migrated from North America into Asia to continue the evolutionary process, dying out in North America.

Once in Asia, *Camelus* radiated through eastern Europe (Rumania and southern Russia), the Middle East, and North Africa as far west as the Atlantic and as far south as Tanzania. It is likely that the dromedary evolved from the Bactrian camel, although the hump(s) may be an acquired characteristic of domestication. Wild camels had become extinct in North Africa before historic times (3000 B.C.). Only *C. bactrianus* now exists in the wild state in one small area in the Trans-Altai Gobi Desert on the border of Mongolia and China, with a limited population of 300–700 animals (5).

Lamoid

The first lamoids migrated to South America at the beginning of the Pleistocene epoch (approximately 3 million years ago) when an open land connection between North and South America developed (10). The major early lamoid genus appearing in South America was *Hemiauchenia* (*Tanupoloma*), which radiated throughout the flatter regions east of the Andes. During the middle Pleistocene, the genera *Palaeolama, Lama,* and *Vicugna* developed from the long-limbed, flatland-adapted *Hemiauchenia.* These genera had shorter limbs, which more adapted them to the mountainous Andes (13, 14).

Various species of *Palaeolama* migrated back to North America. Fossils have been found along the Gulf Coast and Florida in association with North American *Hemiauchenia* (13).

DOMESTICATION

Camels

The precise time and location of domestication of the Bactrian camel is unknown, but it is thought to have occurred some time prior to 2500 B.C. on the border of Turkmenistan and Iran on the east side of the Caspian Sea (5). The name Bactrian is derived from a place name, Baktria, on the Oxus River in northern Afghanistan. Strangely, this is not the place of origin of the domestic two-humped camel, nor is the species even found in this area at present (5).

Domestic Bactrian camels had spread north into southern Russia by 1700–1200 B.C. and were in western Siberia by the tenth century B.C. Bactrian camels were used in China as early as 300 B.C. as the original "silk route" camels but were replaced by crossbreeds of the dromedary and Bactrian camel later on (5).

Domestication of the dromedary occurred prior to 3000 B.C. in the Arabian peninsula. The term "dromedary" is derived from dromos (Greek for road) and thus is only directly applicable to the riding or racing dromedary camel. However, dromedary is the name used throughout the world for this species, which existed in historic times only as a domesticated animal. Dromedaries were first associated with nomadic Semitic cultures and never became important until the rise of the Arabian culture (5).

Dromedaries were reintroduced into North Africa in the third century B.C. More were brought into Egypt during the Roman period, after the third century A.D., but became important domestic animals only with the Moslem conquests of Egypt in the seventh to eleventh centuries A.D.

Llamas and Alpacas

The cradle of llama domestication is the Andean puna (elevation 4000–4900 m), probably around Lake Titicaca, at approximately 4000 B.C. Alpaca domestication probably occurred elsewhere, perhaps near Telarmachay. Alpaca-type incisors have been found in middens at Telarmachay, dated at 4000–3500 B.C. (7). Once domesticated, llama and alpaca herding economies spread beyond the limits of the puna and became important in the economy of the Andean people from sea level to high mountain elevations (7).

The Inca empire was dependent upon the llama and alpaca for food, fuel, clothing, transport of goods, and religious ceremonies. All lamoids were the property of the government, and production of domestic species was rigidly controlled (7). The fiber from vicuñas was for royal usage only. The maximum numbers and broadest distribution of lamoids developed under Inca rule. After the Spanish invasion of 1532 and the introduction of European breeds of livestock, numbers and distribution of lamoids declined. However, llamas and alpacas survived because they are essential to Andean culture. They are the most reliable source of food, fiber, and fuel in the high, cool Andean environment. Lamoid ownership is the primary source of wealth for indigenous people (7).

At present, all llamas and 80% of alpacas in the Andes are under the control of traditional pastoralists (6). Small to moderate herds (30–1000) are grazed on communal lands. The remaining alpacas are managed by large cooperatives (40,000 alpacas), which developed after the agrarian reform program of the 1970s began in Peru.

Lamoids were exported to other countries from South America in the nineteenth century as zoo animals. Peru enacted legislation in 1843 prohibiting the export of live alpacas. Approximately 60 years ago, all the Andean countries banded together to prevent exploitation of lamoids by other countries. No legal exportations occurred from then until the 1980s when the ban was lifted from alpacas and llamas (2).

North American llamas have expanded from the small population imported from South America prior to 1930. A few animals have been imported from other countries. Current numbers of North American llamas are estimated to be between 12,000 and 15,000. Alpaca numbers are small, 500–1000. Sporadic importation of llamas and alpacas from Chile into the United States began in 1984 after the U.S. government periodically recognized Chile as free of foot-and-mouth disease.

Additional biologic information is provided at the beginning of other chapters.

REFERENCES

1. Farb, P. 1964. The Land and Wildlife of North America. Life Nature Library. New York: Time, p. 11.

2. Franklin, W. L. 1982. Biology, ecology, and relationship to man of South American camelids. In M. A. Mares and H. H. Genoways, eds. Mammalian Biology in South America. Linesville, Pa.: Pymatuning Laboratory of Ecology, Univ. of Pittsburgh Spec. Publ. 6, pp. 457–89.

3. Harrison, J. A. 1979. Revision of the Camelinae (artiodactyla, Tylopoda) and description of the new genus *Alforjas.* Paleontol. Contrib., Pap. 95, Univ. of Kansas, pp. 1–27.

4. Kurten, B., and Anderson, E. 1980. Pleistocene Mammals of North America. New York: Columbia Univ. Press.

5. Mason, I. L. 1984. Camels. In I. L. Mason, ed. Evolution of Domestic Animals. London: Longman.

6. Miller, G. S., Jr. 1924. A second instance of the development of rodent-like incisors in an artiodactyl. Proc. U.S. Nat. Mus. 66, Artic. 8, No. 2545.

7. Novoa, C., and Wheeler, J. C. 1984. Llama and alpaca. In I. L. Mason, ed. Evolution of Domestic Animals. London: Longman.

8. Romer, A. S. 1966. Vertebrate Paleontology, 3rd ed. Chicago: Univ. of Chicago Press.

9. Simpson, G. G. 1945. The principles of classification and a classification of mammals. Bull. Am. Mus. Nat. Hist. 84:258–65.

10. ______. 1980. Splendid Isolation. New Haven, Conn.: Yale Univ. Press.

11. Strahler, A. N. 1973. Introduction of Physical Geography, 3rd ed. New York: John Wiley & Sons, p. 356.

12. Vallenas P., A. 1970. (Commentary on the position of South American camelids in systematic classification) Comentarios sobre la posición de los camélidos sudamericanos en la sistemática. Bol. Extraordinario 4:128–41.

13. Webb, S. D. 1965. The osteology of camelops. Bull. Los Ang. Cty. Mus. Sci. 1.

14. ______. 1974. Pleistocene Mammals of Florida. Gainesville: Univ. of Florida Press.

2 Feeding and Nutrition

TO UNDERSTAND the basis for feeding practices and nutritional physiology, knowledge of the anatomy of the digestive system is required. Therefore, study of this discussion should be preceded by a review of llama anatomy of the digestive tract (Chap. 13).

Little has been written on the basic nutrition of lamoids. The energy requirement for animals kept in different habitats and under different feeding regimens is not known. Some information about grazing behavior and feed preferences in South America is available (28, 29, 36, 37, 38, 45), and some experience in managing the feeding of lamoids in zoos and private ownership has been reported (3, 10, 23, 43, 57).

This chapter provides background on the feeding behavior of lamoids in their native habitat, presents a review of the literature concerning digestive physiology as it relates to nutrition, and makes some recommendations for suitable rations based on current knowledge of nutrient requirements.

FEEDING BEHAVIOR

The vicuña is one of two species of wild lamoids. It inhabits the high Andes at elevations of 3700–4800 m. This is a harsh environment, with cold temperatures, sparse vegetation, semiarid grassland, and barren pampas (14). The vicuña is a grazer of forbs and grasses.

The guanaco, also a wild species, has the broadest geographic and altitudinal distribution, ranging from sea level to 4250 m. The guanaco is both a grazer and a browser, inhabiting desert grassland, savanna, and shrub land; it may even be seen in forests. It is found in one of the driest deserts of the world, the Atacama in Chile, and also in the wet archipelago of Tierra del Fuego, where rain falls year around.

The llama is found at moderate elevations of 2300–4000 m. This distribution pattern may be more cultural than biologic, since the llama has shown ready adaptability to diverse altitudinal and geographic habitats in locations outside South America. The llama is both a grazer and a browser, preferring to pasture on dry tablelands and slopes, feeding on the tall coarse bunchgrass community dominated by fescue (*Festuca dolichophylla*), but it also browses available shrubs and trees.

The alpaca is found at elevations of 4400–4800 m and is strictly a grazer, preferring the bottomland vegetation of meadows and marshes collectively called occonales or bofedales (14). A list of highly desirable plants for alpacas, growing in various plant communities, is found in Tables 2.1 and 2.2. The nutrient composition of these plants varies greatly seasonally, altitudinally, and according to soil type (21). In dry seasons the vegetation is sparse and of poor nutrient quality. However, proximate analysis charts for Peruvian plants (Table 2.3) show that at least during part of the year the nutrient quality may be quite high. Even though the lamoids have become evolutionarily adapted to survival in their harsh environment, it is important to recognize that they may grow better and be more fertile if given optimal nutrition, at least for a major portion of the year.

Table 2.1. Preferred plant species for alpacas in marshy meadows (bofedales) in Peru

Grasses	27% of diet
Festuca dolichophylla, fescue	
Calamagrostis antonia, reedgrass	
Sedges and reeds	58% of diet
Juncus sp.	
Eleocharis albibracteata	
Distichia muscoides	
Carex equadorica	
Forbs	14% of diet
Hipochoeris taraxacoides	
Stylites andicola	

Source: Reiner and Bryant 1986.

Table 2.2. Preferred plant species for alpacas in the altiplano area (high grassland) of Peru

Grasses	53% of diet
Festuca dolichophylla	
Muhlenbergia fastigiata	
Sedges and reeds	32% of diet
Eleocharis albibracteata	
Carex equadorica	
Juncus sp.	
Forbs	15% of diet
Alchemilla pinnata	

Source: Reiner and Bryant 1986.

Table 2.3. Composition of Peruvian llama and alpaca pasture plants

Feed – Pasturage South America		Dry matter	Protein	Digestible energy	Fiber	Calcium	Phosphorus	Ca:P
		(%)	(%)	(*Mcal/kg*)	(%)	(%)	(%)	
Muhlenbergia, aerial part, fresh	Early	100.0	6.8	2.60	31.2	0.37	0.13	2.8
Muhlenbergia fastigiata	Mature	100.0	5.8	2.86	27.5	0.41	0.13	3.2
Reedgrass, aerial part, fresh	Early	100.0	6.2	2.59	33.8	0.38	0.11	3.5
Calamagrostis antonia	Mature	100.0	4.6	2.34	32.0	0.64	0.07	9.1
Fescue, aerial part, fresh	Midbloom	100.0	8.3	2.12	41.3	0.09		
Festuca dolichophylla	Mature	100.0	2.5	1.21	44.3	0.20	0.04	5.0
Spikesedge, aerial part, fresh	As fed	21.7	3.4	0.59	7.4	0.07	0.04	1.8
Eleocharis geniculata	Dry	100.0	15.5	2.73	34.1	0.32	0.19	1.7
Plantain, aerial part, fresh	Dry	100.0	14.7	3.05	35.4	0.16	0.26	0.6
Plantago sp.								
Crimson clover, aerial part, fresh	As fed	17.6	3.0	0.49	4.9	0.24	0.05	4.8
Trifolium incarnatium	Dry	100.0	17.0	2.81	27.7	1.38	0.29	4.8
Ladysmantle, aerial part, fresh								
Alchemilla pinnata	Dry	100.0	10.9	2.79	28.9	1.90	0.24	7.9

Source: McDowell et al. 1974.

NUTRITIONAL PHYSIOLOGY

Prehension

All the lamoids have incisor teeth that are firmly fixed in the mandible, similar to the dentition of sheep and goats but in contrast to the loose attachment of bovine teeth. These teeth, pressing against the upper dental pad, shear vegetation. These animals are able to graze short plants and cut them close to the ground, but their general behavior is to move about a feeding area, picking a mouthful here and there, not mowing any one spot clean.

The lips of camelids are unique. The upper lip is split by a labial cleft. Each side of the lip can be manipulated independently to investigate a potential food item and draw it to the teeth. Lamoids rarely consume foreign bodies because of this fastidious checking of feed with the lips.

The tongue does not participate in prehension. Since the tongue rarely protrudes from the mouth, camelids do not, as a rule, lick themselves, their young, or salt blocks. Some may lick at a salt block long enough to obtain some supplement, but usually camelids chew at the block rather than lick it.

Mastication

Initial chewing is cursory, sufficient only to mix feed with saliva to form a bolus to be swallowed. The amount of time required by a lamoid to complete sufficient ingestion of feed will vary with the quality and availability of the forage, but in most cases it will occupy a third of the daylight time. Lamoids are not active in the dark.

Mastication is also a part of the rumination cycle. Koford (24) described the rumination cycle in the vicuña. While resting, the vicuña will bring up a bolus and begin chewing, with the mandible scribing a horizontal figure 8 arc. A deer or a bovine masticates with a unilateral elliptic movement of the jaw. The vicuña retains the cud in the mouth for 15 seconds, during which time it will chew 25–35 times. That bolus will then be swallowed and the process repeated. Other lamoids have a similar pattern.

Saliva

The gross and microscopic anatomy of the salivary glands are similar to those of other artiodactylids. Salivary secretion is necessary to moisten and lubricate feed so that it can be swallowed. In one study (34), the prefeeding flow of the parotid saliva of the alpaca was 140 ml/hr. The pH was 8.6 and the composition was as follows: 121 mEq/L HCO_3, 33.5 mEq/L HPO_4, 164.8 mEq/L Na, and 13.7 mEq/L K.

While feeding, the flow was 202 ml/hr, pH was 8.59, composition was 127.8 mEq/L HCO_3, and other ion concentrations were similar to prefeeding levels. At postfeeding, the flow remained higher than during prefeeding, at 159 ml/hr, and the pH stayed at 8.58. Other parameters returned to prefeeding levels.

Stomach

Even though camelids are not taxonomically classified as ruminants, they are functional ruminants (9, 25, 52, 55). Compartments one and two (C-1 and C-2) of the three-compartmented stomach are anaerobic fermentation chambers, hosting the microbial flora and fauna necessary for utilization of coarse, fibrous herbage (52). Nonetheless, there are numerous and significant differences in the anatomy and physiology of the camelid stomach as compared with the stomach of true ruminants (14, 50, 52, 56).

Stomach motility is markedly different. At rest, three to four contractions of C-1 per minute are average (48, 50). If the animal has eaten recently, the rate is faster. The contraction wave of C-1 is from caudad to craniad, in contrast to the craniad-caudad wave of the true ruminant. It is generally not possible to palpate the contraction in the left paralumbar fossa, as can be done with cattle and sheep; rather, it is necessary to listen with a stethoscope. Since fermentation takes place only in the forestomach of camelids, there should be little gas formation, hence borborygamous, except from the stomach.

In true ruminants, the rumen contents are stratified with a gas layer dorsally, a solid layer of ingesta in the middle, and a more liquid and small particulate matter layer ventrally. In camelids, the ingesta is homogeneous and relatively dry. This causes some difficulty when attempting to aspirate ingesta to transfaunate another animal. Bloat is rare in camelids, and the homogeneity of the ingesta may be a factor in avoiding frothy bloat.

The reticular groove of camelids is not nearly as well defined as it is in cattle, sheep, and goats. Nonetheless, in the neonate camelid, milk is shunted past C-1 into C-2 and then into C-3. In a study by Vallenas et al. (46, 47, 49), the response to chemical stimulation was more like that of a bovine than of an ovine. There was good to fair response with 10% solutions of sodium sulfate, sodium chloride, and sodium bicarbonate, but no reaction to a copper sulfate solution (47).

The same study evaluated glucose absorption in alpacas (47, 49). In the alpaca neonate, the plasma glucose level was 121 mg/dl, whereas in the adult alpaca it is 72–99 mg/dl. In the bovine, it is generally believed that all carbohydrates are acted upon by ruminal microorganisms and converted to volatile fatty acids. This requires a functional rumen. Thus, in the neonate up to about 3 months of age, glucose reaches the abomasum and intestine where it is absorbed as such. In the adult, there is no glucose absorption from the rumen and less available glucose reaches the abomasum and intestine, so plasma levels are lower. In the alpaca a similar situation exists.

Blood glucose levels in llamas (125 ± 38 mg/dl) must be evaluated carefully, because elevated levels may be the result of the excitement caused by restraint necessary for blood collection, stimulating catecholamine release.

Urea metabolism in camelids is similar to that in the ruminant in that urea can be recycled and utilized by stomach microorganisms for the synthesis of protein (17,18). In general, blood urea levels are low in adult ruminants (8–30 mg/dl). This is true in llamas also, with adults at 24 ± 13 mg/dl and neonates at 14 ± 8 mg/dl.

When a llama fasts for 3–4 days, plasma urea elevates because of a significantly lower turnover and transfer of urea to the gastrointestinal (GI) tract (8). Tissue catabolism may also be a factor. The specific mechanism involved is not known, but it is likely that decreased permeability to urea has developed in the stomach mucosa (17). The foregoing has relevance to a llama that is ill and anorectic. Elevated blood urea nitrogen levels may not necessarily indicate a primary renal problem.

In one study, it was noted that llamas were able to hydrolyze more urea per unit of time (m mol/hr/kg) in C-1 than cattle and sheep in the rumen. Therefore, more urea would be available for protein synthesis by microorganisms in the llama (17).

A number of studies have investigated lamoids' superior increased efficiency in extracting energy and other nutrients from coarse forages (2, 5, 35, 49). Some early studies indicated that alpacas were 50% more efficient than sheep in digesting fiber (11). Later and more sophisticated studies demonstrated greater efficiency, but to a lesser degree, in experiments involving poor-quality forage and no difference in those involving high-quality forage (19). Table 2.4 provides data from a study comparing an alfalfa hay and a pelleted complete ration.

A greater efficiency of digestion of fiber and protein may be the result of a number of factors, among which are more rapid forestomach contractions that provide for better maceration, mixing, and absorption (2). Early studies indicated that a more effective buffering system in C-1 neutralizes short-chain volatile fatty acids (VFA), which in turn encourages increased production of VFA (40, 53). More sophisticated studies, using a Pavlov pouch, did not corroborate those findings but rather suggested that the glandular areas provided more complete and more rapid absorption of VFA, thus stimulating further production of VFA (40).

Table 2.4. Percent digestibility of two diets in ponies, sheep, guanaco, and llama

Feed	Nutrient	Pony	Sheep	Llama/guanaco
Alfalfa pellets	Dry matter[a]	64.8	63.8	71.5
	Acid detergent fiber	46.7	50.5	61.0
	Cellulose	51.2	64.8	77.6
	Crude protein	65.7	69.7	74.7
Complete pelleted diet	Dry matter	69.7	71.7	78.0
	Acid detergent fiber	29.3	34.0	38.7
	Cellulose	34.5	39.4	47.2
	Crude protein	68.8	63.1	69.2

Source: Hintz et al. 1973.
[a]The animals consumed between 1.7 and 2% of their body weight in dry matter.

The degree of digestive efficiency may reflect the quality of forage eaten. More studies in a variety of situations and with a variety of forages are needed to establish the facts.

The end products of carbohydrate fermentation in camelids are VFA, just as in the true ruminant. In the llama and guanaco, the peak production of VFA occurs approximately 1.5–2 hours after feeding, and normal levels return within 5–6 hours (51). There is a negative correlation of increase in VFA with pH. In cattle, peak production occurs 2–3 hours after feeding, and the level is maintained longer. The pH drops faster and lower, presumably because cattle lack the more effective absorption system of the lamoid (19).

In a study conducted by Vallenas et al. (54), VFA were found all along the GI tract, but compared with sheep, cattle, and deer, there was a lower concentration of VFA caudal to the stomach in llamas and alpacas, indicating either more efficient absorption of these nutrients from the stomach or less microbial activity beyond the stomach.

The camelid forestomach is characterized by the presence of glandular mucosal areas in all compartments (7, 52). In C-1, in both cranial and caudal sacs, areas of saccules lined with a mucinous glandular epithelium evert during stomach contraction, expelling the contents into the lumen of C-1.

The glandular epithelium of C-2 covers all but the small area of the lesser curvature. The cells are not as deep as those of the saccules of C-1. The reticular pattern of C-2 is superficially like the pattern of the reticulum of the true ruminant, but these structures are not analogous.

STOMACH MICROBIOLOGY. The microflora and fauna of the true ruminant have been intensely studied and found to be highly complex. Hundreds of species of bacteria and protozoa inhabit the rumen and participate in the fermentative process so important to the nutrition of these species. Both Gram-positive and Gram-negative organisms are present, but all are anaerobic. Each species, or perhaps group of species, acts on certain components of the diet. Specific bacteria digest cellulose, hemicellulose, starches, sugars, acids, lipids, and proteins. Other bacteria produce ammonia, or methane, and still others synthesize vitamins. Several bacteria have multiple functions.

The species present and relative proportions of each may be dependent upon numerous factors. Each species has its own special substrate requirement, and any disease-induced or human-induced change in the environment may destroy a specific population of bacteria, upsetting the nutrition of the animal.

In addition to bacteria, dozens of species of ciliated and flagellated protozoa have been found. The species present in a given animal may vary according to diet, season of the year, and geographic location (4).

Few reports have been published of studies of the species of protozoa found in camelids (42). Speciation is a complicated and specialized process. Practically, it is important to know that protozoa are present and that sudden changes in diet should be avoided so as not to destroy the resident population. Camelids are able to adapt to new forages, but introduction should be gradual.

One study compared the volume and variety of protozoan species in goats and guanacos (16). In the goat, from 1 to 2 million cells per gram of ingesta were found. Approximately 90% were in the small protozoa category. In the guanaco, there were about 1.3 million cells per gram of ingesta, and all the protozoa corresponded to the small species found in goats. It was estimated that the total volume of protozoa amounted to 9.4% of the rumen ingesta of the goat (wet weight) and 5.3% of C-1 ingesta in the guanaco. The health of stomach microorganisms is vital to the nutritional status of lamoids. This may have practical relevance when treating a sick llama that has been anorectic over a period of time with stomach atony. It is likely that much of the stomach microflora and fauna have been destroyed. Transfaunation is commonly practiced in true ruminants and has also been performed in llamas.

The question arises as to whether rumen contents from a bovine or ovine would be efficacious, or only the contents of a llama stomach. Given a choice, it is best to transfaunate llamas with llama stomach contents, but bovine ingesta from fistulated donors have been used in llamas with apparent success. No studies have been conducted to determine the efficacy of commercial desiccated rumen microorganisms for reestablishing the flora of a llama stomach. Feces are not recommended for transfaunation, because stomach microorganisms will have been digested in the intestine and not be viable in feces.

Intestinal Function

Intestinal digestion and absorption in the lamoid are apparently similar to the process in true ruminants. Lamoids lack a gallbladder, so bile may flow continuously. The cecum and large colon do not function as primary fermentative chambers. The large intestine forms a spiral colon that diminishes in diameter by two-thirds within the coils. Fecal pellets are formed approximately halfway through the spiral. The diminution of size contributes to the formation of impactions in llamas.

NUTRIENT REQUIREMENTS OF LAMOIDS

The nutrient requirements of lamoids are not known. Few detailed nutritional studies have been conducted. What is known is based on observations from feeding practices and extrapolation from data accumulated by studies of sheep, goats, and cattle (30, 31, 32). Since lamoids may have a more efficient digestive system than ruminants, some of the figures may be in error. However, this purported efficiency may make a greater difference when the diet is poor. In the recommendations being made, a fair- to good-quality diet is assumed, so the margin of error in the recommendations may not be great.

Table 2.5 provides a summary of estimated basic nutrients required by lamoids. Perhaps the most significant column is the final one, which gives the amount of feed required to supply the general needs of a llama of a given weight. Feed amounts must, however, be correlated with forage composition (Tables 2.6–2.8) to assure that adequate levels of all nutrients are provided.

Energy

The only reported study of the energy needs of lamoids was done in Germany (41). The investigators concluded that the daily maintenance digestible energy requirement was $71 \times W_{kg}^{.75}$ = Kcal digestible energy (DE). In order to follow the computations of Table 2.5, a clear understanding of the concept of metabolic weight is needed.

In early studies of metabolism, researchers found that many reactions were not proportional to body mass but rather to body surface area. Smaller animals have a higher proportion of surface to mass than larger animals. The surface to mass ratio was calculated for many spe-

Table 2.5. Estimated basic nutrient requirements for llamas

Body weight		Metabolic weight	Digestible energy, maintenance (Mcal)		Crude protein, maintenance (g) C		Calcium (g)	Phosphorus (g)	Dry matter consumed at 2.5 Mcal DE/kg forage (E)				Feed consumption percent of body weight (F)			
(kg)	*(lb)*	*($W_{kg}^{.75}$)*	A	B	X	Y	D	D	X *(kg)*	X *(lb)*	Y *(kg)*	Y *(lb)*	DM 90% X	DM 90% Y	DM as fed X	DM as fed Y
10	22	5.62	0.48	0.67	15	21	5	3	0.19	0.42	0.27	0.60	1.9	2.7	2.1	3.0
20	44	9.50	0.81	1.15	25	36	6	4	0.32	0.73	0.46	1.01	1.6	2.3	1.8	2.6
40	88	15.91	1.36	1.91	42	59	7	5	0.52	1.15	0.76	1.68	1.3	1.9	1.4	2.1
50	110	18.80	1.63	2.26	51	70	8	6	0.65	1.43	0.90	1.99	1.3	1.8	1.4	2.0
75	165	25.50	2.18	3.06	68	95	9	7	0.87	1.92	1.22	2.70	1.2	1.6	1.3	1.8
100	220	31.60	2.70	3.79	84	118	11	9	1.08	2.38	1.52	3.34	1.1	1.5	1.2	1.7
125	275	37.40	3.20	4.49	99	139	13	10	1.28	2.82	1.80	3.96	1.0	1.4	1.1	1.6
150	330	42.90	3.67	5.15	114	160	16	12	1.47	3.24	2.06	4.54	1.0	1.4	1.1	1.5
175	385	47.50	4.07	5.70	126	177	18	12	1.63	3.59	2.28	5.03	0.9	1.3	1.0	1.4
200	440	53.20	4.55	6.38	141	198	20	13	1.82	4.01	2.55	5.63	0.9	1.3	1.0	1.4
225	495	58.10	4.97	6.97	154	216	21	14	1.99	4.39	2.79	6.15	0.9	1.2	1.0	1.4
250	550	62.90	5.38	7.55	167	231	23	17	2.15	4.74	3.02	6.66	0.8	1.2	1.0	1.3

Note: A = $85.6 \times W_{kg}^{.75}$ = Kcal DE (Schneider, $60.5 \times W_{kg}^{.75}$ = ME, ME × 1.22 = DE + 15% × Schneider's metabolism cage data, for routine living); B = sheep and goat data ($120\ W_{kg}^{.75}$ = Kcal DE); C = 31 g protein/Mcal DE; D = requirements extrapolated from sheep and cattle; E = required Mcal/2.5 = amount of feed required; F = amount required/body weight × 100 = % body weight consumed; X = calculated from A; Y = calculated from B.

Table 2.6. Composition of llama feeds

Feed		Dry matter	Crude protein	Digestible energy	Fiber	Calcium	Phosphorus	Ca:P
		(%)	(%)	*(Mcal/kg)*	(%)	(%)	(%)	
Alfalfa leaves, sun-cured	As fed	89	20.6	2.84	21.0	2.27	0.24	9.5
Medicago sativa	Dry	100	23.1	3.17	24.0	2.54	0.27	9.4
Alfalfa hay, late bloom, sun-cured	As fed	90	12.6	2.06	28.8	1.13	0.20	5.7
	Dry	100	14.0	2.29	32.0	1.25	0.22	5.7
Alfalfa hay, mature, sun-cured	As fed	91	11.7	2.01	34.4	1.03	0.17	6.1
	Dry	100	12.9	2.21	37.7	1.13	0.18	6.3
Oat hay, sun-cured	As fed	91	8.5	2.46	27.8	0.22	0.20	1.1
Avena sativa	Dry	100	9.3	2.69	30.4	0.24	0.22	1.1
Orchardgrass hay, late bloom, sun-cured	As fed	91	7.6	2.16	33.6	0.35	0.32	1.1
Dactylis glomerata	Dry	100	8.4	2.38	37.1	0.32	0.35	0.9
Fescue, early bloom, sun-cured	As fed	92	8.7	1.95	34.0	0.28	0.24	1.2
Festuca sp.	Dry	100	9.5	2.12	37.0	0.30	0.26	1.2
Ryegrass hay, late veg., sun-cured	As fed	86	8.8	2.34	23.0	0.53	0.29	1.8
Lolium multiflorum	Dry	100	10.3	2.73	30.0	0.62	0.34	1.8
Timothy hay, full bloom, sun-cured	As fed	89	7.2	2.27	28.4	0.38	0.18	2.1
Phleum pratense	Dry	100	8.1	2.56	32.0	0.43	0.20	2.2

Source: U.S.-Canadian Tables of Feed Composition, 3rd ed. 1982.

Table 2.7. Composition of mixed alfalfa and grass hays

Feed		Dry matter	Crude protein	Digestible energy	Fiber	Calcium	Phosphorus
		(%)	(%)	(Mcal/kg)	(%)	(%)	(%)
Alfalfa–grass hay, cut 2, 25% grass	As fed	89.1	14.1	2.00	33.1	0.94	0.26
Medicago sativa	Dry	100.0	15.8	2.24	37.1	1.05	0.29
Alfalfa–orchardgrass, cut 1	As fed	92.9	9.8	2.53	29.4	. . .	. . .
Medicago sativa, Dactylis glomerata	Dry	100.0	10.6	2.72	31.7	. . .	. . .
Alfalfa–timothy hay	As fed	89.0	12.2	2.12	30.9	0.79	0.18
Medicago sativa, Phleum pratense	Dry	100.0	13.7	2.37	34.7	0.89	0.20

Source: U.S.-Canadian Tables of Feed Composition, 3rd ed. 1982.

Table 2.8. Composition of North American llama feeds

Feed		Dry matter	Protein	Digestible energy	Fiber	Calcium	Phosphorus	Ca:P
		(%)	(%)	(Mcal/kg)	(%)	(%)	(%)	
Pasturage								
Acacia leaves, fresh	As fed	30	1.5	0.25	6.8	. . .	. . .	. . .
Acacia catechu	Dry	100	5.8	0.84	22.6	. . .	. . .	. . .
Crested wheat grass, fresh, early veg.	As fed	28	6.0	0.92	6.0	0.18	0.07	2.60
Agropyron desertorum	Dry	100	21.5	3.31	21.5	0.45	0.19	2.40
Grama grass, hairy, fresh, late veg.	As fed	55	3.6	1.21	. . .	. . .	. . .	. . .
Bouteloua desertorum	Dry	100	6.7	2.21	. . .	. . .	. . .	. . .
Bermuda grass, fresh	As fed	34	4.1	0.89	8.9	0.43	0.16	2.70
Cynodon dactylon	Dry	100	12.0	2.65	6.4	0.47	0.17	2.80
Orchardgrass, fresh, early bloom	As fed	25	4.0	0.72	7.4	0.10	0.11	0.90
Dactylis glomerata	Dry	100	12.0	2.91	30.0	0.37	0.39	0.95
Rye grass, perennial, fresh	As fed	27	2.8	0.80	6.2	0.15	0.07	2.10
Lolium perenne	Dry	100	10.4	3.00	23.2	0.55	0.26	2.00
Alfalfa, fresh, late veg.	As fed	21	4.3	0.59	4.9	0.48	0.07	6.90
Medicago sativa	Dry	100	20.0	2.78	23.0	1.96	0.30	6.50
Clover, fresh	As fed	19	4.5	0.55	3.3	0.30	0.06	5.00
Trifolium hybridum	Dry	100	24.1	2.91	17.5	1.32	0.28	4.70
High-energy concentrates								
Oats, grain	As fed	89	11.8	3.02	10.8	0.07	0.33	0.20
Avena sativa	Dry	100	13.3	3.40	12.1	0.07	0.38	0.20
Barley, grain	As fed	88	11.9	3.27	5.0	0.04	0.34	0.10
Hordeum vulgare	Dry	100	21.5	3.31	21.5	0.45	0.19	2.40
Acorns, oak fruit, fresh	As fed	64	3.1	1.32	8.8	. . .	. . .	. . .
Quercus sp.	Dry	100	4.8	2.07	13.9	. . .	. . .	. . .
Wheat, grain	As fed	89	14.2	3.45	2.6	0.11	1.22	0.09
Triticum aestivum	Dry	100	16.0	3.88	2.9	0.13	1.38	0.09
Molasses (treacle), blackstrap 80 brix	As fed	75	4.4	2.37	0	0.75	0.07	10.70
Saccharum officinarum	Dry	100	5.8	3.17	0	1.00	0.11	9.10
Sorghum, milo, fresh	As fed	90	11.1	3.40	2.4	0.03	0.28	0.10
Sorghum vulgare	Dry	100	12.4	3.79	2.6	0.04	0.32	0.10
Corn, dent yellow, grain	As fed	89	9.6	3.40	2.6	0.03	0.26	0.10
Zea mays	Dry	100	10.9	3.84	2.9	0.03	0.29	0.10

Source: U.S.-Canadian Tables of Feed Composition, 3rd ed. 1982.

cies and found to generally conform to the body weight in kilograms raised to the .75 power. Therefore, in nutritional calculations, metabolic weight is expressed as $W_{kg}^{.75}$, which simply means that a large animal has a smaller nutrient requirement per unit of body weight than a small animal.

Protein

The protein requirement for any animal has a direct relationship to the requirement for energy. The figure used here is the same as for sheep and goats, 31 g protein/Mcal DE.

Camelids may be able to digest protein and fiber more efficiently than ruminants. Efficiency has been demonstrated in some studies of forage with high-fiber content and low-protein levels, in other words, when a poor ration was consumed. On adequate diets, camelids apparently digest fiber and protein at an efficiency rate similar to that of sheep. In making recommendations for the nutrition of llamas, an optimum ration, not a marginal one, should be the goal.

Dry Matter

All figures in Table 2.5, except those in the last two columns, are based on 100% dry matter. The amount actually fed will depend on the moisture content of the forage eaten. For most sun-cured hay, the moisture content is 10–12% and for pasture plants, 50–75%.

Increased levels above adult maintenance are required for growth, lactation, late pregnancy, work, and inclement weather (Table 2.9). None of these requirements have been ascertained specifically for llamas or alpacas. Extrapolating from the data on goats, the following recommendations may be made. For the last 4 months of pregnancy, 0.093 Mcal DE/$W_{kg}^{.75}$ should be added to maintenance requirements. For growth, based on 8.92 Kcal DE/g gain, the figure is 1.78 Mcal DE/day. For lactation, based on 1533 Kcal DE/kg milk, if a 20 kg cria is consuming 10% of its body weight, the female must produce 2 kg of milk. The added energy requirement for that female would be 3.06 Mcal DE/day. A working pack animal may require a 75% increase in energy over the adult maintenance requirement.

Table 2.5 should be used only until more specific data are reported in the literature. Furthermore, biologic variation among individuals must be considered. Observation and adjustment by the feeder is necessary to maintain a sound nutritional basis for feeding practices.

Water

The drinking behavior of South American camelids (SACs) is to suck in water with the mouth slightly opened. Camelids have learned to drink from all types of waterers and containers but are slow to become accustomed to automatic waterers, especially if it is necessary to press a lever to cause the water to flow. Running streams and ponds are natural for them. They are fastidious and may refuse to drink polluted water. This is interesting, because packing llamas on the trail are inclined to urinate and defecate in a stream while they are drinking. Trail llamas will surprise the novice in that they frequently do not drink during the day, even with ample access to water.

Like all animals, camelids require adequate amounts of good-quality water to sustain life, reproduce, work, and produce fiber and milk. Although Old World camelids are legendary in their ability to subsist on little or no water for long periods, they nevertheless need an adequate balance.

Only limited studies have been conducted on the water requirements of SACs (39). It has been determined that the water content of the body of the llama is approximately 67%, compared with the goat at 60%. This varies with age and body fat content. In the same study, it was found that goats and llamas have similar water requirements. In an indoor experiment in a neutral environment, the water turnover rate (water intake by drinking plus food and oxidative water) was 62.1 ml/$W_{kg}^{.82}$/24 hr in the llama and 59 ml in the goat. The amount of water consumed was 42.5 ml/$W_{kg}^{.82}$ in the llama and 40 ml in the goat. With a 40% reduction in food intake, water consumption of the llama decreased by 18%. When water was restricted, the llama was able to maintain food consumption. In similar studies of llamas on pasture, water turnover rates were double those of the indoor experiments, 122.2 ml/$W_{kg}^{.82}$ (39).

Based on these studies, a basic water requirement for lamoids would be as indicated in Table 2.10. This correlates quite closely with water requirements of other ungulate species. Water requirements can be met by free water consumption, moisture in feed, and water produced by the oxidative processes associated with energy metabolism. Camelids on lush pasture may obtain a majority of the water requirement from feed. Dry feed necessitates greater water intake. Salt and other mineral content of forage may affect the water requirement as well.

Table 2.9. Estimated extra energy to be added to maintenance requirements for special physiologic states in llamas

Body weight	Additional energy required for growth[a]	Additional energy required for pregnancy	Additional energy required for lactation	Additional energy required for work or cold
(kg)	*(Mcal/day)* (F)	*(last 4 mo.)* (G)	*(Mcal/day)* (H)	*(Mcal/day)* (I)
10	1.8			
20	1.8			
40	1.8			
50	1.6			
75	1.6	2.4	3.1	
100		2.9	3.1	
125		3.5	3.1	2.3
150		4.0	3.1	2.6
175		4.4	3.1	2.9
200		5.0	3.1	3.2
225		5.4	3.1	3.5
250		5.9	3.1	3.8

[a]Added to maintenance energy requirement.

Note: F = 8.92 Kcal DE/g gain; G = 0.93 Mcal DE × $W_{kg}^{.75}$; H = 1533 Kcal DE/g milk; I = 50% additional Mcal.

Table 2.10. Water requirements for llamas

Body Weight (kg)	Metabolic Weight ($kg^{.82}$)	Water Intake in a Controlled Environment[a] ($ml/kg^{.82}$)
40	20.59	0.88
50	24.73	1.05
75	34.48	1.47
100	43.65	1.86
125	52.42	2.23
150	60.87	2.59
175	69.07	2.94
200	77.06	3.28
225	84.88	3.61
250	92.54	3.91

Source: Rubsamen and von Englehart 1975.

[a]Actual consumption may be 1.5 to 2.5 times this, depending on weather and activity.

Water is lost through urine, milk, perspiration, and evaporation from the respiratory tract. Situations resulting in an increased production of any of these fluids will increase water needs.

Lactation places a significant demand on water consumption. No studies have been conducted on lamoids, but in the goat, it is recommended that 1.43 L water be provided for each kilogram of milk produced (31).

Elevated ambient temperatures result in extra demands for water in lamoids because they lack the ability of Old World camelids to withstand elevation of body temperature. Old World camelids, particularly the dromedary, have evolved special physiologic mechanisms to deal with water deprivation. The camel can control the water content of feces and the concentration of urine, which reduces excretion of vital fluids during heat stress. Contrary to popular belief, the camel does not store water any more than any other species, but because of its ability to conserve body fluids, it need not drink water for considerable periods.

The dromedary is able to tolerate extreme dehydration and has been known to survive the loss of body water equal to 40% of its body weight. In contrast, a human losing 12% of the body's weight in water would be close to death. The small oval erythrocyte of the camel continues to circulate despite increased blood viscosity. Even after severe dehydration, the camel is able to drink sufficient water at one session to make up the deficit. Immediate intake of this amount of water would cause severe osmotic problems in humans or other animals of temperate climates. In the camel, water is absorbed from the stomach and intestines slowly, allowing establishment of equilibrium. The erythrocytes are able to avoid osmotic problems by swelling to 240% of their initial volume without rupturing. SACs may share this ability with Old World camels. In other species, erythrocytes can swell only to 150%.

Camels are also able to endure a wide range of diurnal fluctuation of body temperature, from 36.5 to 42°C. The body acts as a heat sink during the hot times of the day, thus conserving vital water that would otherwise be lost through evaporative cooling. The excess heat is dissipated by conduction and radiation during the cool desert nights.

SACs should be given access to unlimited free-choice consumption of clean water. Intake will be adjusted to body needs. If water is restricted below requirement, feed consumption will decrease, lactation will slow down or cease, and, in the extreme, hyperthermia may result.

Minerals

In spite of the harsh environment and the sparse vegetation of some areas of the Andes, there are no reports of vitamin and mineral deficiencies or toxicities in lamoids in their native habitat (22). This does not mean that they do not occur or that deficiencies may not develop in locations outside of South America. The problem may be lack of diagnostic facilities, observation, or experience or failure to report. Lamoids evolved with their environment and have developed the ability to cope with native soil types, climates, and forage quality. Out of the native habitat, they may not be able to cope.

CALCIUM AND PHOSPHORUS. Calcium (Ca) and phosphorus (P) levels were extrapolated from sheep (32) and cattle (30) requirements. These are the two most important minerals in all vertebrates; 99% of body Ca and 80% of P are found in the skeletal system (29). In order for Ca requirements to be met, the final diet should contain over 0.3% Ca on a dry weight basis, and the Ca-P ratio (Ca:P) should not be less than 1.2:1 (Table 2.5). Lamoids are usually exposed to sunlight, providing for the necessary vitamin D.

It is unlikely that these minerals will be deficient in animals given free access to pastures or hays in temperate climates, which usually contain ample Ca and P, with a satisfactory Ca:P. In tropical climates, however, P deficiency is common in livestock on pasture (27). Notice from Table 2.8 that grains are deficient in Ca, and the Ca:P is poor. When concentrates are added to the diet, it is necessary to evaluate the diet to assure that adequate Ca and P levels have been maintained.

Ca-P ratios of less than 1:1 and over 7:1 have been shown to decrease growth and feed efficiency in ruminants (27), though ruminants tolerate more variation in Ca:P than other livestock. Excesses of either Ca or P in a ration may inhibit the availability of certain trace elements.

Metabolic bone disease (MBD) is a collective term used to describe the various manifestations of the complex syndrome produced by inadequate Ca, inadequate

P, improper Ca:P, and nonexposure to ultraviolet light or no vitamin D in the diet (13). Other factors that may have an impact on the syndrome include protein deficiency and primary diseases of the kidney, liver, and intestine, which affect the conversion of vitamin D to the active hormone and absorption of minerals from the intestine.

The clinical signs of MBD exhibited by an individual animal depend on age, which component is deficient, duration of the deficiency, and degree of deficiency. Signs include lameness, fractures, deformity of bones, painful joints, and reluctance to move. Anorexia results from painful mastication, caused by loosening of teeth. Growth of young animals will be slowed. In lactating females, milk production decreases. Severe Ca deficiency may result in tetany (12). Some species develop fibrous osteodystrophy, but it is not known if this occurs in lamoids. Any, some, or all of the above signs may be seen in an affected animal.

Some llamas develop angular limb deformities, the etiology of which has not been determined. Considering that this may have a nutritional basis, some owners are finding fault with alfalfa and its high Ca content (1–2.5% on dry matter basis). Granted that this could yield a Ca:P of over 7:1 on pure analysis, other factors must be considered. First, not all of the Ca in alfalfa is available for absorption. Oxalates, found in high levels in alfalfa, tie up Ca into insoluble calcium oxalate. Second, Ca absorption is an active process, requiring 1,25 dihydroxycholecalciferol (the hormone derived from vitamin D) to induce transport of Ca across the intestinal mucosa, whereas P is absorbed by simple diffusion; thus there is more chance for metabolic imbalance to occur with P.

In the ruminant, excess Ca is either passed through the gut in the ingesta or, if absorbed, recycled back through the intestine and excreted in the feces (19). With P, excess must be excreted via urine; thus water is required to flush P from the body.

COPPER AND MOLYBDENUM (27). Copper deficiency is the second most common mineral deficiency observed in tropical climates. Copper (Cu) and molybdenum (Mo) are usually considered together because of their inverse interrelationship. High Mo levels depress Cu levels and vice versa. Numerous other dietary factors, including sulfur, zinc, iron, and protein, may affect Cu and Mo metabolism. Any evaluation of a problem must include consideration of all factors.

Cu is a required trace element, a component of certain body pigments (hair), and essential for hemoglobin production and vital enzyme systems. Although Mo is required in certain enzyme systems, rarely does a deficiency develop; rather, the usual clinical problem seen is toxicity. The clinical signs of Mo toxicity are similar to those of Cu deficiency. It is, however, possible to have an absolute Cu deficiency without concomitant high levels of Mo.

The collective signs of Cu deficiency in ruminants are chronic diarrhea, anemia, roughened and bleached hair coat, and slow growth or loss of weight. Deficient animals may also have fragile bones, predisposing to fractures and lameness. Sudden death has also been reported, apparently when essential cardiac enzyme systems fail (27).

No observations of Cu deficiency or Mo toxicity in camelids have been reported. Cu deficiency in lambs is common in the altiplano of Peru, yet the problem has not been diagnosed in lamoids.[1] However, the clinical signs have been seen in camelids, and deficiency of these minerals should be kept in mind when making a differential diagnosis. There are no camelid-specific diagnostic data that can be used for making a diagnosis. Ruminant data must be used. In cattle and sheep, serum levels of Cu below 0.5 μg/ml are indicative of a deficiency (normal, 0.6–1.5 μg/ml) (Table 2.11). At necropsy, or with biopsy, liver Cu levels below 75 ppm dry weight would be diagnostic.

Both Mo toxicity and Cu deficiency can be treated and/or prevented by either supplying a dietary supplement containing Cu or giving parenteral organic Cu. Mineral supplements used in known trouble sites should

1. W. Bravo, LaRaya, Peru, personal communication.

Table 2.11. Parameters used to evaluate selected mineral deficiencies in cattle and sheep

	Minimum dietary requirements			Laboratory analysis	
Element	Dairy cow	Beef cattle	Sheep	Tissue	Critical levels
Calcium, %	0.54	0.18–0.53	0.21–0.52	Bone (fat free)	29.5%
				Bone ash	37.6%
				Plasma	8 mg/dl
Phosphorus, %	0.38	0.18–0.37	0.16–0.37	Bone (fat free)	11.5%
				Bone ash	17.6%
				Plasma	4.5 mg/dl
Copper, ppm	10	4–10	5	Liver	25–75 ppm dry matter
				Serum	0.65 μg/ml
Zinc, ppm	40	20–40	35–50	Serum	0.6–0.8 μg/dl

Source: McDowell et al. 1983.
Note: Requirements of camelids unknown.

contain 0.1–0.2% copper sulfate. Although it has not been reported in llamas, Cu toxicity could result from over supplementation.

ZINC. Zinc (Zn) is an essential component of specific enzymes and zinc-dependent enzyme systems. The enzymes are involved with nucleic acid and protein metabolism. A Zn deficiency will inhibit cell replication and other functions in which protein synthesis is vital (27).

The primary signs of Zn deficiency in ruminants include reduced feed intake, poor growth rate, and dermatologic disorders. Just as important, but less easily evaluated, are joint stiffness, swollen feet, and impairment of reproductive organs and tissues.

Reproductive disorders may be manifested in the male by impaired spermatogenesis, testicular growth, and development of sexual organs, accompanied by poor libido. In the female, estrus, parturition, and lactation may be inhibited.

Skin lesions may begin as erythema, in appearance, much like a sunburn. The skin subsequently becomes dry and scaly. The basic lesions are parakeratosis and acanthosis. The skin thickens and cracks, and keratin crusts form. Secondary infection is common. When evaluating skin biopsies in llamas, it should be remembered that a cellular infiltrate surrounding the dermal arterioles that would suggest an inflammatory response in other species is normal for this camelid.

Nonspecific dermatitis is a common lesion reported in llamas. An etiologic diagnosis is seldom obtained. Many therapeutic regimens have been tried, some successful, some not. In certain sections of the United States, when such a dermatitis appears in llamas, clinicians are making a tentative diagnosis of Zn deficiency and are treating it as such.

The diagnosis of Zn deficiency in llamas is based on extrapolation of data from ruminants (Table 2.11). Serum levels of less than 0.5 μg/dl in cattle and sheep are considered suspect. Forage analysis studies indicate that a minimum of 40 ppm Zn is required in the total ration.

Zn deficiency in cattle can be corrected by feeding a trace mineral salt mixture containing 0.5% Zn. This may be difficult with llamas that refuse to eat a salt mix. Zn may be incorporated into a sweet feed mixture in a ratio to allow ingestion of an extra 20–30 ppm Zn in the total ration. Commercial trace mineral mixes may not contain sufficient Zn. Even though it is listed on the label, the quantity incorporated may be insignificant. Trace minerals interact with each other, and there may be more need for a certain element at one given period of life than at another. Zn, for instance, is especially needed for growth and reproduction.

SELENIUM (13, 33). Both deficiencies and toxicities of selenium (Se) have been reported in livestock species in North America. There is circumstantial evidence that lamoids are also susceptible, though no clear clinical picture of the effects of Se deficiency has been established. A variety of signs have been reported in various species, making it difficult, if not impossible, to make an antemortem diagnosis. The signs seen in a horse differ slightly from those seen in cattle, sheep, or swine. Young animals exhibit different signs than adults.

In cattle, Se deficiency may cause any of the following: muscle stiffness, paralysis, diarrhea, or sudden death due to cardiac muscle necrosis. In a milder form, there may be retained placentas, abortions, reduced fertility, decreased growth rate, and a decreased immune response.

The clinical signs seen in horse foals include muscle atrophy and sudden death. In adults, reproductive disorders including pyometra, infertility, abortion, and early embryonic death have been reported. Also, both skeletal and cardiac muscles may necrose.

In swine, stress seems to bring on the clinical disease. Swine suffer from cardiac and skeletal muscle damage, decreased resistance to disease, and reproductive problems. In addition, the liver is affected, and the syndrome includes the effects of liver dysfunction.

All of these signs and lesions have been seen at one time or another in llamas. Some of the signs are typical of other diseases as well, making it difficult to single out Se deficiency as the cause.

To summarize, it is evident that Se deficiency affects the reproductive process in all species, causing abortion, early embryonic death, retained placenta, and weakened neonates. Also, muscle damage causes weakness, ataxia, and paralysis. Sudden death will result if cardiac necrosis occurs. Chronic diarrhea with poor growth and a decreased ability to mount an immune response may occur, resulting in decreased resistance to infection and parasites.

The Se content of forage depends on the site of origin. Figure 2.1 provides an overview of the problem in North America. Owners of llamas and alpacas being raised in a known or even suspected deficient area should take steps to supplement the diet or otherwise manage their animals to prevent the problem.

Prevention of Se deficiency through supplementation is practiced by a wide variety of methods. A supplementation routine should be selected after consultation with knowledgeable persons in the area concerned. A program must be tailored to fit the needs of a particular area.

Llamas may learn to eat a mix containing Se, other trace minerals, and salt. This mix must be protected from rain. A number of companies market such prod-

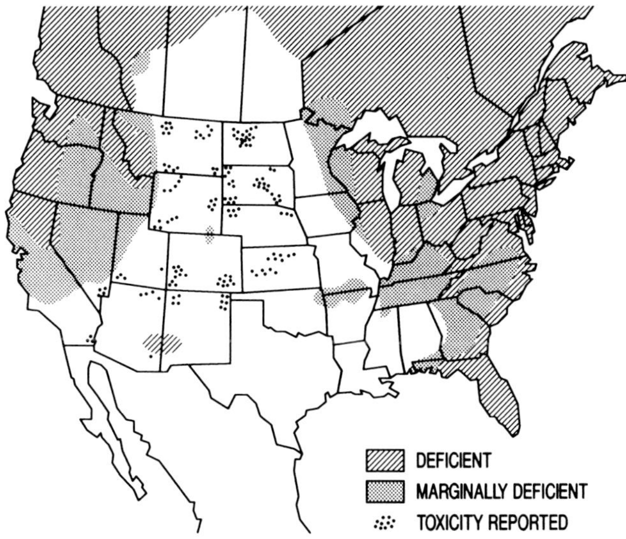

2.1 Regional selenium levels in North American forages.

ucts. Salt blocks can be purchased containing Se and other trace minerals. Some llamas chew at these blocks, but others ignore them completely. If the owner is feeding a pelleted total feed, Se in a premix may be added. The Se concentration should not exceed 0.1 ppm. Feed manufacturers can provide this only within the limits dictated by federal, state, or provincial regulations.

Se can be purchased in bulk, weighed out for each animal daily on a scale calibrated in milligrams, and fed individually in a grain mix. One breeder in a severely deficient area gives each of his animals 1.5–2 mg Se each day.

A final method of supplying Se is by injection with sodium selenite, using one of the commercial products listed in Table 2.12. Although the intramuscular site is recommended by the manufacturer, llamas seem to develop a severe adverse reaction to this method, and subcutaneous injections have proved to be more suitable.

Management of a Se deficiency problem may involve analysis of either forage or blood to determine concentrations. No normal blood levels of Se have been established for llamas, but levels determined for cattle and sheep (Table 2.13) seem to be adequate. Forage should contain at least 0.05 ppm Se, but not more than 1 ppm.

Table 2.13. Selenium blood levels

Condition	Whole blood	Serum
	(μg/ml or ppm)	*(μg/ml)*
Severely deficient, white muscle disease likely	<0.02	0.006
Deficient, no clinical response from treatment	<0.03	0.008
Deficient, no clinical signs	<0.05	0.014
Marginally deficient	0.05–0.08	0.014–0.022
Acceptable	>0.08	>0.022
Excellent	0.1–0.3	0.03–0.08
Toxic	>2	0.56

Note: These levels are for cattle and sheep established by Dr. Ben Norman at the University of California, Davis. They may serve as a guide until similar levels are established for llamas. Samples may be run on whole blood or serum. Selenium is found at different concentrations in different portions of the blood. Assuming that the level in whole blood is 100%, the level in serum would be 28% (this is for sheep and cattle; llamas may or may not be the same).

Selenium Toxicity. The signs of Se toxicity are likewise difficult to evaluate. Interestingly, the signs may be exaggerations of the signs of deficiency. Poor conception rates, abortion, and developmental defects have been reported in cattle along with alopecia and sloughing of the hoofs. In horses, toxicity may cause lameness, dullness, emaciation, and depraved appetite.

OTHER TOXICITIES. Most toxic plants, heavy metals, and insecticides will be ingested in the feed. For a discussion of these problems see Chapter 23. Table 2.14 provides some levels for toxic mineral analysis.

Table 2.12. Injectable selenium products

Concentration of selenium[a]	Company[b] and product	Recommendations for livestock	Suggested dosage for llamas[c] Newborn	Juvenile	Adult
(mg/ml)					
0.25	L-Se	Lambs, newborn, 1 ml Lambs, 2 weeks+, 4 ml Piglet, 1 ml (subcutaneous)	2–4 ml	4–6 ml	Do not use
1.00	Bo-Se	Calves, 3 ml/100[d] Lambs, 2 weeks+, 1 ml/40[d] Sows, 1 ml/40[d]	1–2 ml	2–4 ml	6–8 ml
5.00	Mu-Se	Calves, weaning, 200[d] Cows, 1 ml/200[d] (subcutaneous)	Do not use	0.25/ml 50[d]	1 ml/200[d]
2.50	E-Se	Horses only 1 ml/100[d] (intramuscular)	Do not use	Do not use	Do not use
1.00	Seletoc	Dogs only	Do not use	Do not use	Do not use

[a]All formulations contain 68 IU vitamin E/ml.
[b]Schering Corp., Kenilworth, NJ 07033.
[c]Adapt to regional requirements and situations.
[d]Pounds body weight.

Table 2.14. Parameters used to evaluate selected mineral toxicity in cattle and sheep

	Dietary levels above which toxicity is likely			Laboratory analysis wet or dry	
Element	Dairy cow	Buffalo	Sheep	Tissue	Critical levels of dry matter
(ppm)					
Copper	80	115	8–25	Liver	700
Fluorine	30	30–100	60–200	Bone	4500–7500
Molybdenum	6	6	5–20	Liver	4
Selenium	5	5	>2	Liver	5–15
Zinc	500	500	1000	. . .	. . .

McDowell et al. 1983.

NORTH AMERICAN FEEDING PRACTICES

Pasture

There are nearly as many different pasture feeding practices as there are llama owners. Llamas and alpacas have been grazed on every conceivable type of pasture, from native pastures in Texas or Arizona to improved pastures in Michigan or British Columbia. The tables of composition of feed items indicate relative values of some forages (Tables 2.3, 2.8). Information on feeds not mentioned may be found in the references appended (1, 15, 26, 44). The nutrient content of feeds may vary from region to region, so these figures cannot be considered as absolutes.

Adult llamas may be maintained on most pastures if sufficient forage is available for ingestion within a reasonable amount of time. Some pastures are not of sufficient quality to sustain pregnant and lactating females without weight loss or to supply growing animals with adequate nutrition. Forage quality should be compared with the requirements of different classes of llamas.

As an example, if a llama weighing 100 kg was kept on a rye grass pasture, the animal would have to consume 5.54 kg/day (rye grass contains 0.80 Mcal DE/kg, as fed, and the animal requires 4.43 Mcal/day). This amounts to 5.54% of the body weight. To consume sufficient forage of this type, the animal must graze for much of the day. If this llama were a pregnant female or nursing a baby, the pasture would not provide sufficient nutrients, and supplementation would be necessary to maintain her weight.

It should be remembered that pasturage is all that is available to lamoids in South America. Animals found in particularly harsh areas suffer accordingly. Also, there is considerable seasonal variation in nutrient intake, hence periodic weight gain and loss.

Hay

A large percentage of North American lamoids are fed hay for at least a part of the year. Numerous legumes and grasses may be cured and stored in a variety of ways to preserve the nutrients for feeding at a later time. Climate greatly affects the quality of hay. Hay subjected to rain during the curing process loses much of its nutrients.

Tables 2.6 and 2.7 provide the composition of some of the plants and combinations used for hay in North America. Most of these have been used at one time or another for llamas and alpacas. Probably all of them are satisfactory if appropriate supplementation is provided according to the needs of the animals. Llamas may be considered to be picky eaters. Those who feed alfalfa will know that llamas prefer the leaves and fine stems, avoiding the large stems. This results in significant wastage if unlimited free-choice feeding is practiced.

Some owners subscribe to the theory that if a "cafeteria" of various feed items is provided, a llama will select a diet that meets individual requirements. This is neither economically, behaviorally, nor nutritionally justified. As in all species, llamas eat not to satisfy basic nutrient requirements but to satisfy appetite, i.e., taste and smell. The wise manager will learn the animal's requirements and develop a feeding regimen that coincides with those requirements.

As one example of use of the tables to determine the quality of a hay ration, consider a 100 kg llama with a DE requirement of 4.43 Mcal/day. Alfalfa hay has a caloric density of 2.49 Mcal DE/kg. Therefore, a llama consuming 1.78 kg of alfalfa hay would satisfy the energy requirement. Other nutrient requirements would also be met. As this amount is only 1.78% of the body weight, it would easily be consumed by this animal. If the same llama was kept on a rye grass pasture, the animal would have to consume 5.54 kg/day (rye grass contains 0.8 Mcal DE/kg, as fed) and the animal would have to consume 5.54% of its body weight. To consume sufficient forage of this type, the animal must graze for much of the day. If this llama were a pregnant female or nursing a baby, the pasture would not provide sufficient nutrients, and supplementation would be necessary to maintain her weight.

Processed Feeds

Current agricultural practices supply livestock growers with hays and concentrates in various forms, such as bales, cubes, and pellets. Forages may also be harvested green and preserved as silage or haylage, which have been used to feed llamas but probably do not constitute an important source of feed for llamas.

Pelleted feeds, both simple hay and complete diets, have been fed to camelids in private ownership and in zoos for a long time. This is a somewhat expensive product, but wastage can be kept to a minimum; thus in the long run, it may be less expensive than other types of feed. Camelids seem to deal with pellets satisfactorily. It has been suggested more fiber may be needed in the diet than is provided by pellets. In one study, an increase in soil ingestion by llamas was observed when pellets were fed, even though the pellets were not fed on the ground (20).

Concentrates

Some llamas avoid ingestion of grains or mixed sweet feeds, while others willingly eat them. Individuals may prefer one type of grain over another, but this is probably a learned response, for most of the grains are acceptable. All grains supply increased energy and, in some cases, protein. They are deficient in Ca, P, and trace minerals. Concentrates are usually more expensive than hays and should be used only when needed to supply additional energy. Mixtures of grains, protein supplements, vitamins, and minerals are commonly bound together by blackstrap molasses to form a sweet, palatable, high-energy protein supplement. These are satisfactory for lamoids if the extra nutrients are needed. Camelids are able to metabolize urea as a nitrogen source for synthesis of protein, but suitable levels for inclusion of urea in a ration have not been determined.

Special Feeding Problems

STARVATION/INANITION. There are enough new, inexperienced llama owners that veterinarians may see a starved animal. A thick fiber coat will mask a loss of condition, and unless the owner can and does feel the backbone, there will be little to indicate weight loss. Many large operations regularly monitor the weights of animals. All owners could weigh animals at a public weigh station.

Having found a thin animal, it is necessary to determine if weight loss is caused by a nutritional problem or an infectious or parasitic disease. An evaluation of the feeding practices may help in making a diagnosis. Appropriate remedial measures should be instituted. At necropsy, the starved animal will lack body fat, and serous atrophy of fat around the heart and in the peritoneal cavity may be seen. Bone marrow will be watery rather than gelatinous.

OBESITY. Probably a more frequent problem, especially among new, overly solicitous owners, is overfeeding. This is easily done if concentrates are used routinely without regard to actual requirements. Overfeeding is not only costly, but obese animals are more likely to be infertile and will develop hyperthermia more easily than those of normal weight.

There is no question that some animals become obese more readily than others. The recommended requirements should be adjusted to fit individual needs. If an animal gains undesired weight when fed recommended amounts, the amount of feed given should be decreased until a correct balance is achieved.

WASTING SYNDROME. A number of llamas have been observed to become anorectic, lose weight, and ultimately die. No infectious or parasitic diseases have been identified as the cause. The condition is not always related to a lack of available feed, but certainly the affected animals eat sparingly or, in later stages, not at all. Whether this syndrome will ultimately prove to be related to a nutritional or other metabolic disease is yet to be determined.

POISONS IN FEED. Several poisonous plants have been identified as toxic to llamas (see Chap. 23). In connection with feeding, it is important to recognize that processed feeds present a special hazard for all animals. Given a choice, a llama may not select and eat a toxic plant. However, when included in a cube or a pellet, poisonous plants may be undetectable. Unfortunately, cubes and pellets may be made to utilize poor-quality forage or hay containing poisonous plants. The reputation of the supplier is the only safeguard available.

OTHER DISEASES. Infectious and parasitic diseases place a stress burden on the animal. This may be reflected in increased nutrient requirements, paradoxically, at a time when an animal may be disinclined to eat. Protein and energy requirements may be significantly increased in the febrile state or when an animal is suffering from nutrient-losing diarrhea or pneumonia. Postsurgical wound healing and fracture repair may require 150% of the usual maintenance needs.

Many disease conditions diminish or destroy stomach microorganisms. Without fermentation, the llama will have difficulty in digesting and absorbing nourishment. Hydration and reestablishment of essential flora and fauna may be crucial to recovery.

Special Feeding Situations

FEEDING ON THE TRAIL. Since llamas are popular pack animals, feeding on the trail is necessary. Feeding will be limited to grazing and feed that can be carried in addition to needed items for human participants. Llamas make good use of available plants at rest stops and in camp. They eat all types of forbs, grasses, sedges, shrubs, and small trees without stripping an area clean of all vegetation. Llamas may be hobbled and let run free or tethered to picket lines or, individually, to trees, shrubs, rocks, or stakes.

Poisonous plants may be a hazard. Although llamas in South America may have learned to avoid native poisonous plants, this may not be true of animals in North America. The packer must avoid tethering an animal where there is little to eat but a poisonous plant. A near tragedy occurred when llamas were tied to a mountain laurel shrub, *Leucothoe davisaii.*

Hard working pack llamas may have energy requirements that are double the amount needed for maintenance. Time must be allowed for them to graze and/or consume carried feed.

One successful, experienced packer feeds a mixture of alfalfa pellets and a mixed sweet feed at a rate of approximately 1 pound per animal, night and morning, in addition to permitting as much grazing as possible.

Cold Weather

Lamoids are superbly adapted to cold weather but, surprisingly, not to the degree reached by the extremely cold weather of high elevations in North America. Temperatures rarely dip below −10 to −20° C even at high elevations in the Andes where lamoids live. In North America, temperatures may drop to −40° C (−40°F) and be accompanied with a wind chill factor that drops the effective temperature even lower. Thermoregulatory problems are dealt with in Chapter 9.

REFERENCES

1. Atlas of Nutritional Data on United States and Canadian Feeds. 1972. Washington, D.C.: National Academy of Sciences.

2. Chauca, D., Valenzuela, M. A., and Sillau, H. 1970. (Comparative study of in vitro digestibility of crude fiber between alpaca and sheep) Estudio comparativo de digestibilidad in vitro de fibra cruda entre la alpaca y el ovino. Bol. Extraordinario 4:100–104.

3. Chlarson, N. A. 1986. Hay quality and selection. Llamas 31:58–59.

4. Church, D. C. 1975, 1979. Digestive Physiology and Nutrition of Ruminants, 2nd ed., vols. 1, 2. Corvallis, Oreg.: O & B Books.

5. Clemens, E. T., and Stevens, C. E. 1980. A comparison of gastrointestinal transit times in ten species of mammals. J. Agric. Sci. (Cambridge) 94:735–37.

6. Dougherty, R. W., and Vallenas, P. A. 1986. A quantitative study of eructated gas expulsion in alpacas. Cornell Vet. 58:3–7.

7. Eckerlin, R. H., and Stevens, C. E. 1973. Bicarbonate secretion of the glandular saccules of the llama stomach. Cornell Vet. 63:436–45.

8. Engelhardt, W., and Engelhardt, W. von. 1976. Diminished renal urea excretion in the llama at reduced food intake. In Proceedings, Tracer Studies on Non-Protein Nitrogen for Ruminants III. Vienna: International Atomic Energy Agency, pp. 61–62.

9. Engelhardt, W. von, Rubsamen, K., and Heller, R. 1984. The digestive physiology of camelids. In W. R. Cockrill, ed. The Camelid—An All Purpose Animal. Uppsala: Scandinavian Institute for African Studies, pp. 323–46.

10. Fernandez Baca, S. 1977. New world camelidae diets (natural and synthetic). In M. Rechcigl, Jr., ed. Diets for Mammals. Sect. G: Diets, Culture Media and Food Supplement. Cleveland: CRC Press, pp. 207–11.

11. Fernandez Baca, S., and Novoa, C. 1963. (Comparative study of the digestibility of forages in sheep and alpaca) Estudio comparativo de la digestibilidad de los forrajes en ovinos y alpacas. Rev. Fac. Med. Vet. (Lima) 18:85–96.

12. Fowler, M. E. 1986a. Metabolic bone disease. In M. E. Fowler, ed. Zoo and Wild Animal Medicine, 2nd ed. Philadelphia: W. B. Saunders, pp. 70–90.

13. ______. 1986b. Selenium—friend or foe. Llamas 31:37–43.

14. Franklin, W. L. 1982. Biology, ecology, and relationship to man of South American camelids. In M. A. Mares and H. H. Genoways, eds. Mammalian Biology in South America. Linesville: Pymatuning Laboratory of Ecology, Univ. of Pittsburgh, pp. 457–89.

15. Gohl, B. 1981. Tropical Feeds. FAO Animal Production and Health Series 12. Rome: Food and Agriculture Organization.

16. Harmeyer, J., and Hill, H. 1968. (The volume of protozoa in the rumen of the goat and guanaco) Das Protozoenvolumen in Panseninhalt bei Ziege und Guanako. Zentralbl. Veterinaermed [A] 11(6):493–501.

17. Hinderer, S., and Engelhardt, W. von. 1975. Urea metabolism in the llama. Comp. Biochem. Physiol. [A] 52:619–22.

18. ______. 1976. Entry of blood urea into the rumen of the llama. In Proceedings, Tracer Studies on Non-Protein Nitrogen for Ruminants III. Vienna: International Atomic Energy Agency, pp. 59–60.

19. Hintz, H. F., Schryver, H. F., and Halbert, M. 1973. A note on the comparison of digestion by new-world camels, sheep and ponies. Anim. Prod. 16(3):303–5.

20. Hintz, H. F., Sedgewick, C. J., and Schryver, H. F. 1976. Some observations on digestion of a pelleted diet by ruminants and nonruminants. In P. J. S. Olney, ed. International Zoo Yearbook, vol. 16. London: Academic Press, pp. 54–57.

21. Holgado V., D., Fargan, L. R., and Tapia N., M. 1979. (An evaluation of pasture plants at LaRaya-[Puno]) Evaluation agrostologica de los pastizales de La Raya-(Puno). Rev. Invest. Pecu. 4(1):32–37.

22. Huancapaza, M., and Coasaca, M. 1975. (Use of vitamins A, E, and ADE in pregnant alpaca and their effect on the newborn) Aplicacion de vitaminas A, E y ADE en alpacas gestantes, *Lama pacos,* tipo Huacaya y sus efectos en las crias. Tesis, Fac. Med. Vet. Univ. Nac. Tec. Altiplano (Puno).

23. Hume, C. 1983. On feeding llamas. Llama World 1(4):6–9.

24. Koford, C. B. 1957. The vicuña and the puna. Ecol. Monogr. 27(2):152–219.

25. McCandless, E. L., and Dye, J. A. 1950. Physiological changes in intermediary metabolism of various species of ruminants incident of functional development of rumen. Am. J. Physiol. 162:434–46.

26. McDowell, L. R., Conrad, J. H., Thomas, J. E., and Harris, L. E. 1974. Latin American Tables of Feed Composition. Gainesville, Fla.: Univ. of Florida.

27. McDowell, L. R., Conrad, J. H., Ellis, G. L., and Loosli, J. K. 1983. Minerals for Grazing Ruminants in Tropical Regions. Gainesville, Fla.: Center for Tropical Agriculture.

28. Morley, F. H. W., ed. 1981. Grazing Animals. Amsterdam: Elsevier.

29. Newman, D. M. R. 1984. The feeds and feeding habits of old and new world camels. In W. R. Cockrill, ed. The Camelid—An All Purpose Animal, vol. 1. Uppsala: Scandinavian Institute for African Studies.

30. Nutrient Requirements of Dairy Cattle. 1978. No. 3, Nutrient Requirements of Domestic Animals. Washington, D.C.: National Academy of Sciences.

31. Nutrient Requirements of Goats. 1981. No. 15, Nutrient Requirements of Domestic Animals. Washington, D.C.: National Academy of Sciences.

32. Nutrient Requirements of Sheep. 1975. No. 5, Nutrient Requirements of Domestic Animals. Washington, D.C.: National Academy of Sciences.

33. Oldfield, J. E. 1983. Two faces of selenium. Llama World 1(4):10–11.

34. Ortiz, C., Cavero, J., Sillau, H., and Cueva, S. 1974. The parotid saliva of the alpaca (*Lama pacos*). Res. Vet. Sci. 16:54–56.

35. Oyanguren Perez, F. 1969. (Comparative tests of the digestibility of oat silage and cattails in sheep and alpacas) Ensayo comparativo de la digestibilidad de ensilaje de avena (*Avena sativa*) variedad Mantaro 15 y de totora en ovinos y alpaca. Tesis, Ing. Agr. Univ. Nac. Tec. Altiplano (Puno), pp. 1–33.

36. Raedeke, K. J. 1980. Food habits of the guanaco (*Lama guanacoe*) of Tierra Del Fuego, Chile. Turrialba 30(2):177–81.

37. Reiner, R. J., and Bryant, F. C. 1986. Botanical composition and nutritional quality of alpaca diets in two Andean rangeland communities. J. Range Manage. 39(5):424–27.

38. Reiner, R. J., Bryant, F. C., Farfan, R. D., and Craddock, B. F. 1987. Forage intake of alpacas grazing Andean rangeland in Peru. J. Anim. Sci. 64:868–74.

39. Rubsamen, K., and Englehardt, W. von. 1975. Water metabolism in the llama. Comp. Biochem. Physiol. [A] 52:595–98.

40. ______. 1978. Bicarbonate secretion and solute absorption of the forestomach of the llama. Am. J. Physiol. 235 (1,2):E1–E6.

41. Schneider, W., Hauffe, R., and Engelhardt, W. von. 1974. (Energy and nitrogen turnover in the llama) Energie und Stickstaffumsatz beim Lama. In K. H. Menke, ed. Energy Metabolism of Farm Animals. Eur. Assoc. Anim. Prod., Univ. Hohenheim Dok. 14, pp. 121–30.

42. Sillau, H., Chauca, D., and Valenzuela, A. 1973. (Evaluation of the microbial activity of the ruminal fluid of the sheep and alpaca) Evaluacion de la actividad microbiana del fluido ruminal del ovino y la alpaca. Rev. Invest. Pecu. 2(1):15–21.

43. Ullrey, D. E. 1973. Nutritional management of exotic ruminants and interrelationships. Erkr. Zootiere, Verhandlungsber. Int. Symp., Kolmarden.

44. United States-Canadian Tables of Feed Composition, 3rd ed. 1982. Washington, D.C.: National Academy of Sciences.

45. Valdivia, R., Del Valle, O., and Farfan, R. 1974. (Animal nutrition and pastures) Linia de nutricionanimal y pastos. Bol. Divulg. 15:123–28.

46. Vallenas P., A. 1958. (Preliminary study on the reflex closure of the esophageal groove in alpacas as viewed through a rumen fistula) Estudio preliminar sobre el clerre reflejo del surco esofagico de las alpacas a traves de una fistula abierta en el rumen. Vet. Zootec. (Lima) 10(26):7–12.

47. ______. 1958–59. (Study of some chemical substances which produce closure of the groove of the esophagus in alpacas) Estudio de algunas substancias quimicas que peuden provocar el clerre del surco esofagico en alpacas. Rev. Fac. Med. Vet. (Lima) 13–14:49–65.

48. ______. 1960. (Some aspects of the motility of the stomach of alpaca) Algunos aspectos de la motilidad del rumen de alpaca. Rev. Fac. Med. Vet. (Lima) 15:69–79.

49. ______. 1965. Some physiological aspects of digestion in the alpaca (*Lama pacos*). In R. W. Dougherty et al., eds. Physiology of Digestion in the Ruminant V. Washington, D.C: Butterworth.

50. Vallenas P., A., and Stevens, C. E. 1971a. Motility of the llama and guanaco stomach. Am. J. Physiol. 220(1):275–82.

51. ______. 1971b. Volatile fatty acid concentrations and pH of llama and guanaco forestomach digestion. Cornell Vet. 61:239–52.

52. Vallenas P., A., Cummings, J. F., and Munnell, J. F. 1971. A gross study of the compartmentalized stomach of two new world camelids: The llama and guanaco. J. Morphol. 134:399–424.

53. Vallenas P., A., Esquerre, J., Valenzuela, A., Gandela, E., and Chauca, D. 1973. (Volatile fatty acids and pH in the forestomach of the alpaca and sheep) Acidos grasos volatiles y pH en los dos primeros compartimentos del estomago de la alpaca y del ovino. Rev. Invest. Pecu. 2(2):115–30.

54. Vallenas P., A., Llerena, L., Valenzuela, A., Chauca, D., Esquerre, J., and Candela, E. 1973. (Concentrations of volatile fatty acids in the gastrointestinal tract of alpacas and llamas) Concentracion de acidos grasos volatiles a lo largo del tracto gastrointestinal de alpacas y llamas. Rev. Invest. Pecu. 2(1):3–14.

55. Vallenas P., A., Sillau, H., Cueva, S., and Esquerre, J. 1974. (Advances in the study of the digestive physiology of American camelids) Avances en el estudio de la physiologia digestiva de los camelidos Americanos. Bol. Divulg. 15:118–22.

56. Van Soest, P. J. 1982. Nutritional Ecology of the Ruminant. Corvallis, Oreg.: O & B Books.

57. Williams, R., and Williams, T. 1983. Buying alfalfa hay. Llama World 1(4):5.

3 Restraint and Handling

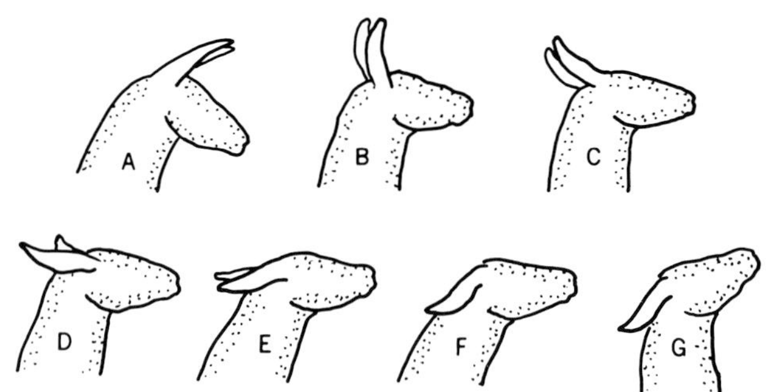

3.1 Ear positions in llamas: (A) alert or alarm, (B) normal, (C–G) various degrees of aggression. Modified from Franklin 1982.

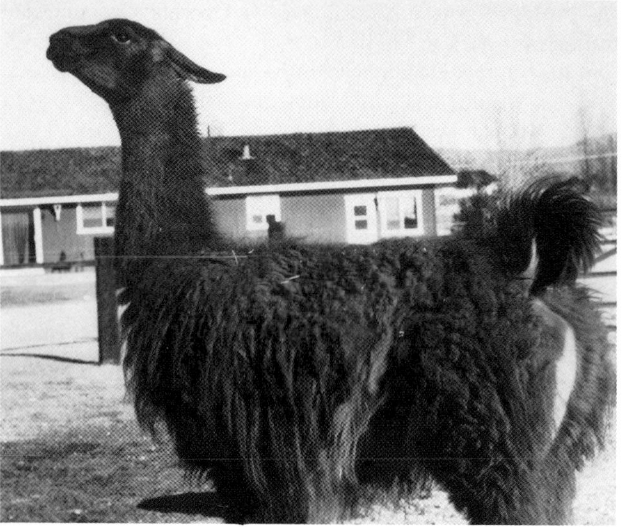

3.2 Dominant or aggressive stance of a female llama.

LLAMAS AND ALPACAS have been domesticated for thousands of years. When accustomed to being handled, they are docile and pleasant. Only the rare individual is aggressive or a "spitter." Guanacos and vicuñas are wild animals and cannot be as easily handled, i.e., chemical immobilization may be necessary. However, guanacos can be tamed and handled similarly to llamas if procedures are carried out slowly and quietly.

Effective restraint requires a knowledge of lamoid behavior. All four species of South American camelids (SACs) are social animals, an advantage when moving groups of animals into a small enclosure for close observation or capture. Alpacas are generally more flock oriented than llamas. Alpacas are also shy, more easily frightened and less inquisitive than llamas.

COMMUNICATION

Lamoid ear position conveys important social information (Fig. 3.1). Handlers should understand these signals in order to minimize stress for both animals and humans. The ears of a contented, unaroused lamoid are in a vertical position and turned forward. In the alarmed animal, the ears are cocked forward. The degree of incipient aggressive behavior is signaled by ears positioned from barely behind the vertical to flattened on the neck (Fig. 3.2).

Tail position also communicates social information (Fig. 3.3). In the unaroused lamoid, the tail lies flat against the perineum. If the animal is alarmed, the tail rises to horizontal or as much as 45 degrees above horizontal. Intense, aggressive behavior is signaled when the tail is elevated to the vertical. Basically, the higher the tail the higher the level of aggression.

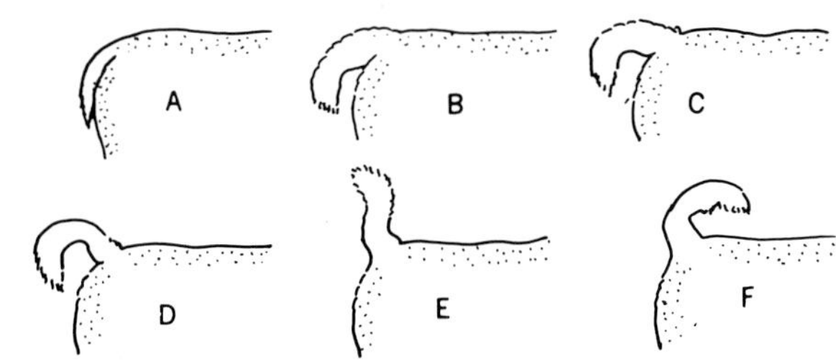

3.3 Tail positions in llamas: (A) normal, (B–D) alert to alarm, (B-E) various degrees of aggression, (F) forward curl (submissive). Modified from Franklin 1982.

Ears, tail, and other body language are generally coordinated to transmit signals. For instance, submissiveness in the llama, guanaco, and alpaca is indicated by curving the tail forward over the back, with the head and neck held low, the ears in a normal to above horizontal position, and the front limbs slightly bent (Fig. 3.4). This behavior is frequently seen in llamas that become imprinted on humans. The submissive crouch of a vicuña is with the tail curved forward but with the head curved back over the body.

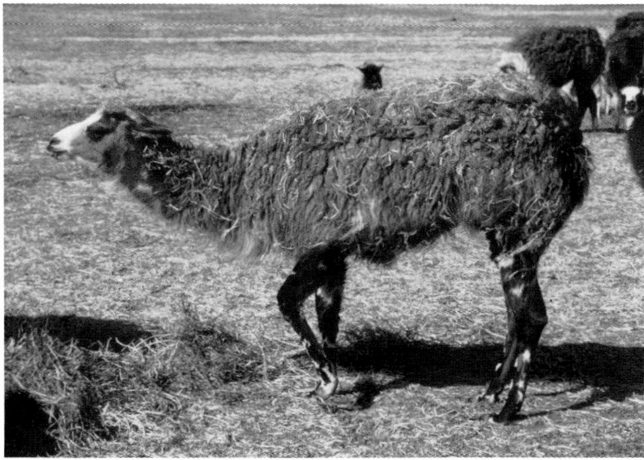

3.4 Llama in a submissive stance.

Lamoids are not highly vocal, but they do have a repertoire of sounds (2). A gradient of sounds has been described as *humming* (bleating). This sound provides auditory contact between animals and is especially important between a female and her cria. Humming also occurs when highly socialized animals are separated for a time and then reunited.

Llamas emit a *snort* characterized by a short burst of air through the mouth with loose lips (2). The snort indicates mild aggression. A *clicking* sound can be made with the tongue, which also indicates mild aggression. A *grumbling* threat is emitted when a feeding animal is approached too closely by another.

Screaming indicates extreme fright. Some llamas scream continuously when restrained for diagnostic or therapeutic procedures. The angry llama may emit a loud squealing sound called *screeching*. This sound is heard when males fight.

The lamoid *alarm* call is emitted when a male or female perceives danger to be near. The approach of strange dogs or other predators may trigger an alarm call. Male llamas, alpacas, and guanacos emit a guttural sound called *orgling* while copulating. Vicuñas may or may not orgle.

Further details on lamoid behavior may be found in Franklin's paper on lama language (2) and various field behavioral ecology studies.

OFFENSE AND DEFENSE

Llamas and alpacas are generally placid. The most common behavioral response to annoyance is the spewing of stomach contents at the offender (restrainer). The ears are laid back against the neck prior to the onset of defensive action (Fig. 3.2). A gulping or gurgling sound will be heard in the throat region, and a bolus of ingesta will be regurgitated from compartment one of the stomach. Ingesta is spewed out of the mouth in a diffuse pattern and may spray as far as 1 or 2 m. The unfortunate recipient will find that the obnoxious odor persists until after a shower and shampoo.

Offensively, male llamas bite, charge, chest butt, and rear up and strike down on another male. Properly reared and trained, male llamas are as safe and as easy to handle by humans as female llamas. Imprinted (rogue) males are a different matter.

Lamoids generally "cowkick" by arching a rear limb forward and outward. However, they also kick with a quick jab directly backward. The padded foot mitigates the sharpness of a kick, but the potential for injury from a large llama should not be underestimated. Fortunately, lamoids are not as agile kickers as their Old World cousins, the camels. The safest place to stand when handling a lamoid is near the shoulder. Not so for camels, since they can reach far forward of the shoulder to strike a handler. Adult llamas rarely strike with a front limb. They may rear to escape an unpleasant situation, but usually without directed striking.

Biting is usually reserved for aggression between intact males, but llamas have been known to bite humans on occasion. Mature males have one lower and two upper canine teeth on each side of the mouth. Unless blunted or cut short, these teeth are as formidable as sabers. The canines of females and early-castrated males are usually small or may even be absent.

CAPTURE

In Large Enclosure or Pasture

Experienced llama owners recommend that a small catch pen be associated with a pasture. This area can incorporate a shed or feeding area so that llamas become accustomed to entering it. Designs of such facilities are as variable as the mind can imagine. If advising a client about the design of future facilities, appropriate principles of design for catch pens for cattle and sheep may provide guidance.

If no catch pen is available, it is relatively easy to restrict one or many llamas with ropes, poles, or even humans with outstretched arms. Two or more people can corner a llama by approaching it slowly with arms outstretched and waving slightly (Fig. 3.5). Only one person should signal the team to move forward or retreat.

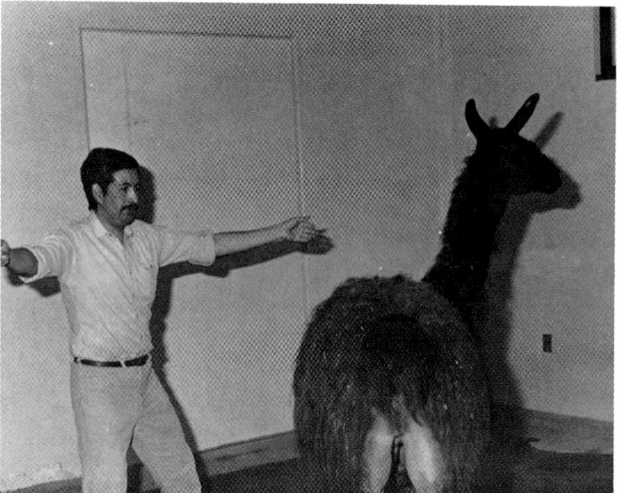

3.5 Directing and containing with outstretched arms.

Two people can hold a rope (minimum of 10 m) taut between them 1 m above the ground (Fig. 3.6). The intended captive should be moved along a fence line to a corner. Most llamas will not challenge the rope. Occasionally, an individual will run under the rope or try to charge through it. It is easier to contain all members of a group at once. If one llama in a group escapes capture, others will attempt to escape also. When the group is cornered, the rope should be shortened until the animals are completely restricted. One end of the rope may be tied to the fence to free a handler to move among the llamas to place a rope or halter on the one(s) selected.

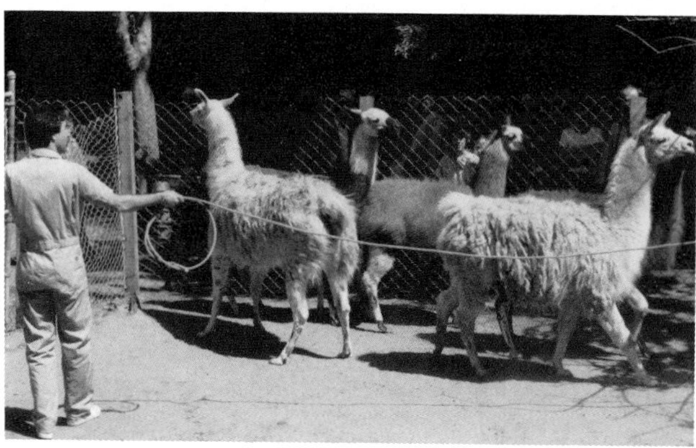

3.6 Containing llamas with a rope.

In a large pasture, with more help, two ropes may be used in a crisscross pattern. With this, a llama group can be restricted along a fence row instead of in a corner. A modification of this technique employs long bamboo poles or plastic pipes, each carried by a single individual in the manner of a tightrope walker (Fig. 3.7). Two or more of the poles are used to herd and contain the llamas.

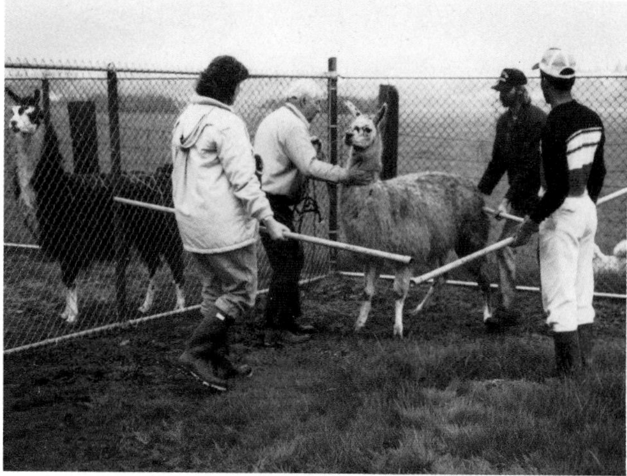

3.7 Containing a llama with plastic pipe.

The method used by "llameros" (handlers) in the Andes to load packs is as follows: pack llamas are driven in a group; llameros surround the group with llama fiber ropes (Fig. 3.8). While the rope ring is in place, other llameros work their way into the herd and with a shorter rope tie three animals together by their necks (Fig. 3.9). The rope is looped around the neck of the first llama, the ends given one or two twists, then looped around

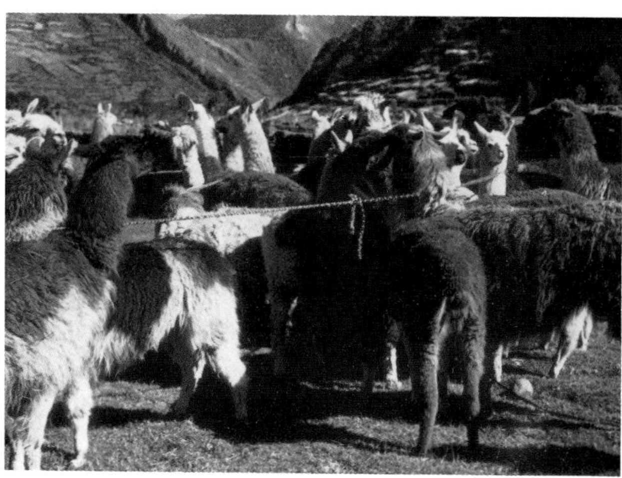

3.8 Rope corral around Peruvian llamas.

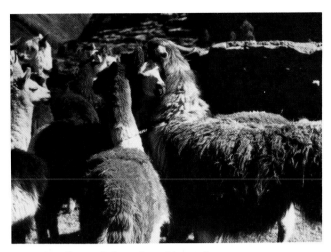

3.9 Three llamas tied together with a neck rope.

another and twisted, and finally a third llama is included before the ends are tied together. Once all the triads are roped up, the perimeter rope is dropped. Since three llamas tied together will not all go in the same direction, they stand still. Packs may then be placed on their backs.

A handler may not be able to enter an enclosure housing an aggressive, imprinted male. It may be necessary to rope such an animal to gain initial contact. A halter may then be placed or a temporary rope halter fashioned from the loop around the neck (Fig. 3.10).

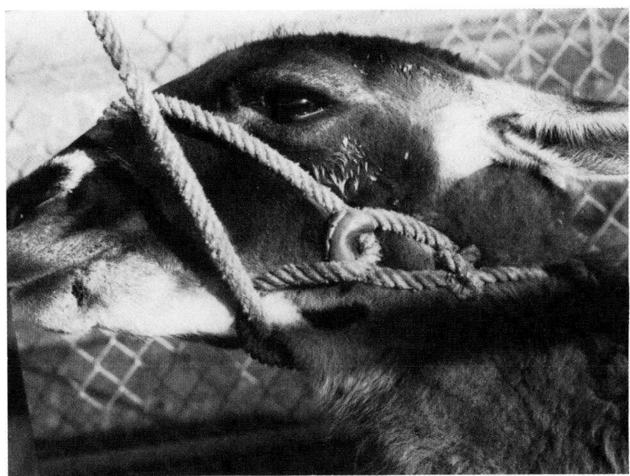

3.10 Temporary rope halter constructed from a lariat.

Llamas dislike having their heads touched or scratched. To place a halter, the llama should be approached from the left side at the withers. The right arm should reach over the neck while the halter's poll strap is pushed under the neck to be grasped with the right hand. The nose loop should be slowly moved up and positioned over the nose. The llama may try to dodge this action. With the nose loop in place, the poll strap can be buckled or snapped to the cheek ring.

Halters used on llamas resemble pony-sized horse halters. Most llama owners prefer not to leave a halter on a llama when it is free in a corral or pasture for fear a strap may catch on something and the llama could be injured. Some llama owners leave a leather or fiber neckband in place to facilitate capture.

In Restricted Area

Several approaches may be used. The first is to slowly approach the llama and place one arm around the chest and neck while the opposite hand grasps the tail. This is similar to the way a sheep is handled. It may be difficult to hold a llama weighing over 150 kg in this manner unless it can be quickly pushed against a wall or fence.

Another method is to approach the llama as before, reach over the back with one arm, grab a handful of the fleece with each hand on either side of the shoulder region, and at the same time place downward pressure over the back (Fig. 3.11). A third method is for the handler to reach across the back with both hands, grasp the fleece low on the opposite side, and pull upward (Fig. 3.12).

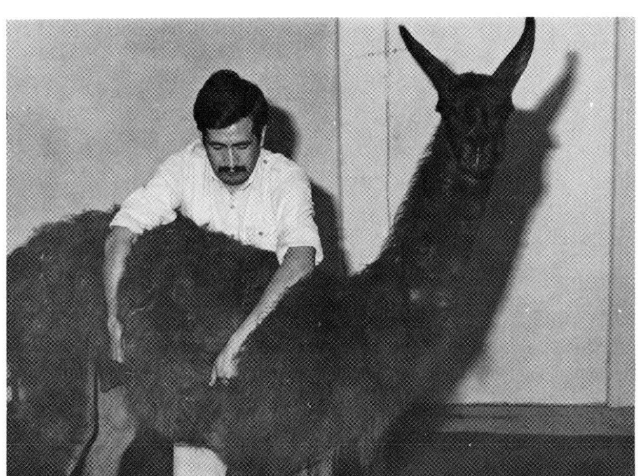

3.11 Restraining a llama by reaching over the back and grasping the fleece.

None of the foregoing techniques are suitable for single-handed containment of a spitter, since the llama can easily turn its head and spray the handler. With a spitter, a second handler must quickly grasp the head or ears to direct the spray away from the handlers, then place a "spit rag" over the muzzle.

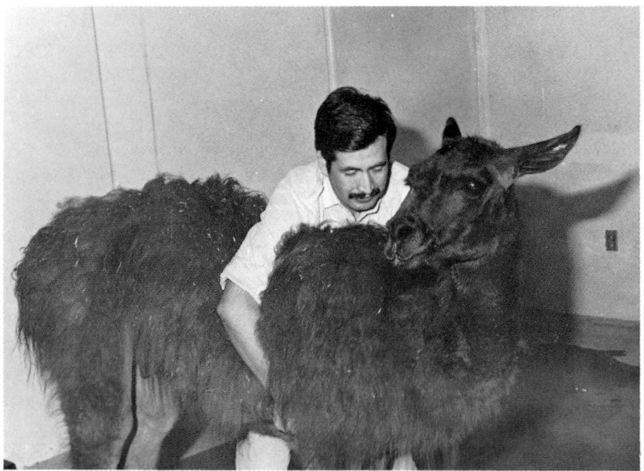

3.12 Restraining a llama by grasping fleece on both sides of the body.

EARING

The llama responds to "earing" like a horse. Llamas do not like to have their ears touched; alpacas are less sensitive. If this hold is applied correctly, the llama will not become "ear shy" or be more difficult to capture another time. Before grasping an ear, a handler should explain the procedure to the owner and inquire if this is acceptable. Some owners do not understand the process and may resent the "rough" handling.

The procedure for earing a llama is similar to that for earing a horse (1). The handler should stand on the left side of the withers, place the right arm over the neck, and work the opened palm of the hand up the neck to surround the base of the ear (Fig. 3.13). Squeeze firmly, because the llama may try to pull free at this point. Frequently, the llama will jerk its head toward the left and the handler to escape pressure on the right ear, using its head as a battering ram. One handler suffered a broken nose when an obstreperous llama slammed its head into her face. The left ear may be grasped for additional restraint.

An individual llama in a herd can be restrained for quick procedures by one handler grasping the ears and another grasping the tail. Greater restraint is achieved by pushing the llama against a fence or wall. Care should be taken to assure that the llama does not put a foot or leg through a net fence or under or through a wooden fence or wall.

CHUTES AND STOCKS

Tractable llamas can be crosstied in a narrow alleyway or in a conventional equine stock. Semipermanent pipe stocks are available. Animals must be trained to being handled in a pipe stock. A number of injuries to llamas and handlers have occurred in such facilities. Stout, aggressive llamas are able to lift the stock if it is not bolted to a floor or platform. Once, such a stock was lifted and dropped on a handler's foot, fracturing the metatarsal bone. The jaws of the llama may be traumatized when anchored to the padded yoke of such stocks. Both back bands and bellybands may be used, but one llama ruptured its bladder while struggling against such restraint. Too often, a novice llama handler uses maximum rather than the minimum restraint needed to accomplish a task. The pipe stock is frequently used to clamp a llama so tightly that it can't move instead of using more appropriate sedation or anesthesia.

Many homemade stocks function admirably. Some provide more flexibility in use than others, and there is wide variation in cost and ease of construction. A few designs are illustrated.

Fowler Design

This is a simple, easily constructed chute/stock. The neck is readily accessible for blood collection. Reproductive tract examinations can be conducted with the squeeze applied, and other examinations may be carried out with the squeeze released.

Figures 3.14–3.17 illustrate the construction and actual use of this chute. A narrow space is allowed through which the head and neck may pass but which holds the shoulders. The head should be pulled forward and upward and secured to a recessed ring on a wall or post placed forward of the shoulder poles, as indicated.

The chute may be constructed against the solid wall of a barn (Fig. 3.17), or both sides may be left free to swing on hinges at the shoulder posts. Sheets of 1 in. × 4

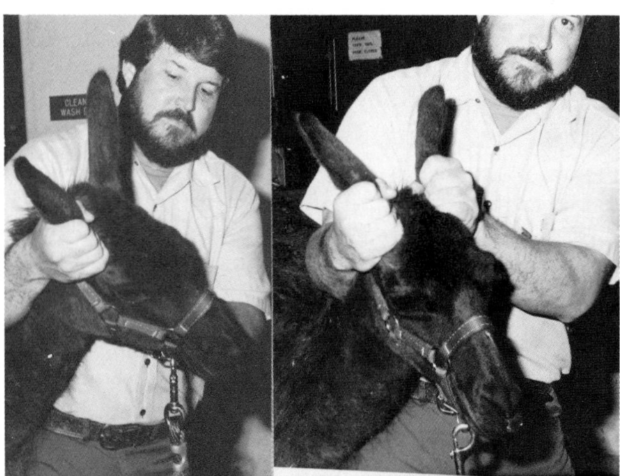

3.13 Earing a llama.

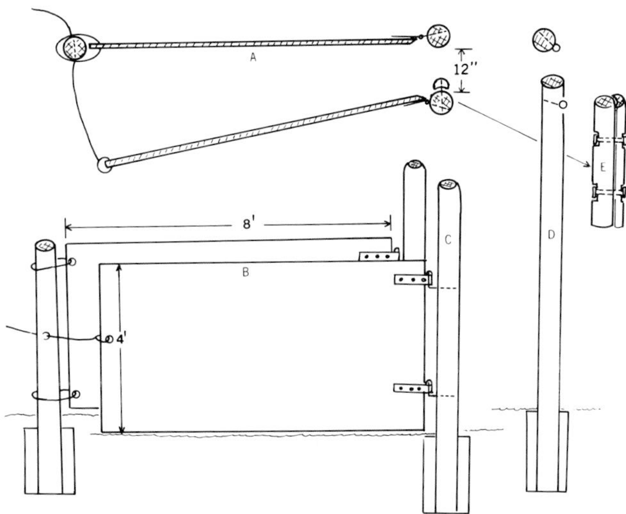

3.14 Diagram of the Fowler-designed squeeze chute for llamas: **(A)** top view, **(B)** side view, **(C)** shoulder post, **(D)** tie post, **(E)** shoulder post with detachable scab for small llamas.

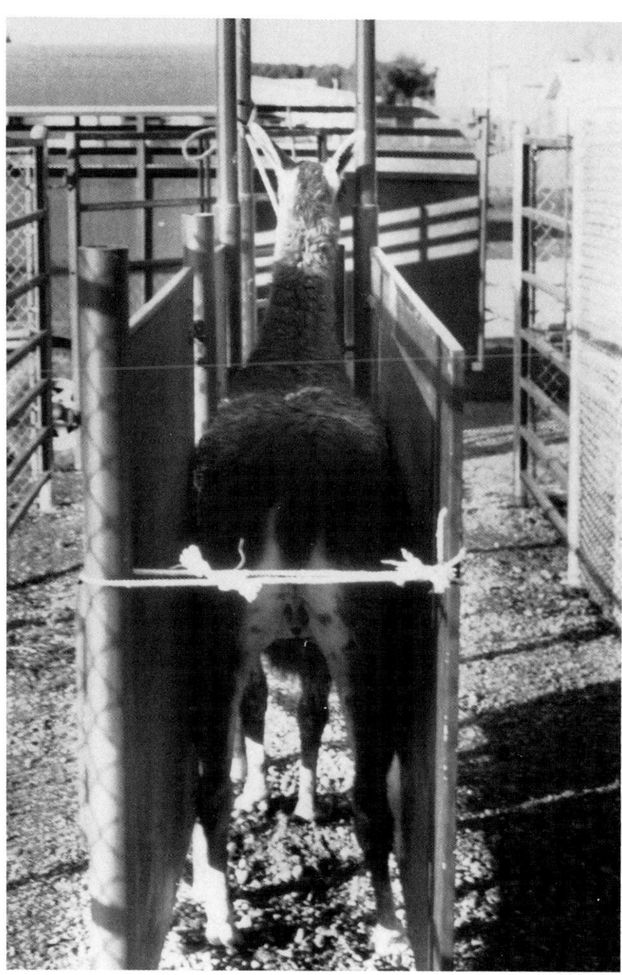

3.16 Fowler-designed llama chute, rear view.

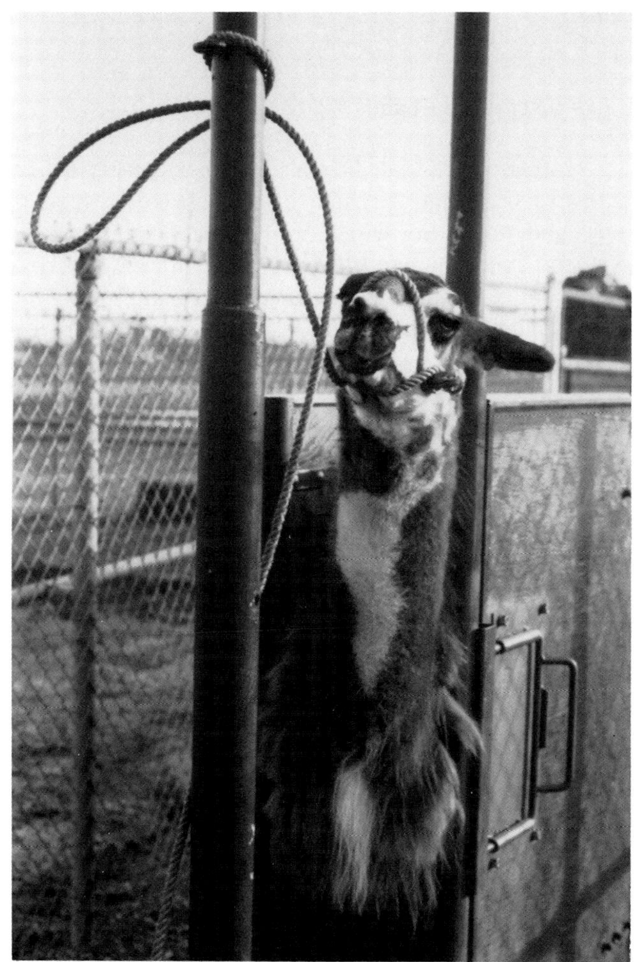

3.15 Fowler-designed llama chute, front view.

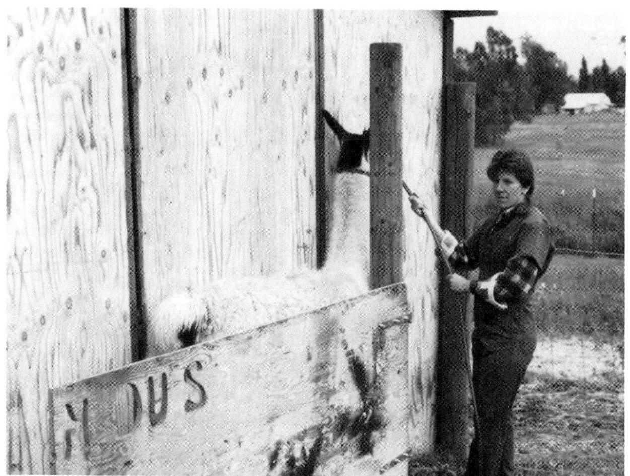

3.17 Fowler-designed llama chute constructed at the side of a barn.

ft × 8 ft plywood are hung on heavy-duty hinges. A back band may be used to prevent rearing, but the llama is able to lie down if necessary or desirable.

Ebel Design

This is an excellent, versatile design (Fig. 3.18). It requires more space for construction than the above, but may be portable. Basically, this is a three-sided, reinforced plywood box, open on the top and at both ends. Adjustable shoulder poles prevent the llama from moving forward. The head is crosstied to the sides of the box. Access is provided to both sides, the front, and the back of the llama (3).

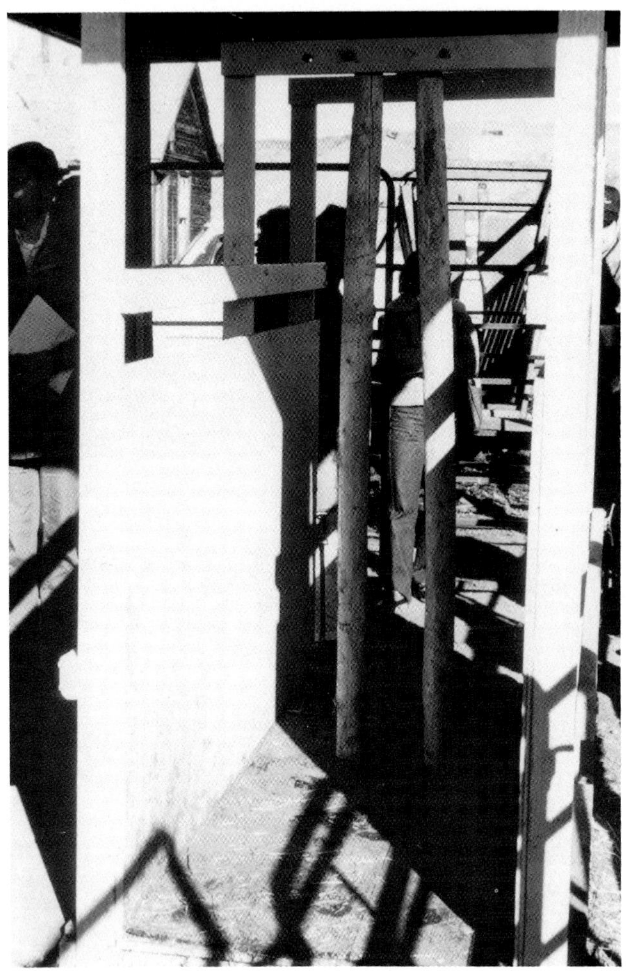

3.18 Ebel-designed llama chute.

Christensen Design

A third design uses a double-hinged pipe frame to restrict both forward and sideways movement (Fig. 3.19). The llama is secured to the ring, and the frame is used to move the animal into a desired position. Animals having a tendency to rear may become entangled in this chute, but it is flexible and easily used. Either side of the animal is available by reversing the direction of the frame.

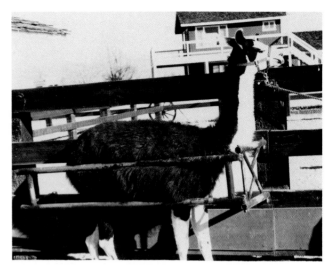

3.19 Christensen-designed llama chute.

IMPRINTED MALE

Mother-reared male llamas are usually no more difficult to handle than females, in contrast to bulls, stallions, and rams. Bottle-fed orphan males or neonates given too much human attention may imprint and develop a dangerous behavioral pattern. Essentially, an imprinted male treats a human as if he or she is another male llama.

This behavior may be anticipated in the male youngster that approaches and pushes its nose into a person's face or gallops up and pushes the owner around with its neck or chest. Peculiarly, overt aggression may not manifest itself until maturity, and then a particular person may bear the brunt of the aggression. A number of people have been severely injured by vicious attacks of otherwise handleable males.

In a full attack, the ears will be laid back against the llama's neck. He will charge and attempt to knock a person down by butting with his chest. If this fails, he may rear up and slam down on the person. A person who falls will be trampled with the llama's forefeet and bitten. A victim who remains standing may be bitten at the neck, knees, or any other spot within reach. When male llamas fight with other males, they bite the neck, hind limbs, and scrotum.

Several anatomic adaptations in male lamoids protect against fatal injuries during such encounters. The skin of the upper cervical region is as much as 1 cm thick. Instead of lying superficially in a jugular furrow, the lamoid jugular vein lies deep, in juxtaposition to the carotid artery. Finally, a ventral projection of the transverse process of the cervical vertebrae forms an inverted U channel that protects vital cervical structures.

Aggressive males are ferocious, uttering loud vocalizations and attempting to climb fences to get at intended victims. Once this behavior has been exhibited, contact with that llama is no longer safe for any person. A few individual animals have been deconditioned with negative stimulation, but usually safety has been achieved only for the individual deconditioning them. Others remain at risk.

Not all imprinted males develop aberrant behavior, and some may become obnoxious but not dangerous. Castration of adult males is not effective in changing behavior, as it is in bulls and stallions. It is recommended that orphaned males given extensive human attention be castrated by 2 months of age or, at the latest, before weaning.

DEALING WITH A SPITTER

The initial catch of a spitter is difficult. It may be roped, or if it is to be caught by hand, the catcher may protect against ingesta spewing by wearing a plastic garbage sack with cutout arm and face holes.

A spitter can be dealt with by several methods once it is in hand. The head can be directed away from the handlers, or a towel or rag may be tucked into the nose piece of the halter and draped over the nose and mouth (Fig. 3.20). The accumulation in the towel of stomach contents seems to deter further spitting, since the llama seems to dislike contact with the ingesta as much as humans.

A more permanent muzzle can be fashioned that will snap into the cheek rings of the halter (Fig. 3.21). Such muzzles are often fitted on camels that have a propensity to bite. Once a spitter is caught, the upper and lower lips can be grasped and held together (Fig. 3.22), much as a hand nose twitch is applied to a horse. Since the llama is unable to clear the ingesta from its mouth, it ceases to spit.

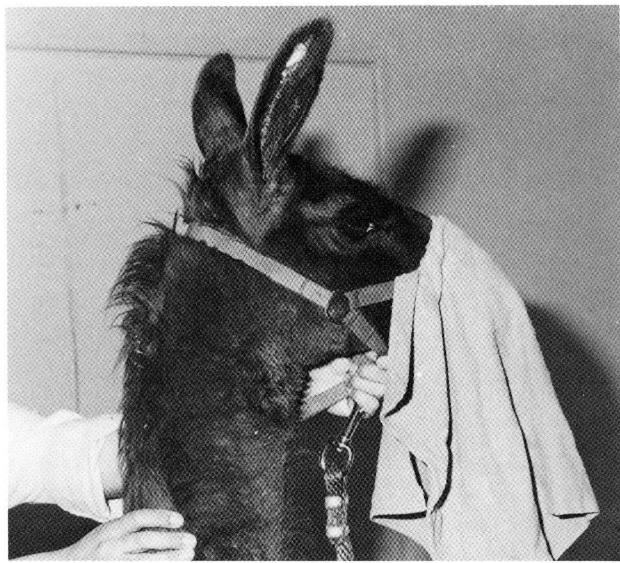

3.20 Spit rag.

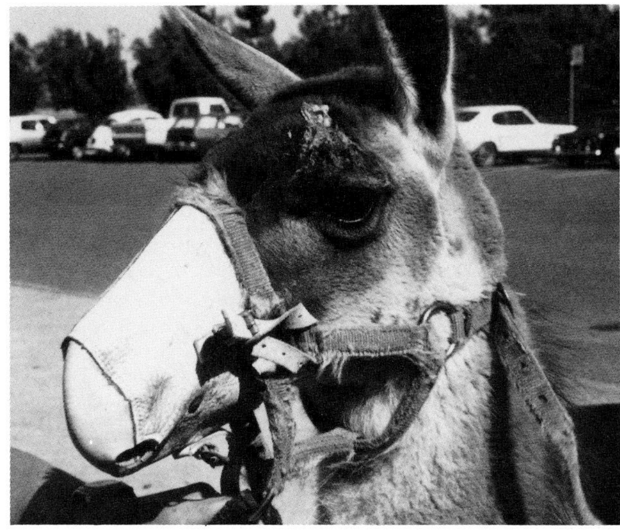

3.21 Muzzle for a llama.

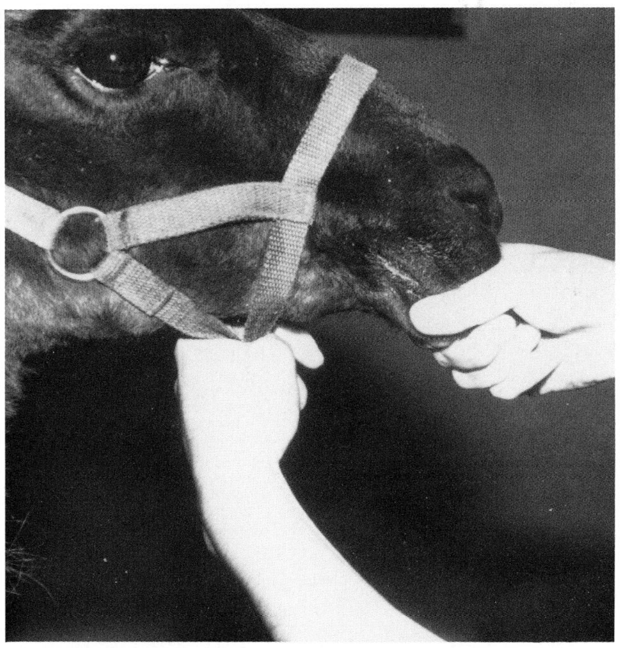

3.22 Hand-held nose twitch.

ROPING

Once a llama or alpaca feels a rope around its neck, it usually submits to handling. It has been necessary on occasion to rope the head and hind limbs ("head and heel") and stretch some llamas. It should be mentioned that in a group including an adult male, the male will attempt to mount the recumbent llama.

Llamas quickly learn to dodge a tossed lariat. They may also stand close to a fence, making it difficult to lay the loop over the head. Even an experienced roper may be unable to catch some llamas.

TRAILERING

Llamas and alpacas travel well. The majority lie down soon after the beginning of a journey and remain recumbent while moving. Llamas do not need to be tied within a truck or trailer. At least two fatalities have been associated with trailering tied llamas. In the first accident, a person borrowed a llama to use in a parade. The borrower disregarded instructions and tied the llama in the trailer with a lead rope. The llama became entangled in the rope and suffocated.

In the second accident, the llama was tied in a trailer constructed with a horizontal bar across the front, at a height corresponding to the midcervical region on the llama. The llama was tied with a rope over the bar. At the destination, the llama was found dead, partially hanging from the bar. At necropsy, a massive hematoma was located in the pharynx, which obstructed the glottis. Apparently the llama had bumped against the horizontal bar at some point in the journey, rupturing a vessel in the pharynx. As the llama pulled back on the rope and halter, the mouth was forced shut so that blood in the pharynx could not flow out the mouth or nostrils.

Special care should be taken when trailering llamas in cold weather. The floor of the trailer should be heavily bedded with straw. Since the underside of the llama is relatively fiberless, a recumbent llama may become chilled by the cold penetrating the floor.

A mother and baby may be trailered together, but it is dangerous to trailer llamas in large groups, unsegregated by size. Infants may easily be crushed by larger animals during a quick stop.

LEADING

It is surprising how quickly an untrained llama may learn to be led. In the beginning, it is helpful for a second person to walk behind, encouraging forward progression. A single person may encourage the llama to lead by pulling forward on a loop over the rump, a technique often used to teach a foal to lead (Fig. 3.23).

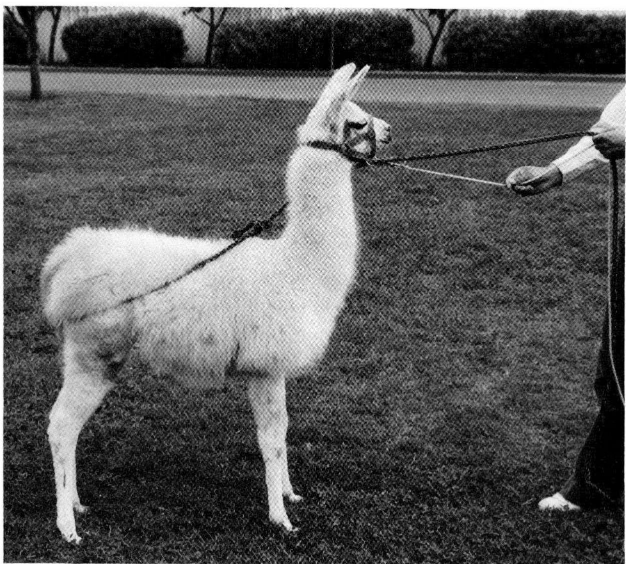

3.23 Tail loop used to teach a cria to lead.

Llamas can be trained to jump into and out of high-level trailers and even pickup trucks. Some caution is necessary, particularly if transporting a sick llama to a clinic, since it may not have normal coordination. Even healthy llamas have fallen as they jumped out of a truck bed.

HANDLING

Neonates

The lamoid neonate may be handled by methods similar to those used for a foal or calf. One person working alone can easily handle a neonate. One arm is placed around the chest while the tail is grasped with the opposite hand (Fig. 3.24). Prolonged pressure on the tail will cause the neonate to slump to the ground.

A cria of less than 20 kg (45 lb) may be lifted with one arm around the chest and the other behind the rear legs (Fig. 3.25). Larger crias may struggle and push themselves from the handler's arms. An arm in front of the rear legs has a natural calming influence on the neonate and reduces struggling (Fig. 3.26).

The neonate may be restrained in lateral recumbency by casting as illustrated in Figure 3.27 and then by laying an arm over the neck, grasping the arm of the down forelimb. The other arm should pass over the body in front of the hips to grasp the thigh of the down rear limb (Fig. 3.28). Folding the limbs and straddling the

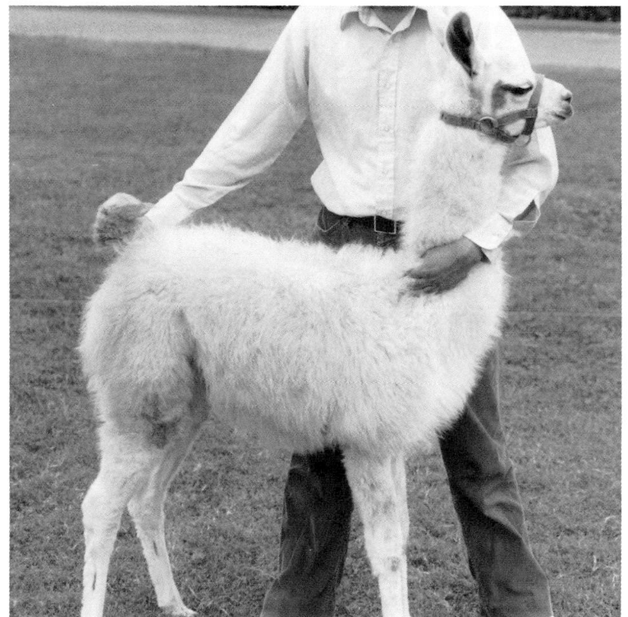

3.24 Restraining a cria by holding the neck and tail.

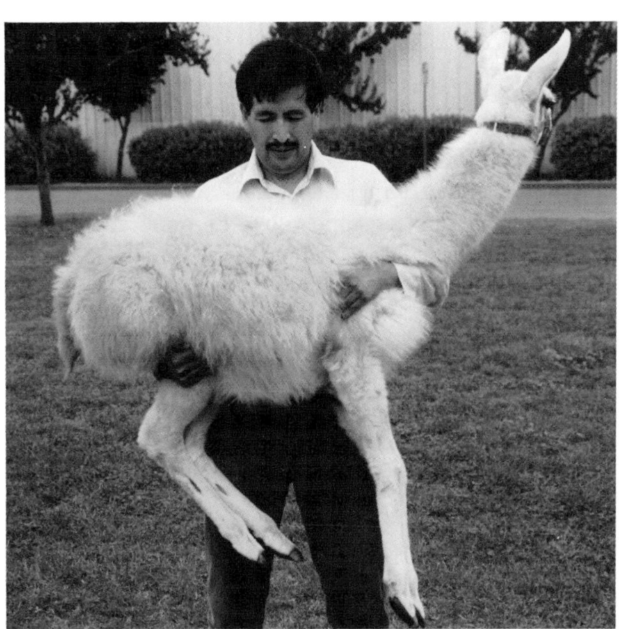

3.25 Lifting a neonate incorrectly by grasping behind the legs.

body in a kneeling position will force the neonate into sternal recumbency. Pressure can be adjusted as appropriate (Fig. 3.29).

From the sternal position a single person can perform venipuncture, pass an orogastric tube, or give an enema (see Chap. 21 for details).

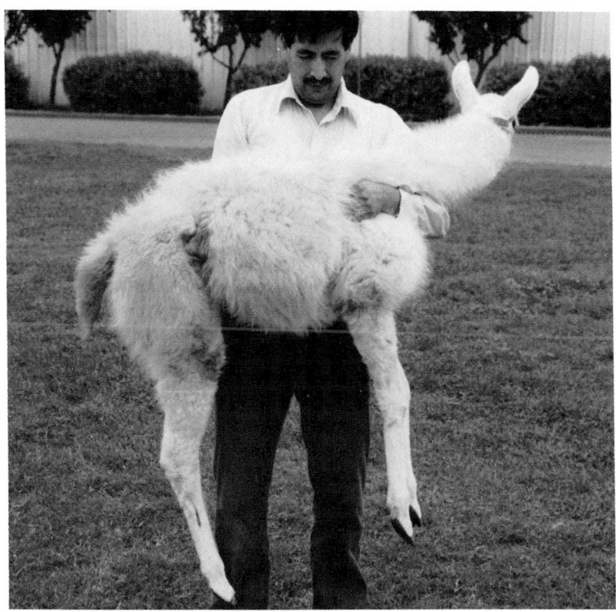

3.26 Lifting a neonate correctly.

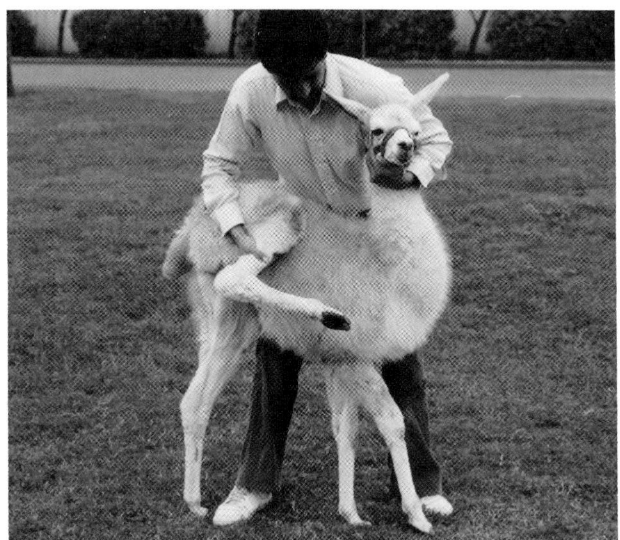

3.27 Method used to place a cria into lateral recumbency.

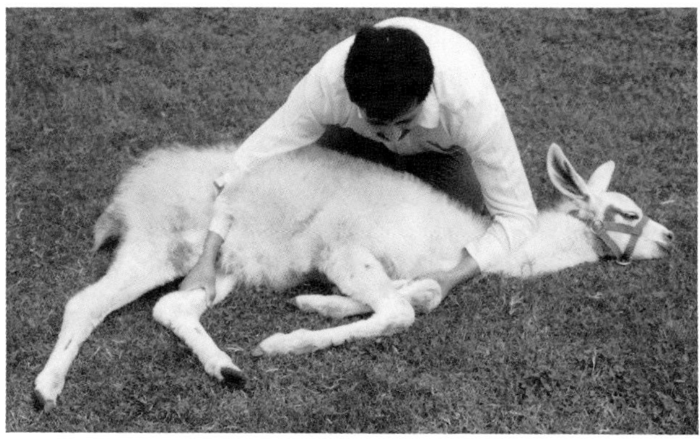

3.28 Holding a cria in lateral recumbency.

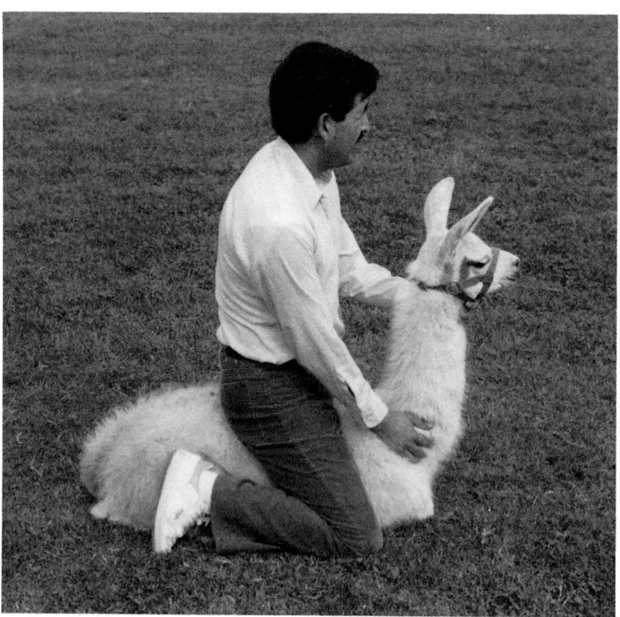

3.29 Restraining a neonate in sternal recumbency.

Weanlings and Yearlings

This age group is the most difficult to restrain for blood collection, general examination, passing an orogastric tube, or other diagnostic or therapeutic procedures. These animals are too large to force into sternal recumbency, as described for neonates, and too small to put into one of the described chutes.

Many animals of this age group have not been halter trained and may struggle excessively if tied for the first time. Some llamas have suffered neck injuries, sustained while "fish tailing" on the end of a lead rope. The most satisfactory method is to hold the youngster with one arm under the chest, grasping the tail with the other hand (Fig. 3.24). Even with this mild restraint, animals of this age are inclined to jump.

Guanacos and Vicuñas

Guanacos may be tamed if reared in association with humans and handled during maturation. Such animals may be handled in a similar manner as llamas or alpacas, recognizing that guanacos may be more easily frightened or excited.

Wild guanacos or vicuñas require more vigorous manual restraint. Two or more persons may be needed to catch an animal within a restricted space such as a small stall. Most of these animals will not tolerate being tied with a halter and will fight if placed in one of the chutes designed for their domestic cousins.

A less traumatic and stressful method of restraint is intramuscular chemical sedation via a blow gun or stick pole syringe (see Chap. 5). Neither the guanaco nor the vicuña has a heavy fleece to obstruct insertion of the needle into the muscle mass of the upper rear limb or triceps. The stick pole syringe method may also be used to sedate an extremely aggressive male llama. For more specific handling and training procedures, the reader is advised to consult training texts.

HOSPITALIZATION

Lamoids use communal dung heaps for defecation and urination. It may be difficult to induce them to defecate in strange surroundings. If trailered to the hospital, the lamoid will usually have a full bladder and rectum. The animal should be given access to a dirt or grass area for voiding before confinement in a concrete or wood-floored stall.

Many types of bedding may be used for stalls. Wood shavings and sawdust work into the fleece and are extremely difficult to remove. A healthy animal unaccustomed to straw may consume more of it than is desirable, causing indigestion. However, straw is more satisfactory than shavings.

When automatic waterers are used in a stall, an alternative water source should be provided until it is certain that the animal is using the automated source.

REFERENCES

1. Fowler, M. E. 1978. Restraint and Handling of Wild and Domestic Animals. Ames: Iowa State Univ. Press.

2. Franklin, W. L. 1982. Llama language. Llama World 1(2):6–11.

3. Johnson, L. 1987. Llama restraining chutes. Llamas 11(5):30–32.

4 Clinical Diagnosis: Examination and Procedures

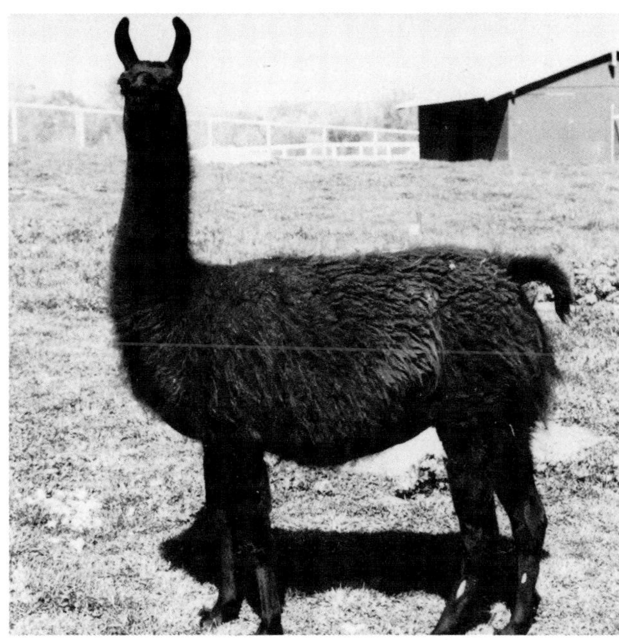

4.1 Llama with neck held in the normal vertical position.

THE BASIC PROCEDURES of clinical diagnosis in camelids are similar to those used in livestock, horses, and even small animals, but anatomic differences necessitate some modifications. Unique characteristics and normal data are discussed.

PHYSICAL EXAMINATION

Conformation

All species of South American camelids (SACs) are similar in conformation, with differences primarily in size. Veterinarians conducting soundness examinations and evaluations for lameness should have an understanding of the morphology of the animal. See Chapter 22 for details and illustrations. The high head carriage is immediately noticeable, and it contributes to the functional balance of these unique animals.

In a healthy individual, the neck is held almost vertical (Fig. 4.1). With weakness or depression, the head is held lower, and in a sick, laterally recumbent animal, the head and neck are usually positioned back over the thorax in what would be considered opisthotonos in other species.

GAITS OF LLAMAS. Llamas have three natural gaits: the walk, pace, and gallop. The walk is common to all quadrupeds and the gallop to other ungulates. The pace is not unique to camelids, but in this group, more than any other, the pace is the preferred medium-speed gait, in contrast to most ungulates in which the trot is preferred.

The pace is physically demanding, and certain anatomic modifications make this an efficient gait for camelids. Natural pacers, such as camelids, have relatively long legs. Each limb is longer than the trunk, allowing the animal to develop a long stride. The forward area of the thorax is narrow, allowing the upper forelimbs freedom to move forward and back. The hind limbs of camelids have a narrow attachment to the pelvis, and the abdomen is less rounded than in other species, allowing the hind limbs free motion.

It is advantageous to the pacer for the limbs to be set closely to the midline, minimizing the side-to-side rolling that occurs when the center of body gravity is changed with each stride. Camelids are ideally conformed in this regard.

The pace is an unstable gait. Lateral stability is significantly decreased. Strong, straight legs are needed to overcome this disadvantage. Furthermore, in the pace, maneuverability is reduced, since direction cannot be changed as readily as with the trot. The pace is designed to permit an animal to cover ground swiftly in open country.

It is possible that the unique foot of camelids is an adaptation developed to increase the stability of the animal for the pacing gait. All other two-toed ungulates have a ligamentous structure that ties the toes together. Not so in lamoids, which have a splay-toed foot (not to be confused with splay footed). The spread of the toes provides a stronger base of support. This, combined with the padded foot, makes the camelid one of the more sure-footed ungulates.

Body Condition

An accurate evaluation of body condition cannot be made visually, since the fiber coat covers the body and upper limbs. Muscle mass can be evaluated only by palpation. Evaluation of body condition should not be based on palpation of the pelvis or loin of a llama. The bony prominences of those areas can always be felt. Instead, the muscle mass over the thoracic vertebrae, just behind the withers, is a good indicator. The muscles should be filled out but firm. A fat layer in this location will feel soft, almost fluctuant.

Llamas easily become obese, with significant fat layers laid down in subcutaneous tissues, retroperitoneal, omental, and pelvic fat deposits. As in all species, excessive fat deposits are detrimental to sound health and especially affect reproductive performances.

The propensity to store heavy fat layers may be an evolutionary adaptation to the harsh conditions of feast/famine in South America. Researchers in Peru[1] indicate that llamas and alpacas used for meat develop the same types of fat deposits as are recognized in North America. Apparently, these fat deposits are a reservoir for supplying energy during the periods of drought that are integral in the normal seasonal cycle these animals have been subjected to for thousands of years.

Since North American feeding practices do not include a feed-shortage cycle, animals accumulate fat with no opportunity to rid themselves of the burden. Individual differences in the propensity to accumulate fat make it crucial for a herd manager to identify and limit feed for animals that have a tendency toward obesity. An accurate scale is important to good management of a llama herd.

Table 4.1 shows comparative weights for the camelids. There are marked variations in size among domestic camelids. Male and female SACs vary little, but this is not true of Old World camelids. It is a widely believed myth that North American llamas are 20–40% larger than their South American counterparts, but large llamas may be found in Peru and small or even dwarfed llamas may be seen in the United States.

Body Temperature

The resting body temperature of adult llamas and alpacas varies from 37.5 to 38.9°C (99.5–102°F) when in a neutral or moderately extreme ambient temperature environment. Normal body temperatures of neonate llamas fluctuate in a wider range because thermoregulatory mechanisms are not yet as sophisticated as those of adults. SACs evolved in harsh, cool climates and are well able to adapt to cold. Extremely hot and humid climates are less well tolerated and special cooling systems should be incorporated into management programs to help them cope with heat stress (see Chap. 9).

During hot summer seasons, some llamas are able to allow body temperatures to elevate and remain at 40°C (104°F). It is disconcerting to see a heavily fleeced llama lying peacefully in full sunshine on a hot summer day. However, it should be remembered that fleece insulates from heat as well as from cold.

The llama that is forced to remain recumbent because of trauma or disease is more subject to heat stress, even in neutral environments, because the underside is a fleece-free area of the body and the site for heat dissipation. If the llama is continually recumbent, neither normal nor fever-induced body heat can be dissipated.

The dromedary is able to endure diurnal fluctuations of body temperature, from 36.5 to 42°C (97.7°–107.6°F). The body acts as a heat sink during the heat of the day, thus conserving vital water that would otherwise be lost through evaporative cooling. During the cool night, body heat is dissipated by conduction and radiation. It should be obvious that evaluation of a fevered state in the dromedary is difficult.

1. Antonio Ramierez, Lima, Peru.

Table 4.1. Weights of camelids

Common name	Scientific name	Male		Female	
		(kg)	*(lb)*	*(kg)*	*(lb)*
Bactrian camel	*Camelus bactrianus*	500–690	1100–1520	450–550	992–1213
Dromedary camel	*Camelus dromedarius*	500–750	1100–1650	400–550	881–1213
Llama	*Lama glama*	130–243	286–536	108–200	238–441
Alpaca	*Lama pacos*	60–80	132–176	55	121
Guanaco	*Lama guanicoe*	100–150	220–330	100–120	220–264
Vicuña	*Vicugna vicugna*	40–65	88–143	30–40	66–88

Cardiac Assessment

The heart rate of a resting adult llama is 60–90 beats per minute. Pulse evaluation is not utilized in camelids, since there are no readily accessible arteries. The heart is accessible for auscultation as in other mammals. By reaching under the fleece at the elbow, the stethoscope may be placed on a fleece-free area caudal to the triceps, which allows for both cardiac and thoracic auscultation.

A number of congenital cardiac anomalies may persist into adulthood (see Chap. 22). A thorough assessment of the heart should be made in every physical examination.

Thoracic Cavity Assessment

The resting respiratory rate of an adult llama varies from 10 to 30 per minute. The thoracic area is bound by the caudal border of the triceps muscle, a line extending caudally for 20–25 cm (8–10 in.) below the top of the ribs and triangled back to the olecranon. The line of diaphragmatic reflection is more caudal than this area, but lung sounds are not heard in the caudal thorax.

Normal lung sounds are muted in llamas and may be difficult to hear. With excitement and more rapid breathing, the sounds will be vesicular rather than bronchiolar. Respiratory rate is best established by placement of the stethoscope over the trachea at the thoracic inlet.

Abdominal Auscultation

The major fermentative process of lamoid digestion takes place in compartment one (C-1) of the stomach, which occupies the entire left side of the abdomen. Since gastrointestinal sounds are primarily associated with gas/liquid churning, usually sounds are heard only on the left side.

Gastric motility in camelids differs from that in the ruminant (see Chap. 13). Palpation is usually not possible, and a stethoscope is required to hear the subdued sounds. Normal gastric motility rate is 3–4 per minute, which will increase slightly after feeding. A fleece-free abdominal area is located just cranial to the thigh muscles of the hind limb. To expose the area for auscultation, it is necessary to reach under the fleece in what would be the flank area in other species and lift it up.

Eye

One of the more attractive features of the llama and alpaca is the large expressive eyes with long eyelashes. The iris has a large corpus nigrum (granula iridica) on the dorsal aspect and a smaller one on the ventral, the function of which is unknown. Unilateral or bilateral nonpigmentation of the iris, (blue eye, glass eye, wall eye, or watch eye) has been seen. The retina is characterized by a pronounced vascular pattern and no fovea. There is no tapetum or eyeshine.

The nasolacrimal duct originates approximately 5–7 mm from the medial canthus of both the upper and lower lids. The duct terminates within the nares on the cutaneous side of the mucocutaneous border, a centimeter or two dorsal to the floor of the ventral meatus on the lateral wall over the ridge formed by the premaxilla. The orifice is 2–3 mm in diameter.

A slight ectropion of the lower eyelid may be seen on some individuals when they are excited, frightened, or agitated. This condition should not be confused with anatomic ectropion, which may be either congenital or acquired.

Ear

Llamas usually have long, variably shaped pinnae that are used to express mood (see Fig. 3.1). Alpacas have shorter ears. Close inspection of the pinna and the external ear canal is difficult, since llamas resent having the ear touched.

The external ear canal is small (3–5 mm in diameter), and a bend along the course of the canal precludes visualization of the tympanic membrane in most adults (see Chap. 19). Foxtails (*Hordeum* sp.) have become lodged in the canal and in one case penetrated the tympanic membrane, middle ear, and temporal bone to lodge in the base of the brain. Facial paralysis is usually seen with ear infections. Spinose ear ticks, *Otobius megnini,* and other species of ticks have been seen in the ear.

Lacerations of the ear are frequently observed when multiple males with intact canines are housed together. Frostbite, with variable shortening of the ear, has been seen, but so also has congenital absence of the pinna.

Mouth

Lamoids are unable to open the mouth wide enough to make possible a more than cursory examination of the oral cavity. The incisor and canine teeth can be viewed and should be checked in every physical examination, especially to check for over- or underbite. Congenital malocclusion is prevalent in lamoids (see Chap. 22). The tongue rarely protrudes from the mouth. Nonpigmented gingiva may be used to determine a capillary refill time.

DIAGNOSTIC PROCEDURES
Hematology and Serum Biochemistry

BLOOD COLLECTION. Blood analysis is vital to differential diagnosis of many diseases. Venipuncture and collection of blood is not as simple a task in lamoids as it is in most other domestic animals. Lamoids have evolved a number of protective mechanisms to prevent exsanguination from bites by males fighting with one another. In all locations of the neck, extreme caution must be exercised to prevent accidental cannulation of the carotid artery when taking blood samples.

Two major sites are suitable for jugular venipuncture: low on the neck near the thoracic inlet and high, near the ramus of the mandible. The site selected may depend on restraint facilities, assistance available, desires of the client, and experience of the operator. Both locations have advantages and disadvantages.

An understanding of the anatomy of the vessels of the cervical region is necessary. The jugular vein is formed by the confluence of the lingual, facial, and maxillary veins, approximately 1 cm caudad to the ramus of the mandible. Superficially, the vein is covered by the skin and platysmas muscle. This junction and the first few centimeters of the jugular vein are embedded within the ventral border of the parotid salivary gland. The jugular vein will, at this point, be on the lateral surface of the sternomandibularis muscle tendon as it inserts on the mandible. The vein then courses slightly dorsal around the tendon to go deeper into the neck, medial to the sternomandibularis muscle (Figs. 4.2, 4.3).

The jugular vein lies superficial to the omohyoideus muscle, which separates the vein from the carotid artery.

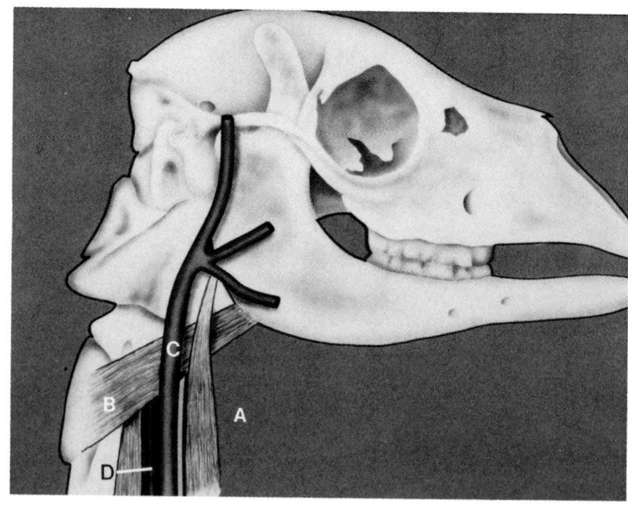

4.2 Diagram of the anatomy of the jugular vein: **(A)** sternomandibularis muscle, **(B)** omohyoideus muscle, **(C)** external jugular vein, **(D)** common carotid artery.

The omohyoideus muscle and its extended fascia form the deep border of the jugular furrow in horses and cattle, which extends throughout most of the cervical region. In lamoids, the muscle lies in a different position (Fig. 4.4). It is narrow (10 cm) and serves as a separation between the artery and the vein for a distance of only 14 cm caudal to the ramus of the mandible.

The jugular vein continues on toward the thoracic inlet, coursing deep to the sternomandibularis muscle, and is incorporated in the same fascial sheath with the carotid artery and the vagosympathetic nerve. All these structures lie on the ventrolateral surface of the trachea. There is no jugular furrow in lamoids.

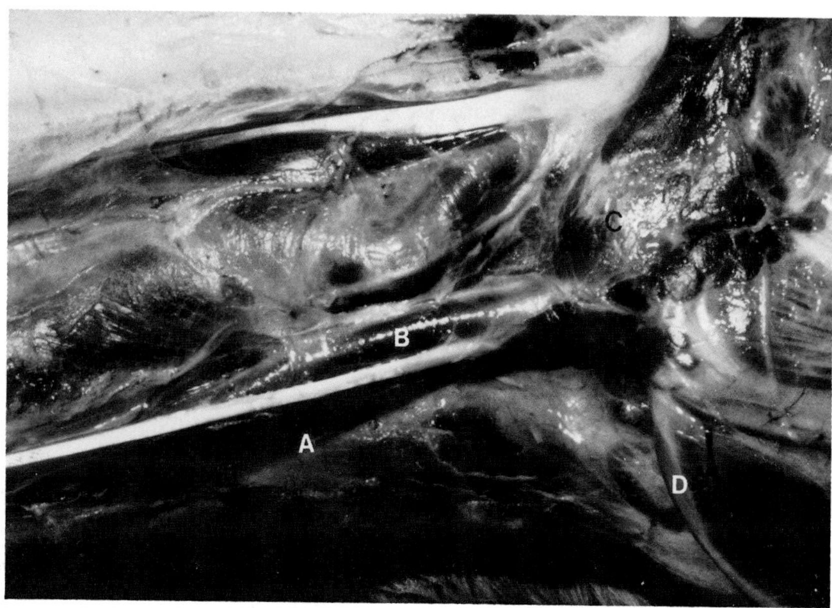

4.3 Anatomic dissection of the jugular vein: **(A)** tendon of the sternomandibularis muscle, **(B)** jugular vein, **(C)** parotid gland, **(D)** mandible.

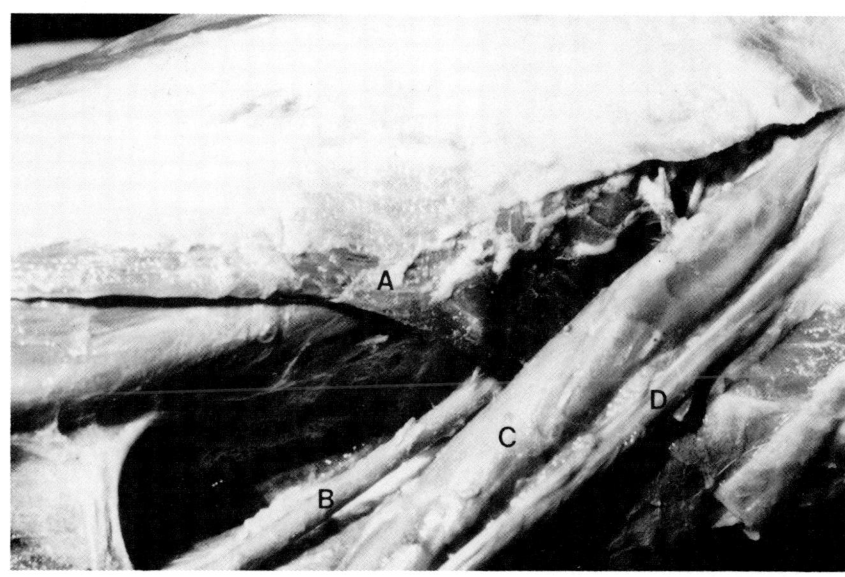

4.4 Anatomic dissection of the jugular vein: **(A)** omohyoideus muscle, **(B)** common carotid artery, **(C)** jugular vein, **(D)** tendon of the sternomandibularis muscle.

The vessels are further protected from accidental laceration by the ventral projection of the transverse process of the cervical vertebrae, which forms an inverted semi-U-shaped channel (Fig. 4.5). The jugular vein lies just medial to this projection. The ventral projections on the 6th cervical vertebra are prominent and easily palpated, serving as landmarks for venipuncture low on the neck. In the male, the thickness of the skin of the neck varies from 1 cm near the mandible to 0.5 cm near the thoracic inlet.

In long-necked animals such as horses, giraffes, and camelids, valves in the jugular veins prevent backflow of blood to the head when it is lowered for feeding and drinking. In the llama, four or five of these valves are distributed from the confluence of the veins that form the jugular to the thoracic inlet. The valves may be bicuspid or tricuspid.

A set of valves is sited just caudad to the major veins that form the jugular, approximately 1 cm from the angle of the mandible. Another valve is located 5 cm caudal to the first, at the level of the thyroid vein (Fig. 4.6). This valve may interfere with venipuncture when the upper site is selected. The remaining valves are spaced 15–20 cm (6–8 in.) apart along the jugular vein (Fig. 4.7). One of the valves may be located near the ventral process of the 6th cervical vertebra (the site for a low venipuncture).

High-Neck Venipuncture

Advantages. The jugular vein is more superficial at this location and is separated from the carotid artery, thus there is less likelihood of arterial penetration.

Disadvantage. The skin is thickest at this location, and visualization is not possible in adults, making it necessary to rely on landmarks and ballottement of the vein for venipuncture.

Technique. An imaginary line should be scribed along the ventral border of the mandible onto the neck,

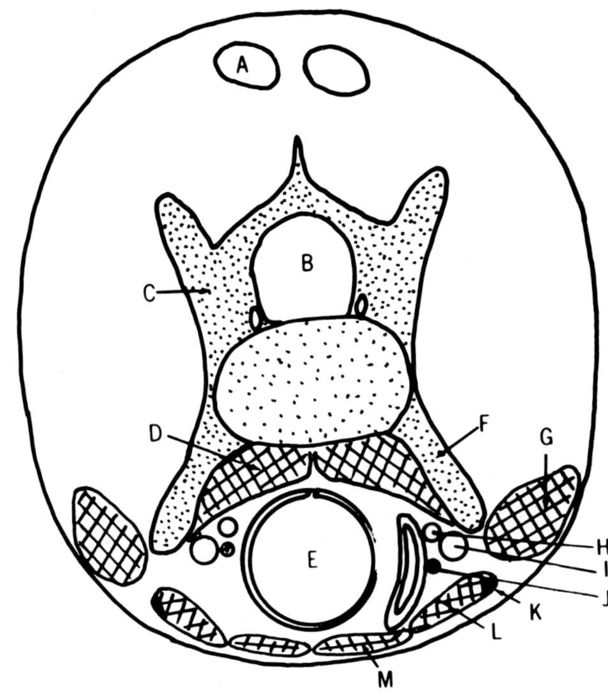

4.5 Cross-sectional diagram of the lamoid cervical region at the level of the 6th vertebra: **(A)** ligamentum nuchae, **(B)** vertebral canal, **(C)** vertebra, **(D)** muscle, **(E)** trachea, **(F)** ventral extension of the transverse process of the vertebra, **(G)** brachiocephalicus muscle, **(H)** carotid artery, **(I)** jugular vein, **(J)** vagosympathetic trunk, **(K)** sternomandibularis muscle, **(L)** esophagus, **(M)** sternothyrohyoideus muscle.

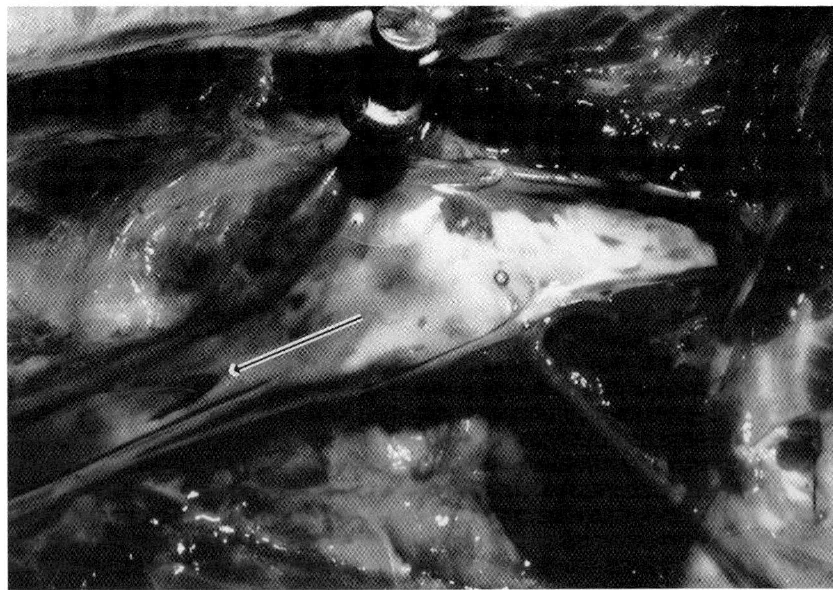

4.6 Valves in the jugular vein in the upper neck.

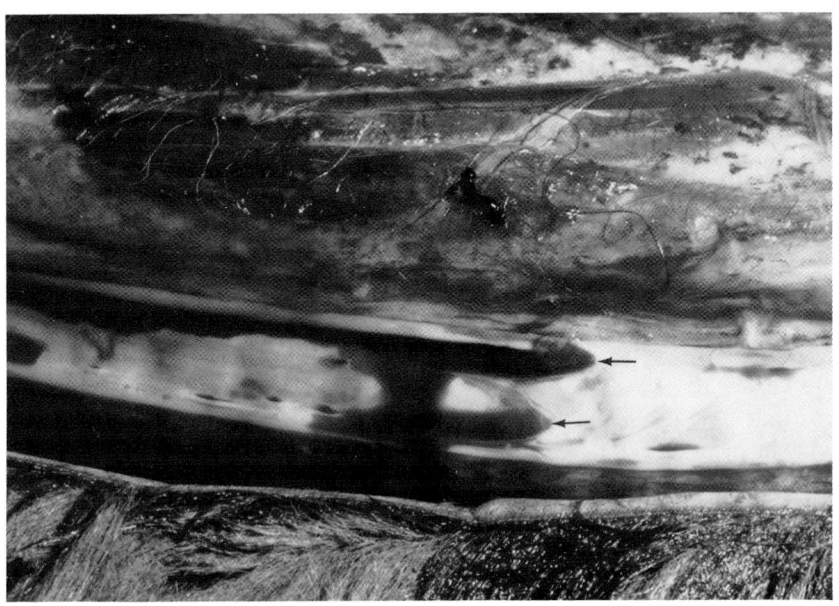

4.7 Valves in the jugular vein low on the neck.

with the head held in a slightly flexed position. The tendon of the sternomandibularis muscle should be palpated to locate the site of penetration, just dorsal to the intersection of those two lines (Fig. 4.2). The vein should be occluded by deep, firm pressure at the ventrum of the vertebrae. By stroking the area of the vein toward the occluding hand, a wave may be felt against the fingers. Alternatively, correct selection of the site may be tested by placing a finger over the suspected location of the vein and releasing the occlusion to see if the dilated vessel empties.

Positioning of the head and neck is important to achieve success with this procedure. The author prefers to perform venipuncture from the right side. An assistant should stand on the left to grasp the right ear while pressing his or her body against the left neck to produce a slight bow, with the convex side toward the operator. The nose should also be pulled toward the left, making certain that the halter straps do not press on the vessels proximal to the penetration site.

Low-Neck Venipuncture

Advantages. The skin is thinner, and movement of the head is less disruptive.

Disadvantages. The lower neck is usually more heavily fleeced. Since the jugular vein and carotid artery are in juxtaposition at this location, there is a greater chance of arterial cannulation. Some type of a stock or chute is necessary to fix the head upward to prevent the llama from pushing forward.

Technique. The head should be elevated. The operator should palpate for the ventral projection of the transverse process of the 6th cervical vertebra and occlude the vessel at this site by wrapping the fingers around the projection. The pulsation of the carotid artery may be felt. The needle should be inserted slightly medial to the projection, toward the center of the neck.

Restraint for venipuncture in a neonate up to 4 months of age may be difficult. Fortunately, the skin of the neonate is thin, and the jugular vein can usually be distended and visualized. A simple method for a single person to perform venipuncture begins with straddling of the neonate, folding the front legs with the hand as the baby is pushed down (Figs. 4.8, 4.9). Select a clean, dry location and place a clean towel beneath a newborn to protect the umbilicus. The head should be pushed down with the other hand. As the baby lies down on the forehand, a slight pressure on the rump encourages it to assume sternal recumbency. The baby should never be collapsed by sitting on it. Alternatively, it may be lifted off its feet and tipped to lie on its side. Then the legs will fold up beneath it as the handler straddles it. While kneeling over the baby to keep it in sternal recumbency, the left arm should be placed on the right side of the neck to push the head and neck to the left. The left hand should also be used to occlude the vessel while the right hand inserts the needle to collect blood or give medication (Fig. 4.8). Venipuncture may be accomplished at either the low or high position.

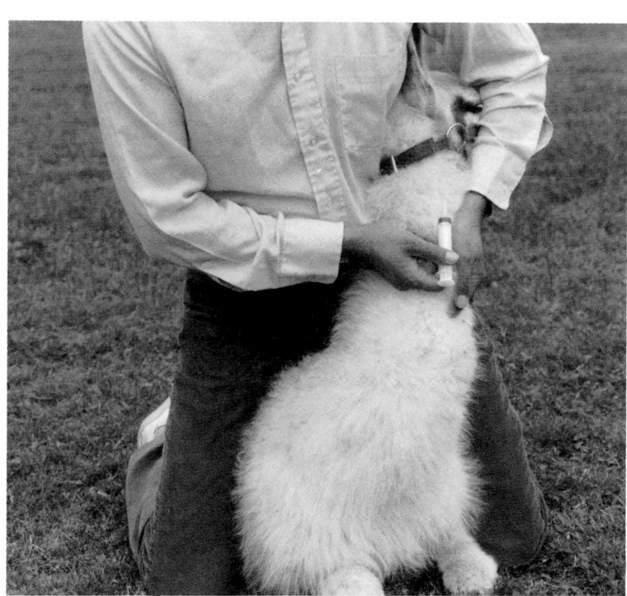

4.8 Position for venipuncture in a cria.

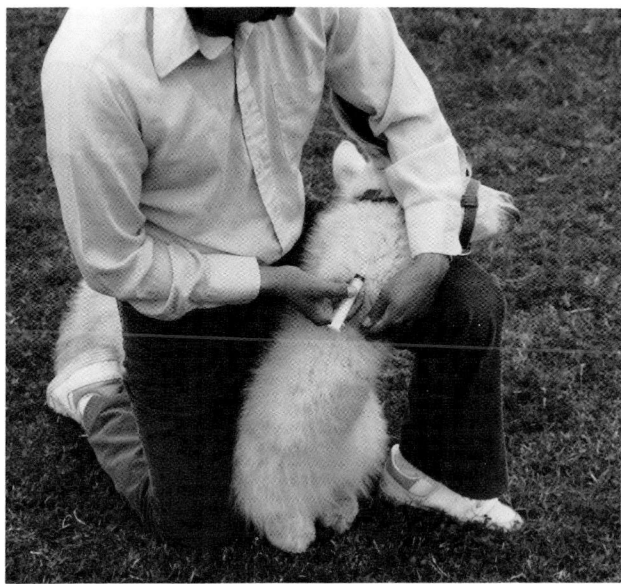

4.9 Alternate position for venipuncture in a cria.

Yearlings are often more difficult to restrain for venipuncture than neonates or adults. Many are not accustomed to being tied or having their heads restrained. They will frequently rear up and struggle vigorously. Chutes and stocks are not usually designed for animals smaller than adults. Nonetheless, the basic principles apply.

Venipuncture may be performed at other locations as well. The saphenous vein is superficial and easily palpated on the medial aspect of the stifle in a recumbent animal. The artery and vein lie contiguous to each other, with the vein more craniad.

Small volumes of blood may also be collected from the middle coccygeal vein on the ventrum of the tail. In the llama, the coccygeal vein is superficial, lying just beneath the skin. The tail should be elevated, but pushing it too hard up over the back should be avoided, since this will occlude the venous return. The procedure for blood collection from the tail of a lamoid is easier than it is in the bovine, in which the vein is situated deep, near the body of the coccygeal vertebrae. It is unwise to administer medication in the coccygeal vein because the long bevel on most needles may span the vessel and allow perivascular deposition of the medication.

There are also accessible veins on the ear (Fig. 4.10). Llama owners may nick the caudal border of the ear to collect small samples for progesterone analysis. A vein can also be cannulated with a 23 gauge needle for a pediatric catheter. The largest vein is located on the outer caudal border of the pinna. A temporary tourniquet (heavy elastic band) may be placed at the base of the ear to raise the vein.

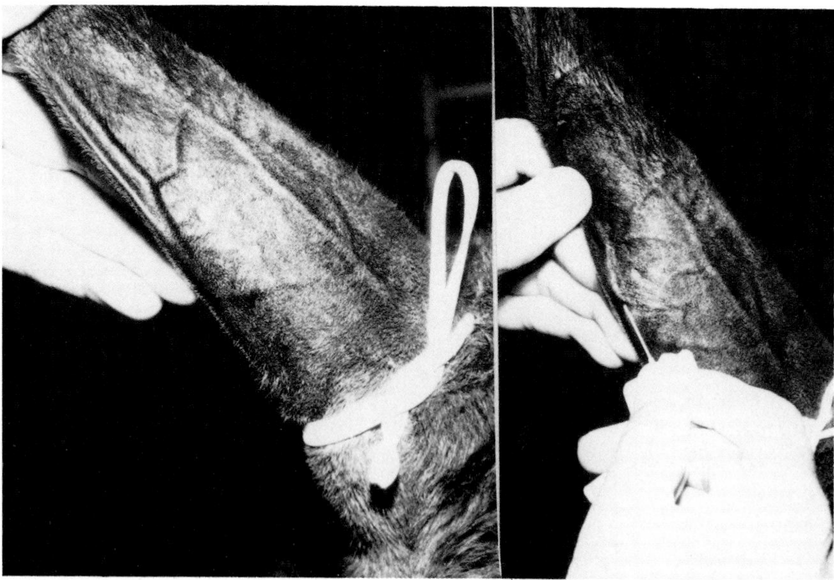

4.10 Ear veins on a llama.

HEMOGRAM. Hematology and serum biochemistry parameters are discussed in Chapter 15.

Abdominocentesis

An evaluation of peritoneal fluid is a vital component of differential diagnoses of digestive and other abdominal disorders. Peritoneal fluid aspirate is best obtained from the midline, just caudal to the umbilicus. Llamas may have a retroperitoneal fat layer as much as 6 cm (3 in.) thick and 14 cm (6 in.) broad lying on either side of the linea alba (Fig. 4.11). Only on the precise midline or 16–20 cm (7–8 in.) lateral to the midline is it possible to penetrate the peritoneal cavity with certainty (Fig. 4.12). The sample may be obtained from either the standing or recumbent llama. The site should be clipped and surgically prepared and local anesthesia injected. A stab incision should be made with a No. 12 scalpel blade for insertion of a 6 cm (3 in.), 14 gauge teat cannula with a quick thrust.

In adult lamoids, the glandular saccule area of C-1, covered by the greater omentum, is located on the ventral midline craniad to the umbilicus. As the omentum may occlude the ports of a teat cannula, it is recommended that abdominocentesis be performed caudal to the umbilicus.

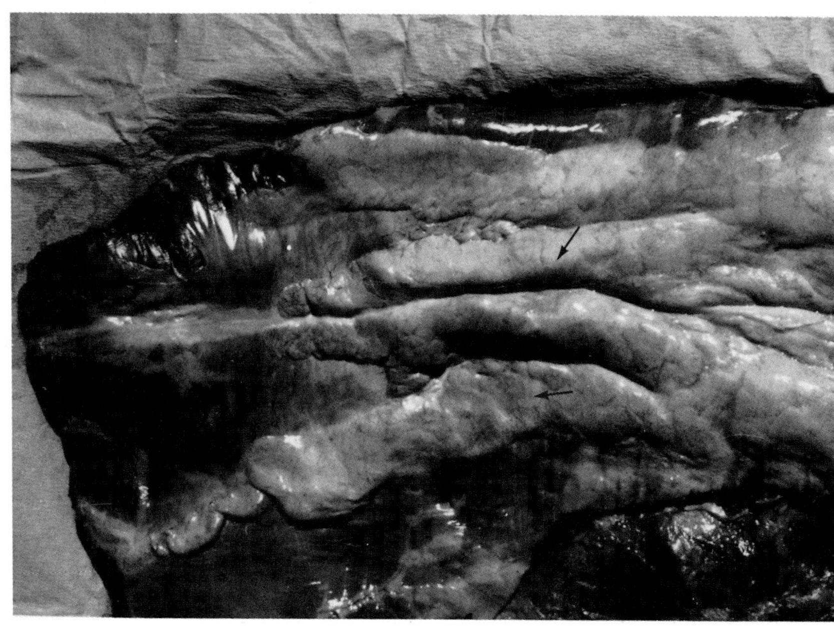

4.11 Abdominal fat lying on the ventral midline.

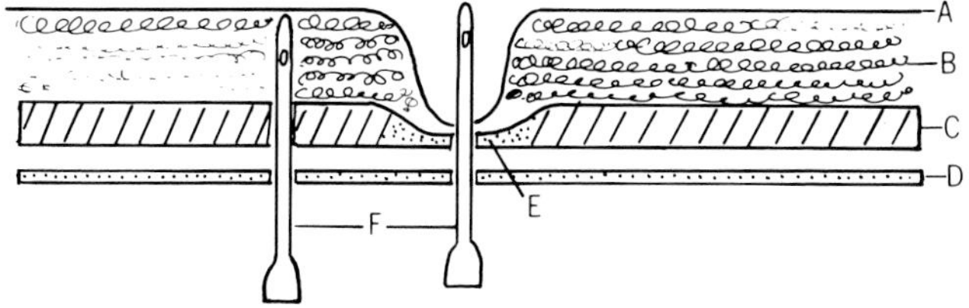

4.12 Diagram of the abdominocentesis location: **(A)** peritoneum, **(B)** abdominal fat, **(C)** abdominal muscles, **(D)** skin, **(E)** linea alba, **(F)** teat cannula.

In a normal animal, insufficient abdominal fluid may preclude collection. Unless there is 150 ml or more of fluid in the cavity, it will not flow freely. If it does not, attaching a syringe and establishing slight negative pressure while repositioning the needle tip in the cavity may yield a sample. If the fluid accumulation is localized, successful aspiration will be fortuitous. Table 4.2 provides data on abdominal fluid.

Orogastric Intubation

Gastric intubation is accomplished via the oral cavity. The nasal cavity is narrow and precludes passage of any except tiny tubes (see Chap. 12 for description of the nasal cavity). Passage of the orogastric tube differs little from the procedure in cattle and sheep. The cheek teeth are sharp, so a speculum is necessary to guide the gastric tube through the oral cavity and into the oropharynx. A standard cattle Frick speculum is too large except for the largest llama. A 20–25 cm (8–10 in.) segment of rubber garden hose slightly larger than the orogastric tube makes an excellent guide. A similar length of polyvinyl chloride pipe, wrapped with adhesive tape to prevent accidental shattering, is also suitable. Neonates may be intubated while in sternal recumbency (Fig. 4.13).

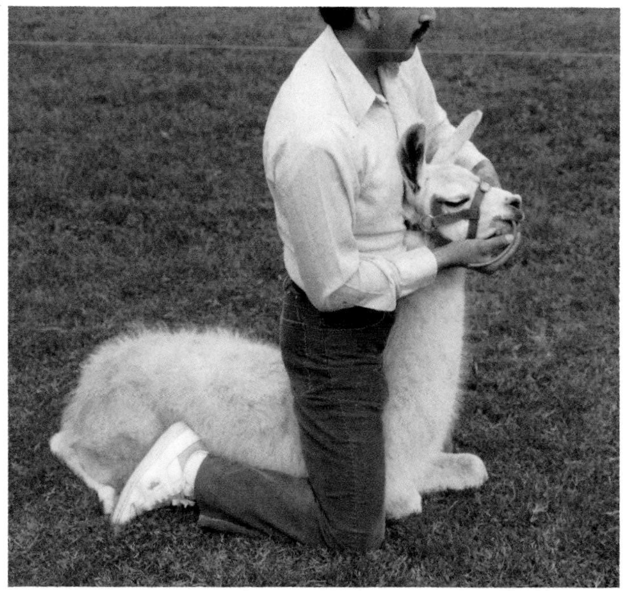

4.13 Positioning for gastric intubation of a neonate llama.

Table 4.2. Abdominal fluid analysis in selected diseases

	Normal	Infectious peritonitis	Ascites, cardiac failure	Rupture of bladder	Perforated bowel	Intestinal incarceration	Intraabdominal hemorrhage
Amount	±	±	+ + + +	+ + + +	+ to + + +	+ to + + +	+ +
Odor	None	None to foul	None	Ammonia	Ingesta	None to fetid	None
Gross appearance	Clear to slightly yellow	Yellowish-gray, cloudy	Clear	Colorless to cloudy, light yellow	Cloudy	Hemorrhagic	Hemorrhagic ±
Supernatant transparency	Clear, colorless to slightly yellow	Clear	Yellow, clear to slightly cloudy	Clear	Clear	Clear to reddish	Clear, reddish ±
Specific gravity	<1.0110	. . .	. . .	1.024	1.0185	1.0178	. . .
Foreign matter	None	Exudate	None	None	Fecal material	Blood	Blood
Refractive index	<1.3390	↑	↑ ±	↑ ±	↑	↑	↑ ±
Total protein (g/dl)	<3	3–18	<3	<3	4–8	Slight to significant increase	Normal to slight increase
Erythrocytes	None	±	–	–	±	+ +	+ + + +
Total nucleated cells	2000–5000	. . .	. . .	. . .	. . .	. . .	. . .
Type/μl	Mononuclear	Neutrophils	Mononuclear	Erythrocytes	Neutrophils	Mononuclear	Mononuclear
Count/μl	1000	5000–10,000	100–5000	Low	5000–100,000	5000–100,000	0–100
Bacteria	None	+ +	None	None	+ + +	None	None
Potassium (mmol/L)	4.9 ± 0.7	4.9	4.9	185–400	4.9	4.9	4.9
Coagulation	–	±	–	–	+ +	±	. . .

The head should be secured with a halter that will allow opening of the mouth sufficiently to insert the speculum over the base of the tongue. The head should be slightly flexed. Once the tip of the tube is in the oral pharynx, gentle pressure should be exerted to stimulate the animal to swallow. Indiscriminate jabbing should be avoided, but gently rotating the tube or adjusting the position of the head will encourage the llama to swallow the tube. There should be a slight resistance to passage of the tube.

The tube should be palpated as it transverses the left ventral cervical region to ensure intubation of the esophagus rather than the trachea. Alternatively, the free end of the tube may be placed into a container of water to check for bubbles. The tube may be inserted into the lumen of C-1. However, if it is desired to bypass disposition of fluid or medication into C-1, the tube should be kept within the esophagus. This is particularly important when feeding orphan neonates via stomach intubation. Milk deposited in C-1 may remain and ferment rather than be digested in C-3.

Gastric intubation may stimulate regurgitation (Fig. 4.14). This is not serious, but it does make the process disagreeable and may necessitate starting over again.

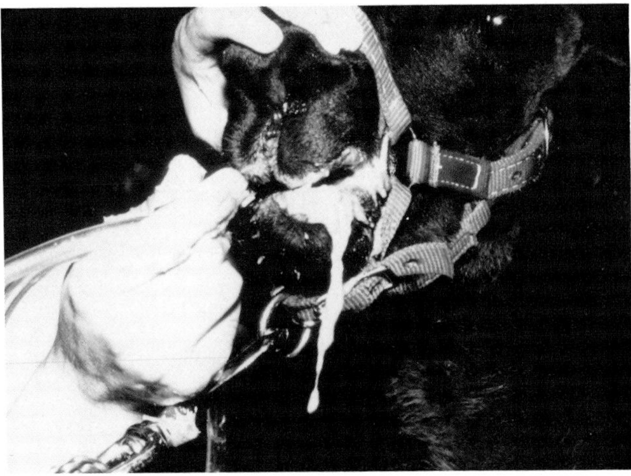

4.14 Regurgitation accompanying gastric intubation.

Urinary System

URINE COLLECTION. The easiest way to collect a urine sample is to make a free catch while the animal is urinating. Lamoids use a communal dung heap for both urination and defecation. Both the male and female eject urine caudally from a partial squat position. Unless extremely wild, most llamas will permit an approach to catch the urine in an open cup. Complete urination requires 30–60 seconds, allowing ample time to obtain a sample.

A free catch is the only available method of obtaining a urine sample in an adult male, because a recess, located dorsal to the urethra at the ischial arch, makes catheterization virtually impossible (Fig. 4.15). It would be most difficult to prevent insertion of the catheter into the diverticulum, even if digital pressure is applied through the wall of the rectum to aid direction of the catheter into the pelvic urethra.

It is possible to catheterize the female. The external urethral orifice, a groove, is easily palpated on the floor of the vulva at the region of the hymen. However, a suburethral diverticulum in the female may also complicate catheterization (Fig. 4.15). After the vulva has been cleansed, a sterile gloved finger should be inserted into the vulva to palpate the orifice. Withdrawing the finger slightly and inserting the catheter dorsal to the finger will aid in avoiding penetration into the more ventral blind diverticulum. A 1/67 mm (#5 French) polypropylene catheter is suitable for urine collection. The bladder should be found at a depth of 25 cm from the lips of the vulva. For urinalysis data see Chapter 18.

Thoracocentesis

Thoracocentesis may be indicated to obtain samples of pleural fluid for diagnostic purposes, removal of excess fluid or exudate, or removal of air from the pleural spaces. Penetration can be made from either side. The preferred site is at the 6th or 7th intercostal space (there are 12 ribs), 10–15 cm (4–6 in.) dorsal to the ventrum of the sternum or 2–4 cm dorsal to the costochondral junction of the ribs. The area should be clipped and prepared for aseptic surgery.

Selection of the needle or cannula to be used will be determined by the purpose for the thoracocentesis. If fluid is expected, a 14–16 gauge, 5 cm (2 in.) needle should be inserted near the cranial border of the rib to avoid the intercostal vessels. The pleural cavity may be penetrated at an approximate depth of 2–3 cm (1–1.5 in.). Fluid should flow from the needle. A spinal needle and stylet may be selected if air is to be removed.

If the lung has collapsed, a more dorsal and caudal position should be selected. Entrance should be made at the 8th or 9th intercostal space, approximately 25 cm from the dorsum of an adult llama. Distances for smaller individuals must be reduced proportionately. An indwelling catheter may be placed within the pleural space, using a standard technique.

Penis

The penis is situated in the ventral pelvic area and has a sigmoid flexure similar to that of other artiodactylids. The prepuce is directed caudally in the unaroused

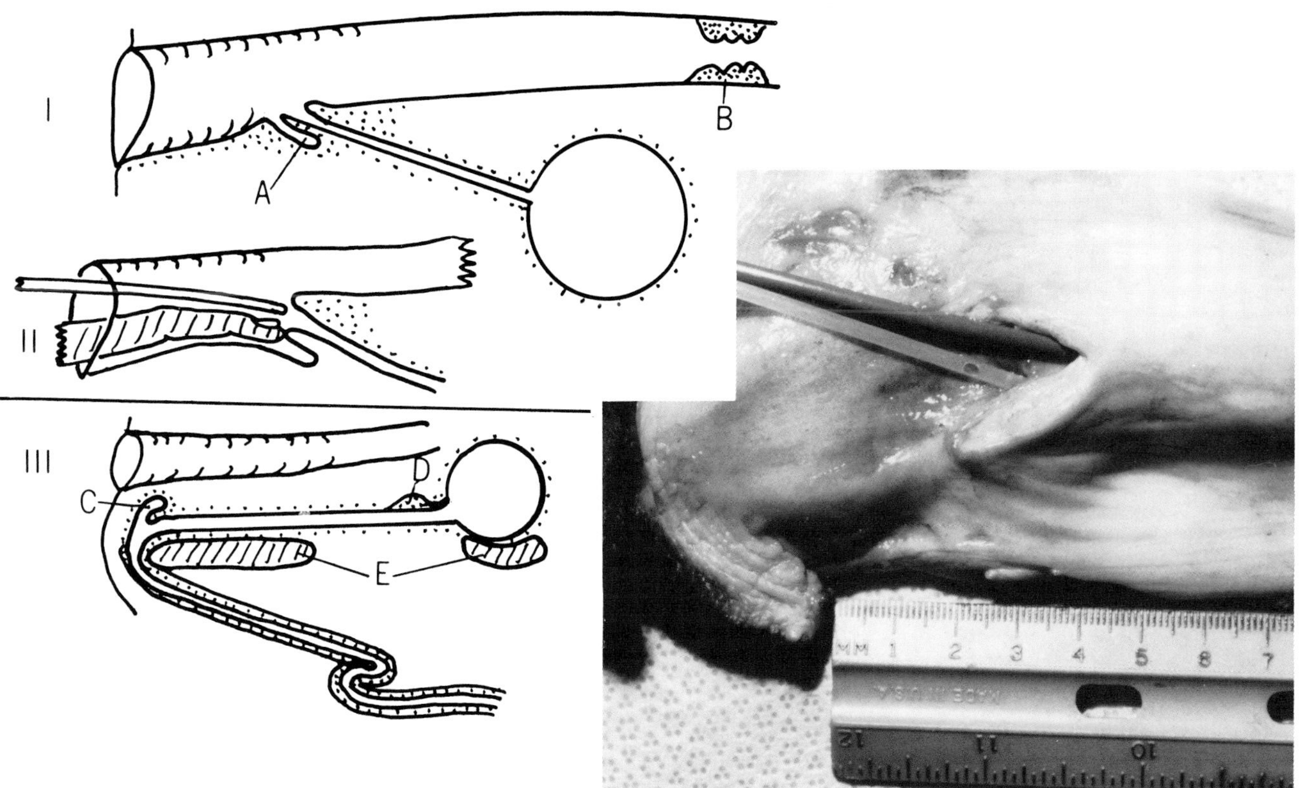

4.15 (Left) Diagrams of the urethra. I. Schematic of the female urethra: (A) suburethral diverticulum. II. Covering the suburethral diverticulum to catheterize the female. III. Schematic of the male urethra: (C) urethral recess, (D) prostate gland, (E) pubic bones. (Right) Dissected specimen, with top catheter in urethra, bottom in suburethral diverticulum.

male. The orifice of the prepuce is under the control of two sets of muscles: the cranial prepucial muscle, which pulls the prepuce cranially, and the caudal prepucial muscle, which pulls it caudally. When urinating, the male squats to spread the rear limbs.

The accessory sex glands include a small prostate gland and a pair of bulbourethral glands but no seminal vesicle. The erect penis is less than 2 cm in diameter and has a cartilage at the tip of the glans. The urethral opening lies alongside the process (see Fig. 17.2). The terminal urethra is only 3–5 mm in diameter, allowing passage of only a #5 French catheter. Urinary stones have been found lodged approximately 6–10 cm from the tip of the glans.

Foot

The foot of the llama is unique, with two digits on each foot (see Chap. 6 for a full discussion). The bearing surface of each digit has a soft, pliable sole and a digital cushion that is composed of fibroelastic tissue similar to the tissue of the digital cushion of the equine. Between the sole and the digital cushion is a layer of undifferentiated fibrous tissue that is thinnest near the toe and thickest at the bulb of the heel. The suborder name for camelids is Tylopoda, meaning "padded foot."

A small, true nail tips each digit, and phalanx 2 and 3 lie horizontally above the cushion. Old World camels have a single sole and pad beneath the digits, while SACs have a pad beneath each digit.

Bone Marrow Aspiration

Bone marrow is collected from one of the sternebrae. The wing of the ilium is too thin to allow penetration of the marrow cavity, and the rib marrow is less consistent in its location than the marrow of the sternebrae. An appropriate site is approximately 3–4 cm dorsal to the callosity on the ventrum of the sternum (Fig. 4.16). The needle[2] should be directed medially and slightly dorsally to engage the bone. Significant pressure exerted on the needle is required to enter the bone. A grating may be felt with the thrust. The needle should not be twisted during the insertion or the bevel will be damaged.

2. Monoject bone marrow biopsy needle, 5 cm (2 in.), 16 gauge, Sherwood Medical, St. Louis, MO 63103.

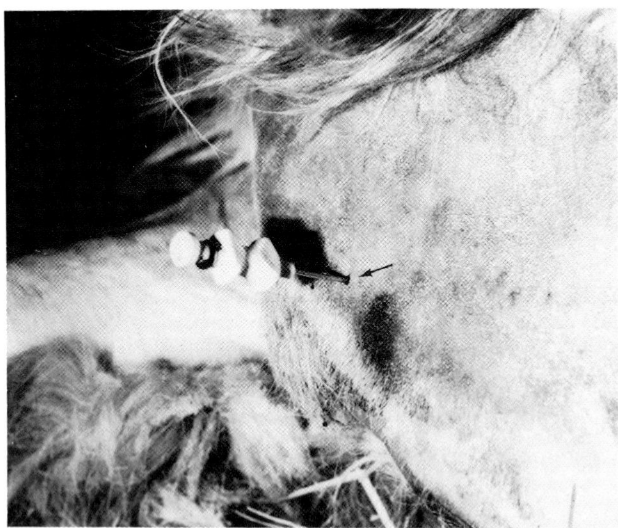

4.16 Needle position for collection of a bone marrow sample.

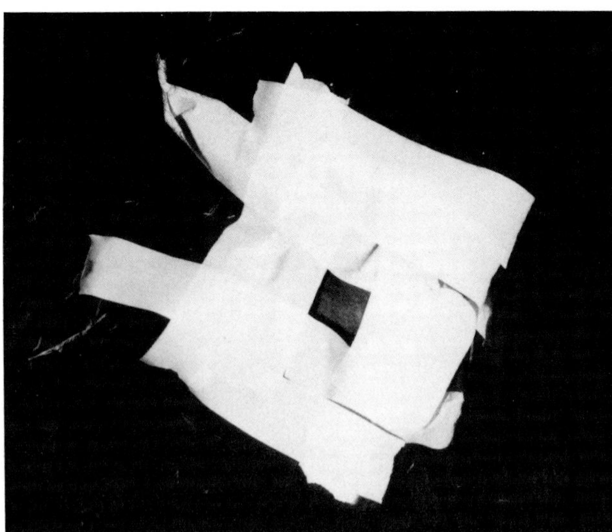

4.17 Masking a small area for sterile collection of a liver biopsy.

Marrow may be obtained at a depth of approximately 2.5 cm in an adult. After penetration, the stylet should be removed and a 12 ml syringe attached. Withdrawing the plunger with a pumping action should yield a sample. Marrow in the llama will be diluted with blood and is more fluid than that of cattle and horses. A smear made of marrow will show fat droplets. Smears may be made directly or the sample may be placed in an anticoagulant vial. The sample must be mixed thoroughly with the anticoagulant before the needle is removed from the vial to ensure collection of a proper sample.

If no marrow is obtained, the stylet should be replaced and penetration continued. After two or three unsuccessful attempts at aspiration, the needle should be withdrawn and moved 2–3 cm cranial or caudad, assuming that the initial insertion was made into an intersternebral space.

Liver Biopsy

In the camelid the liver lies entirely on the right side of the abdomen. The technique for obtaining a biopsy entails penetration of the caudal thorax, through the pleural space and the diaphragm, into the liver. Clipping a large area may be avoided by parting the fibers and fixing them out of the operative site with masking tape. An area 1 cm^2 should be clipped and prepared for aseptic surgery (Fig. 4.17). Liver biopsy may be done with the animal in either a standing or sternally recumbent position, using local anesthesia.

The recommended site for performing a liver biopsy is at the 9th intercostal space and approximately 20–22 cm (9–10 in.) from the top of the back. The needle should be directed toward the midline, caudally and slightly ventrally (Fig. 4.18). The chest wall is thin. The diaphragm is located immediately adjacent to the chest wall. To check proper siting, remove the hands from the needle. If the needle is in the diaphragm, it will move forward and back in synchrony with respiration. Since the liver lies immediately medial to the diaphragm, pushing the needle 2–3 cm deeper will penetrate the liver. The sample should be collected as indicated for the type of needle being used.

If the sample is desired for histologic examination, a wide choice of needles[3] is available. Disposable needles

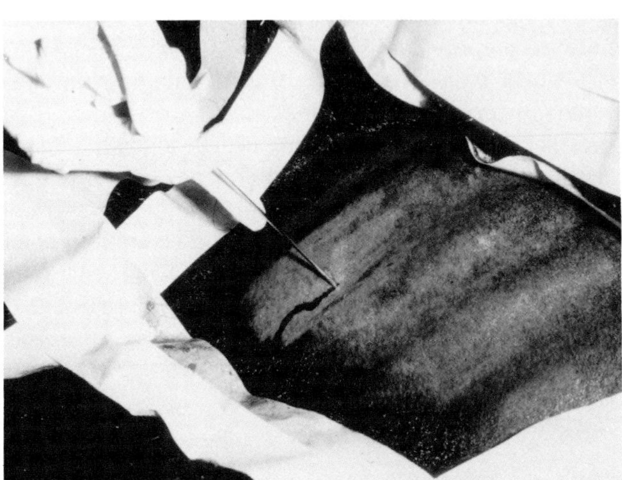

4.18 Insertion of needle for collection of liver biopsy.

3. Tru-cut disposable biopsy needle, 15.2 cm (6 in.), 14 gauge, Travenol Laboratories, Deerfield, IL 60015; ABC actuated biopsy needle, 15.2 cm (6 in.), 14 gauge, Monoject (Sherwood Medical), St. Louis, MO 63103; Silverman biopsy needle, 15.2 cm (6 in.), 14 gauge, many medical suppliers.

used in human medicine are satisfactory (Fig. 4.19). If larger samples are required for nutritional studies, special types of trocars and cannulas are required.

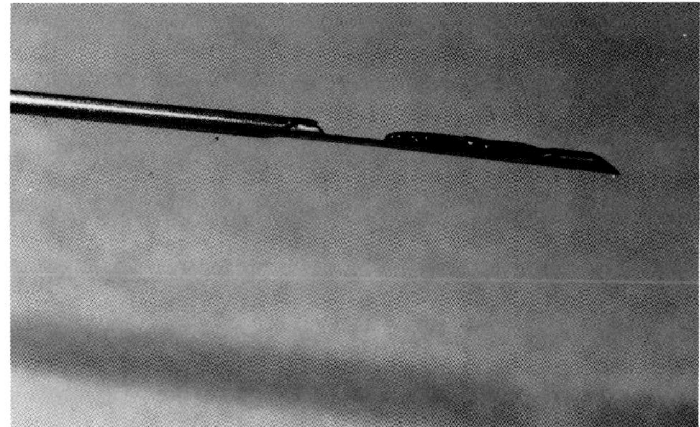

4.19 Liver biopsy sample collected with True-cut needle.

Collection of Cerebrospinal Fluid (1)

INDICATIONS. Penetration of the subarachnoid space is performed to collect cerebrospinal fluid (CSF) for laboratory analysis, for conducting a myelogram, and to ascertain CSF pressure.

ANATOMY. The subarachnoid space may be entered either at the lumbosacral space or at the atlantooccipital space. The relationship of the subarachnoid space to the meninges, vertebrae, and spinal cord is the same in camelids as in livestock and horses (Figs. 4.20, 4.21). In the llama, the spinal cord ends at the level of the 2nd sacral vertebral segment. The site should be prepared for aseptic surgery and appropriately draped.

ANESTHESIA. The type of anesthesia should be determined by the site and the procedure to be carried out. Myelography requires general anesthesia. Collection of fluid from the lumbosacral space may be done under local anesthesia, but collection from the atlantooccipital space should be done under general anesthesia to avoid uncontrolled movement and possible trauma to the spinal cord.

ATLANTOOCCIPITAL SPACE. With the head in a flexed position, the wings of the atlas should be palpated to locate the narrowest width at the cranial border (Fig. 4.22). An imaginary line from wing to wing should be established and the skin penetrated directly on the midline, perpendicular to the cervical vertebrae.

The needle will penetrate the funicular ligamentum nuchae and then the dorsal atlantooccipital membrane.

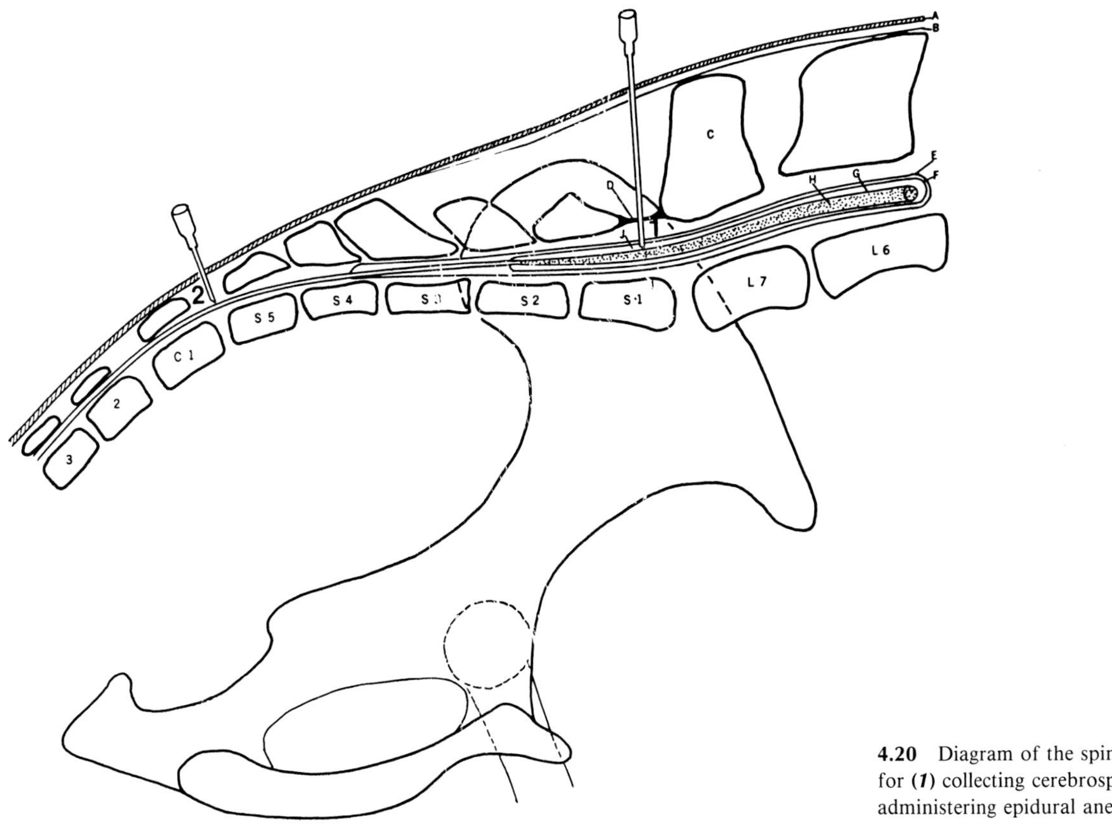

4.20 Diagram of the spine, with locations for (*1*) collecting cerebrospinal fluid and (*2*) administering epidural anesthesia.

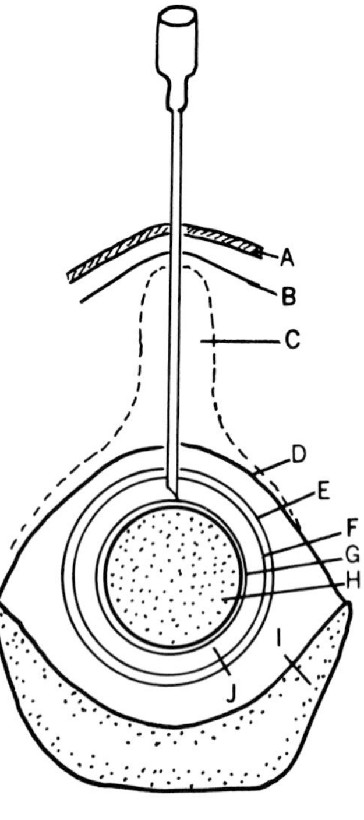

4.21 Diagram of a cross section at the lumbosacral space to illustrate layers penetrated to collect cerebrospinal fluid or administer spinal anesthesia: **(A)** skin, **(B)** lumbodorsal fascia, **(C)** dorsal spine of the 6th lumbar vertebra, **(D)** interarcuate ligament, **(E)** dura mater, **(F)** arachnoid meningeal layer, **(G)** pia mater, **(H)** spinal cord, **(I)** body of the vertebra, **(J)** subarachnoid space.

The cervical dura mater lies closely adjacent to the membrane, and with the head held in tight flexion, the membrane and dura will be tense. The needle should penetrate the subarachnoid space with an audible or palpable "pop."

The stylet should be withdrawn to check for fluid. If none is present, the stylet should be reinserted and the needle rotated 90 degrees and again a check made for fluid. If still no fluid is encountered, the stylet should be reinserted again and the needle advanced 1 or 2 mm deeper. This may be continued until fluid can be withdrawn. The needle should never be manipulated without the stylet in place, otherwise the spinal cord may be lacerated or a plug of neural tissue removed.

A 6.35 cm (2.5 in.), 20 gauge spinal needle is appropriate for this location. The depth of the subarachnoid space in an adult llama is approximately 4 cm (2 in.).

LUMBOSACRAL SPACE. The landmarks for this location are formed by the tuber sacrale of the pelvis and the dorsospinous process of the last lumbar vertebra (L-7). It is not difficult to palpate the dorsospinous proc-

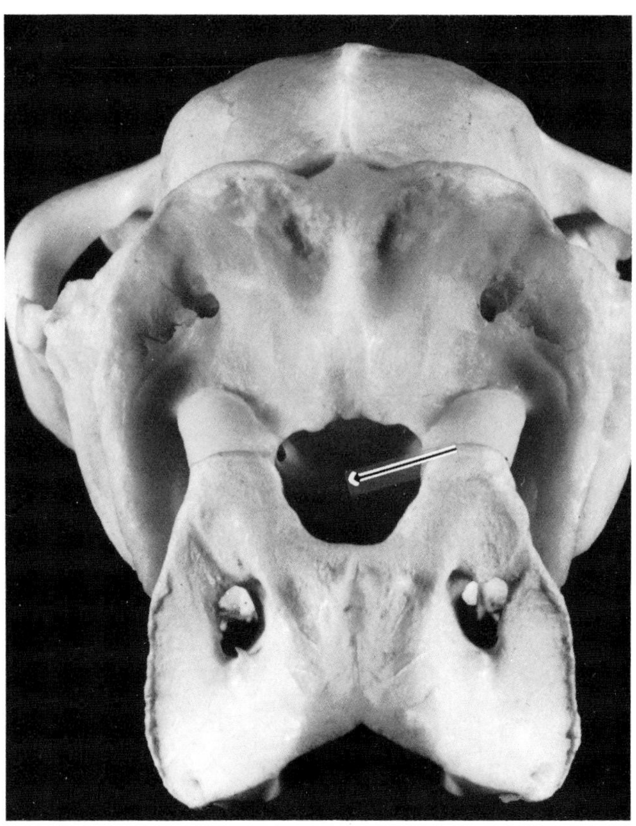

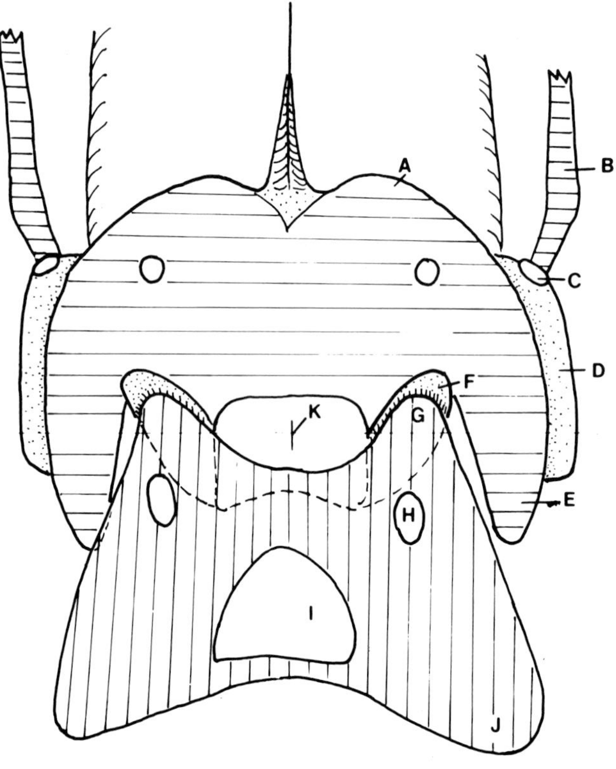

4.22 (Left) Atlas and occipital region of the skull illustrating the anatomy of the site for cerebrospinal fluid collection. (Right) Diagram of the atlantooccipital space for cerebrospinal fluid collection: **(A)** nuchal crest, **(B)** zygomatic arch, **(C)** osseous ear canal, **(D)** mastoid process, **(E)** jugular process, **(F)** occipital condyle, **(G)** cranial wing of the atlas, **(H)** alar foramen, **(I)** vertebral foramen, **(J)** caudal wing of the atlas, **(K)** site for needle insertion.

ess of L-7 because the dorsal processes of the sacrum are short. The correct site is 2 cm caudal to the dorsospinous process of L-7 on the midline, perpendicular to the vertebral column. The interarcuate space between L-7 and the 1st sacral vertebra (S-1) is large (2 cm cranial caudal and 4 cm wide) (Fig. 4.23).

The tissues penetrated by the needle will be the skin, thoracolumbar fascia, interspinous ligament, interarcuate ligament, dura mater, and the arachnoid (Fig. 4.21). A pop will not be felt when passing through the interarcuate ligament as in the atlantooccipital position, but decreased resistance should be noted.

A check for fluid should be made with each change of resistance. As previously indicated, the needle should never be moved without the stylet in place. If no fluid flows, the jugular may be occluded to increase intraspinous pressure (Fig. 4.24). If still no fluid is encountered, the needle may be advanced through the conus medullaris of the cord to the floor of the spinal canal. Then the needle should be withdrawn, a millimeter at a time, until fluid flows.

The depth of the subarachnoid space is 6–6.5 cm in an adult and 2–2.5 cm in a neonate. The floor of the spinal canal is approximately 8 cm in an adult and 3.5 cm in a neonate. An 18–20 gauge, 9 cm (3.5 in.) spinal needle is necessary to reach the subarachnoid space in an adult llama.

Table 4.3 lists the normal values for CSF along with a differential for various disorders.

Arthrocentesis

Arthrocentesis should be performed under strict asepsis. Anesthesia may be either sedation with xylazine HCl (0.1–0.4 mg/kg) or the use of a local anesthetic. A needle with a short rather than a regular bevel should be

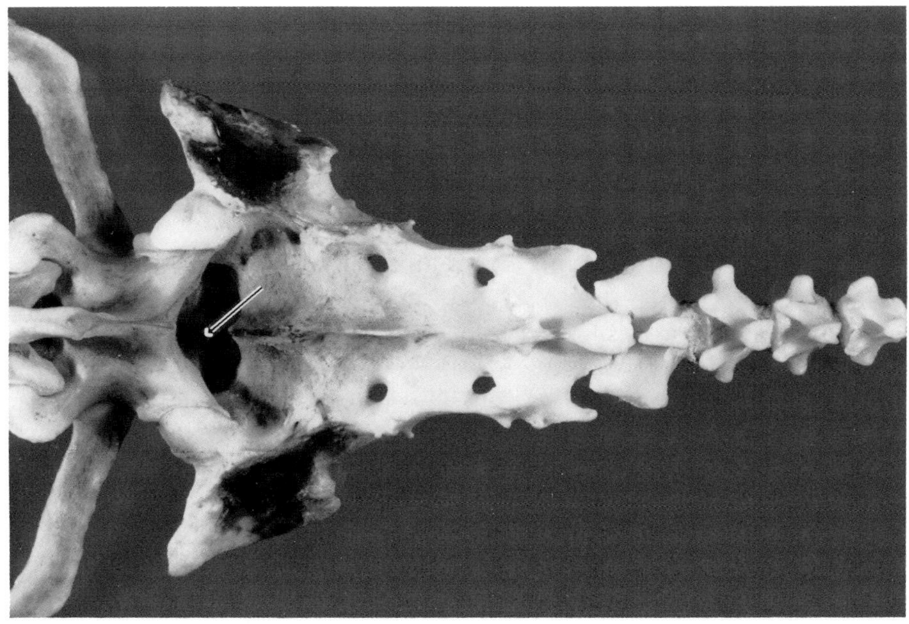

4.23 Lumbosacral space, dorsal view.

Table 4.3. Cerebrospinal fluid analysis in selected diseases

	Normal	Nonpurulent encephalomyelitis	Purulent encephalitis
Pressure	<250 mm H_2O	Normal to elevated	>250
Transparency	Clear	Clear to cloudy	Cloudy with strings, coagulates
Color	Colorless	Colorless, whitish	White to reddish
Specific gravity	1.005–1.010	↑	↑
Refractive	<1.3350	↑	↑
Erythrocytes	<35	?	?
Nucleated cells	<20	30–400	200–600
Neutrophils	None to few	±	+ + +
Lymphocytes	95% + + +	+ +	±
Protein (mg/dl)	<80	<200	>200–1000
Glucose (mg/dl)	<70	?	?

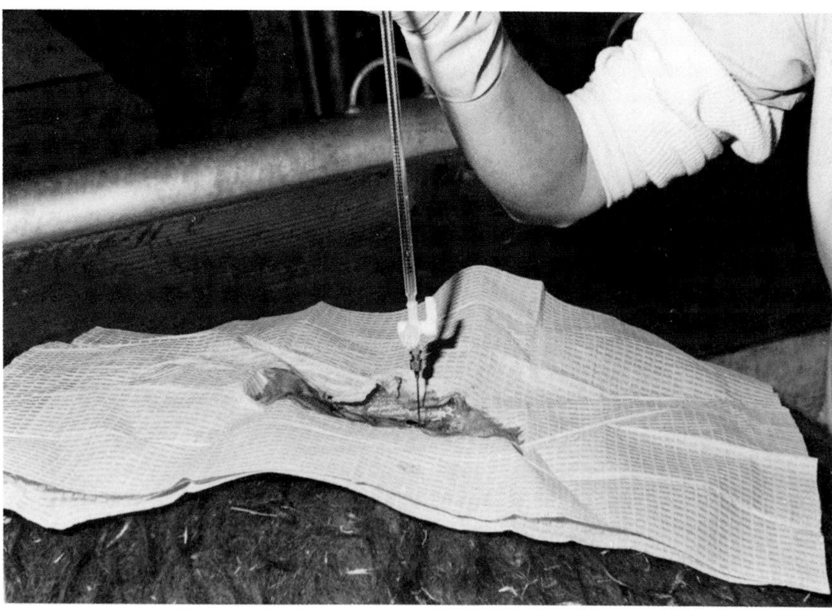

4.24 Evaluation of cerebrospinal fluid pressure at the lumbosacral space.

used. It may be difficult to obtain synovial fluid from a normal joint.

SHOULDER. To aspirate the shoulder joint, palpate the acromion process of the scapula and the tendon of the infraspinatus muscle as it attaches to the greater tubercle of the humerus. The greater tubercle has a notch just cranial to the tendon. The needle should be inserted through the notch horizontally and slightly caudal to the vertical axis of the body.

ELBOW. The needle should be inserted on the lateral side of the olecranon and directed ventrally in a line on the axis of the olecranon. The needle should be kept close to the olecranon.

CARPUS. Either the radiocarpal or carpal metacarpal articulation can be palpated by flexing the carpus and separating the carpal bones. Insertion of the needle through the extensor tendons should be avoided. They may be palpated on the dorsal surface of the carpus. A 3–4 cm, 20 gauge needle should be used.

STIFLE. Aspiration of the stifle joint capsule may be accomplished from three locations. It is unknown at the present just how these complicated joint capsule compartments intercommunicate, but joint fluid may be removed from an obviously distended compartment. The distal compartment may be entered by insertion of the needle just proximal and slightly lateral to the tibial tuberosity. This requires at least an 8 cm needle. The interfemoral tibial fat pad is freely moveable and may inhibit penetration of the joint capsule unless the joint is distended.

As in the horse, another site for aspiration is alongside the lateral digital extensor muscle tendon as it passes over the tibial groove on the craniolateral border of the proximal end of the tibia.

A third location for aspiration is from the dorsolateral aspect of the patella. The needle should be inserted beneath the patella. The femoral patella compartment is large and, if excessive fluid is present, provides the easiest access to stifle joint fluid.

The anatomy of the stifle is unique in the llama. The tendons of the vastus lateralis and vastus medialis muscles form a sheet that inserts partly on the dorsal aspect of the patella, but, also, a free portion extends around the patella to insert on the tibial tuberosity. Instead of one, two, or three patellar tibial ligaments, there is a sheet of tendons composed of a combination of the quadriceps group plus the tendons of the biceps femoris muscle.

HOCK. The needle should be inserted ventral to the lateral malleolus of the tibia and directed medially and ventrally to enter the tibiotarsal joint sac.

The metacarpal, tarsal, phalangeal, and interphalangeal joints should be penetrated on the dorsolateral or medial aspect in areas devoid of tendons, vessels, and major nerves, all of which can be easily palpated beneath the skin.

REFERENCE

1. Mayhew, I. G. 1975. Collection of spinal fluid from the horse. Cornell Vet. 65:50.

5 Anesthesia

LOCAL ANESTHESIA (3)

In the llama, infiltration of a surgical site with a local anesthetic agent is a routine practice for lancing abscesses, suturing lacerations, laparoscopy, abdominocentesis, and thoracocentesis. Local anesthesia may also be used in combination with mild sedation in such surgical procedures as castration or a standing exploratory laparotomy.

Regional nerve blocks are less often selected because the course of the nerves is not well documented in the llama, but what is known indicates wide variation from other livestock species (22). For instance, the major nerve supply to the foot is located only on the medial aspect of the metacarpus and metatarsus rather than bilaterally, as in the equine and bovine. An inverted L local block is appropriately used for a flank laparotomy incision to avoid interference in wound healing as a result of anesthetic agent infiltration of the operative site.

Any of the standard local anesthetic agents are suitable. Selection may depend on the rapidity of onset and duration of anesthesia desired or the experience of the operator (Tables 5.1, 5.2). Any local anesthetic agent may be toxic if the administered dose is excessive.

A 2-month-old llama was sedated with xylazine at 0.4 mg/kg and the surgical site for an umbilical herniorrhaphy was infiltrated with 40 ml of 2% lidocaine. The neonate died while exhibiting respiratory distress and tachycardia (15). Assuming that the baby llama weighed approximately 25 kg at 2 months, the dose of lidocaine was 32 mg/kg. The lethal dose reported for horses is 4.5 mg/kg.

Overdosage of lidocaine, and most other local anesthetic agents, causes central nervous system (CNS) stimulation, with muscle twitching and convulsions in dogs. Additional signs may be hypotension, nausea, vomiting, tachycardia, and dyspnea (3).

EPIDURAL ANESTHESIA (3, 17)

Indications

Epidural anesthesia is indicated for any type of perineal surgery (suturing lacerations, penetration of a persistent hymen), replacement of a prolapsed rectum or vagina, and prevention of excessive straining during rectal palpation.

Preparation

Epidural anesthesia should not be performed without surgical preparation of the site, which requires clipping the fiber. This may distress a client. Minimal disfigurement results if a 1 cm^2 patch around the site is clipped with scissors. The remaining fibers may be parted and taped away from the site with masking tape. The site should be scrubbed and disinfected.

Technique

The tail should be grasped with one hand and rocked up and down to locate the sacrococcygeal intervertebral space. The 5 sacral vertebrae (S-1 to S-5) are fused in most individuals, so the first moveable intervertebral space would be between S-5 and coccygeal 1 (C-1) (see Fig. 4.20). In a few individuals, S-5 is free and moveable. The space available between S-4 and S-5 for penetration into the neural canal is minimal. If difficulty is encountered when attempting an epidural, move caudally to the second moveable space to facilitate the procedure.

A 1.5 in., 20 gauge needle should be inserted perpendicularly or slightly cranial to the slope of the tailhead, directly on the midline. The depth of the spinal canal is 1.5–2 cm in a 130 kg animal. If the needle is positioned properly, the fluid should flow and drain from the hub of the needle when the syringe is detached and a drop of the anesthetic agent is put on the hub. The needle should be left in position until motor control of the tail is lost, in approximately 1–2 minutes.

Solutions containing preservatives should not be used for epidural or spinal anesthesia. One to two ml 2% lidocaine HCl, without epinephrine, will provide anesthesia for over an hour and allow the animal to remain standing. Higher volumes may allow cranial migration of the agent, involving the nerves to the hind limbs, resulting in incoordination and recumbency.

In a study conducted in Peru, 2% lidocaine HCl was used epidurally in doses of 1–5 ml. Anesthesia was accomplished within 5 minutes, persisting as long as 5 hours. Higher doses may cause paralysis of the hind limbs (17).

Analgesics

PHENYLBUTAZONE[1] (BUTAZOLIDIN). Oxyphenbutazone is similar (4).

Pharmacology. The analgesic effect of phenylbutazone is produced by its antiinflammatory action. It has been used extensively in a variety of species, including humans, to treat musculoskeletal disorders and reduce soft tissue inflammation. It also has an antipyretic effect.

1. Butazolidin, Burroughs-Wellcome, Kansas City, MO 64141.

Indications. Phenylbutazone is recommended for the same types of conditions for which it is useful in horses and livestock. The oral or intravenous (IV) dose is 2–4 mg/kg once daily. Perivascular injections of phenylbutazone may result in phlebitis and an adjacent skin slough.

There has been insufficient usage of phenylbutazone to enable drawing of conclusions as to its efficacy in various disorders. In general, however, it seems to be more effective in relieving musculoskeletal pain than for soft tissue and colicky pain.

Phenylbutazone is supplied in 50 and 100 ml bottles (200 mg/ml); as 1 g, 2 g, and 4 g boluses; in 8 g packages of granules; and as a paste that can be measured in grams of phenylbutazone.

Side Effects and Precautions. Phenylbutazone has been reported to be ulcerogenic in the equine. There are no convincing reports of ulcers in llamas following its use, but as a precaution, the author simultaneously administers cimetidine (2.2 mg/kg parenterally) once daily when treating with phenylbutazone. There has been no evidence of hematologic disturbance in lamoids, as has been reported in humans.

Table 5.1. Comparison of injectable local anesthetic agents

Agent	Trade names	Company	Formulation	Onset	Duration	Single-dose toxicity
				(min)	*(hr)*	
Procaine HCl	Procaine, Novocaine	Various, Winthrop	1–2% sol. 1% and 10% sol.	2–5 (2% sol.)	0.25–0.50 (2% sol.)	
Lidocaine HCl	Lidocaine, Xylocaine	Various, Astra	1–2% sol. 2% sol.	0.5–1 (1% sol.)	0.5–1 (1% sol.)	>4.5 mg/kg
Lidocaine HCl with epinephrine	Lidocaine	Various	1% sol.	0.5–1	2–6	>7.0 mg/kg
Mepivacaine	Carbocaine	Winthrop	1–2% sol.	3–5	0.75–1.5	
Bupivacaine	Bupivacaine, Marcaine	Abbott, Winthrop	0.25–0.75% sol.	5 (0.25% sol.)	2–4 (0.25% sol.)	

Note: Facts and comparisions are from Drug Information Service, J. B. Lippincott, St. Louis, MO 63246.

Table 5.2. Topical local anesthetic agents

Agent	Trade name	Company	Formulation	Indications
Proparacaine HCl	Ophthaine, Ophtheltic proparacaine	Squibb Allegram, various	0.5% sol.	Ophthalmic
Tetracaine HCl	Tetracaine, Pontocaine	Various, Astra	0.5% sol. 0.5% ointment	Ophthalmic
Lidocaine HCl	Lidocaine, Xylocaine	Various, Astra	5% ointment 2% jelly 10% solution	Mucous membrane, endotracheal intubation, urethral catheterization, mucous membrane
Benzocaine HCl	Benzocaine, Americaine	Various, American	20% gel 20% gel	Oral and laryngeal, mucosa, endotracheal intubation, endoscopy

Note: Facts and comparisons are from Drug Information Services, J. B. Lippincott, St. Louis, MO 63246.

FLUNIXIN MEGLUMINE[2] (BANAMINE)

Pharmacology. Flunixin (4) is a nonsteroidal antiinflammatory agent that has analgesic and antipyretic effects. It has proven to be an effective analgesic for colicky pain.

Indications. Flunixin has been used extensively in llamas and alpacas for analgesia in musculoskeletal disorders. It seems to be more effective than phenylbutazone in the relief of gastrointestinal (GI) spasms. However, automatic administration of this drug early in a colicky disorder may mask clinical signs, delaying differential diagnosis and selection of appropriate therapy.

Flunixin is supplied in granular form in 250 mg packets and as a solution in a concentration of 50 mg/ml. The recommended IV dosage for llamas is 1.1 mg/kg, given once daily.

Side Effects and Precautions. Although never reported in lamoids, intraarterial injection of flunixin has resulted in ataxia, rapid breathing, muscle weakness, and hysteria in other species. As stated before, flunixin may mask critical signs. As flunixin has been reported to be ulcerogenic, cimetidine is usually administered simultaneously.

ASPIRIN (formerly acetylsalicylic acid)

Pharmacology. Aspirin is a nonsteroid antiinflammatory analgesic. It is often administered to animals but is not used as extensively as it is in humans. Aspirin has a variety of pharmacologic actions that have little relevance to lamoids.

2. Banamine, Schering Corp., Kenilworth, NJ 07003.

Indications. The primary indications for use of aspirin are to relieve mild musculoskeletal postsurgical pain when the cost of more potent analgesics is prohibitive or if therapy is contemplated for a long time.

There are no studies upon which to base a sound dosage regimen. Extrapolating from cattle, an oral dose of 5–100 mg/kg given twice daily may be appropriate (4).

Side Effects. None reported.

Sedation, Tranquilization, Chemical Immobilization

Many procedures can be carried out on nervous or apprehensive lamoids by dulling the sensorium with tranquilizers or low doses of injectable anesthetic agents (Table 5.3). In some instances the animal remains standing, at other times recumbency may be necessary. Chemical immobilizing agents are routinely used to render wild, dangerous zoo animals immobile. Immobilization of obstreperous or vicious male llamas may be necessary to carry out even such minor procedures as nail trimming. Chemical immobilization of vicuñas or untrained guanacos may be preferable to physical restraint.

Individual drugs will be described, followed by a discussion of applications, either individually or in combination.

ETORPHINE HYDROCHLORIDE (M99)

Pharmacology. Etorphine (10) is a highly potent narcotic analgesic, producing pharmacologic effects similar to those of morphine, namely, depression of the respiratory and cough centers, decreased GI motility, elevated blood pressure, tachycardia, and behavioral

Table 5.3. Drugs used for sedation, injectable anesthesia, or immobilization in camelids

		Sedation		Immobilization		Anesthesia		Comments: special uses,
Agent	Concentration	IM dose	IV dose	IM dose	IV dose	IM dose	IV dose	untoward reactions
Xylazine HCl Rompun	20 mg/ml or 100 mg/ml		0.1–0.2 mg/kg	0.3–0.4 mg/kg	0.25 mg/kg	Not suitable by itself		Reversal of yohimbine 0.25 mg/kg
Ketamine HCl	10 mg/ml or 100 mg/ml		5–8 mg/kg	5 mg/kg, rarely used alone		Not suitable by itself		
Butorphanol-xylazine	B–10 mg/ml X–100 mg/ml		B–0.05–0.1 mg/kg X–0.1 mg/kg					Not suitable for general anesthesia
Xylazine-ketamine	X–100 mg/ml K–100 mg/ml			X–0.35 mg/kg K–5–8 mg/kg	X–0.25 mg/kg K–3–5 mg/kg	X–0.35 mg/kg K–5–8 mg/kg	X–0.25 mg/kg K–3–5 mg/kg	
Diazepam-ketamine	D–5 mg/ml K–100 mg/ml			D–0.2–0.3 mg/kg K–5–8 mg/kg	D–0.1–0.2 mg/kg K–3–5 mg/kg			
Etorphine HCl	1% or 1 mg/ml			2–3 mg total	2mg total administration, slow to effect			Reversal with diprenorphine HCl Dose: double dose of etorphine

changes. In camelids, low doses of etorphine cause CNS stimulation with muscle rigidity, tremors, and possibly convulsions. At higher doses, paradoxically, the CNS is depressed.

Administration. Etorphine is readily absorbed from an intramuscular (IM) site. Onset of anesthesia occurs 5–15 minutes after IM injections. If no antidote is administered, recovery is slow, requiring up to 3 hours. When the antidote is injected, the animal becomes ambulatory within 2–10 minutes. Etorphine should not be mixed with atropine, since atropine reduces its solubility.

Side Effects. Inhibition of respiratory centers may directly or indirectly influence blood gases and acid-base balances. Etorphine is extremely dangerous to humans. If injected accidentally, medical help should be sought immediately. Naloxone or the specific antidote, diprenorphine (M50-50), should be administered intravenously. Equipment for artificial respiration should be kept available to deal with possible respiratory arrest.

Etorphine is readily absorbed through mucous membranes and may be absorbed through the skin. It is important to avoid inhalation, ingestion, or contamination of the skin, particularly of the hands, which might touch the mouth.

Antidote. Diprenorphine (M50-50) is a specific antidote for etorphine. The standard dose is double the amount of etorphine injected. If diprenorphine is unavailable, naloxone may be used.

Application in Lamoids. Etorphine has been recommended for llamas, but the author has not been favorably impressed with its use. In one trial, a 135 kg llama gelding was given 0.5 mg etorphine HCl intramuscularly. In 5 minutes the llama began to stiffen and fell onto its side. The llama was rigid, the legs stiffly outstretched with some jerking. The head was raised, as if the llama were trying to rise. The preinjection heart rate (HR) was 62 and the respiratory rate (RR) was 20. Ten minutes after the first injection, another 0.5 mg M99 was given intramuscularly. Additional relaxation was achieved, but it was not complete. At minute 15, the HR was 66 and the RR was 4. At minute 20, the HR had increased to 110, with the RR remaining at 4 or 5.

In another trial, 1 mm etorphine was administered to a 130 kg llama. The animal became recumbent in 10 minutes but remained rigid. This dose was insufficient to completely immobilize the llama. Diprenorphine was administered, and within 2 minutes the llama was standing.

Heck (16) immobilized adult guanacos with etorphine at 1.4 mg total dose and adult llamas with 1.5 mg total dose. No mention was made of rigidity as a complication. Merilan (20) used 1.5 mg etorphine combined with 20 mg xylazine in adult lamoids for electroejaculation (see Chap. 17).

Prior experience with numerous zoo species has led the author to believe that the dosage being reported for camelids is low and that a minimum of 2 mg should be given to an adult llama. Also, as in many other species, such as the equines, it would be preferable to combine etorphine with xylazine or acepromazine to minimize the CNS stimulation effected by etorphine.

KETAMINE HYDROCHLORIDE (KETALAR, VETALAR, KETAJECT, KETANEST)

Pharmacology. Ketamine (5, 10) is a nonbarbiturate dissociative anesthetic agent. The animal usually retains normal pharyngeal-laryngeal reflexes. This desirable effect minimizes accidental aspiration of food or ingesta. However, endotracheal intubation is difficult when ketamine is the only agent used.

Ketamine produces an increased RR with a decrease in the tidal volume. If ketamine is given intravenously at a too-rapid rate, apnea may be produced.

Ketamine does not produce skeletal muscle relaxation, rather a catatonia. There is profound analgesia at medium to high dosages, although analgesia of the visceral peritoneum may be less than optimal. Excessive salivation can be alleviated with atropine.

Animals experience transitory pain upon IM injection of the solution. Since ketamine crosses the placenta, anesthetic effects are noted in the fetus when ketamine is used as a sedative for cesarean section or dystocia.

Ketamine produces a fixed expression in the eyes. The eyelids stay open, yet the cornea usually remains moist. Occasionally, corneal ulceration has resulted from prolonged exposure. Palpebral reflexes persist. Ketamine is detoxified in the liver, and metabolites are excreted via the urine.

Administration. Ketamine is supplied as a solution in 20 mg/ml and 100 mg/ml concentrations.

Side Effects. Tonic-clonic convulsions are produced in some species but have not been observed in lamoids except upon accidental intracarotid injections. Ketamine is not known to produce abortion. Regurgitation has occurred following ketamine usage in camelids. It is difficult to say whether this was an effect of the drug or simply passive regurgitation from immobilization. Ketamine is rarely used as the sole immobilizing or anesthetic agent in camelids. Side effects are generally ameliorated by the combined drug.

Antidote. There is no known clinical antidote for ketamine.

XYLAZINE (ROMPUN, BAYER 1470)

Pharmacology. Xylazine (2, 10, 19, 23) is not a narcotic; it is a sedative, analgesic, and muscle relaxant, producing its effect by stimulating both central and peripheral presynaptic alpha 2 adrenoceptors. Under the influence of xylazine, animals appear to be sleeping. Other actions include depressed thermoregulation; hyperglycemia; decreased heart rate, cardiac output, and aortic flow; temporary increase in blood pressure followed by hypotension; and respiratory depression (6).

Administration. Xylazine is supplied in 20 mg/ml and 100 mg/ml solutions and may be given intravenously or intramuscularly. Immobilization occurs within 3–5 minutes following IV injection or 10–15 minutes after IM injection. Analgesia lasts from 15 to 30 minutes, but the sleeplike state is maintained for 1–2 hours. Painful procedures should not be performed after 30 minutes.

Side Effects and Precautions. Stimulation during the induction stage may prevent optimum sedation. Seemingly sedated animals have roused explosively, negating the sedation. Occasionally, muscle tremors, bradycardia, and partial atrioventricular block occur with standard doses. Salivation is pronounced in lamoids; atropine (0.04 mg/kg) should be given to counter cardiac effects and diminish salivation.

Intracarotid administration produces transient seizures and collapse.

Xylazine has been used extensively in llamas at all stages of pregnancy with no apparent abortions, as have been reported in the bovine.

Antidote. Yohimbine HCl (0.125–0.25 mg/kg) reverses the effects of sedation in lamoids, presumably by blocking alpha 2 adrenoceptors, as it does in experimental animals (25).

ACEPROMAZINE MALEATE

Pharmacology. Acepromazine maleate is a potent tranquilizing agent that depresses the CNS. It produces muscular relaxation and reduces spontaneous activity, exhibiting antiemetic, hypotensive, and hypothermic properties.

Indications. Acepromazine maleate is rarely used singly but is usually combined with ketamine or etorphine. Its muscle-relaxing characteristic is of particular value when combined with ketamine. Acepromazine maleate has been used in llamas. A dose of 0.15 mg/kg quieted an aggressive male that was subsequently anesthetized using mask induction with halothane. Barrie (2) reported that an adult female guanaco (approximately 100 kg) was tranquilized for an eye examination with 3 mg (0.03 mg/kg).

Administration. Acepromazine is supplied in solution in a 10 mg/ml concentration that may be injected intravenously, intramuscularly, or subcutaneously.

When given intravenously, effects are noted within 1–3 minutes. Intramuscularly, 15–25 minutes are required for full effect. Reports of usage are insufficient to establish a standard dose in camelids.

Side Effects and Precautions. Acepromazine should be used cautiously in combination with other hypotensive agents. Occasionally, instead of producing CNS depression, it acts as a stimulant, and hyperexcitability ensues. Acepromazine is a phenothiazine derivative and may potentiate the toxicity of organophosphate parasiticides, so inquiry should be made about the prior use of these products before administration. Acepromazine is contraindicated for the control of convulsions in progress. While the drug may prevent convulsions, it also reduces the threshold for convulsion stimuli.

Antidote. There is no known antidote.

DIAZEPAM (VALIUM, TRANIMAL, TRANIMUL)

Pharmacology. Diazepam acts on the thalamus and hypothalamus, inducing calm behavior. It has no peripheral autonomic blocking action, unlike some other tranquilizers. Transient ataxia may develop with higher doses as muscle relaxation progresses. Spinal reflexes are blocked. Diazepam is an effective anticonvulsant.

Indications. Diazepam prevents the convulsive effect of ketamine. If injected intravenously, it effectively controls convulsive seizures in progress. It can also be used as preanesthetic medication to calm an excited animal.

Administration. Diazepam is supplied in solution in a concentration of 5 mg/ml and administered at a dose of 0.1–0.5 mg/kg. Onset is within 1–2 minutes when given intravenously. If given intramuscularly, it takes effect in 15–30 minutes, depending on the dose. Diazepam is metabolized slowly in the normal liver. Usually, clinical effects disappear within 60–90 minutes.

Side Effects and Precautions. Diazepam may be chemically incompatible with other immobilizing agents and it should not be mixed with them in the same syringe nor in IV solutions. Some pain is associated with IM injection, and a transient inflammatory reaction may develop at the site. Diazepam is contraindicated in patients with suspected glaucoma.

Antidote. There is no known antidote.

Muscle Relaxants

SUCCINYLCHOLINE CHLORIDE (SUSCOSTRIN, ANECTINE)

Pharmacology. Succinylcholine chloride is a depolarizing muscle relaxant, with no analgesic or anesthetic properties.

Indications. Although the drug has been reported as having been used as an immobilizing agent for capturing guanacos (24), it is not recommended as a drug for dealing with llamas, alpacas, or captive wild lamoids. Its use should be restricted to an anesthesiologist during general anesthesia to provide additional muscle relaxation for orthopedic procedures.

Side Effects. This drug suppresses respiration, and suffocation will ensue without assisted respiration.

GUAIFENESIN. Guaifenesin (Gecolate, guaiphenesin, glycerol guaiacolate) is a muscle-relaxing agent that is usually combined with the short-acting barbiturates xylazine or ketamine to provide analgesia and/or anesthesia. These combinations are used extensively in equine anesthesia. An anesthetist accustomed to working with equine species may prefer these combinations for injectable anesthesia. It has been found to be safe and effective in llamas. The dosage currently recommended in the llama is 100–150 mg/kg (1–1.5 ml/kg of a 10% solution). A short-acting barbiturate such as sodium thiamylal or sodium thiopental at a dose of 4.5 mg/kg may be added to the solution before administration to provide 15–20 minutes of anesthesia, which may be supplemented if the llama begins to awaken.

A disadvantage to the use of guaifenesin is the volume required to induce and maintain anesthesia. An IV catheter should be placed in the jugular vein before attempting to use this agent.

GENERAL ANESTHESIA

General anesthesia may be accomplished by the use of higher than sedation doses of some drugs used for sedation and immobilization (18). Gaseous agents may be used to induce and maintain anesthesia. It is difficult to stabilize the depth of anesthesia in llamas (1). When general anesthesia is selected for a lamoid, the patient must be continuously monitored by an anesthetist.

Preanesthetic Considerations

For elective surgery, the llama should be fasted for 24–48 hours and water withheld for 8–12 hours. This will not completely empty compartment one (C-1) of the stomach but will decrease the volume and diminish gas production. To remove feed debris the mouth should be irrigated immediately before applying a mask or attempting tracheal intubation.

Both passive and reflex regurgitation are potential sequelae to general anesthesia in llamas. The primary factors predisposing to passive flow of ingesta from the stomach are relaxation of the gastroesophageal sphincter, surgical positioning, pressure buildup in the stomach (either gaseous or external), and a large volume of ingesta in the stomach.

In an anesthetized lamoid, continuing contraction of C-1 of the stomach moves ingesta toward the cardia. In a normal cycle, the cardia relaxes and ingesta is propelled to the mouth for rechewing. This cycle is a hindrance during anesthesia. These mechanisms are under parasympathetic control, thus atropine may diminish stomach contractility.

Laryngeal stimulation will result in reflex closure of the glottis, which in turn causes high negative intrathoracic pressure during inspiration. This induces passage of ingesta into the esophagus. It is essential that the laryngeal reflex be abolished before attempting endotracheal intubation.

Positioning for Anesthetic Procedures

Lamoids may be placed in any conceivable position for surgery, but selection should be made after consideration of various factors. Regurgitation is more likely in left rather than right lateral recumbency. Prolonged surgery in either right or left lateral recumbency may produce postsurgical radial paralysis. However, paralysis can be prevented by properly padding the shoulder and by pulling the lower limb forward to avoid direct pressure from the rib cage on the midhumeral region.

Dorsal recumbency should be avoided unless it is possible to place an endotracheal tube. If regurgitation has occurred during the surgery, special care must be taken while removing the tube. The head should be lowered and the mouth gently irrigated to remove any particulate matter remaining in the oropharyngeal cavity. The cuff should remain inflated while withdrawing the tube from the trachea, though if resistance is noted at the larynx, it may be necessary to deflate the cuff slightly. The inflated cuff will scoop any fluid or particulate matter out of the trachea. Excessive coughing may be noted in an animal that has inhaled fluid or feed particles.

Dorsal recumbency also shifts the weight of the abdominal viscera toward the diaphragm and the lungs, restricting inflation, which causes decreased functional residual capacity and closure of the small airways. Pressure is also applied to the greater abdominal vessels. There is decreased cardiac output and change in pulmonary blood-flow patterns, especially in the dependent areas of the lung. All these cardiopulmonary changes may lead to hypoxemia.

A suitable method for maintaining a llama in dorsal recumbency is the simple cradle illustrated in Figure 6.14. Alternatively, the llama could be supported between two bales of straw or hay. Overflexion or overstretching of the limbs when clearing the limbs from the operative site with ropes should be avoided.

A llama may be kept in sternal recumbency to facilitate perineal surgery. However, keeping an anesthetized animal in this position for 2 or more hours may result in ischemia of the limbs. Ischemia does not occur in a conscious animal, even one that is down and unable to rise for various reasons.

In one instance of scrotal surgery, the llama was draped over the end of the table with the hind legs hanging. This animal was unable to get up after surgery. Considerable edema and hemorrhage at the stifle area were seen at necropsy.

Often, the forequarter is tilted downward during abdominal surgery to allow the viscera to drift out of the caudal abdomen and give better exposure. A lamoid should be positioned like this only if an endotracheal tube is in place, because passive regurgitation is likely to occur.

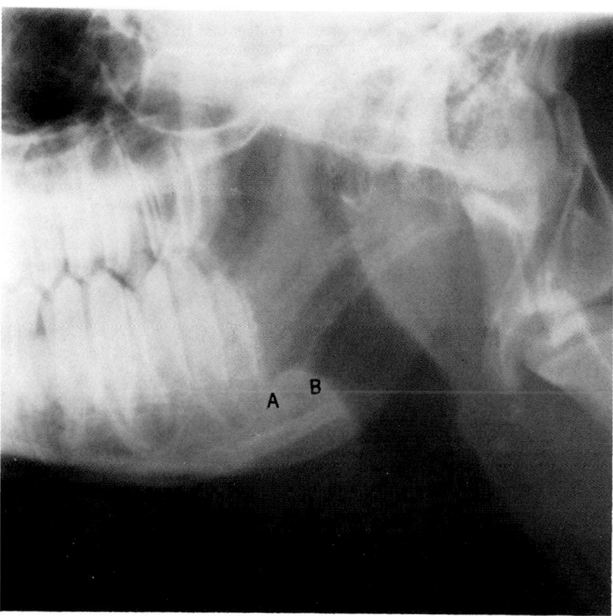

5.1 Lateral radiograph of the oropharyngeal region of a llama with the soft palate dorsal to the epiglottis. **(A)** Soft palate, **(B)** epiglottis.

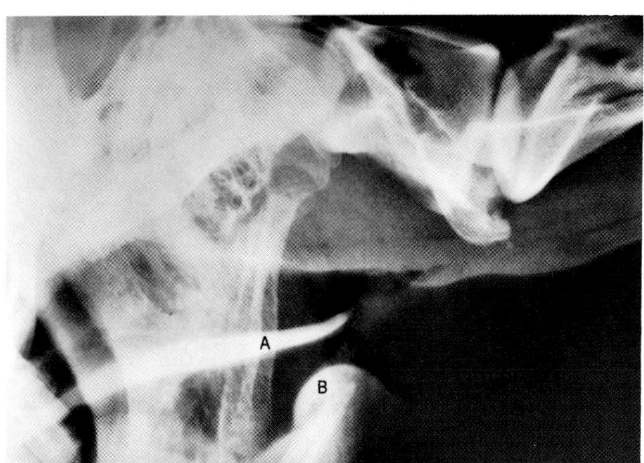

5.2 Lateral radiograph of the oropharyngeal region of a llama. The soft palate is ventral to the epiglottis. **(A)** Soft palate, **(B)** epiglottis.

Tracheal Intubation

To provide positive support for respiration and avoid complications if the lamoid should regurgitate, tracheal intubation is recommended whenever general anesthesia is selected. Intubation is also necessary to inflate a collapsed lung and to correct pulmonary edema.

Endotracheal intubation is difficult in lamoids because the restricted space in the oropharynx impairs visualization of the glottis with a laryngoscope while the endotracheal tube is manipulated into position (11). The restricted space is the result of a combination of factors, including the narrow space between the rami of the mandible, inability to open the mouth widely, the elevated mound on the dorsum of the caudal aspect of the tongue, and the elongated soft palate that may be situated either ventral or dorsal to the epiglottis (Figs. 5.1, 5.2).

Tubes designed for small animals are too short for use in llamas. Tubes designed for cattle and horses are too long. In adult llamas, the tube should be 50 cm long, with a diameter appropriate to the size or weight of the animal (Table 5.4).

To prevent reflex regurgitation, chewing and swallowing reflexes must be abolished before attempting to insert an endotracheal tube. Relaxation may be accomplished by use of a xylazine-ketamine or guaifenesin-barbiturate combination or by masking the animal for induction with an inhalant agent.

PLACEMENT. There are three methods of tube placement. Blind insertion, which is a technique commonly employed with horses, has been used on llamas but is not consistently applicable because the soft palate may become hooked ventral to the epiglottic cartilage, directing the tube into a blind pocket. If this method is chosen, the head should be extended maximally and, with the mouth opened slightly, the tube should be inserted between the rami of the mandible, over the base of

Table 5.4. Endotracheal tubes for llamas

Body weight		Inside diameter	Outside diameter	Length	French
(kg)	*(lb)*	*(mm)*	*(mm)*	*(cm)*	*(size)*
9–60	20–132	3	4.7	30	14
		4	6.0	30	16
		5	7.0	35	22
		6	8.7	35	26
65–160	143–350	7	10.0	50	30
		8	11.0	50	33
		9	12.3	50	37
		10	14.7	50	44
		11	15.3	50	46
		12	17.0	50	51
160	350	14	19.0	50	57
		16	21.0	50	63

the tongue. The larynx should be grasped from the exterior and fixed while pressing the tube up against the glottis with the other hand.

A second method is to insert the endotracheal tube while visualizing the larynx with a laryngoscope (Fig. 5.3). Some anesthetists prefer this method, even though visualization is impaired. In some animals, the limited space makes it impossible to visualize the laryngeal opening and insert the endotracheal tube at the same time. The mouth should be held open with gauze loops and the head extended maximally. The laryngoscope blade should be inserted and the epiglottic cartilage depressed. An aluminum rod stylet should be placed in the endotracheal tube to keep the tube rigid. The tube may be inserted through the laryngeal opening at the time of maximum opening. The stylet should be removed and a check made for air flow through the tube.

The third and preferred method is the insertion of a small catheter into the larynx over which the endotracheal tube is threaded (11). To do this, two 8–10 French, 50 cm stiff polyethylene catheters should be coupled with tape. A long-bladed (45 cm) laryngoscope is desirable, but a 19 cm blade can be used if the unit is inserted up to the commissure of the mouth.

The head should be extended maximally. It may be desirable to hold the mouth open with gauze loops and gently pull the tongue rostrally. The laryngoscope blade may be inserted and the epiglottic cartilage depressed (Fig. 5.4). If the epiglottic cartilage is not visible, the soft palate may be lifted from beneath the epiglottis with the tip of the blade. The polyethylene catheter is inserted into the trachea (Fig. 5.5) and the laryngoscope blade removed. The endotracheal tube should be threaded over the catheter and pushed gently between the cheek teeth into the trachea (Fig. 5.6).

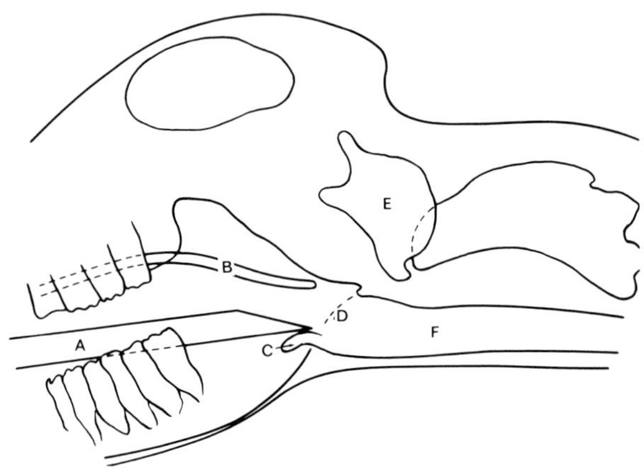

5.4 Diagram of placement of laryngoscope blade: **(A)** laryngoscope blade, **(B)** soft palate, **(C)** epiglottis, **(D)** glottis, **(E)** atlas, **(F)** trachea.

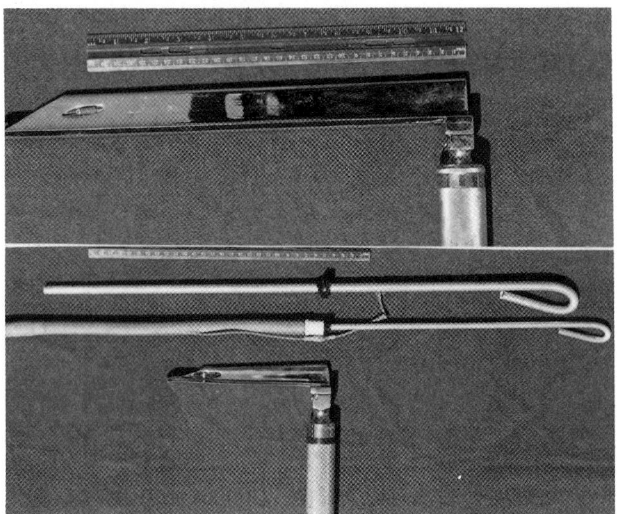
5.3 Laryngoscopes used for endotracheal intubation in lamoids.

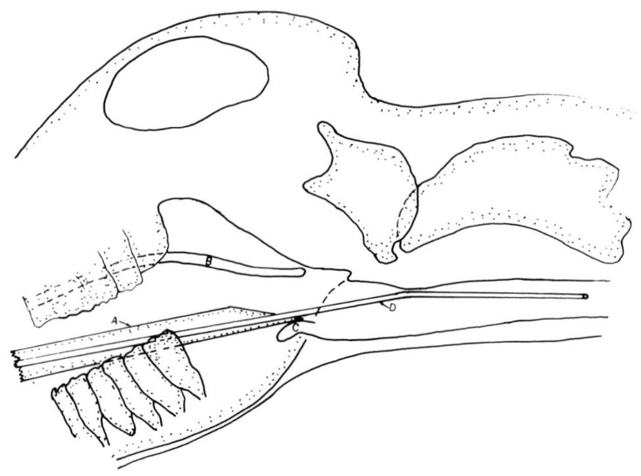
5.5 Inserting catheter into trachea.

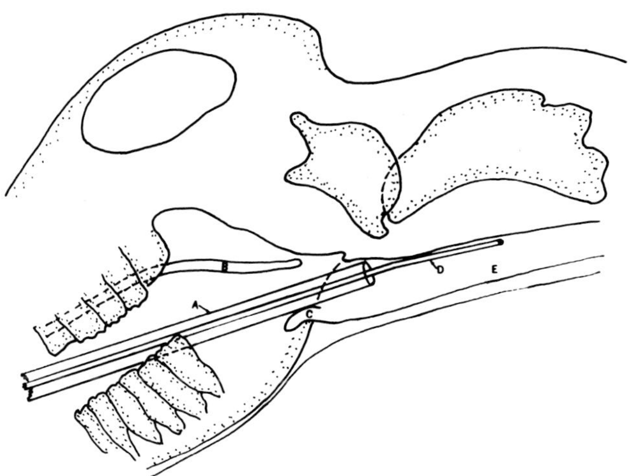

5.6 Threading endotracheal tube over catheter.

Some difficulty may be experienced in threading the endotracheal tube through the laryngeal opening. If anesthesia is too light, there will be reflex closure of the laryngeal opening as the tube touches the epiglottic or arytenoid cartilage. The endotracheal tube should be gently pressed against the larynx. The head may be repositioned slightly, or it may be of assistance to fix the larynx from the exterior. If these adjustments fail, a slightly smaller tube should be tried.

A check should be made for air movement through the endotracheal tube before the catheter is removed. The cuff should be inflated and the tube tied or taped to the lower jaw.

Evaluating Depth of Anesthesia

The use of multiple drug combinations makes assessments of certain reflexes and parameters difficult. The HR of a normal llama is 60–90 beats per minute. Neonate and juvenile lamoids have higher HRs. The rate accelerates during induction, gradually slowing toward normal. Xylazine, given as a preanesthetic agent, induces bradycardia (45–60 beats per minute), while the administration of atropine may cause acceleration of the HR. The HR remained relatively stable in experimental halothane anesthesia (14).

Although assessment of the pulse is not a usual clinical parameter, superficial arteries may be palpated in the anesthetized individual. The largest and most accessible artery is the saphenous, which lies on the medial aspect of the stifle, but the caudal articular and digital arteries can also be palpated.

Ocular reflexes are utilized to assess depth of anesthesia. The ventral eyelid palpebral reflex is suppressed when anesthesia is adequate, but the upper lid will likely retain the response to tactile stimulation. Nystagmus rarely occurs. The administration of ketamine may complicate assessment of ocular reflexes until the inhalant anesthetic agent takes effect.

Neonate Anesthesia

General anesthesia is usually reserved for invasive orthopedic procedures, correction of choanal atresia, and laparotomy. The neonate will be less stressed if physical restraint and mild sedation or local anesthesia is selected whenever possible. For general anesthesia, inhalation anesthesia is preferred, with mask induction being the simplest. Regurgitation is not a major problem in the neonate, as it is in the adult llama.

Injectable Anesthesia

Numerous injectable anesthetic agents or combinations of agents have been used in llamas (Table 5.3). Refer to the pharmacodynamic discussions of the agents for details. In this section, applications for use in lamoids are described.

XYLAZINE. Doses of 0.1–0.2 mg/kg xylazine HCl provide sedation, enabling excited or wild animals to be examined or certain special procedures to be carried out. A higher dose (0.25 mg/kg) will induce calm animals to lie down, especially if administered intravenously. This dose, in conjunction with a local anesthetic, provides sufficient analgesia to lance abscesses and suture lacerations.

The author's standard immobilizing dose is 0.25 mg/kg intravenously or 0.35–0.45 intramuscularly. Many diagnostic procedures may be performed under this degree of sedation and analgesia. Induction occurs within 5 minutes and lasts for no more than 20 minutes. Procedures that may be performed include abdominocentesis, thoracocentesis, bone marrow aspiration, radiography, and blood collection.

Some have recommended that higher doses of xylazine (0.4–0.7 mg/kg) may permit longer procedures, but the author prefers to combine drugs or shift to an inhalant anesthetic for more prolonged procedures.

XYLAZINE IN COMBINATION WITH OTHER AGENTS. Following are combinations that have been used by the author:

1. Xylazine (0.25 mg/kg) and ketamine (2–5 mg/kg) (12, 13, 20). A similar combination has been successful in the equine, but Heath (15) has seen difficulties with this combination in goats and thus does not recommend it for llamas. The author, on the other hand, finds this

combination useful for minor surgery, dental procedures, preanesthetic induction, and endotracheal intubation. This combination has been used experimentally in our laboratory with extensive monitoring and has been found to be a safe anesthetic combination.

Supplemental doses of either drug may be given intravenously without complicating recovery. Supplemental IM doses will prolong recovery and should not be administered.

2. Xylazine (0.1 mg/kg) and butorphanol (0.05–1 mg/kg). This combination will allow most llamas to remain standing.

3. Wiesner used his Hellabrunner Mischung (Hellabrunn mixture) to immobilize vicuñas (27). The mixture contains 125 mg/ml xylazine and 100 mg/ml ketamine. His dose was 0.2–0.5 ml/animal. Assuming a 50 kg vicuña, the dose administered was 0.5–1.25 mg/kg xylazine and 0.4–1 mg/kg ketamine. He reported satisfactory immobilization.

DIAZEPAM AND KETAMINE. If use of xylazine is not desired, a combination of diazepam (0.2–0.5 mg/kg) and ketamine (2–5 mg/kg) provides adequate anesthesia for procedures in a variety of domestic and wild ungulates, including the llama.

BARBITURATES. In two different studies of anesthesia in alpacas, sodium pentobarbital was used in a 6.5% solution (65 mg/ml). In one, the IV dose was 14 mg/kg and in the other, 20 mg/kg (7). Induction occurred in 3–4 minutes and lasted for approximately 1 hour. Both investigators considered the anesthesia to be excellent. The author recommends a lower dose of pentobarbital (10 mg/kg) (18). Ultrashort-acting barbiturates such as sodium thiamylal or sodium thiopental may be used as a single anesthetic agent in a dose of 8–11 mg/kg given only intravenously. This dose provides anesthesia for only 10–15 minutes.

Inhalation Anesthesia

INDICATIONS. Inhalation anesthesia has many advantages. With this type, it is possible to control the depth of anesthesia, provide respiratory support, and reduce the risk of toxicity to the patient. The disadvantages are the cost of the agent, the expense of specialized equipment for administration, and the requirement for an anesthetist.

EQUIPMENT. Llamas weighing up to 140 kg (300 lb) may be managed on a small animal anesthetic unit with a 5–6 L rebreathing bag. The soda lime canister must be monitored constantly to assure that the system is not overburdened with carbon dioxide. Larger animals require a rebreathing bag of up to 7–8 L in size and a correspondingly larger soda lime system. A large animal anesthetic unit is preferred for larger llamas.

AGENTS. Halothane, methoxyflurane, and isoflurane are all suitable agents for use in inhalation anesthesia of lamoids (Table 5.5).

Table 5.5. Inhalant anesthetic agents for lamoids

Generic name	Commercial name	Source
Isoflurane	Arrane	Anaquest, Madison, WI 53713
Methoxyflurane	Metofane	Pitman Moore, Washington, NJ 08560
Halothane	Fluothane	Halocarbon Labs, Hackensack, NJ 07601

Halothane (Fluothane). Halothane is the most commonly used inhalant anesthetic agent (8, 9, 14). It depresses many cardiopulmonary functions, so the patient should be carefully monitored. The degree of depression is dose related or depth of anesthesia related. Functions affected include cardiac output, stroke volume, arterial pressure, and muscle blood flow. The rate and depth of breathing may also be depressed, and respiratory acidosis develops after prolonged anesthesia.

Oxygenation is poorest when the patient is in dorsal recumbency. Hypoxemia is common during the recovery stage, so administration of supplemental oxygen is desirable for 10–15 minutes.

Isoflurane. Isoflurane has been used on numerous cases in the author's clinic. The flow rates for oxygen are the same as for halothane. The vaporizer settings have been approximately 3.4% for the first 5 minutes and 1–1.5% for maintenance.

Nitrous oxide has been used in combination with other inhalant gases in llamas, but the author does not recommend it because of its propensity to accumulate in obstructed loops of bowel, one of the more common indications for general anesthesia.

Atropine (0.04 mg/kg) may be given, but some anesthesiologists do not use atropine for fear of secondary paralysis of peristalsis.

PROCEDURES. The tidal volume of an adult llama is 10 ml/kg/min. Oxygen flow rates of 20 ml/kg/min are recommended for induction. In a controlled ventilation system, this can be reduced to 10–12 ml/kg/min for maintenance (2 L/min for a 175 kg llama). Flow rates for nonbreathing systems are three times the foregoing (6 L/min).

In a study inducing llamas with xylazine and ketamine followed by halothane maintenance, both spontaneous and controlled ventilation were used (13). After initial induction and endotracheal intubation, general anesthesia was accomplished while the llama was breathing spontaneously by setting the halothane vaporizer at 4.5% for 5 minutes and at 3–3.5% for the remainder of a 120-minute experiment. The actual end tidal alveolar halothane concentration was measured at 1.21–1.28%.

A lower concentration of halothane was required when the llama was under controlled ventilation with a respirator. The setting was 3% for the first 5 minutes and 1.75–2.25% for the remainder of the procedure. The end tidal alveolar concentration was 0.68–0.72%.

In these same studies, cardiovascular and pulmonary function parameters were measured using intravascular catheters and blood gas analysis. Parameters of cardiovascular function such as the HR, mean arterial pressure, and cardiac output were satisfactorily maintained when the animal was breathing spontaneously, while parameters of pulmonary function such as $PaCO_2$ and arterial pH were markedly altered. Conversely, with controlled respiration, parameters of cardiovascular function changed more. It was concluded that the safest physiologic state was maintained with controlled ventilation.

The mean arterial blood pressure of an unanesthetized llama varies from 130 to 170 mm of mercury (Hg). Intraarterial catheters may be placed in an auricular or saphenous artery. Measurement of blood pressure, using a Doppler unit, can be made over the medial aspect of the distal metacarpus or metatarsus or on the ventrum of the tail. Doppler measurements should be considered only approximations of the actual pressure, but are sufficiently accurate to indicate changes.

During both spontaneous and controlled–ventilation halothane anesthesia, arterial blood pressure dropped from 140 to a low of less than 60 mm Hg at approximately 1 hour into surgery. Then the pressure steadily climbed back to about 110 after 2 hours.

Recovery time from halothane anesthesia varies with the physiologic state of the patient. Debilitated animals remain affected longer than vigorous patients. In general, a llama should be able to remain in sternal recumbency within 60 minutes following cessation of administration of the agent and be able to stand within 90 minutes but be depressed for several hours.

The body temperature of a llama will drop during general inhalation anesthesia. In experimental 2-hour procedures, body temperature dropped from 38.3 to 36.5°C (100.9–97.7°F). Body temperature did not return to normal for 1–3 hours after recovery from surgery. These animals were kept in a thermoneutral environment, and no steps were taken to warm the llamas.

SUPPORTIVE THERAPY DURING ANESTHESIA. HR, RR, and body temperature should be assessed periodically during anesthesia. Hypothermia may be countered by the application of heating pads to the inner thighs, abdomen (if accessible), and axilla. In extreme cases, administration of warm IV fluids or warm water enemas is indicated.

An IV catheter should be placed and appropriate fluids administered during the procedure. An arterial catheter is desirable if facilities for arterial pressure assessment or blood gas analysis are available.

The head should be positioned to avoid overextension in order that saliva and stomach contents may be appropriately drained. Artificial tears should be instilled into the conjunctival sac and measures taken to protect the prominent eye from positional trauma.

If an injectable anesthetic is used, body and head positions are of even greater importance. If a procedure is prolonged, the patient would benefit from supplemental oxygen, administered by placement of a small tube up a nostril and at a flow rate of 1 L/min.

Sophisticated electrocardiographic monitoring is desirable but not required, especially if an anesthetist is continually monitoring the patient.

Anesthetic Support Drugs (Table 5.6)

ATROPINE SULFATE

Pharmacology. Atropine is a parasympatholytic drug with action equivalent to blockage of the parasympathetic autonomic nervous system. It decreases salivation, sweating, gut motility, bladder tone, and gastric and respiratory secretions. Vagal blockage produces tachycardia. Mydriasis occurs.

Indications. Atropine diminishes excessive secretions induced by ketamine. It is also commonly used as a preanesthetic medication to prevent reflex vagal stimulation of the heart (cholinergic bradycardia) during induction.

Administration. Large animal formulations are supplied as solutions at 2 mg/ml and small animal formulations at 0.5 mg/ml. Atropine can be given orally or parenterally at dosages of 0.04 mg/kg. Atropinization occurs within 1–15 minutes, depending on the route of administration.

Side Effects and Precautions. Dilated pupils should be protected from direct sunlight to prevent retinal damage. Atropine is contraindicated for patients with glaucoma.

Table 5.6. Miscellaneous drugs used in llama anesthesia

Generic name	Commercial name	Concentration	Dosage	Route of administration	Indications
Atropine sulfate	Atropine	0.1 mg/ml	0.04 mg/kg	SC, IV, IM	Sinus arrhythmia, bradycardia, sinus arrest control salivation
Epinephrine	Adrenalin	1:10000 (1 mg/ml) 1:1000 (0.1 mg/ml)	0.1 mg/kg	IV, IM	Cardiac arrest, anaphylaxis
Doxopram	Dopram	20 mg/ml	2 mg/kg	IV, IM	Respiratory depression
Dexamethasone $NaPO_4$	Azium	4 mg/ml	4 mg/kg	IV	Shock
Lidocaine HCl	Xylocaine	20 mg/ml	1 mg/kg	IV	Ventricular arrhythmia
Diazepam	Vallium	5 mg/ml	0.5 mg/kg	IV, IM	Seizures
Calcium gluconate	Invenex	10% solution 0.465 meq/ml	100 mg/kg	IV	Hypocalcemic tetany
Naloxone	Narcan	0.4 mg/ml	0.04 mg/kg	IV, IM	Antidote for narcotics
Diprenorphine HCl	M50-50	2 mg/ml	Twice dose of M99 etorphine	IV, IM	Antidote for etorphine
Yohimbine	Yohimbine	5 mg/ml	0.25 mg/kg	IV, IM	Reversal of xylazine

Antidote. Parasympathomimetic drugs may aid in counteracting the effects of atropine, but atropine is difficult to reverse.

DIPRENORPHINE (M50-50)

Pharmacology. Diprenorphine is a narcotic antagonist used to reverse the effects of etorphine. It acts as a depressant on the CNS and, if used in excessive dosages, may complicate recovery from etorphine administration.

Administration. Diprenorphine is injected intravenously if possible, otherwise, intramuscularly. The recommended dose is double the injected dose of etorphine. When injected intravenously, reversal occurs within 1–4 minutes. IM injection requires 15–25 minutes to accomplish reversal.

Antidote. Naloxone acts as an antidote for diprenorphine.

NALOXONE HYDROCHLORIDE (NARCAN)

Pharmacology. Naloxone is a narcotic antagonist. In the absence of narcotic or agonistic effects of other narcotic antagonists, it exhibits little or no pharmacologic activity.

Euthanasia in Llamas

The same methods used in cattle, sheep, and horses are suitable for euthanasia in lamoids. The most often used method currently is IV injection of T-61 euthanasia solution.[3] This solution contains three complex chemicals that provide rapid muscle relaxation, local anesthesia, and general anesthesia. General anesthesia is followed by respiratory arrest, cerebral death, and circulatory collapse. This solution is indicated only for euthanasia.

METHOD. Solution T-61 should be administered rapidly intravenously at a minimum dose of 0.1 ml/kg. If the heart continues to beat for more than 2 minutes, a second dose should be injected. Experience has varied on the reliability of this agent for rapid euthanasia. In one instance, 20 ml T-61 was given to an adult male llama. He became unconscious in 30 seconds and the heart stopped in 1.5 minutes. In another instance, 20 ml T-61 was given to a 55 kg female llama. She became immobile in 1 minute, but heart and respiratory patterns were unaffected. Five minutes later, another 10 ml T-61 was given with no apparent effect. In each case, the drug was administered intravenously. Finally, a 20 ml dose was administered as a quick bolus intravenously and within 15 seconds, respiration and heart stopped.

3. T-61, American Hoechst, Sommerville, NJ 08876.

REFERENCES

1. Barrie, K. P., Jacobson, E., and Pfeiffer, R. L., Jr. 1978. Unilateral cataract with lens coloboma and bilateral corneal edema in a guanaco. J. Am. Vet. Med. Assoc. 173:1251–52.

2. Bauditz, R. 1972. (Sedation, immobilization and anes-

thesia of zoo and wild animals with Rompun) Sedation, Immobilization und Anasthesie von Zoo und Wildtieren mit Rompun. Veterinaermed. Nachr. 3:204–30.

3. Booth, N. H. 1982a. Local anesthesia. In N. H. Booth and L. E. McDonald, eds. Veterinary Pharmacology and Therapeutics, 5th ed. Ames: Iowa State Univ. Press, pp. 353–68.

4. ______. 1982b. Nonnarcotic analgesic. In N. H. Booth and L. E. McDonald, eds. Veterinary Pharmacology and Therapeutics, 5th ed. Ames: Iowa State Univ. Press, pp. 297–320.

5. Candela Velasco, D. E. 1970. (Use of a new general anesthetic in alpacas [Ketamine]) Uso de un nuevo anestesico general ("Ketalar") en alpacas, *Lama pacos.* Tesis, Fac. Med. Vet. Univ. Nac. Mayor San Marcos (Lima), pp. 1–56.

6. Custer, R., Kramer, L., Kennedy, S., and Bush, M. 1977. Hematologic effects of xylazine when used for restraint of Bactrian camels. J. Am. Vet. Med. Assoc. 171:899–901.

7. Diaz Navarro, A. 1964. (General anesthesia in alpacas with sodium pentobarbital) Anestesis general en alpacas con pentobarbital sodico. Tesis, Fac. Med. Vet. Univ. Nac. Mayor San Marcos (Lima), pp. 1–49.

8. Esquerre, C. J., and Vallenas P., A. 1968. (General anesthesia by inhalation with fluothane in alpacas and llamas) Anestesia general por inhalacion con fluothane en alpacas y llamas. Rev. Fac. Med. Vet. (Lima) 22:86–99.

9. Fowler, M. E. 1978. Camelids and South American camelids. In M. E. Fowler. Restraint and Handling of Wild and Domestic Animals. Ames: Iowa State Univ. Press, pp. 249–51.

10. ______. 1984a. Restraint and handling of llamas. 3 L Llama (No. 20):1113.

11. ______. 1984b. Clinical anatomy of the head and neck of the llama, *Llama glama.* In O. A. Ryder and M. L. Byrd, eds. One Medicine. Berlin: Springer, pp. 141–49.

12. ______. 1986. Camelids. In M. E. Fowler, ed. Zoo and Wild Animal Medicine, 2nd ed. Philadelphia: W. B. Saunders, pp. 969–81.

13. Gavier, D., Kittleson, M., Fowler, M. E., Johnson, L., Hall, G., and Nearenberg, D. 1989. Evaluation of the combination of xylazine/ketamine HCl and halothane for anesthesia in llamas. Am. J. Vet. Res. In press.

14. General anesthesia in alpacas and llamas with fluothane. 1963. Lame, IVITA, Inf. Trimestr. 2(5):22–23.

15. Heath, R. B. 1986. Anesthetic programs. Proc. Llama Med. Short Course Colorado State Univ., p. 64.

16. Heck, H., and Rivenburg, E. 1972. Dosages of M-99 used on hoofed mammals at Catskill Game Farm. Zool. Gart. 2(5):282–87.

17. Iparraguirre, G. M. 1969. (Evaluation of sacrococcygeal and intercoccygeal anesthesia in alpacas) Evaluacion de la anestesia sacrococcigea y intercoccigea en alpacas. Tesis, Fac. Med. Vet. Univ. Nac. Mayor San Marcos (Lima), pp. 1–23.

18. Jennings, S. 1971. General anesthesia of ruminants and swine. In L. R. Soma, ed. Textbook of Veterinary Anesthesia. Baltimore: Williams & Wilkins, p. 350.

19. Knight, A. P. 1980. Xylazine. J. Am. Vet. Med. Assoc. 176:454–55.

20. Kock, M. D. 1984. Canine tooth extraction and pulpotomy in the adult male llama. J. Am. Vet. Med. Assoc. 185:1304–6.

21. Merilan, C. P., Sikes, J. D., Read, B. W., Boever, W. J., and Knox, D. 1979. Comparative characteristics of spermatozoa and semen from a Bactrian camel, dromedary camel and llama. J. Zoo. Anim. Med. 10:22–25.

22. Nunez, Q., Sato Sato, A., and Guzman Chavez, J. 1966. (Anatomic considerations in anesthetizing the foot of the alpaca) Consideraciones anatomicas para el bioqueo anestesico del pie de la alpaca. An. Congr. Panam. Med. Vet. Zootech. (Venezuela, Quito) 2:834–44.

23. Peshin, P. K., Nigam, J. M., Singh, S. C., and Robinson, B. A. 1980. Evaluation of xylazine in camels. J. Am. Vet. Med. Assoc. 177:875–78.

24. Raedeke, K. J. 1976. (Immobilization of the guanaco [*Lama guanicoe*] with succinylcholine chloride) La immobilizacion de guanacos (*Lama guanicoe*) con cloruro de succinilcolina. An. Inst. Patagonia 7:185–88.

25. Riebold, T. W., Kaneps, A. J., and Schmotzer, W. B. 1965. Reversal of xylazine-induced sedation in llamas, using doxapram or 4-aminopyridine and yohimbine. J. Am. Vet. Med. Assoc. 189:1059–61.

26. Tasher, J. B. 1980. Fluids, electrolytes and acid-base balance. In J. J. Kaneko, ed. Clinical Biochemistry of Domestic Animals, 3rd ed. New York: Academic Press, p. 424.

27. Wiesner, H. 1977. (Anesthesia of zoo animals: Practical experiences with a blowpipe gun) Zur Narkoseprazis mit dem "Blasrohrgewehr." Kleintierpraxis 22(8):327–30.

6 Surgery

SURGERY IN THE LAMOID is fundamentally the same as surgery in other livestock. Variations in anatomy that have surgical implications will be emphasized in this chapter (9, 13, 17). Though details of every surgical procedure that has been performed or may be performed will not be discussed, unique conditions will be described, including indications for surgery, pertinent anatomy, clinical signs, diagnosis, presurgical recommendations, anesthesia, positioning, method, postsurgical care, and complications. Occasionally, the reader will be directed to appropriate standard surgical texts (10, 18, 26).

HEAD

Abscesses

INDICATIONS. Abscesses of the head and neck are common clinical entities (Fig. 6.1). In the author's practice, the organism most often isolated from camelid abscesses is *Corynebacterium pyogenes.* However, streptococci, staphylococci, bacteroides, actinomyces, and *Escherichia coli* have also been isolated. It has been suggested that these organisms may be present in the normal flora of the oral mucosa and skin of camelids and opportunistically invade the tissue via a break in the epithelium. Two isolates of *Nocardia asteroides* have been made in the author's clinic.

Pathogens may also be introduced via the hematogenous route, in which case, infection is likely to be found in a lymph node. Abscesses may be located in the oral and pharyngeal submucosa, any lymph node of the head and neck region, the salivary glands, or the subcutaneous tissues of the head and neck.

When male llamas fight, they bite the throat and neck. Abscessation may be a sequel to such encounters. Lacerations of the labial mucosa may result from sharp enamel points on the teeth. Grass awns and other harsh forages may traumatize the mucosa, providing a portal of entry for opportunistic bacteria.

CLINICAL SIGNS. Signs vary with the anatomic site of the abscess. Swelling usually calls attention to an external abscess (Fig. 6.1). Other swellings that may be confused with abscesses include hematomas, tumors, cellulitis, and edema.

Oral or deep pharyngeal abscesses may not be observable without the aid of a laryngoscope or endoscopic equipment. Usually, impairment of prehension or deglutition resulting in anorexia has been observed.

Though localized abscesses rarely produce a febrile

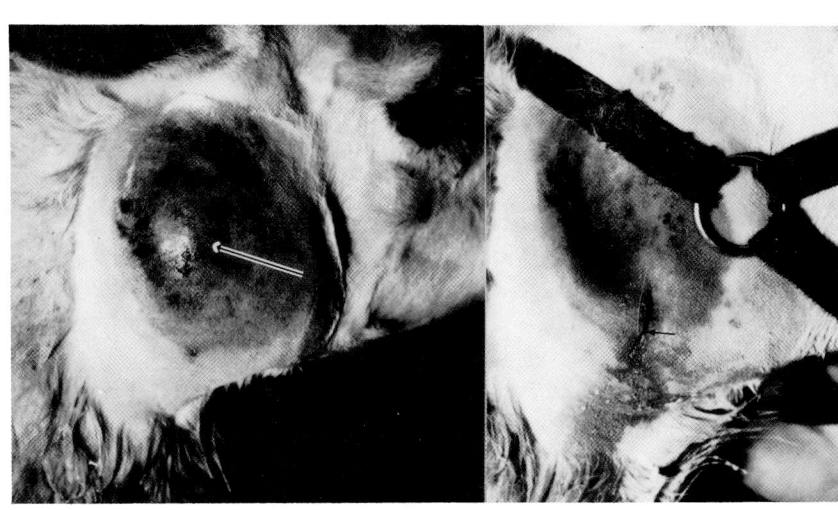

6.1 (Left) Abscess of the parotid area; (Right) abscess lanced for drainage.

response or a change in the hemogram, progressive enlargement of a developing abscess may obstruct venous drainage, causing edematous swelling. Some abscesses develop slowly over a period of days or weeks; others mature in 2–6 days.

The degree of fluctuation of an abscess depends on its stage of maturity and the extent of encapsulation. *Corynebacterium* sp. and streptococcal organisms tend to produce minimal encapsulation, while abscesses caused by *Actinomyces* sp. develop a thick capsule and little lumen.

Abscesses located on the lateral face may impinge on the facial nerve or the parotid salivary duct. Special care must be taken to isolate and reflect these structures from the incision site when an abscess is lanced or extirpated.

POSITION. Unless the animal is extremely fractious, lancing an abscess can be accomplished in the standing position, utilizing a combination of physical restraint and local anesthesia. The use of a stock is recommended to better control the head, but it should not be employed to overpower the animal or to omit appropriate sedation or anesthesia.

PRESURGICAL PREPARATION. The area should be clipped and cleansed. Surgical asepsis is superfluous, but it is important to collect the exudate upon opening the abscess. Even though the infective organism may be ubiquitous and opportunistic, the exudate should be collected or drained onto a surface that can be cleansed and disinfected. Gloves should be worn by the operator to prevent self-infection.

ANESTHESIA. If the abscess has fully matured, to the point of forming a head (producing mucosal necrosis or a necrosed spot of skin), anesthesia is not necessary. If a deep abscess is suspected, infiltration of the intended incision site with a local anesthetic agent is recommended. If the skin is closely adhered to the capsule of the abscess, diffusion of the anesthetic agent may be impeded or prevented. If cellulitis has developed, the local anesthetic agent may be neutralized by a change in pH of the inflamed site. If extirpation of the abscess and its capsule are anticipated, especially in the region of such vital structures as nerves, vessels, or salivary glands, sedation or general anesthesia is indicated.

SURGERY. Surgery is frequently preceded by aspiration with a diagnostic needle to confirm the presence of an exudate or other fluids. The point of insertion of the needle should be selected to avoid vital structures and should be as ventral as possible. The needle should be left in place while a vertical incision is made through the skin, alongside the needle. Further penetration may be accomplished by blunt dissection with either a finger or Mayo scissors, inserted closed, but opened as they are withdrawn. If the capsule is thick and fibrous, it may be necessary to stab with a scalpel, guided by the shaft of the needle. This incision should be small enough to allow insertion of a hemostat or needle forceps to bluntly enlarge the incision and avoid the risk of lacerating a vessel or nerve.

The lumen of the abscess should be explored with forceps or finger. The orifice should be enlarged sufficiently to establish good drainage. If the initial incision site lies far dorsal, it may be appropriate to establish a more ventral second drainage site, again avoiding vital structures.

The exudate may be viscous or inspissated to the degree that it must be removed by curettage. The lumen should be irrigated thoroughly with dilute povidone-iodine solution. Acute abscesses may require no further treatment to induce healing. Chronic abscesses with thick capsules may produce an inner abscess membrane that inhibits healing, similar to the inner lining of a fistula. In such cases, the lumen of the abscess should be treated with caustic solution, such as 7% tincture of iodine, to destroy the inner lining and allow healing to commence.

Extirpation is possible only if the abscess is accessible, with a well-developed capsule and no surrounding cellulitis. For this procedure, surgical asepsis is desirable in order that the wound may be closed following surgery.

POSTSURGICAL CARE. The wound should be irrigated with a disinfectant solution once a day until granulation tissue fills the lumen and it is no longer possible to insert an irrigator. If two incisions were made, a seton may be placed using 2 in. or 3 in. gauze. This will keep the incisions open, and irrigation should be continued. An ointment such as zinc oxide should be applied to prevent maceration of the skin ventral to the incision.

Antibiotics are not indicated for either nonsurgical or postsurgical management of localized abscesses. Though the action of antibiotics may slow development of an abscess, it will rarely halt such development. Encapsulation prevents penetration of the abscess by parenterally administered antibiotics, and locally applied antibiotics are immediately washed out by the exudate. Healing must proceed by granulation from within, outwardly. Once this begins, the process should not be inhibited by excessive cautery. The lumen may be kept free of exudation by maintaining patency and irrigation.

COMPLICATIONS. Multiple abscesses may be seeded in an area in various stages of development. Initial lancing of a large abscess may miss some of the smaller seeds, which will continue to develop. If incisions are too small or they close prematurely, the abscess may recur. The most serious complication is damage to vital contiguous structures, either as a result of the inflammatory process or from trauma during surgery.

Lacerations

Lacerations may occur on the lips, cheeks, or face. A large male may bite a smaller male, inflicting lacerations anywhere on the head, ears, or neck. Aggressive males may traumatize themselves in a frenzy to reach an opponent. Lacerations may also result from dog bites. Severe disfiguring as a result of dog bites has occurred; e.g., the lower lip has been stripped away from the mandible.

Restraint or transport of lamoids may result in lacerations from sharp obstructions. The tongue may be lacerated by sharp enamel points of the teeth or by rough manipulation when the tongue is pulled out for tracheal intubation.

PRESURGICAL PREPARATION. The wound area should always be clipped or shaved and cleansed as thoroughly as possible. Clipping tends to deposit short fibers in the wound unless a moist compress is applied over the laceration before beginning. Alternatively, lubrication jelly may be applied to the wound.

ANESTHESIA. Once the wound is cleansed, subcutaneous infiltration along the margins of the laceration with a local anesthetic agent usually provides sufficient analgesia. General anesthesia may be necessary to repair multiple lacerations or lacerations of the lips or eye structures.

SURGERY. Debridement of a wound is a basic essential surgical procedure for removing foreign material or devitalized tissue from the wound. The wound should be irrigated with povidone-iodine solution, diluted 1:10. A water pick may be improvised, using a 20–35 ml syringe and a 22–25 gauge needle. A pulsating spray can be achieved by periodic pressure on the plunger. The spray penetrates the recesses of the wound, flushing out particulate matter.

The skin of lamoids is relatively thicker than that of other species; thus infolding is not a serious problem. However, there is less flexibility in lamoid skin, and it is more tightly adhered to the underlying structures than in other species, making reconstructive surgery more difficult. Tension sutures may be used as appropriate.

An attempt should be made to replace the torn gingiva and labial mucosa when repairing an injury in which the lower lip has been stripped away from the mandible. Little gingival tissue may be left to which the labial mucous membrane may be reattached. If this is the case, a nonabsorbable suture may be laced around the roots of the incisors to form a latticework to which sutures may be attached. If the wound is fresh and thoroughly cleansed and debrided, the subcutaneous tissue may heal to the periosteum and minimize the potential defect from such a laceration.

POSTSURGICAL CARE. Antibiotics are indicated only if vital structures (such as articulations) are exposed, in puncture wounds (as a precaution against tetanus), or when devitalized tissue must be left in a wound for fear of traumatizing vessels, nerves, or ducts during debridement. Otherwise, routine postsurgical care should be followed.

DENTAL DISEASE

Dental anatomy is dealt with in Chapter 13. That section should be studied before considering dental surgery.

Malocclusion

Malocclusion is a term describing abnormal positioning of a tooth or teeth that prevents appropriate fitting and wear with corresponding teeth in the opposite jaw. Both superior and inferior brachygnathism frequently occur in llamas and alpacas (see Chap. 22), resulting in either elongated incisors or excessive pressure and wear on the dental pad.

CAUSES. Malocclusion may be caused by trauma to the teeth, the bones supporting the teeth, or the temporomandibular articulation. Chronic pain in any of these tissues may result in chewing abnormalities, which, in turn, cause asymmetric wear of the teeth and, ultimately, malocclusion.

A more frequent cause of malocclusion in South American camelids (SACs) is congenital anomaly: shortening of the premaxilla, lengthening of the mandible, or a combination of both. Bustinza (6) and Sumar (21) believe that these are hereditary conditions (see Chap. 22). A third cause may be fluorine poisoning, which causes softening of the enamel and uneven wear of the teeth.

CLINICAL SIGNS. It is easy to determine whether or not the incisors are aligned. In the normal animal, the incisors fit against the rostral tip of the dental pad. It is more difficult to ascertain the occlusion of the cheek teeth. Gross abnormalities may be palpated through the buccal membrane. Camelids have a narrow mouth, which cannot be opened widely enough to allow clear visual inspection without great difficulty. A thorough inspection of the mouth necessitates sedation or anesthesia.

Sharp enamel points on the buccal surface of the upper and lingual surface of the lower cheek teeth are normal in SACs. This condition should not be confused with malocclusion. However, if either upper or lower jaw is shifted rostrally in relation to the other, the end cheek teeth will not wear against their opposites and will become elongated.

Animals with malocclusion suffer from varying degrees of dysfunction in prehension and chewing. Severe malocclusion may result in malnutrition and poor body condition. Neonates with severe malocclusion will be unable to nurse.

INDICATIONS. Radiographic evaluation of the dental structures may help in making a diagnosis. A detailed film series, including oblique studies, is required to visualize each jaw without superimposition of the opposite jaw.

The condition should also be evaluated in terms of potential genetic transmission. Congenital malocclusion should be viewed as a hereditary defect until proven otherwise, and such animals should not be included in breeding herds. It is unethical for a veterinarian to surgically correct such a defect on an animal intended for sale as a breeding animal. Otherwise, appropriate action should be taken to correct interference with prehension and chewing.

POSITION. SACs do not tolerate oral examination or submit to dental work without resistance. It may be possible to file off a small tooth projection with the unsedated animal in a standing position, but most dental work will necessitate sedation, recumbency, and, perhaps, general anesthesia. Lateral recumbency is the recommended position.

ANESTHESIA. As appropriate.

SURGERY. Minor dental elongations may be leveled using standard equine dental floats. The enamel points on the cheek teeth should *not* be leveled as in the horse. If a cheek tooth has been lost, with corresponding elongation of the opposing tooth, the elongated tooth should be shortened. Teeth at both ends of each dental arcade should be checked carefully and leveled to that of the rest of the arcade.

A Hauptner bovine dental speculum, set on the narrowest opening, is suitable for holding the mouth open for inspection and surgery. A narrow wooden block, inserted between the cheek teeth of the jaw opposite to the jaw being corrected, makes a satisfactory substitute for a speculum.

Elongated incisors may be cut off with obstetric wire, a Gigli surgical wire saw, a hacksaw, a Stryker orthopedic saw, or a circular saw mounted on a hobby drill unit (Dremel Mototool). In a correctly trimmed incisor, the pulp cavity is not opened and the nerve is neither exposed nor stimulated. However, the nerve is affected by the vibration and heat generated during the cutting, making this a painful procedure that should not be performed without administration of appropriate analgesia.

It should be reiterated that the incisor teeth of the vicuña and, to a lesser extent, the alpaca continue to erupt until late adulthood. Incisor malocclusion will preclude even wear, resulting in a chronic problem of overgrowth of the incisors.

Retained Deciduous Incisors

In the normal eruption process, the permanent tooth bud begins development at the base of the deciduous tooth and pushes it out as eruption progresses. The permanent tooth bud for a single tooth, or for each of the incisors, may develop in an abnormal position and fail to push out the deciduous tooth, resulting in a double set of incisors.

CLINICAL SIGNS. A double set of teeth is readily apparent. The permanent set is on the lingual surface (see Fig. 22.26). The deciduous teeth are usually smaller, worn on the occlusal surface, and may be loose in the jaw, attached only by a short root.

ANESTHESIA. Usually sedation and analgesia are all that are necessary.

SURGERY. Retained incisors may be so loose in the jaw that they can be removed with the fingers. If not, the attachment of the gingiva to the tooth should be loosened with a dental elevator. The alveolar periosteal membrane may also be broken down with the elevator, if necessary. Damage to the attachment of the permanent tooth is a hazard. The tooth may be grasped with small animal dental forceps and rotated gently on its vertical axis while exerting slight traction. As the tooth loosens, the degree of rotation and the traction should be increased until the tooth is extracted.

POSTSURGICAL CARE. The alveolar sockets may be left open. Hemorrhage is usually minimal, and neither antibiotics nor disinfectants are recommended for use in the mouth. The mouth may be inspected for 2–3 days following surgery to remove any feed material that is trapped in the socket. Otherwise, the wounds should be allowed to heal by second intention. Usually, the animal will continue to eat, with no evidence of discomfort.

Disarming the Canine Teeth

All of the camelids have canine teeth, which are especially well developed in the male. It is a common practice in North America to blunt these teeth in some manner to avoid severe lacerations of the ears, throat, limbs, and scrotum when two males fight.

The essential anatomy of the canine teeth is described in Chapter 13. Additional anatomic considerations for surgery follow: (1) The most ventral curve of the mandibular canine is immediately adjacent to the mental foramen and nerve. Manipulation in that area should be avoided. (2) The alveolus of the third incisor is immediately adjacent to the rostral border of the mandibular canine. Rough elevation and leverage may damage the root of the incisor. Roots of the canine are located rostral to the caudal border of the mandibular symphysis (Fig. 6.2). This site provides added structural strength for applying leverage to the canine or when it is necessary to remove the bony plate. Even here, application of too much force may fracture the mandible or cause separation of the symphysis.

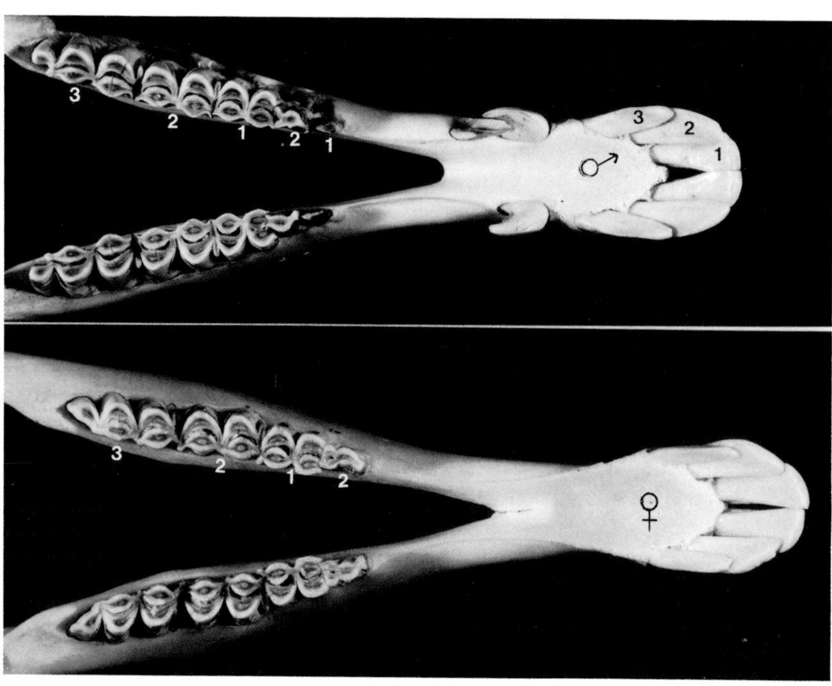

6.2 Inferior cheek teeth, lower incisors, and lower canine teeth of a male and female llama, dorsal view.

Four methods are recommended to disarm canine teeth: total extraction, pulpotomy after cutting off the crown, cutting off the crown above the gingiva, and cutting off the crown at the mandible and covering the stub with the gingiva. The advantages and disadvantages of each of these alternatives will be described. Other procedures have been reported by Kock (12) and Taylor (25).

EXTRACTION

Indications. This procedure is not recommended for routine disarming, because the roots of the canines are curved and large (Fig. 6.3). However, a fracture of the tooth and subsequent infection of the pulp cavity may necessitate extraction. Extraction is also indicated if a pulp cavity abscess has developed following removal of the crown.

Surgery. The gingiva should be incised rostrally and caudally to the crown. A second incision should be made diagonally from the crown toward the root apex. The gingiva may be reflected from the bone and the crown with a dental elevator or chisel.

A plate of bone should then be removed from the lateral aspect of the upper canine tooth root and the dorsolateral aspect of the mandibular canine. The bony plate may be carefully chiseled off or cut with a surgical saw. Once the plate is removed, the root may be separated from the alveolus with a dental elevator.

The crown should be grasped with a small animal dental forceps and a gentle rocking motion, medial to lateral, used to further loosen the tooth. It is not possible to rotate canine teeth on the vertical axis because of the curved root. The gentle elevation and forceps movements should be continued until the tooth is released. This

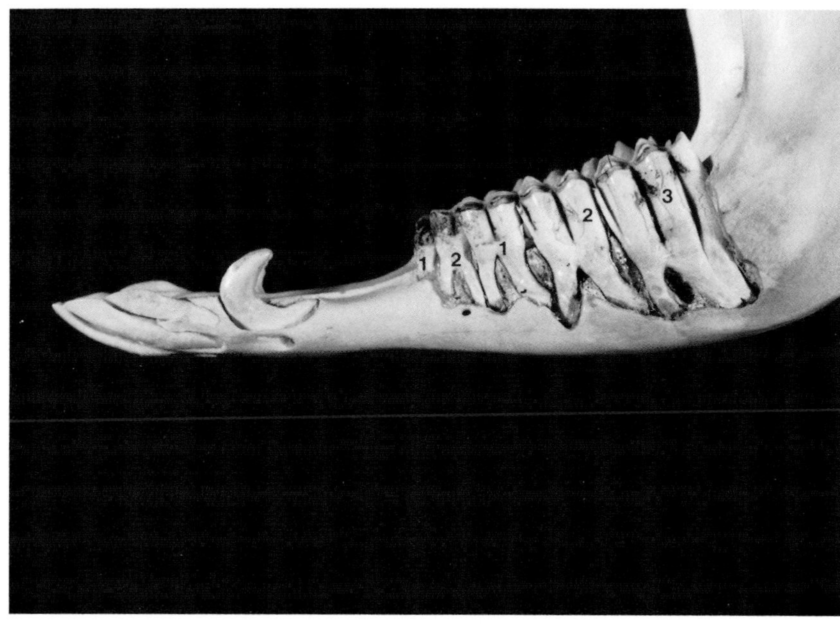

6.3 Sculptured mandible exposing the roots of the cheek teeth, incisors, and canine tooth of a male llama, lateral view.

process should not be hurried, since some time is required to loosen the root. Excessive torque may fracture the root, complicating complete extraction.

The extracted tooth should be closely examined to ascertain that the entire root has been removed. Any spicules of the alveolar plate or fractured segments of the root should be removed with a small curette.

PULPOTOMY

Indications. Pulpotomy would be the method of choice for disarming canines, except that the procedure requires special instruments and materials. It is the most sophisticated of the recommended procedures and most surgically sound. It may be completed more quickly than extraction but requires more time than the other two procedures.

Surgery. The crown should be cut off 2–3 mm above the gingiva, using the circular saw of an electric hobby drill, a hacksaw, or an obstetric wire, to expose the pulp cavity. A hole should be drilled vertically into the pulp cavity with a No. 35 carbide burr for a distance of 4 mm and the canal undermined to create a pocket. Small cotton pledgets impregnated with epinephrine should be inserted into the cavity to stop hemorrhage. When hemostasis is complete, all cotton pieces should be removed and the cavity allowed to thoroughly air dry. A cotton pledget, soaked in formacresol with the excess removed, should be inserted into the pulp cavity to sterilize it. If hemorrhage recurs at this point, the epinephrine, air drying, and formacresol treatments should be repeated.

Zinc oxide powder should be mixed with liquid eugenol and a drop of formacresol to produce a dry but malleable putty, which should be firmly packed into the cavity with a dental condenser. The cavity is then redrilled to a depth of 2 mm, with an undercut. A dental restorative resin (Johnson & Johnson Adaptic Kit), mixed according to directions, should then be packed into the cavity. Firm finger pressure should be applied for 30 seconds and the resin allowed to air dry. The resin should not extend above the surface of the cut crown. The procedure must be repeated on each canine tooth.

CUTTING OFF THE CROWN ABOVE THE GINGIVA

Indications. This procedure requires the least amount of time, instrumentation, and materials. It is especially applicable when it is desired to blunt the tip of the canines while they are still erupting. Also, if the deciduous canines are particularly long and sharp and the young male is overly aggressive with penmates, the tips of these teeth can be blunted with this technique.

Anesthesia. The procedure has often been performed by the breeder by securing the head in a stock or over a yoke and cutting off the teeth without anesthesia. Omitting anesthesia may be acceptable if no more than the tip is to be cut off, but if the tooth is to be cut off near the gingiva, the pulp cavity and nerves will be exposed. It is not justifiable to subject an animal to that degree of pain simply because the animal can be physically overpowered.

Intravenous (IV) xylazine HCl (0.4 mg/kg) will sedate the animal and provide analgesia for the short time necessary to complete the surgery.

Surgery. The mouth should be held open with a speculum. A surgical wire saw (Gigli wire) or an obstetric wire may be used to cut off the tooth. The cut should begin 2–3 mm above the gingiva. A rapid sawing motion with the wire will generate heat, searing the pulp cavity as the crown is removed. Less pressure should be exerted on the wire as the cut nears completion to avoid fracturing the edge of the tooth.

If only the tip is cut off, the pulp cavity will not be exposed. With a deeper cut, exposing the pulp cavity and development of pulpitis and/or apical abscess are risks, but hundreds of llamas have been operated on by owners and veterinarians using this technique with only a few reports of postsurgical infection. Apparently, the pulp cavity usually seals itself, with a dentine layer forming quickly at the exposed surface. Nonetheless, if the pulp cavity and nerves are exposed, discomfort is associated with this procedure. No postsurgical care is necessary.

CUTTING OFF THE CROWN AND COVERING THE ROOT WITH A GINGIVAL FLAP

Indications. This is the author's preferred method. It is more time consuming than simply cutting off the crown, but it requires less time than extraction or pulpotomy. The only special instrument needed is the circular saw of a hobby drill.

This procedure should be used only on fully erupted, permanent canine teeth. Otherwise, as the growing tooth continues to erupt, it will again protrude through the gingiva.

Anesthesia. IV xylazine HCl (0.25 mg/kg), followed 10 minutes later by IV ketamine (3–5 mg/kg), provides suitable anesthesia. It may be necessary to periodically supplement anesthesia with half doses of IV ketamine if the procedure is unusually prolonged.

Surgery. The gingiva is incised approximately 1 cm rostrally and caudally to the canine, elevating the gingiva away from the crown down to the bone with a dental elevator. The gingiva should be reflected and held out of the surgical site with a sterile wooden tongue depressor. The crown should be cut off at the level of the bone with a circular saw. The cut surface should be palpated for sharp borders, which should be smoothed. The gingival flaps should be drawn over the stub and closed with vicryl or other absorbable suture.

Postsurgical Care. No special postsurgical care is necessary; however, the mouth should be examined every other day for a week to check for dehiscence or infection. Usually, the animal will resume eating as soon as it recovers from anesthesia.

Anatomy of the Cheek Teeth

SUPERIOR CHEEK TEETH. Each upper arcade has one or two premolars and three molars (Fig. 6.4). These are frequently designated as "cheek teeth" and are numbered 1 to 5 cranial to caudal. Cheek tooth 1, when present, is small and triangular shaped (1 × 1 × 1 cm),

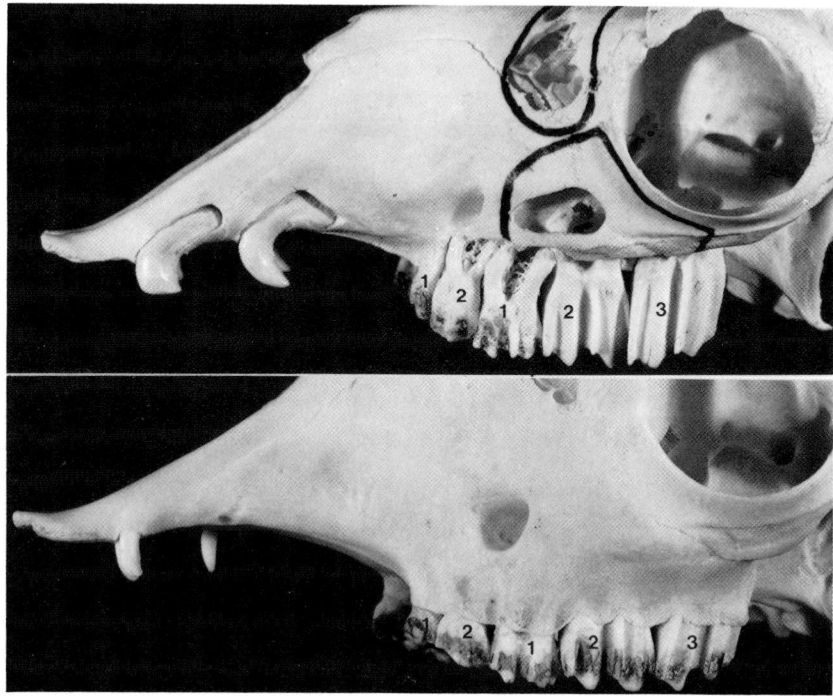

6.4 (Top) Sculptured upper jaw exposing the roots of the canine teeth and superior cheek teeth, lateral view. (Bottom) Canine teeth and maxillary cheek teeth, lateral view.

with three roots and no infundibulum, but the occlusal surface is folded on its caudal border (Fig. 6.5).

Cheek tooth 2 is rectangular (1.5 × 1 cm), with one medial and two lateral roots and one infundibulum. The roots of this tooth are immediately ventral to the infraorbital foramen.

Cheek tooth 3 (molar 1) is rectangular (2 × 1.5 cm), with four roots and two infundibuli. Cheek tooth 4 is the largest tooth in the mouth (2.5 × 1.5 cm), rectangular in shape, with four roots and two infundibuli. Cheek tooth 5 is slightly smaller than the 4th but also has four roots and two infundibuli. The roots of the upper molars (cheek teeth 3–5) lie within the maxillary sinus.

INFERIOR CHEEK TEETH. The inferior cheek teeth are narrower than the superior cheek teeth and the mandibular arcades are closer together. In a normal resting position, the upper arcade extends approximately 1 cm labially to the lower arcade and the lower arcade extends 3–4 mm lingually to the upper arcade. This fosters the development of sharp enamel points on the lingual surfaces of the lower cheek teeth and the buccal surfaces of the upper cheek teeth. Development of such points is normal, and unless they become exaggerated or cause labial lacerations, the enamel points need not be floated.

The inferior cheek teeth have the following characteristics (Figs. 6.2, 6.3, 6.6, 6.7): lower cheek tooth 1 (premolar 1), if present, is conical in shape (0.8 × 0.5 cm), with two roots lying closely together and no infundibulum. Cheek tooth 2 (premolar 2) is triangular (1 × 0.6 cm), with two divergent roots and no infundibulum. Cheek tooth 3 (molar 1) is rectangular (1.7 × 1 cm), with two roots and two infundibuli. Cheek tooth 4 (molar 2) is rectangular (2.4 × 0.2 cm), with two divergent roots and two infundibuli. Cheek tooth 5 (molar 3) is rectangular (3 × 1.2 cm), with three roots, the caudal two fused, and two infundibuli.

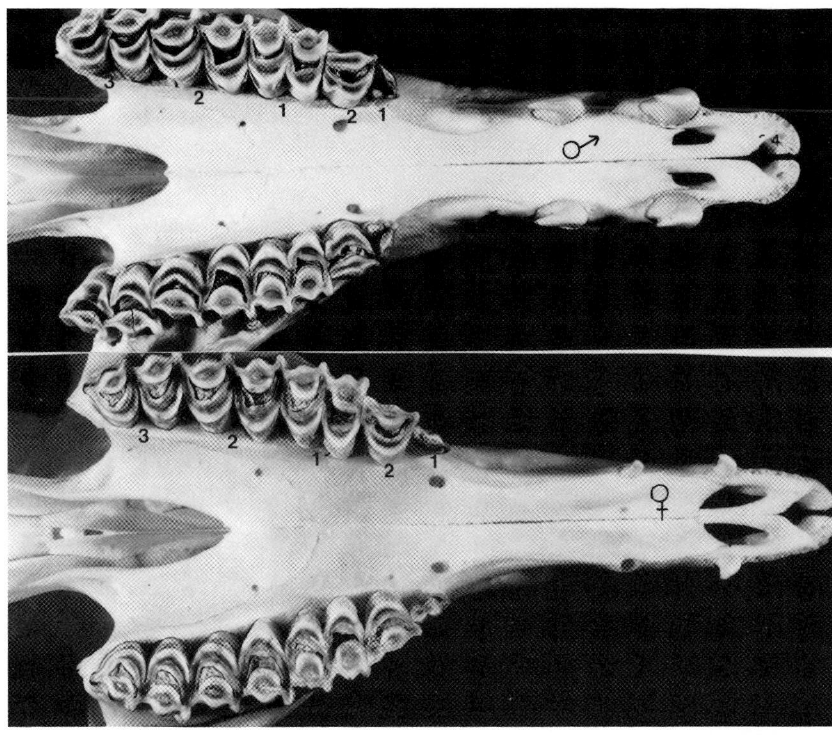

6.5 Superior cheek teeth and canine teeth, ventral view.

Infection of the Cheek Teeth (premolars and molars)

Pulpitis and alveolar periostitis or osteitis may result from infection of the alveolar space through a break in the gingiva, fracture of a tooth exposing the pulp cavity, or decay within the infundibulum. A compound fracture of the mandible or maxilla may also provide a portal of entry for infection. Various species of opportunistic bacteria may be involved.

CLINICAL SIGNS. The classic signs of an infected tooth are swelling over the root; retraction of the gingiva from the crown; reluctance to eat or peculiar chewing behavior, indicating an attempt to avoid pressure on the tooth; and with involvement of the upper molars a malodorous unilateral nasal discharge, smelling

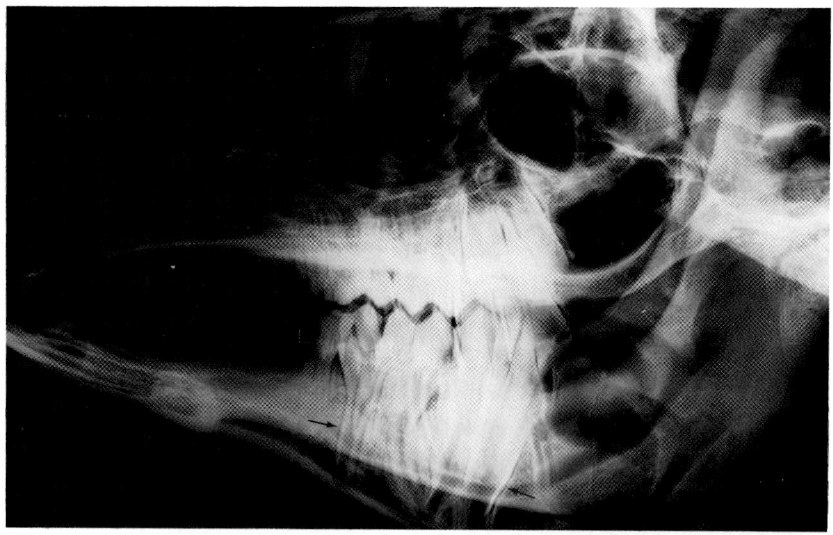

6.6 Lateral oblique radiograph of a mature normal llama mandible.

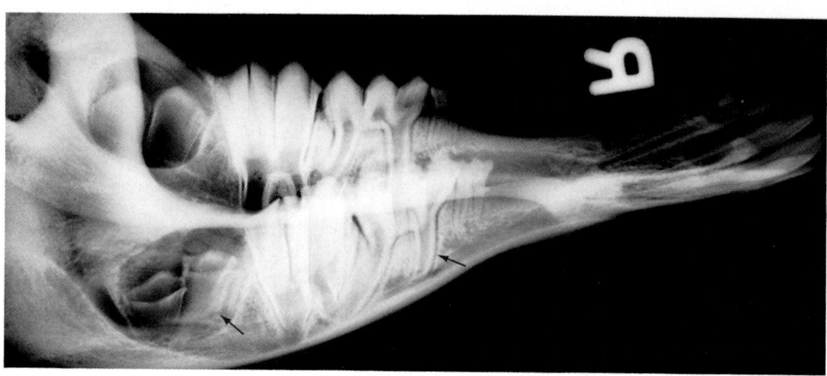

6.7 Lateral oblique radiograph of an immature llama mandible with erupting molars.

like necrotic bone, emanating from the maxillary sinus.

Chronic periosteal infection of the inferior arcades usually proceeds to osteitis. Ultimately, a fistulous tract will break through to the exterior, with exudation from the ventral border of the mandible. This exudate also has an odor like that of necrotic bone. Any drainage from the ventral border of the mandible should be considered to be associated with a dental infection until proven otherwise.

DIAGNOSIS. A detailed examination of the cheek teeth via the oral cavity will necessitate sedation or anesthesia. Although clinical signs may be suggestive, a definitive diagnosis should be based on radiographic evaluation. Radiographs must be of high quality, and right and left oblique views must be taken so that roots in both arcades can be evaluated without superimposition of the roots of the opposite arcade (Figs. 6.6–6.10).

ANESTHESIA. General anesthesia is required and inhalant anesthesia is preferred, even though an endotracheal tube will diminish the space available for oral manipulation. With a cuffed endotracheal tube in place, there will be less chance for aspiration of blood from the oral cavity or ingesta from regurgitation. If IV anesthesia is used, an IV catheter must be placed for the administration of supplemental doses of anesthetic agent, should it be necessary. Controlling the depth of anesthesia is difficult with IV agents, and inhalation of foreign material is a possible complication.

SURGERY. Endodontic procedures are rarely indicated to save infected lamoid teeth. If a definitive diagnosis of an infected tooth is made, the tooth should be removed by extraction or repulsion.

Extraction of Cheek Teeth

Dental surgery in SACs presents some special challenges. The mouth does not open widely, and the interarcade space is narrow. Further, these animals are too small for the efficient use of equine dental instruments and too large for the effective use of instruments designed for small animal dentistry. Both sizes may be required.

Both upper and lower cheek teeth 1 are accessible

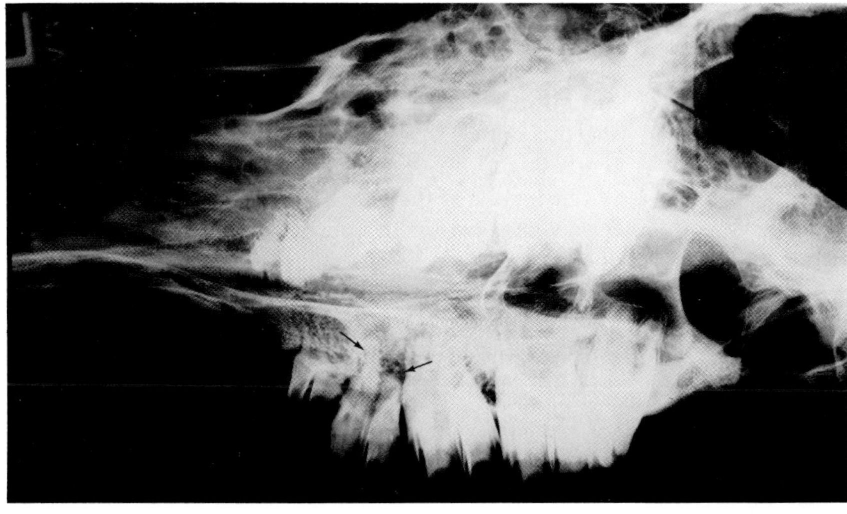

6.8 Lateral oblique radiograph of maxillary alveolar periostitis.

and may be loosened with a dental elevator and grasped with a small animal right-angle dental forceps to rock the tooth medially and laterally or rotate the tooth on its vertical axis, beginning with minimal torque. When the tooth loosens, a slooshing noise may be heard as the alveolar membrane begins to break down. Tooth extraction is a laborious process and should not be hurried lest, with the leverage of an equine extractor, the crown be broken from the root.

To extract cheek tooth 2, the mouth should be held open with a dental speculum (a Hauptner bovine speculum works well) and the gingiva separated from the crown with a sharp dental pick or scalpel. The tooth may be grasped with a small animal right-angle dental forceps and manipulated as described for tooth 1.

Extraction of the remaining teeth is difficult. The extractor will occupy nearly all of the space between the

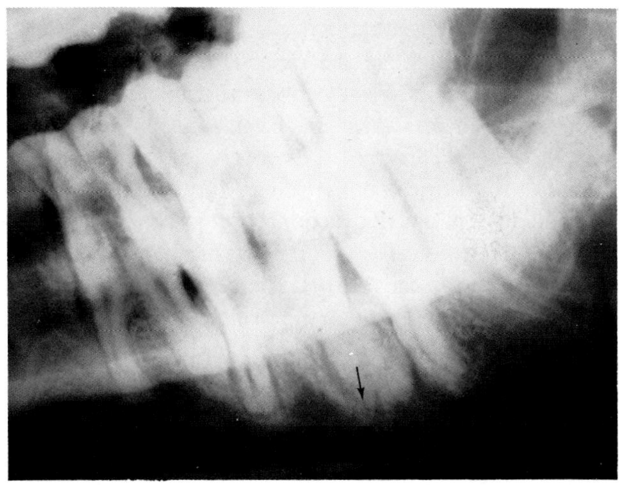

6.9 Lateral oblique radiograph of mandibular alveolar periostitis.

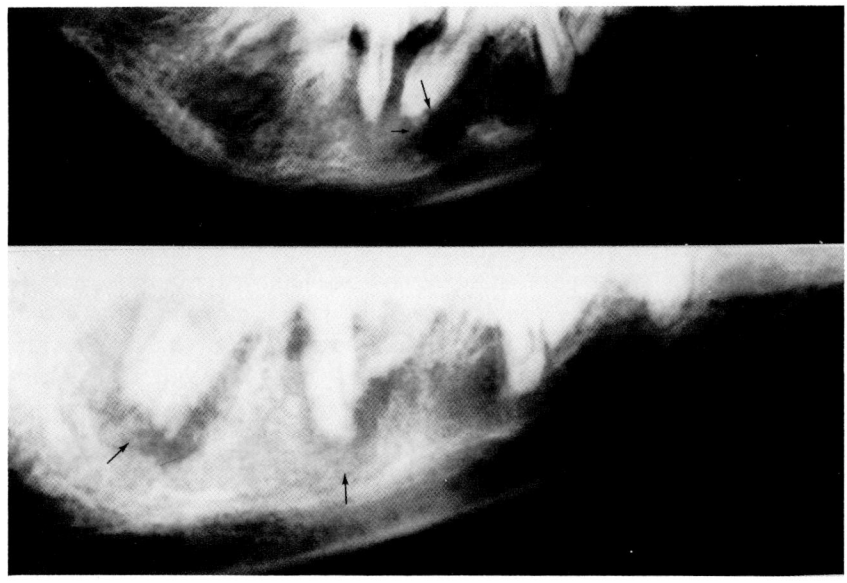

6.10 Lateral oblique radiograph of mandibular alveolar periostitis.

opposing jaws, even with the mouth fully opened, leaving little room to apply sufficient leverage to pull a tooth from its socket. If the tooth is loose, it may be possible to manipulate the forceps to either the labial or lingual side of the opposing arcade and apply slight tension. Otherwise, rotation must be continued until the entire alveolar membrane has been broken down and the tooth may be lifted from the socket with fingers or a small canine forceps.

Repulsion of the Cheek Teeth

A trephine opening for repulsion of the upper teeth should be made just dorsal to the facial crest and below a line scribed from the medial canthus of the eye to the infraorbital foramen. This will place the operative site ventral to the osseous lacrimal canal and the canal for the infraorbital nerve.

Even with the trephine opening properly located, it is possible to damage the osseous canal of the infraorbital nerve, since it lies between the medial and lateral roots of the molars. The punch must be carefully placed over the lateral aspect of the roots.

The third upper molar (cheek tooth 5) is extremely difficult to remove. Extraction is impossible because of space limitations. The roots lie within the maxillary sinus, but so far caudad that the alveolus for the tooth forms the ventral floor of the orbital socket. Repulsion can be done only through a small trephine opening through the malar (zygomatic) bone just ventral to the facial crest and at the lowest point of the orbit. It is necessary to separate the masseter muscle from the facial crest to make the trephine opening.

Once the anatomic site for the trephine hole is located, a circular incision the approximate size of the trephine should be made in the skin. Muscles, blood vessels, nerves, and the parotid duct should be reflected and the incision continued through the periosteum. The parotid duct enters the buccal cavity at the level of the junction between upper cheek teeth 2 and 3. Caution must be exercised to avoid injury to the duct when operating in this area.

A 13 or 16 mm (½ or ⅝ in.) Galt trephine is generally used, but a 9 mm (⅚ in.) Michelle trephine may also be satisfactory. The center bit of the Galt trephine should be extended 2 mm past the circular saw in order to fix the trephine to the bone. As the trephine is swiveled back and forth, a circular groove is cut into the bone. The center bit may then be retracted and the cut through the bone continued to remove a disc. Excessive pressure on the trephine should be avoided to prevent fracturing the bone, especially when opening a sinus. If a trephine is not available, a window can be cut in the bone over the root of the tooth with a small osteotome, a sterilized wood chisel, or a bur on a surgical drill.

A speculum should be used to open the mouth to identify the affected tooth. The gingiva may be cut from the crown of the tooth with a sharp dental pick, a curved sharp bistoury, or a curved scalpel blade. The affected tooth should be grasped with the thumb and forefinger of one hand and the punch directed with the other hand. It may be necessary to improvise the punch. It should be about 6 mm (¼ in.) in diameter. The punch should be carefully placed over the root(s) of the tooth encased in the alveolar bone plate. A mallet is used to strike the punch gently to break down the alveolar bone. As solid pressure is exerted on the tooth, the vibrations will be felt on the tooth crown within the mouth. It is important to align the punch with the vertical axis of the tooth. The punch should be struck with gradually increasing intensity until the tooth begins to erupt past the table surface of the arcade. Thereafter, gentle strikes of the punch will finish repelling the tooth.

The removed tooth must be examined to ascertain the completeness of the repulsion. Any remaining segments of the alveolar plate or roots should be removed with a curette or small bone chisel.

POSTSURGICAL CARE. The socket must be plugged to prevent feed from packing into the site and inhibiting healing. Traditional postsurgical care is to insert a gauze pack into the tooth cavity and tie it to another gauze pack at the external trephine opening. This is accomplished as follows: start with a roll of 1 in. gauze bandage. Measure the rostral/caudal length of the tooth and cut the gauze to fit the space snugly. Unwind the gauze until the bandage will not project above the table surface of the arcade when pressed into the socket. Attach either a double strand of 65 mm (¼ in.) umbilical tape or 0.71 mm (0.028 in.) stainless steel wire to the gauze roll using a lark's head hitch (Fig. 6.11). Reach through the trephine opening into the mouth with a forceps, grasp the strands, and pull the gauze roll snugly into the socket. Tie the strands around a folded 4 × 4 in. gauze sponge using a bow knot.

During the first week postsurgery, the pack should be changed daily and the socket flushed with a mild disinfectant such as povidone-iodine solution. To replace the pack, untie the bow and remove the outside pack. Tie a new double strand, using the bight end to attach to the free end of the existing strands. Open the mouth with a speculum and grasp the socket pack with a curved forceps. Pull the new strands into the mouth. It is important that the strands be sufficiently long to allow the necessary manipulation. A new socket plug is attached, again using a lark's head, and pulled into position. After a week, the packs need be changed only every third day. When the socket begins to fill with granulation tissue, the outside/

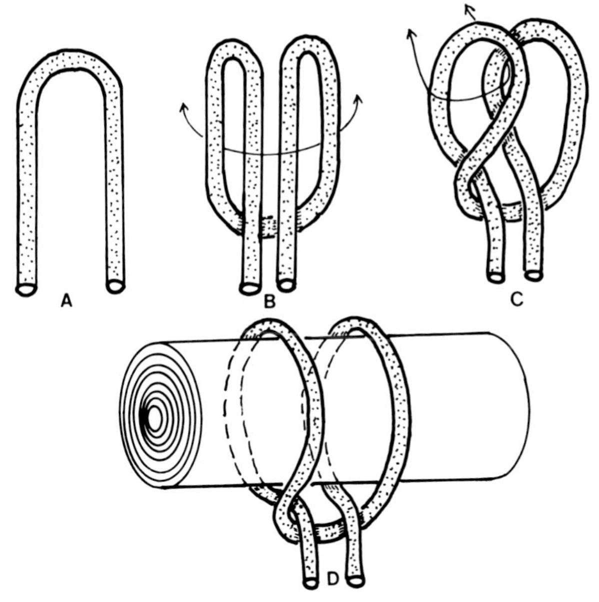

6.11 Lark's head knot used to attach strands to the dental pack.

inside packs may be replaced with dental wax or dental acrylic.

An alternate material for plugging the socket is methylmethacrylate, hoof acrylic, or dental impression material (Optisil) applied at the time of the initial surgery (14). In this method, wire is placed around the teeth contiguous to the socket and a cross strut is strung between the wires to help form a latticework to support the acrylic. The softened acrylic is placed in the defect between the teeth and extended approximately 5 mm past the gingiva into the socket (14). The hardened acrylic plug will prevent feed penetration and allow granulation to fill in the socket. Irrigation and drainage of the socket is accomplished through the trephine opening.

COMPLICATIONS OF TREPHINATION AND TOOTH REPULSION. Trephination and repulsion are not without hazard. Improper placement of the punch may result in penetration of the hard palate; damage to contiguous tooth roots; fracturing of either the medial or lateral aspect of the mandible or maxilla; and/or damage to the infraorbital nerve, facial nerve, nasolacrimal duct, or parotid salivary duct.

Tracheostomy

INDICATIONS. The SACs are primarily nasal breathers, thus any lesion causing obstruction of the nasal or nasopharyngeal airways produces dyspnea and may warrant a tracheostomy. Surgery performed in the region of the nasal cavity, such as for correction of choanal atresia (see Chap. 22), requires that a preoperative tracheostomy be done first.

POSITION. The surgeon should be prepared to perform this surgery in all conceivable positions (standing, sternal, lateral, or dorsal recumbency).

PRESURGICAL PREPARATION. In an elective tracheostomy, standard surgical asepsis should be practiced. A site on the ventral midline of the cranial third of the neck should be prepared with sufficient fiber clipped off to preclude the remaining fiber from dangling over the orifice of the tube. In a heavily fleeced llama or alpaca, this may require feathering away from the site.

ANESTHESIA. An emergency tracheostomy may be performed on a semiconscious or unconscious patient without anesthesia or surgical preparation. In an elective tracheostomy, either infiltration of the incision site with local anesthesia or sedation with xylazine HCl is appropriate.

SURGERY. To avoid hemorrhage, the incision should be made on the midline. The paired sternohyoideus muscles should be separated by blunt dissection. The underlying fascial layer may be separated with blunt Mayo scissors or may be incised with a scalpel. Care should be taken to avoid scoring the tracheal rings.

The trachea of the llama or alpaca lies deeper within the cervical structures than it does in ruminants or horses. The external jugular veins, common carotid arteries, vagosympathetic trunks, and the esophagus (on the left side) are in close apposition to the trachea. Nonetheless, if strict adherence to a midline approach is used, hemorrhage will be minimal.

The trachea should be opened by incising the anular ligament between two tracheal rings. Avoid incising more than half the circumference. Additional space for insertion of a tube may be obtained by removing a half-moon-shaped segment from adjacent rings, but the rings should not be transected.

Various types of tracheostomy tubes may be inserted; the most satisfactory are those consisting of an outer sleeve and an inner tube that may be removed for cleaning.

The inside diameter of the trachea is approximately 1 cm in a neonate and 3 cm in a 175 kg adult. The procedure followed at this point will be determined by the type of endotracheal tube chosen and the objective of the surgery. For long-term placement, the skin should be sutured around the tube and the tube itself may be sutured to the skin. For short-term placement, the incision may be left open.

POSTSURGICAL CARE. It is extremely important to monitor the patency of the tube at frequent intervals to prevent obstruction from exudate or mucus. Exudate or dried blood and mucus should not be pushed into the trachea. When the tube is no longer needed, it should be removed and the wound allowed to heal by granulation. The wound should be debrided twice daily with a povidone-iodine–soaked gauze sponge until healing is complete.

Tracheostomy tubes should be removed, cleaned, and replaced as often as necessary to maintain patency. Alternatively, the tube can be cleaned by suction.

LAPAROTOMY

Anatomy

To perform abdominal surgery, the anatomy of the abdominal musculature must be understood. The cutaneous trunci muscle is limited to the specialized preputial muscles in the male and a few fibers on the ventral midline in the female. The abdominal tunic (deep fascia) is less well developed in SACs than in the horse or cow. It is composed of fibroelastic tissue that adds support to the muscles and their aponeuroses. The tunic covers the external abdominal oblique muscle dorsally and cranially and is an integral part of the aponeurosis of the external oblique muscle ventrally and caudally. The abdominal tunic extends into the inguinal area and helps to form the superficial inguinal ring.

A specialized section of the abdominal tunic becomes the medial suspensory ligament of the mammary gland. The suspensory ligaments of the mammary gland are paired, but the right and left halves are not as easily separated at surgery as they are in cattle.

The external abdominal oblique muscle is the most superficial of the abdominal muscles. Its fibers are directed caudad to slightly ventrad. This muscle originates on the caudal border and lateral aspect of the last few ribs and the fascia over the intercostal muscles. The body of the muscle is composed of short fibers and is approximately 1 cm thick. An extensive aponeurosis inserts onto the tuber coxae, prepubic tendon, and linea alba.

The internal abdominal oblique muscle lies beneath the external abdominal oblique muscle (Fig. 6.12). Its fibers are directed ventrad, craniad, and mediad. This muscle has its origin on the tuber coxae and the deep lumbar fascia. The body of the muscle is composed of short fibers and is 1–2 cm thick. Ventrally and cranially an aponeurosis blends with the aponeurosis of the external oblique muscle. These combined aponeuroses (abdominal tunic, internal and external abdominal oblique muscles) insert on the caudal border of the last rib and the linea alba and are the main fibrous support for the abdominal organs. They form the outer sheath of the rectus abdominis muscle.

The fibers of the transversus abdominis muscle are directed ventrad and mediad (Fig. 6.13). The aponeuroses of the transversus muscle lie dorsally and ventrally. The dorsal aponeurosis originates in the deep lumbar fascia and the transverse processes of the lumbar vertebrae and the costal arch; it is 10 cm long cranially and 4 cm long caudally. The length of the body of the

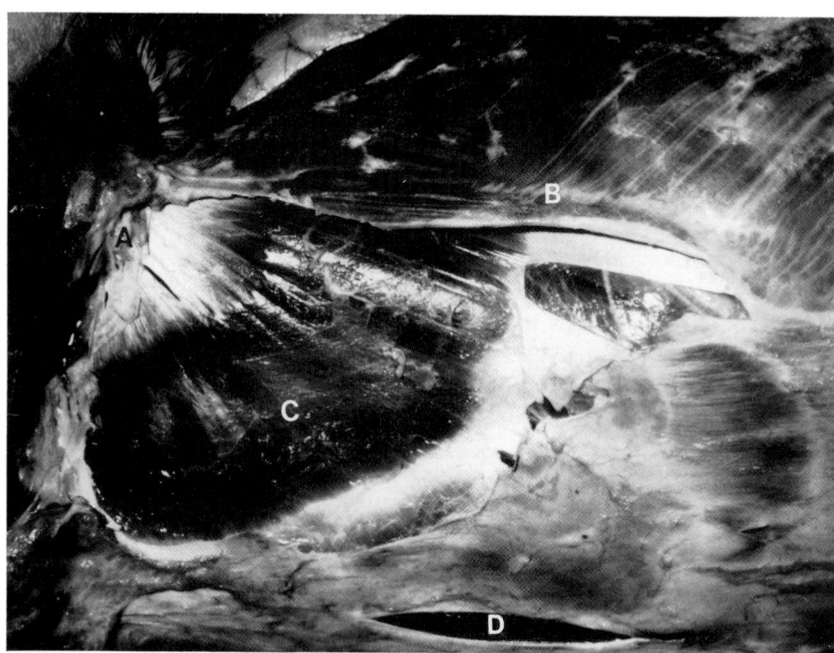

6.12 Position of the internal abdominal oblique muscle: **(A)** tuber coxae, **(B)** external abdominal oblique muscle, **(C)** internal abdominal oblique muscle, **(D)** rectus abdominis muscle.

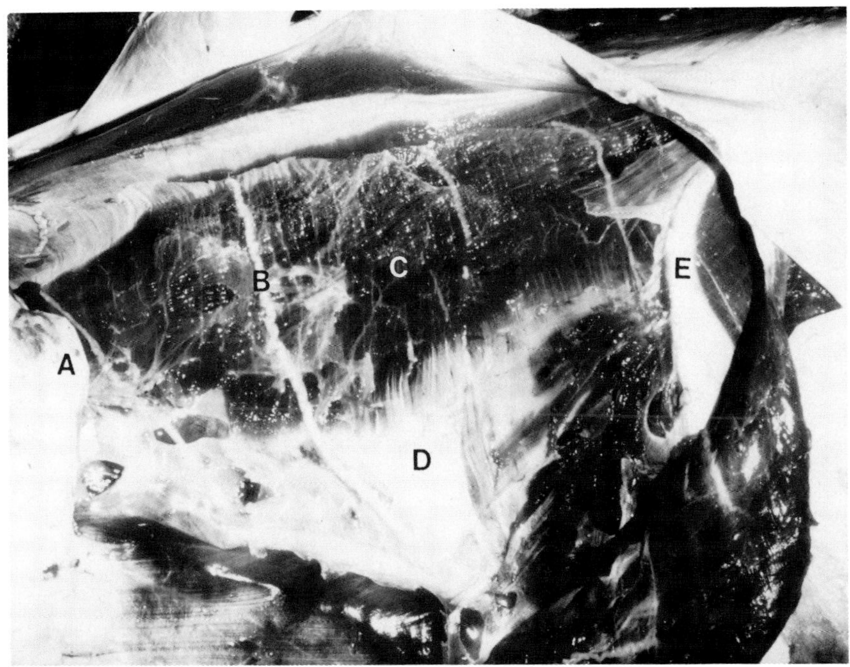

6.13 Position of the transversus abdominis muscle: **(A)** tuber coxae, **(B)** lumbar spinal nerve, **(C)** body of the transversus muscle, **(D)** ventral aponeurosis of the transversus muscle, **(E)** costal arch.

muscle is only 9 cm, continuing on as the ventral aponeurosis, which inserts on the linea alba deep to the rectus abdominis muscle.

The abdominal wall of the camelid has unique features. There is no flank. The paralumbar fossa is not prominent. The only muscle fibers over the area bordered by the last rib, the transverse processes of the lumbar vertebrae and the tuber coxae, are those of the external abdominal oblique muscles at the cranial aspect and some of the internal oblique muscle fibers caudally. Immediately dorsal and lateral to the rectus abdominis muscle, caudal to the costal arch, there is no muscle fiber, only aponeurosis. Therefore, in the camelid, this area is not suitable as a site for an abdominal incision.

In the female camelid, the mammary gland is situated cranial to the pubic attachment of the rectus abdominis muscle. A caudal ventral midline incision to perform ovariohysterectomy will necessitate elevation and reflection of the gland caudally to allow adequate exposure.

In the male camelid, the prepuce and penis are located in a similar area. The external preputial orifice of a 175 kg male is located 15 cm cranial to the rim of the pelvis. The prepuce opens caudally in a sexually unaroused male. The prepuce is under the control of two pairs of muscles that are modifications of the cutaneous trunci muscle (Fig. 6.14). The cranial preputial muscle pulls the preputial orifice forward when the male is aroused sexually. The caudal preputial muscle pulls the preputial orifice caudally as arousal subsides.

It is necessary to transect one of the cranial preputial muscles when making a ventral midline approach to the caudal abdomen for cystotomy. The muscle segments must be accurately reapposed and sutured during closure to avoid subsequent malfunction.

The umbilicus is located slightly cranial to the midpoint of the distance between the xiphoid cartilage and the pubis. The linea alba is indistinct in the llama, particularly caudal to the umbilicus.

Position

A ventral midline approach requires dorsal recumbency. Although elaborate surgical tables are employed in university and private clinics, a simple cradle may suffice to hold a llama in the correct position (Figs. 6.15, 6.16). The llama may be lifted onto an elevated platform composed of bales of straw to avoid back strain in the surgeon from bending over and working on the floor. Bales of hay or straw may also be used to brace the llama, but they have the disadvantage of diminishing exposure.

The llama should be in lateral recumbency for a high–abdominal wall approach.

Presurgical Preparation

Feed should be withheld for 24–36 hours and water for 12 hours prior to elective surgery on an adult SAC. Feed and water should not be withheld from neonates. Precautions should be taken to deal with regurgitation, which is common when the patient is in dorsal

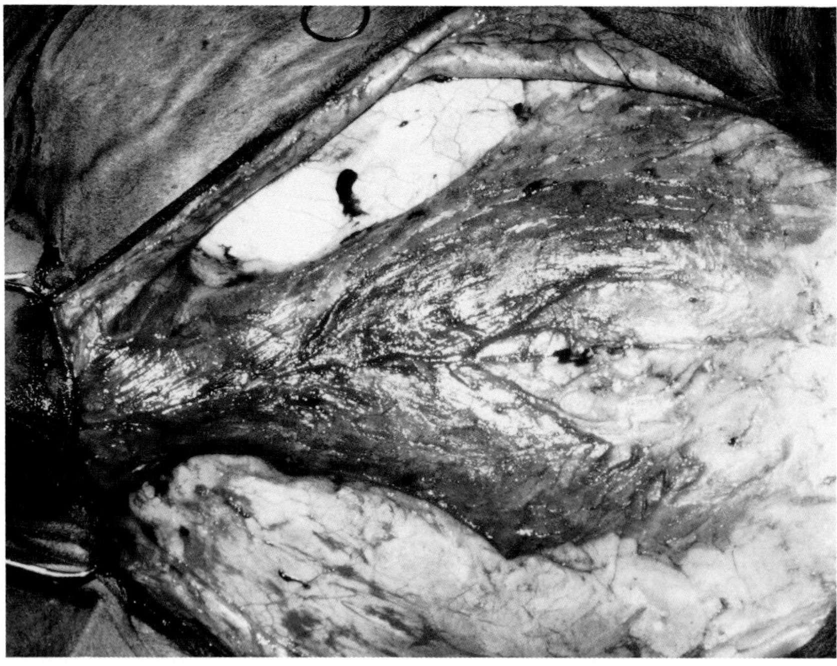

6.14 Preputial muscles of the llama.

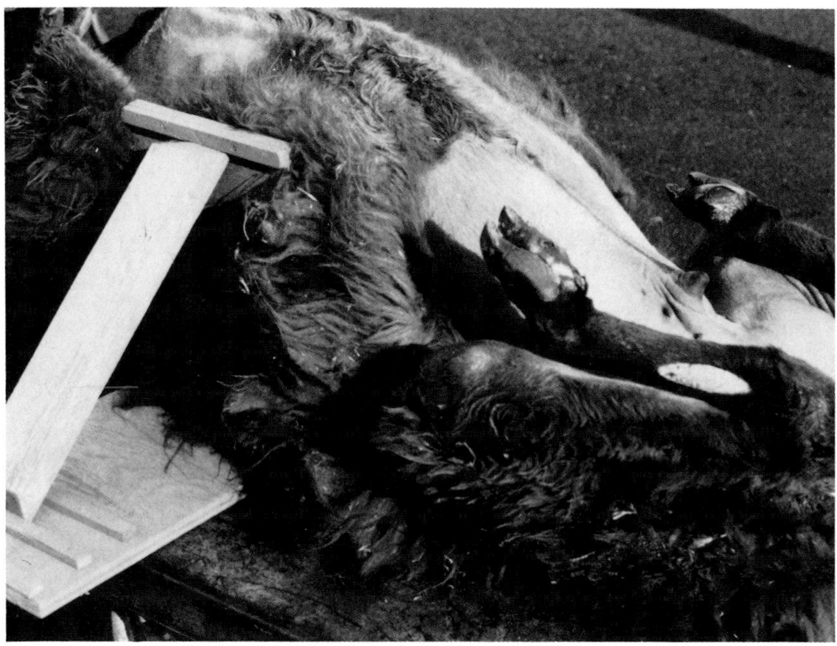

6.15 Cradle used to restrain llama in dorsal recumbency.

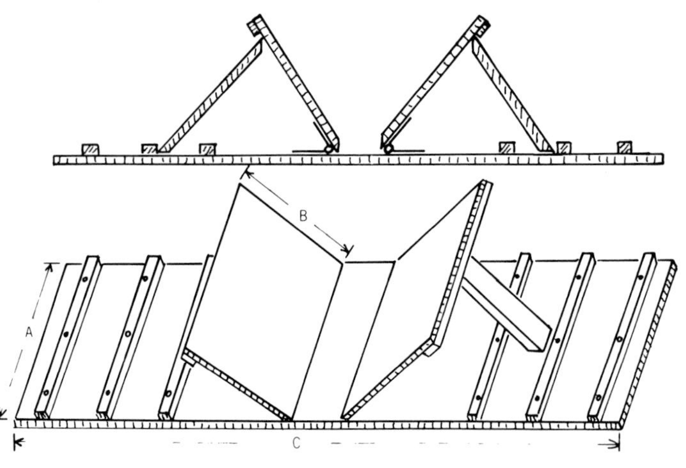

6.16 Diagram of lamoid cradle: **(A)** 30 cm, **(B)** 38 cm, **(C)** 125 cm.

recumbency but which may also occur in other positions.

Anesthesia

General anesthesia is usually necessary.

Midline Approach

The tissue layers penetrated will vary with the site of the incision. Cranial to the umbilicus, the layers encountered are the skin, subcutaneous areolar tissue, a single layer of fascia composed of the aponeuroses of the abdominal muscles, deep abdominal fat, and the peritoneum.

Caudal to the umbilicus, the layers found are the skin, subcutaneous tissue, cutaneous trunci muscle, superficial fascia (aponeuroses of the external and internal abdominal oblique muscles), deep fascia (thin aponeurosis of the transversus abdominis muscle), deep abdominal fat, and peritoneum. Lateral to the midline, the two fascial layers are separated by the paired bodies of the rectus abdominis muscle. The incision must be made directly on the midline to avoid incising the muscles. In addition, deep abdominal fat will complicate entrance if the incision is off the midline.

Closure also varies with the incision site. Cranial to the umbilicus, the suture layers include the peritoneum, fascia, and skin (Fig. 6.17). Caudal to the umbilicus, it is important to assure inclusion of all the fascial layers into one or more suture layers.

The body of the rectus abdominis muscle is usually included in the suture of the deep fascia, but it should be understood that the fascia is the tissue that provides support for the abdominal wall.

The author prefers placement of a cruciate pattern tension suture, using sutures of No. 2 polyglactin 910 (vicryl) on the fascial layers. Postsurgical dehiscence and herniation are more frequent complications with the more caudal midline incisions than when alternate surgical sites are selected.

Vicryl or gut is suitable for buried sutures. Any nonabsorbable suture or polyglactin 910 is suitable for suturing skin.

Mid- to High-Flank (paralumbar fossa) Approach

INDICATIONS. The paralumbar approach is recommended for first compartment gastrotomy from the left side. A vertical incision should be made midway between the tuber coxae and the last rib and 6–8 cm ventral to the transverse processes of the lumbar vertebrae. If maximal intraabdominal exposure is required, the horizontal fibers of the external abdominal oblique muscles must be incised. The internal oblique and transversus muscles are separated longitudinally in the direction of their muscle fibers. The deep abdominal fat layer, which should not be too thick at this location, may be bluntly dissected and the peritoneum picked up with thumb forceps. The peritoneum should be held taut while it is penetrated with a digit or a Mayo scissors.

The peritoneum may be closed with either a continuous or simple interrupted pattern, using absorbable sutures. If a grid incision was made, the muscle layers may be closed with simple interrupted sutures. If the muscle masses were incised, they should be accurately apposed and the outer muscle fascial layer included to provide more strength for the suture to optimize healing.

A third alternative site for a laparotomy incision is cranial and slightly ventral to the tuber coxae. This approach is indicated for simple ovariohysterectomy or intraabdominal orchidectomy.

A diagonal incision should be made 6–10 cm ventral to the tuber coxae, ventrad and craniad in the direction of the fibers of the internal abdominal oblique muscle. The fibers of the external abdominal oblique muscles will be minimal or absent at this site. The incision will penetrate the abdominal tunic, the fibers of the internal abdominal oblique muscle (blunt dissection), the aponeurosis of the transversus abdominis muscle, and the peritoneum. Closure should follow the same sequence as for the high-flank approach.

Herniorrhaphy

All types of hernias that occur in other species have been seen in SACs, but umbilical hernias are most often

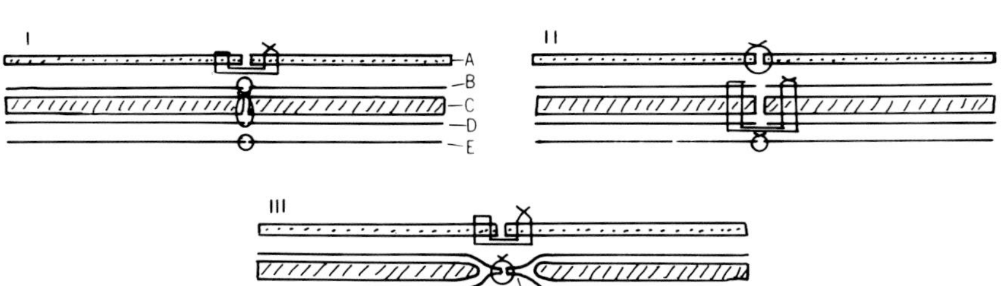

6.17 Diagrams of ventral midline abdominal incision closure: I. Layers caudal to umbilicus, II. layers caudal to umbilicus using tension suture in muscle and fascial layers, III. layers cranial to umbilicus. **(A)** Skin, **(B)** superficial abdominal fascia, **(C)** rectus abdominis muscle, **(D)** deep abdominal fascial layers, **(E)** peritoneum, **(F)** linea alba, fusion of the superficial and deep fascia.

seen. Although not yet proven in SACs, a congenital umbilical hernia is likely to be of genetic origin (see Table 22.5). Appropriate recommendations should be made to owners who ask about breeding-affected individuals.

Temporary patency of the abdominal wall around the umbilical vessels is normal in many neonate SACs. Usually, the tip of a finger can be inserted through the ring. This ring should be closed within a month after birth. Rings allowing insertion of two or more fingers or persisting for longer than a month are unlikely to close and should be regarded as hernias. Herniorrhaphy may be delayed for 2–3 months until the abdominal wall has become firmer to provide better retention for sutures.

Ventral hernias may be caused by trauma. One male adult llama eviscerated itself on a metal post while rearing in an attempt to reach another male. Such hernias may be complete, as in this case, or result only in a rent through the muscle and fascial layers.

Iatrogenic hernias occur from failure of suture lines to hold following laparotomy. Although rare, postcastration inguinal herniation may be prevented by transfixion ligation of the entire spermatic cord.

ANESTHESIA. General anesthesia is appropriate for this surgery.

SURGERY. Techniques, including clamps, appropriate for this surgery in large domestic animals are applicable to SACs. All of the methods illustrated in Figure 6.18, I–V, have been successfully employed. If the defect is less than 4 cm in diameter, the peritoneal cavity should not be opened; the edges of the ring in the abdominal musculature should be scarified and mattress sutures placed to approximate the edges of the ring.

If the size of the ring is 5–10 cm, the closure illustrated in Figure 6.18A is recommended. The hernial sac may be excised with caution to avoid adhered viscera. The author has rarely chosen the technique depicted in Figure 6.18C, since there is usually insufficient slack in the abdominal wall to allow pulling one side over the other. However, this technique provides the most security against recurrence.

Incarceration of a loop of bowel complicates the surgery. Reference to standard surgical texts is suggested for methods of dealing with this rare complication.

The organ most likely to be found immediately adjacent to an umbilical hernia in the adult llama is compartment one (C-1) of the stomach. Although the greater omentum is small in lamoids, it is present at the region of the umbilicus and may protrude into the hernial sac. In neonates and nursing infants, the small intestine may occupy the ventralmost position, and it is possible for a loop of bowel to pass into the hernial sac.

Inguinal hernias are less common than umbilical hernias in SACs. Techniques recommended for cattle or swine are satisfactory for repair.

Iatrogenic hernias present varying problems unique to each situation. It may be necessary to deal with infection, adhesions, lack of tissue orientation, or fragmented tissue.

Incorporation of a teflon mesh is recommended to close a defect when it is impossible to appose the abdominal wall. If possible, heavy tension sutures should be placed, anchored well lateral to the incision line. No. 2 polyglactin 910 placed in a cruciate pattern is recommended. If appropriate, the suture may be doubled. Some or all of the sutures should be placed loosely before tightening. Excessive tension on individual sutures may be avoided by pulling several sutures taut at the same time, minimizing the chance that a tension suture

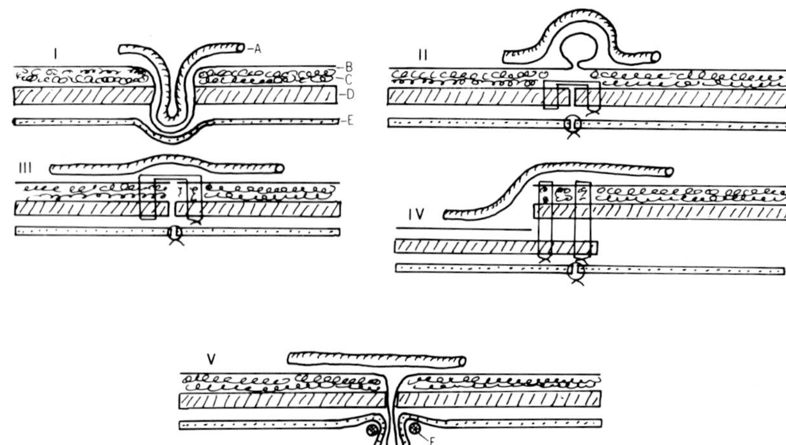

6.18 Diagrams of closure techniques used in herniorrhaphy: I. Intestinal loop in hernial sac, II. closure without entering peritoneal cavity, III. apposition of muscle-fascial ring, IV. overlap of abdominal wall, V. clamp closure. **(A)** Intestine, **(B)** peritoneum, **(C)** deep abdominal fat, **(D)** muscle and fascial layers, **(E)** skin, **(F)** clamp or constricting band.

may pull out. A second row of simple interrupted sutures of gut or vicryl should be placed between the tension sutures to make a tighter closure.

It is not necessary to attempt to close the peritoneum when correcting an iatrogenic hernia. Subcutaneous fascia should be approximated, as appropriate, to eliminate dead space. Finally, the skin may be closed with either simple interrupted or vertical mattress pattern sutures. Absorbable vicryl or nonabsorbable sutures are appropriate for closing the skin.

Diaphragmatic hernia has been reported in llamas. Description of the technique for surgical correction of an operable diaphragmatic hernia is beyond the scope of this book. Standard surgical texts should be consulted.

POSTSURGICAL CARE. Generally, antibiotics are not indicated for postsurgical care of a routine herniorrhaphy. In iatrogenic or complicated hernial repair, administration of antibiotics is necessary.

During recovery, the animal should be kept where the footing is secure to avoid slipping, stretching, or falling. An attendant may soothe the animal to keep it in sternal recumbency until all effects of the anesthesia have dissipated.

Dressings, including elastic body support bandages (elastoplast), may be appropriate. A temporary support bandage, applied while the animal is recumbent, may provide security while it is gaining its feet. In the recumbent animal, relationships of body surfaces are different than in the standing animal, so a permanent support bandage should be applied only while the llama is standing. The abdomen of a llama narrows toward the rear, making it difficult to keep a support bandage in place. Vetrap tends to gather, making it unsuitable. A clean piece of muslin or bed sheeting laid over the top of the fleece before application may avoid difficulty in removing the elastic bandage.

While healing, the llama's activity should be restricted to a small, clean enclosure or box stall. Some movement should be encouraged to aid in the dispersement of edema.

DIGESTIVE SYSTEM

Gastrotomy

A gastrotomy is indicated to remove foreign objects (hair balls, concretions, pieces of plastic) from C-1 or to relieve a concentrate overload. The immediate emptying of C-1 may be crucial to the recovery of a llama that has consumed oleander, *Nerium oleander* (see Chap. 23), or other toxic substances.

This surgery is usually performed under general anesthesia, using a ventral midline approach, but it is also possible to perform a C-1 gastrotomy via a left paralumbar fossa approach. This procedure is similar to a rumenotomy in a cow (9).

Llamas have a tendency to lie down when they are in pain. The llama may be quieted with butorphanol[1] (0.05–0.1 mg/kg intramuscularly) and the incision site desensitized with local anesthetic, using an inverted L block or local infiltration.

A 15 cm incision should be made in the left flank beginning 15 cm (6 in.) ventral to the transverse processes of the lumbar vertebrae, midway between the last rib and the tuber coxae, to avoid the pleural reflection, which may extend 2–3 cm caudal to the last rib. The incision should penetrate the abdominal tunic, and the fibers of the external oblique muscle should be separated as they traverse the incision diagonally, ventrocaudad. If present, the fibers of the internal abdominal oblique muscle should also be separated in the direction of the fibers. The fibers of the transversus abdominis are vertical and should be separated in that direction. The peritoneum may be penetrated with a finger or Mayo scissors.

The rings and shrouds used to perform rumenotomies in cattle are too large for use in llamas. A more adaptable but more time-consuming technique is to suture C-1 to the skin prior to incising the wall of the compartment. This technique precludes contamination of the peritoneal cavity while exploring and evacuating C-1.

Ingesta should be removed as appropriate. In the case of ingestion of oleander, C-1 should be washed out with water to remove all ingesta possible. Even small particles of leaves may be sufficient to produce toxicity.

The exposed wall of C-1 should be thoroughly cleansed with physiologic saline and povidone-iodine solution, diluted 1:10. The compartment wall incision should be closed with a Cushing or Connel pattern before the skin/wall stay sutures are released. The abdomen should be closed as for a laparotomy.

Permanent C-1 Fistulation

This surgery is usually done as an experimental procedure for basic nutrition studies, but it may also be indicated for maintenance of a donor animal for transfaunation of other llamas with digestive disorders (9). The basic incision is made as for gastrotomy. A half circle should be removed from the skin on each side of the incision. The resultant circular opening should be the size of the plastic fistula to be inserted later.

The dorsal aspect of the caudal sac of C-1 should

1. Torbugesic—Bristol, Syracuse, NY 13221-4755.

be pulled up into the skin incision and the serosa of the stomach sutured to the skin with a single continuous suture. The seal at the ventrum must be secure. It may be appropriate to scarify the serosa of C-1 prior to the suturing. This will enhance the adhesion of the stomach wall to the skin.

The exposed serosa of C-1 should be covered with a moist dressing to preclude drying. One to two weeks should be allowed for healing before the stomach is incised for insertion of the plastic fistula.

Surgery of the Spiral Colon

The spiral colon is a frequent site of intestinal impaction. If obstruction of the spiral colon is encountered during an exploratory laparotomy, it should be evaluated and treated as follows. The spiral colon may be seen near a ventral midline incision unless it is displaced by gaseous or fluid distention of other segments of the intestine or by torsion of the mesenteric root.

Intestinal coloration will vary with the severity of the lesion, ranging from normal in a simple impaction or mild ulceration to congested and cyanotic in torsions or other conditions with vascular compromise. Necrosis of the bowel wall may also be encountered. The proximal colon and the distal small intestine may become distended in colonic impaction.

If a torsion is found, the direction and degree of the twist should be established and the appropriate correction made. The spiral colon may be exteriorized through the incision to aid in evaluating torsion or impaction.

It may be possible to gently knead a semisolid impaction and reduce it to particles small enough to be moved through the remainder of the intestine by normal peristalsis. However, if the wall is ischemic and friable, more harm may be done by using this technique than by performing an enterotomy.

Before an enterotomy can be performed, the segment of colon containing the obstruction must be isolated from other segments of the spiral. The centrifugal coils are deeply embedded within the mesentery that binds the segments of the spiral together. Blood vessels should be avoided, but adequate exposure is necessary to allow manipulation of the colon to achieve a simple enterotomy or intestinal resection.

It will usually be necessary to decompress loops of bowel distended by gas or fluid prior to complete examination of the digestive tract and, surely, before enterotomy or resection (14). One of two methods may be chosen for decompressing the bowel. Gas and fluid may be withdrawn via a large-gauge needle or a rubber tube inserted through a stab incision and surrounded by a purse-string suture. A more rapid and thorough decompression can be accomplished using a technique frequently employed in equine colic surgery. In this technique, the distended bowel is laid on a sterile tray inclined to a collecting basket that, in turn, is connected to the surgery's drainage system. A longitudinal incision is made along the antimesenteric border of the bowel. Regular culinary water may be used to wash ingesta down the tray and to wash the surface of the intestine. A common cause of ileus is failure to adequately decompress the intestinal segments before closure. This intestinal incision should be closed using an inverting pattern, preferably a Cushing pattern, before progressing further with surgery.

If enterotomy is necessary, a small longitudinal incision should be made over the mass, which is then withdrawn with forceps and discarded. The incision should be closed with a single-layer inverting pattern. Infolding of the bowel wall should be strictly limited to minimize the potential for future stricture. All exteriorized loops of intestine should be rinsed with sterile physiologic saline and replaced in the normal position. The abdominal wall should be closed as for any laparotomy.

Rectal Prolapse

CAUSE. Chronic enteritis resulting in persistent diarrhea is the primary cause of rectal prolapse. However, the rectum may also evert during tenesmus associated with prolapse of the vagina or uterus. A weak or relaxed anal sphincter may allow a few folds of the rectal mucosa to prolapse, especially while a female in an advanced stage of pregnancy is lying down.

CLINICAL SIGNS. The protrusion of the mucosa and wall of the rectum is evident. A protrusion of 5–15 cm may not compromise the vascularity of the rectum, but if the prolapse is 20–30 cm, ischemic necrosis of the bowel may occur from compression of the vessels. The protruded rectum will exhibit varying degrees of edema, trauma, and necrosis of the mucosa.

POSITION. The standing position is most desirable, but since camelids have a propensity to lie down, it may be necessary to operate with the animal in that position.

ANESTHESIA. Epidural anesthesia (see Chap. 5) will provide analgesia and relaxation sufficient to replace the prolapse.

SURGERY. The mucosa must be cleansed and all foreign material physically removed. The cleansed tissue may be cupped in the palms of the hands and the prolapse gently replaced. If edema is severe, it may be desirable to wrap the prolapse tightly with a moistened towel or sheet until the swelling is reduced. Internal telescoping may be reduced by gentle insertion of a lubricated plastic or cardboard vaginal speculum.

A purse-string suture should be placed in the anus. Four or five loop sutures should be placed approximately 2–3 cm peripheral to the center of the anal orifice (Fig. 6.19). The loops may be laced through with 3 mm (⅛ in.) umbilical tape, which is tied in a bow, leaving sufficient space for feces to be passed.

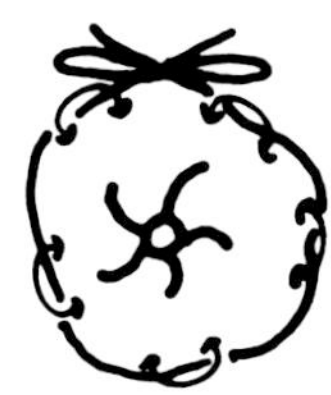

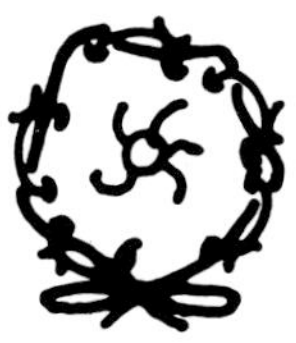

6.19 Placement of purse-string suture for prolapsed rectum.

The author has not had occasion to perform a submucosal resection or amputation of a necrotic segment of the rectum in a camelid, but presumably this could be done with techniques recommended for cattle or sheep (10).

POSTSURGICAL CARE. The patient should be observed for passage of feces and persistent tenesmus. The bow may be released when straining ceases, but the loops should be left in place in case the prolapse recurs.

COMPLICATIONS. Stricture of the rectum or anus may occur from trauma to the mucosa, but stricture more frequently develops following amputation. Peritonitis, resulting from dehiscence of the suture line, is a possible complication.

Rectal Laceration

CAUSES. Laceration of the rectal mucosa or of the entire wall usually occurs during rectal palpation. Veterinarians with large hands or arms have difficulty in conducting a thorough rectal examination because of the small size of the pelvis, rectum, and colon of SACs. Llamas are not as prone to laceration as equine species nor as resistant to rectal trauma as cattle. Incidents of rectal laceration and perforation have been reported at meetings.

In one instance, an epidural had been given to allow a more thorough examination. While the operator's hand was in the colon, a spasm of the colon clamped the wall around the wrist. Any attempt to withdraw the hand met with resistance, and had force been applied, the mucosa would surely have split. Ten minutes elapsed before the spasm relaxed.

Strong peristaltic waves may push against the hand. The palpator must give and take with these waves. A sudden movement of the animal, such as falling or rearing, when the rectum is under tension may result in a perforation.

CLINICAL SIGNS. The palpator may be able to feel the split occur, but usually the first indication is when the hand is withdrawn and a large quantity of blood is seen on or in the hand. It is not unusual or dangerous to see a few streaks of blood on the back of the wrist when the hand is withdrawn, especially with a large hand. The anus may be the limiting orifice, and if a rectal examination proceeds without adequate lubrication or relaxation with an epidural, the anal epithelium may be stretched beyond its flexibility, resulting in tiny fissures. After a prolonged examination, the mucosa may be slightly abraded and a small quantity of blood will be seen on the fingers. Neither of these conditions should be confused with the large quantity seen if a laceration has occurred.

If the laceration is not detected at the time of palpation, the progression of the syndrome will depend on the severity of the lesion. A small mucosal laceration may heal without incident, or streaks of fresh blood may be seen on some of the fecal pellets. In mares, a mucosal laceration may enlarge and penetrate both the muscularis and the serosa. Insufficient numbers of llamas have been studied to know if this occurs in llamas.

If the laceration perforates the colonic or rectal wall, peritonitis will ensue. Signs indicative of peritonitis will appear within 24–36 hours. Without treatment the animal will die in 5–7 days.

If a laceration is suspected, it is unwise to reenter the rectum to investigate. An epidural and an equine plastic or cardboard vaginal speculum may be used to visualize the rectum without imposing excessive further stretching of the mucosa.

PRESURGICAL PREPARATION. Rectal laceration is an emergency. Parenteral administration of broad-spectrum antibiotics should be begun as soon as a laceration is suspected.

ANESTHESIA. Evaluation and suturing via the anus will necessitate epidural or general anesthesia.

SURGERY. The peritoneal reflection is located approximately 10–15 cm from the anus. A penetration caudad to that location will be retroperitoneal. The rectum and colon cranial to the reflection have an outer serosal layer.

Fecal pellets should be gently removed from the rectum and the rectum packed cranially with cotton or gauze to avoid subsequent contamination of the field. The mucosa should be carefully but gently cleaned with physiologic saline, taking precautions to avoid enlarging the laceration. A dilute (1:10) povidone-iodine solution may be used to provide some degree of asepsis.

If it is determined that the laceration penetrates only the mucosa and is less than 1 cm in length, no treatment may be needed other than parenteral administration of broad-spectrum antibiotics for 7–10 days. Lacerations longer than 1 cm or penetrating the muscle layers should be sutured. It will be difficult to obtain exposure via the anus. If the laceration is within 10–15 cm of the anus, a human plastic vaginal speculum, with a spoon length of 10 cm, may provide access to the surgical site.

A mucosal laceration may be closed with simple interrupted sutures using swedged, taperpoint needles and vicryl suture. Picking up the underlying muscle layer will add strength to each suture.

If the laceration has penetrated the bowel wall, a laparotomy should be performed. Since this is an emergency procedure, it will not be possible to fast the llama to partially empty the stomach. Exposure of the surgical site will be the major problem. A high-flank incision would put the surgeon in the closest proximity to the colon and rectum, but unless both the external and internal abdominal oblique muscles are transected, there will not be sufficient exposure to operate. If the patient is a pregnant female, especially if she is in advanced pregnancy, the flank approach will be mandated.

The caudal colon and cranial rectum may be approached from a ventral midline incision. If there is extensive fecal contamination or peritonitis is already present, the prognosis is unfavorable.

Any fecal contamination should be alleviated before closure is attempted. The defect should be closed with an infolding Lembert or Cushing pattern using absorbable suture. Particulate matter should be removed manually and the abdominal cavity flushed with physiologic saline in sufficient quantities to remove any residual contamination. A final flushing with povidone-iodine solution (diluted 1:10) is important. Placing an intestinal clamp (carmalt) on the laceration may prevent further contamination.

Broad-spectrum antibiotics should be administered for 7–10 days postsurgery. The abdominal wall may be closed as for any laparotomy.

POSTSURGICAL CARE. Little can be done to soften the stool without giving a laxative, which is contraindicated, since it would stimulate increased peristaltic activity. Enemas are also contraindicated, since the fluid could seep through the incision and the pressure would be detrimental to healing.

The patient should be monitored for signs of peritonitis. A hemogram should be performed at least every other day for 6 days.

COMPLICATIONS. Peritonitis is the most serious sequel. A rectal stricture is also possible.

Atresia Ani/Coli

Atresia ani or coli is a congenital/hereditary defect of the neonate in which the anal opening is lacking or there is a stricture in the rectum or colon. Both forms have been reported in llamas and alpacas. Since this may be a hereditary condition, the implications should be discussed with the client. These animals should not be used as breeders.

CLINICAL SIGNS. Abdominal distention and straining to defecate are the primary signs. In atresia ani, the absence of the anal opening is apparent and there is usually a bulge at the anus. The signs will be noted within a few days of birth.

Atresia coli is more difficult to detect, depending on how far cranially the lesion is located. Digital palpation may locate a lesion in the rectum, but a barium enema may be required to determine the site of a lesion farther forward in the colon. It is possible for an older animal to acquire a rectal or anal stricture and develop the same clinical signs.

ANESTHESIA. Sufficient anesthesia for the correction of atresia ani may be achieved by infiltration of local anesthetic into the operative site. General anesthesia is required for repair of atresia coli, which necessitates a laparotomy.

SURGERY. With atresia ani, a circular disc of skin approximately 2 cm in diameter should be removed from the center of the bulge. Feces may be allowed to escape by puncturing the rectal mucosa. The opening may be enlarged as seems appropriate. The mucosa should be sutured to the skin using vicryl or chromic gut.

Strictures within the rectum are difficult if not impossible to reach surgically. Strictures farther forward in the colon may be corrected by laparotomy and intestinal resection.

POSTSURGICAL CARE. To maintain patency the orifice should be stretched at least every other day for 2 weeks.

COMPLICATIONS. Colonic or anal stricture is the most important adverse sequel. If there is no anal sphincter, the animal will be incontinent.

REPRODUCTIVE SYSTEM (19)

Cesarean Section

INDICATIONS. A cesarean section is indicated when the fetus is unable to traverse the birth canal. The fetus may be enlarged (emphysema or anasarca) or malformed (ankylosis of carpus or tarsus, schistosomas reflexus).

If an immature female is bred accidentally (cases are on record in which a female has become pregnant at 5 months), parturition will occur before the pelvis and the genital tract have reached maturity. The cervix may fail to relax and dilate properly, or the uterus may clamp around the fetus so tightly that forced extraction will rupture the uterine wall. A fetal mummy lacks flexibility, and the cervix may not relax sufficiently to allow expulsion of a mummified fetus.

Narrowing of the birth canal may occur as a result of previous trauma, causing fibrosis and stenosis, or from pelvic tumors. Uncorrected uterine torsion mandates a cesarean section. In addition, prolonged manipulation may jeopardize the life of the fetus, and a cesarean may be appropriate to obviate the threat.

CLINICAL SIGNS AND DIAGNOSIS. There are no unique clinical manifestations or diagnostic procedures.

POSITION. Dorsal recumbency is required for the ventral midline approach. For a flank incision, lateral recumbency with the animal lying on its left side is appropriate.

PRESURGICAL PREPARATION. A cesarean section is usually an emergency operation, thus preparation will be limited by time and available facilities. The best possible standard of surgical preparation should be followed.

ANESTHESIA. General anesthesia is necessary for a cesarian section.

SURGERY

Right- or Left-Flank Approach. The low-flank area is devoid of muscle mass and should be avoided. A midflank incision is appropriate. The laparotomy technique has been described earlier. There is no greater omental sling to bypass, so it is easy to grasp and exteriorize the pregnant uterine horn. Ninety percent of SAC pregnancies will be in the left uterine horn.

The uterine wall should be incised on the greater curvature, avoiding large vessels. The fetal membrane arrangement in camelids differs from that of other artiodactylids (see Chap. 17). With a cranial presentation, the hind limbs will be encountered first in the uterus; they may be grasped to deliver the fetus. A clamp should be placed on the umbilicus. The uterine-chorial attachment is minimal, and it may be possible to deliver the placental membranes through the uterine incision. If much pressure must be exerted to free the placenta, it should be left in situ for later vaginal delivery. The second horn of the uterus should always be examined for the presence of a twin. Any uterine torsion should be corrected and the uterus palpated externally for possible uterine rupture.

The uterine incision may be closed with one or two layers using a Lembert or Cushing infolding suture pattern and any absorbable suture. The uterus should be replaced in the abdominal cavity and the cavity flushed with physiologic saline if there has been contamination with infected fetal fluids. The presence of uninfected amniotic or allantoic fluid in the peritoneal cavity is not harmful.

The abdominal wall may be closed as for a laparotomy.

Ventral Midline Approach. The initial incision should be made from the cranial border of the mammary gland forward for a distance of 30 cm. The operation may then proceed as for the flank approach.

POSTSURGICAL CARE. If dystocia was prolonged, or significant manipulation occurred before the decision to perform a cesarean section was made, it may be necessary to treat for endometritis or metritis. Oxytocin (30 units) should be administered intravenously to stimulate uterine contraction, expel the placenta, and assist in hemorrhage control. Oxytocin should not be administered until the uterus has been sutured and replaced inside the abdomen; 1–2 g tetracycline powder may be inserted in the uterine horn at the time of surgery. Boluses are contraindicated, since these may stimulate straining. Excessive soft-tissue trauma or microbial contamination may indicate the administration of parenteral antibiotics for 5 days postsurgery.

COMPLICATIONS. Retained placenta, metritis, endometritis, peritonitis, and herniation at the incision site are potential complications.

Ovariohysterectomy

INDICATIONS. A uterine rupture with severe trauma to the uterus may be an indication for hysterectomy. In one case, small fetal mummies were identified by rectal palpation. A hysterotomy was performed and three partially developed fetal mummies were found firmly embedded in the uterine mucosa. These were removed with difficulty. Postsurgically, this female suffered from a prolonged chronic metritis and, ultimately, hysterectomy was required.

One of the more common congenital anomalies of the reproductive tract of llamas and alpacas is segmental aplasia of the tubular tract anywhere along its length, preventing egress of normal uterine secretions. In such cases, uterine fluids accumulate, resulting in enlargement of the uterine horn, simulating pyometra. Eight to ten liters of milky fluid have been drained from some long-standing cases. See Chapter 22 for a more detailed discussion of this condition. Ovariohysterectomy is indicated to enable use of the animal for a pet, packer, or fiber production.

Various experimental protocols may require either ovariectomy or ovariohysterectomy.

POSITION. Dorsal or lateral recumbency may be appropriate, but dorsal recumbency is required if the cervix is to be extirpated.

PRESURGICAL PREPARATION. As in other elective procedures, the animal should be fasted for 24–48 hours.

ANESTHESIA. General anesthesia is required.

SURGERY. Surgery should be from the ventral midline approach. The skin incision should begin just cranial to the mammary gland and extend forward 30–40 cm. The mammary gland should be reflected caudally for better exposure for penetration of the abdominal wall as close to the pelvis as possible. Both uterine horns should be exteriorized.

Fluid may be drained from the uterus with a large-bore needle attached to a flexible tube for gravity drainage or attached to a suction apparatus. More rapid drainage may be accomplished by insertion of a suction head through an incision in the uterine wall. For this procedure, a purse-string suture is placed at the intended site. With the suction head ready, a stab incision is made and the head quickly inserted through the opening. The purse string should be tightened around the suction head with a single throw and the tension held with a hemostat. Following removal of the uterine contents, the suction head should be removed and the purse-string suture pulled tight.

The uterus may then be manipulated to isolate vessels and the cervix. The ovarian and cranial uterine arteries must be identified and double ligated. Other uterine vessels will be found in the broad ligament and on the ventral aspect of the uterus (Fig. 6.20). These arteries and veins should also be secured by double ligation.

Following ligation of the vessels, the uterine ligaments may be transected to expose the vagina just distal to the cervix. Even with marked enlargement of the uterus, the cervix will lie close over the brim of the pelvis or within the pelvis. Visualization of the vagina will be enhanced if the animal can be tilted forward by

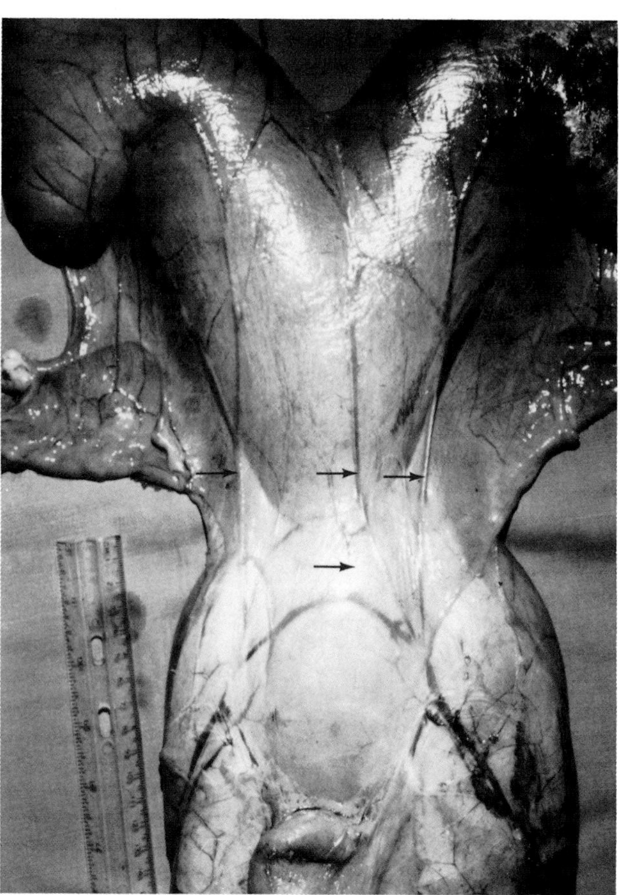

6.20 Mucometria, ventral view, emphasizing vascular distribution.

raising the hindquarters, but it is difficult to achieve the desired exposure.

The vagina should be closed with overlapping mattress sutures and No. 2 or 3 gut or other absorbable sutures of a similar size. Amputation of the reproductive tract proximal to the mattress sutures is best. Simple interrupted sutures may be used to approximate the serosal surfaces of the stump. A final check for hemorrhage should be made before closing the abdomen as described previously.

Routine monitoring during surgery is necessary, since shock may ensue from the removal of such a large organ.

POSTSURGICAL CARE. Standard postsurgical regimens are recommended, as for any laparotomy. Since uterine fluid is not infected, there is no indication for parenteral antibiotics if surgical asepsis is maintained.

Persistent or Imperforate Hymen

DIAGNOSIS. It is critical that this condition be differentiated from segmental aplasia of the vagina. A persistent hymen may be only one manifestation of a continuum of congenital anomalies of the tubular genital tract of the llama and alpaca. Since, in certain breeds of cattle, such anomalies are considered to be hereditary (19), the veterinarian should consider the ethical implications of performing surgery to permit breeding, especially if it is likely that the female is to be sold as a breeder.

Persistence of a segment of hymen may present a stricture at the vulvovaginal junction. This may be discovered by digital palpation. The orifice may be enlarged by gentle finger pressure. The urethral opening on the floor of the vulva should be identified either by digital palpation or inspection with a vaginal speculum before the hymen is manipulated. A small heifer speculum may then be used to enlarge the orifice further to visualize the cervix.

An imperforate hymen may be indicated by a bulge in the vulva caused by the accumulation of fluid in the vagina and uterus. On palpation, this may resemble palpation of a fluid-filled balloon. It may be thought that the hymen should break at breeding, but the male llama does not have a vigorous pelvic thrust, and penile penetration may be easily deterred by even a slight obstruction. In at least one case, the penis was deflected into the urethra. When penetration by the male was checked for by the breeder, it was noted that the urethra was markedly dilated. The female lacked a vagina; there was no passageway beyond the hymen.

INDICATIONS. An imperforate hymen will result in the accumulation of uterine secretions, just as in segmental aplasia of the vagina. Rupture of the hymen and maintenance of patency allows drainage of the fluid and avoidance of the complications of a prolonged distention of the uterus.

POSITION. The animal should be standing, with the tail secured up over the back or to the side, out of the perineal area.

ANESTHESIA. Usually, none is necessary, but an epidural using 1–2 ml 2% lidocaine will provide anesthesia if required.

SURGERY. The membrane may be easily ruptured by a quick thrust with a finger. A membrane too thick to rupture with finger pressure requires surgical intervention. The lips of the vulva may be spread, or a short speculum may be used to allow visualization of the hymen. A stab incision, enlarged with a finger or forceps, is recommended. Palpation proximal to the hymen should ascertain the size of the lumen. The orifice may be enlarged by lateral incisions in the form of a cross or by a circular incision to remove a segment of the hymen.

POSTSURGICAL CARE. It is important to maintain the patency of the orifice by continual stretching during the healing process. Otherwise, contraction and scarring will negate the benefits of the surgery. Stretching may be accomplished by insertion of a heifer vaginal speculum once or twice daily for 10 days.

COMPLICATIONS. Reclosure and stenosis of the vulvovaginal junction are the major complications. It may be possible to make an opening in the tract large enough to allow penetration by the male to inseminate the female. If, however, stenosis develops at the hymenal area, dystocia is probable.

Prolapse of the Vagina

CAUSE. Vaginal prolapse is usually associated with pregnancy. In cattle, it often occurs at 2–3 months of pregnancy, at about the stage in which the placenta begins to secrete estrogens, inducing relaxation of the pelvic structure (19). Insufficient records have been kept to correlate similar happenings in camelids.

Prolapse occurs more frequently in multiparous females, indicating that stretching or injury to the pelvic structures as a result of a previous birth may predispose to vaginal prolapse. In cattle and some other species, it is thought that a hereditary factor may be involved and also that some animals may produce more estrogens than others (19).

Obesity, with excessive pelvic fat, may produce increased abdominal pressure while an animal is lying down. A preexisting relaxation of the pelvic structure could also contribute to vaginal prolapse.

Vaginal prolapse is a complication of parturition, particularly if dystocia has resulted in excessive manipulation of the fetus.

CLINICAL SIGNS. A slight prolapse of the mucous membrane of the vagina is sometimes seen during pregnancy near term, especially when the female is lying down. The membrane is usually pink, moist, and glistening, with no evidence of pathology. If the bulge disappears when the female rises, no treatment is indicated. However, a continually exposed membrane may become traumatized by the tail or become dry and necrotic.

The entire vagina may be exteriorized by persistent tenesmus. Edema or pressure may obstruct the urethra and cause urine retention. Other caudal abdominal organs may prolapse through the vulva via rents in the uterine or vaginal wall.

POSITION. The llama should be standing, if possible, with the hindquarters elevated.

PRESURGICAL PREPARATION. An extensively prolapsed vagina should be wrapped with a moistened bath towel and encased in a plastic bag to keep the membrane moist and avoid trauma and infection.

ANESTHESIA. Epidural anesthesia is recommended.

SURGERY. The extent of the prolapse and degree of trauma to the mucous membrane will determine treatment. The membrane should be thoroughly cleansed with physiologic saline and povidone-iodine solution (diluted 1:10). Any foreign material must be physically removed, and obviously necrotic tissue should be debrided. The vagina may be cupped in the hands and gently pushed back into place with the palms. Point pressure with the fingers should be avoided. The invagination must continue past the lips of the vulva. A person with small hands may be able to push beyond the vulva with bent fingers. A plastic or cardboard mare speculum may be gently inserted to complete the inversion process if the operator's hand and arm are too large to enter the female.

It is usually necessary to suture the lips of the vulva closed to prevent recurrence until the edema and inflammatory response have dissipated. The vulva is small, and a simple purse-string suture may be sufficient. However, the author prefers a lacing technique similar to those used on cattle.

In this technique, two or three loop sutures are placed on either side of the vulva, 2 cm lateral to the vulvar slit. Excessive slack should not be left in these loops (Fig. 6.21). The loops are threaded like a shoe is laced, using 3 mm (⅛ in.) umbilical tape, and tied in a bow. The animal will be able to urinate. The threaded strand may be loosened or even removed to ascertain the degree of healing but can be easily replaced if the prolapse threatens to recur.

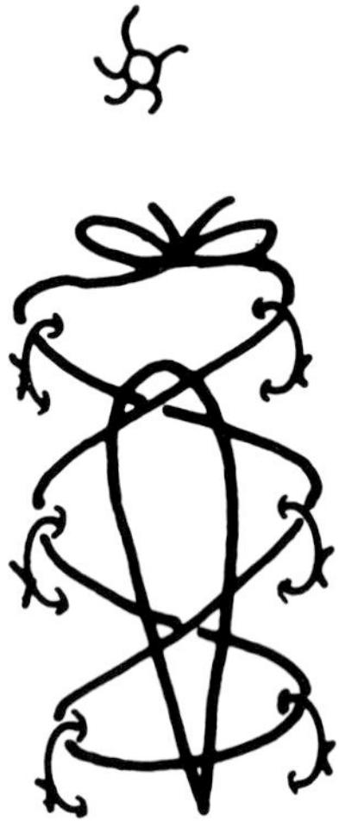

6.21 Truss (shoelace) pattern for retention of vaginal prolapse.

If this procedure is carried out on a pregnant female who is nearing the end of term, the female must be closely observed so that the lacing can be removed as parturition begins.

Sprinkling the swollen membrane with sugar to reduce edema of a prolapsed vagina is a time-honored practice, and there is little doubt that fluid can be removed in this manner. However, theriogenologists believe that as well as being hygroscopic, the sharp sugar granules traumatize the friable mucous membrane, allowing the escape of vital fluid (19).

It may be desirable to insert a catheter and instill a solution containing powdered tetracycline into the vagina, but an antibacterial bolus should not be inserted, since it may stimulate tenesmus.

POSTSURGICAL CARE. The animal should be observed closely for signs of continuing tenesmus or significant exudation.

COMPLICATIONS. The major complication is recurrence of the prolapse; however, vaginitis and even metritis may follow a prolapse. If tenesmus persists, the vagina should be reexamined to assure that the prolapse was completely repositioned.

Prolapse of the Uterus

CAUSE. Much of the discussion relative to vaginal prolapse applies to uterine prolapse. Prolonged and intense tenesmus induced by a retained placenta is a common cause. The uterus has also been known to prolapse during attempted delivery of the placenta immediately following parturition. Following an exhausting dystocia, a completely atonic uterus may prolapse through the relaxed vagina.

CLINICAL SIGNS. The protrusion of the inverted uterus is obvious. In camelids, there are no cotyledons on the placenta. It may be somewhat difficult to differentiate uterine from vaginal mucosa, but it should be possible to identify the cervical rings.

POSITION. Same as for vaginal prolapse.

ANESTHESIA. Same as for vaginal prolapse.

SURGERY. The procedures outlined for vaginal prolapse should be followed. However, it may first be necessary to deliver the placenta. Any portion of the placenta that remains should be delivered. The attachment is minimal, and delivery should not be difficult. It is more difficult to reduce the telescoping, because of the small size of the canal, but immediately after parturition, even a person with large hands can manually reposition the uterus, taking care to evert both horns. If the prolapse occurs at any other time, it may be repositioned only by a person with small hands and arms. As soon as the uterus is replaced, 30–50 units of oxytocin should be administered intravenously or intramuscularly to stimulate contraction of the uterine muscle.

A truss suture pattern may be employed to ensure retention of the uterus, but in many cases this will not be necessary. The animal should be observed closely for tenesmus and reexamined if it persists.

Rupture of the Uterus

CAUSE. In SACs, rupture of the uterus is usually associated with dystocia. Prolonged, hard contractions of the uterine musculature against an immovable fetus may result in a rent in the wall of the uterus. Other causes include uterine torsion and an oversized fetus. A limb may be pressed through the wall if a carpus or tarsus has become ankylosed and inflexible. Chronic peritonitis associated with uterine adhesions may result in a tear in the uterine wall when the contractions of parturition begin. Severe trauma to the abdomen near term may cause a rupture of the uterus.

CLINICAL SIGNS. External signs may be minimal and consist only of knowledge that dystocia has occurred. Frequently, the rent will be palpated after the fetus has been delivered and the uterus is being checked for a twin. If the rupture is not detected at parturition, it may be indicated as signs of peritonitis develop.

POSITION. Dorsal recumbency is the preferred position for surgery.

ANESTHESIA. General anesthesia is required.

SURGERY. The surgical approach to correct a uterine tear is similar to that used for hysterectomy. Hemorrhage in the peritoneal cavity or peritonitis may be present. Since the tear may be in the body of the uterus near the cervix or in the uterine horn, careful palpation is necessary. A tear in the body is more difficult to visualize and suture.

A Lembert or Cushing infolding suture, as in a cesarean section, is satisfactory for closing the tear. The abdominal cavity should be lavaged with physiologic saline and treated as appropriate to prevent or alleviate peritonitis. The abdominal incision is closed as described previously.

A novel technique for suturing a uterine tear in cattle has been described but not yet tried in a llama. With this technique, if the rent is detected during or immediately following parturition, a hand and arm is inserted into the tip of the lacerated horn. An assistant administers 4–6 ml 1:1000 epinephrine HCl intravenously to induce relaxation of the uterine musculature. When the surgeon feels relaxation begin, the tip of the horn is grasped by the fingers and slowly everted and pulled through the vagina. The laceration may then be sutured outside the body and the uterus returned to its proper position. Oxytocin (20 units) should be administered to stimulate contraction of the uterus following the surgery.

POSTSURGICAL CARE. Standard laparotomy protocol is appropriate. A 5- to 10-day course of antibiotics, given parenterally, is indicated to prevent or treat metritis and peritonitis.

COMPLICATIONS. If one of the large uterine arteries is ruptured concurrently, intraabdominal hemorrhage may result in exsanguination or severe anemia.

Anemia would not be detectable via a hemogram for a few days after the incident. Peritonitis is a common sequel, along with metritis.

Laparoscopy

INDICATIONS. To date, laparoscopy has been used only as an experimental tool to observe ovarian function (24). However, it may have application in diagnosis of chronic infertility in conjunction with ultrasonography, rectal palpation, and hormone profiles.

POSITION. Laparoscopy in North America is usually conducted in the standing position from the right flank. In South America, experimental animals are physically restrained in dorsal recumbency on a surgical table that can be tilted vertically, with the animal in a head-down position. With the llama in dorsal recumbency, the penetration site is on the ventral midline near the umbilicus or 3–5 cm cranial to the mammary gland (24). Two penetration sites may be necessary, one for the fiberoptic scope and the other to admit forceps to manipulate structures.

ANESTHESIA. Mild sedation with xylazine HCl (0.1 mg/kg), followed by butorphanol (0.05–0.1 mg/kg), will quiet the animal yet allow it to remain standing. The insertion site for the laparoscope should be infiltrated with a local anesthetic.

SURGERY. For the standing approach, the right flank is selected because C-1 of the stomach would obscure the field on the left side. The appropriate site is 10–15 cm ventral to the transverse processes of the lumbar vertebrae and 10–15 cm cranial to the tuber coxae. The kidney may be traumatized if the penetration site is too far dorsal to the recommended site. The insertion site should be clipped and aseptically prepared for surgery.

Standard laparoscopy procedures are employed, which will vary with the instruments available. The anatomy of the camelid reproductive tract should be reviewed before initiating laparoscopy (see Chap. 17). The camelid ovary is enveloped within a bursa that must be lifted from the ovary before it can be visualized.

Observation of the left ovary is more difficult but is possible from the right side. In dorsal recumbency, the ovaries are equally accessible.

Castration

INDICATION. In addition to the usual indications for castration as seen in livestock, castration is highly recommended for llama male crias that must be hand raised. Bottle-raised crias or crias having close human contact may be imprinted on humans and become aggressive as adults. These animals should be castrated before sexual maturity, preferably before 2 months of age. The gonads are usually present in the scrotum at birth, and castration may be performed as early as 2 weeks of age and any time thereafter.

POSITION. For a right-handed surgeon, lateral recumbency with the right side up is recommended. The upper leg should be tied to the neck and the tail tied to the fleece over the back.

ANESTHESIA. Xylazine (0.3 mg/kg intravenously), with local anesthetic infiltration of the skin 3–5 cm cranial to the scrotum on either side of the median raphe, is satisfactory. If sedation is insufficient, IV ketamine (2–5 mg/kg) may be administered.

SURGERY. Numerous methods have been employed in castrating llamas (23). Any standard method recommended for livestock is suitable. The author's preferred method will be described first, with variations of the technique to follow.

With the animal in lateral recumbency, two 4 cm incisions should be made 3–5 cm cranial to the scrotum and 1 cm to the right and left of the median raphe. Blunt dissection may be used to isolate the spermatic cord. The penis should be palpated to avoid exteriorizing it. A finger may be placed under the cord to lift it out of the incision, pulling the testicle forward from the scrotum. The testicle should be grasped in one hand and the fat stripped from the tunic as far craniad as possible (toward the external inguinal ring).

A transfixation ligature should be placed around the tunic near the external ring and the cord transected with either an emasculator or a scalpel. Alternatively, an incision may be made through the common tunic longitudinally to isolate the vessels and the ductus deferens, which should be ligated separately, transected, and released. Then the common tunic should be ligated.

After both testicles have been removed, the incisions should be plucked to remove any strings of fat that may protrude from the incisions after the animal rises. Any pockets may be eliminated to assure unimpaired drainage. Incisions are not sutured.

POSTSURGICAL CARE. Administration of antibiotics is unnecessary, and equine-origin tetanus antitoxin serum is not recommended. Swelling is rare. Since llamas do not lie in their own feces, the incision remains clean. It is recommended that the llama be returned to pasture or kept in a clean, straw-bedded box stall.

ALTERNATIVE TECHNIQUES

1. The same procedure may be followed, except incisions are sutured as in a canine castration. Surgical asepsis must be employed throughout.

2. The initial incision may be made through the scrotum. Using a closed technique, the testicle and surrounding tunics are isolated and separated from the surrounding fascia as far craniad as possible. An open technique may also be performed, in which case the common tunic is incised, freeing the testicle, epididymis, and ductus deferens. The ductus deferens and other vessels should be ligated prior to transection. The common tunic is left in situ.

3. Standing castration. The llama should be placed in a narrow stock or squeeze chute, with the tail held or secured up over the back. The area should be surgically prepared, with local anesthesia administered subcutaneously over each scrotal sac. Additional local anesthetic may be injected into the spermatic cord, craniad to the scrotum. An open procedure is employed, with incisions left unsutured.

Cryptorchid Castration

Cryptorchidism is one of many genetic malformations of the llama and alpaca male reproductive system (see Table 22.5). Only rarely has the cryptic gonad been retained in the abdominal cavity. More frequently, the gonad has been located in the fascia, anywhere from the external inguinal ring to near the scrotum and alongside the penis. In a few cases, the gonad has been located in the subcutaneous fascia on the medial aspect of the rear limb. The cryptic gonad may be difficult to palpate, since it may be only 0.5–1 cm in diameter.

Since cryptorchidism is a genetic trait, such an animal should not be used for breeding, and both the cryptic and normal testicles should be removed. Bilateral cryptorchidism is extremely rare.

SURGERY. The cryptic gonad should be located and an incision made where necessary to amputate. If the gonad is intraabdominal and the side can be identified, a paralumbar fossa grid approach may be used after incising the skin. If it is impossible to determine the appropriate side, the abdomen may be entered via the ventral midline approach.

Vasectomy

INDICATIONS. The primary purpose for vasectomy is to facilitate study of reproductive physiology. Vasectomized males can be used to check females for pregnancy or to induce ovulation without fertilization.

SURGERY. Since the scrotum is not pendulous, the spermatic cord is not as accessible as it is in the bull or ram. An incision is made cranial to the scrotum, similar to a castration incision. The spermatic cord is isolated and exteriorized. The tunic is incised and the ductus deferens isolated. Ligatures are placed 2 cm apart, and the segment between the sutures is excised. The tunic should be sutured with simple interrupted observable sutures.

Alternatively, a 2 cm segment of the ductus deferens may be excised via standard laparoscopy using a forceps scissors (22).

URINARY SYSTEM

Ruptured Urinary Bladder

INDICATIONS. A rent in the wall of the urinary bladder may result from overdistention of the bladder, usually caused by partial or complete obstruction of the urethra. This is most likely to occur in the male and has been diagnosed in male llamas as young as 6 weeks of age as well as in adults. It is not known whether seepage of urine from a grossly distended bladder occurs in llamas as it does in cattle.

Another major cause of bladder rupture is trauma, especially if it occurs when the bladder is full. Two instances have been reported. In the first, a female llama had been transported in a trailer for a considerable distance and immediately used as a model to demonstrate a portable restraining stock, without being given an opportunity to urinate. The stock included two belly bands and a band over the back to prevent the llama from rearing or lying down. During the course of the demonstration, the llama struggled vigorously against the restraint. The llama died two days later despite treatment for depression and a supposed digestive disturbance. At necropsy, a rent in the bladder wall was observed.

The second instance of bladder trauma occurred during rectal palpation for fertility evaluation. On initial entry, it was determined that the bladder was distended, making it difficult to palpate the genital tract. Digital pressure was exerted over the dorsal surface of the bladder through the rectum in an attempt to manually express urine. The clinician felt the distention suddenly dissipate and immediately realized that the bladder had ruptured. Almost instantaneously, the llama became extremely disturbed, began to vocalize, climbed out of the restraining stock, and threw herself to the floor, jumping up again after rolling. The clinical signs were those of violent colic; apparently, the rapid flow of urine into the peritoneal cavity was excruciatingly painful.

In retrospect, it seems possible that the violent struggling of the llama, restrained by bands in the stock, occurred after the bladder had ruptured, not before.

DIAGNOSIS. Uremic signs in the llama are not definitive. Except at the initial flush of urine into the peritoneal cavity, as previously described, signs of colic have not been seen. Depression and anorexia, with cessation of stomach motility, may be seen. Blood urea nitrogen levels become elevated to 50–100 mg/dl as the condition worsens. The abdomen is not likely to be distended, but fluid will be obtained by abdominocentesis, if done correctly.

The most precise method of determining the presence of urine in the peritoneal cavity is by analysis of fluid aspirate for potassium. Normal peritoneal fluid or exudate has a potassium concentration of 4–5 mEq/L, similar to that of serum. Urine has a concentration of 50–150 mEq/L. Odor and color are not sufficiently precise indicators, but urea nitrogen determinations are indicative. Another positive indication is detection of urate crystals in the peritoneal fluid.

POSITION. The animal should be placed in dorsal recumbency. Although the distended bladder is intraabdominal, the contracted bladder will lie partially within the pelvis or at the brim of the pelvis. A caudal midline approach is necessary to expose all surfaces of the bladder.

PRESURGICAL PREPARATION. Standard surgical asepsis should be practiced. The patency of the urethra must be determined either preceding or during surgery. See Chapter 18 for descriptions of anatomy and catheterization.

ANESTHESIA. General. The uremic patient is an anesthetic risk and should be monitored closely. Hyperkalemia may predispose the development of cardiac arrhythmia, particularly if halothane inhalation anesthesia is chosen. IV fluid should be saline rather than Ringer's solution.

SURGERY. The abdominal wall should be penetrated as near the pubis as possible. All surfaces of the bladder must be inspected for rents, since multiple rents are possible. The rents previously described were found on the dorsal aspect of the body of the bladder, but experience in other species indicates that ruptures may occur at the neck or elsewhere in the body of the bladder.

Before closing the defect, the patency of the urethra should be established via retrograde catheterization of the external urethral orifice or by passing a catheter distally through the bladder. A double layer, continuous infolding suture pattern, using 00 gut, is recommended to close the bladder wall.

The abdominal cavity should be irrigated with warm physiologic saline to remove all traces of urine. Unless secondarily infected, urine will not cause peritonitis.

The abdominal incision should be closed as previously described. This surgical procedure is also recommended for removal of cystic calculi and tumors.

POSTSURGICAL CARE. Postsurgical care is routine. Urine output should be monitored.

Urethral Obstruction

CLINICAL SIGNS. The severity of the clinical signs associated with obstruction of the urethra will be determined by the duration of the obstruction. In early stages, with distention of the bladder, the animal will strain as if to defecate (Fig. 6.22). The posture for urination and defecation are essentially the same in a llama. Other colicky signs may be noted as well.

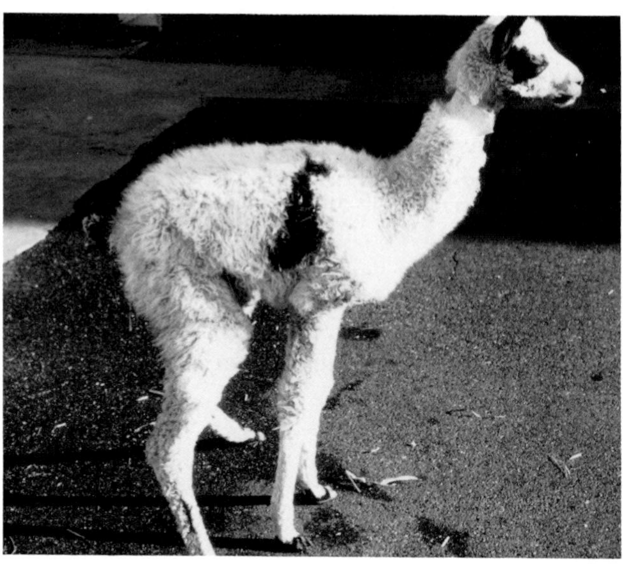

6.22 Stance of a llama cria with urethral obstruction from a urolith.

On rectal palpation, the enlarged, tense bladder should be obvious. It is not likely that obstructions of the urethra can be palpated. If the bladder has ruptured, initial signs of severe colic will be followed by general uremia.

DIAGNOSIS. Urethral obstruction is primarily a male disorder. In animals less than 6 months of age, it will be difficult to locate the urethral opening because of preputial adhesions to the glans penis. Catheterization will be difficult.

The hemogram in early stages of the disorder is normal. If the obstruction persists, creatinine and blood urea nitrogen levels will become elevated and a leukocytosis and left shift may be evident in the differential cell count.

Radiography of the pelvic area is indicated, but some uroliths are not radiopaque. In one of the author's cases, the stone was composed of urate salts and could not be seen on radiographs, either of the animal or when the stones were placed on a cassette after removal from the urethra. In addition to the urate stone, the author has also removed a stone composed of unoriented crystals of 90% hydroxyl apatite and 10% struvite and silicate.

Stones may be located in the sigmoid flexure of the penis, but a more frequently encountered site is at the point where the urethra narrows near its distal end. In a 3-month-old llama, this point was 7 cm from the external urethral orifice, while in an adult male it may be as much as 12 cm from the orifice. This location coincides with the area of preputial reflection, not where the urethra enters the glans. To the author's knowledge, there have been no reports of obstruction in the short urethral process of the penis. If the obstruction is located in the pelvic urethra, it will not be possible to pass a catheter around the ischial arch and on into the bladder.

In a 6-week-old neonate, a 3.5 French catheter was passed to the ischial arch but could not be forced beyond it. Radiographs were taken, but no urolith was seen. A laparotomy was performed and a rupture of the bladder detected and closed. Signs of urinary obstruction recurred. A pelvic urethrostomy was performed. Urine flowed freely from a catheter placed in the bladder. A 3.5 French catheter was passed distally past the external urethral orifice, followed by passage distally of a 5 French catheter. Resistance was noted as the larger catheter reached the location of the narrowing of the urethra, but it was possible to continue on to the orifice. In the process, a urate urolith was pushed out of the urethra. The 3.5 French catheter had passed around the urolith.

PRESURGICAL PREPARATION. The perineal area over and ventral to the ischial arch should be prepared for aseptic surgery.

ANESTHESIA. In cattle and sheep, this procedure is usually performed under epidural anesthesia, supplemented with local infiltration if necessary. This technique could be attempted in the llama, but general anesthesia is more suitable to permit the various manipulations necessary for location and surgical correction of the obstruction.

SURGERY. If the obstruction is located in the distal urethra, the incision should be made directly over the urethra. A catheter should be inserted up to the obstruction to identify the approximate incision site. If the bladder has ruptured or become atonic, urine flow may not resume immediately following removal of the obstruction. The catheter should be passed as far as possible to preclude the possibility of multiple uroliths. The urethra should not be sutured, to avoid inducing a urethral stricture.

Ischial urethrostomy may be performed as a temporary measure to aid in diagnosis or removal of a stone, or a permanent opening may be established if the urethra is severely traumatized and strictured distally. The incision must be made directly on the midline beginning at the ischial arch, extending ventrally 6 cm. The paired retractor penis muscles should be separated. The paired ischiocavernosus muscles are united on the midline by a firm fibrous layer that must be incised directly on the midline to minimize hemorrhage.

Insertion of a polypropylene catheter (5 French) as far as the ischial arch may be helpful in locating the urethra. At this point, the urethra is surrounded by the bulbospongiosus muscle and the corpus spongiosum urethra. The incision should continue into the lumen of the urethra, staying on the midline and fixing the urethra with fingers or forceps to avoid incising alongside the urethra into the corpus cavernosum.

A catheter may then be inserted into the bladder or passed distally to locate the site of the obstruction. If necessary, an additional incision may be made over the distal obstruction to remove a urolith that will not pass with gentle catheter manipulation.

If the obstruction can be relieved, the urethrostomy should be considered temporary and not sutured. The skin incision must be more ventral than the opening into the urethra so as to avoid accumulation of urine in the subcutaneous tissue.

If the urethrostomy must be kept open, either for a period of time or permanently, the urethral mucosa should be sutured to the skin. If urine flow resumes, the urethra/skin sutures can be removed to permit healing.

POSTSURGICAL COMPLICATIONS. The condition(s) allowing formation of the urolith(s) may not have been corrected, or be correctable, with the result that obstruction may recur. Urethral stricture is a common ailment in SACs.

In all cases, it is important to establish whether or not the bladder is intact. If rupture has occurred, a laparotomy, with appropriate surgery, must be performed. Peritonitis is always a possible result of urinary leakage, especially if there is a concurrent bacterial cystitis. Urine may or may not be sterile, so leakage from a stretched or ruptured bladder may or may not initiate peritonitis.

POSTSURGICAL CARE. Urine scald of the skin may be prevented by daily cleaning and application of zinc oxide ointment surrounding the incision or in the direction of urine flow. Systemic antibiotics may be indicated. Close monitoring of urine flow and observation for signs of reobstruction and uremia are recommended.

Patent Urachus

INDICATIONS. Persistent patent urachus may be congenital, characterized by failure of the urachus to close at the time of birth. However, it may also be caused by reopening of the urachus as a result of omphalophlebitis (19). This distinction is critical to the prognosis. Perhaps it should be assumed that omphalophlebitis is present, with the patient treated accordingly with systemic antibiotics.

ANATOMY. The urachus connects the fetal bladder with the allantoic cavity of the fetal membranes, which serves as the receptacle for fetal urinary excretory products until after birth. The urachus is a thin-walled duct lined with columnar epithelium. Within the umbilical cord, the urachus is surrounded by two arteries and two veins. All four vessels are equally thick walled, and it is not possible to differentiate them grossly except by dissection to their origin within the neonate body.

POSITION. Both lateral and dorsal recumbency are appropriate.

PRESURGICAL PREPARATION. The umbilical stump should be cleansed and disinfected with povidone-iodine solution.

ANESTHESIA. This procedure is frequently performed with physical restraint only. Infiltration of local anesthetic agents will produce edema and possibly obstruct details of the surgical site. Furthermore, inflammatory response at the surgical site may negate the effects of local anesthetic agents.

Sedation with xylazine, or even general anesthesia, may be necessary if the umbilical stump has ruptured close to the body wall and it is necessary to explore into the abdominal cavity to locate and ligate the urachus.

SURGERY. If the urachus remains patent at birth it is possible to ligate the entire umbilicus or localize the urachus and ligate it directly. A patent urachus that develops a few days after birth is an indication that an umbilical infection has reopened the urachal stump. Vigorous therapy and surgery is then necessary to avoid the complications of omphalophlebitis and septic arthritis.

The neonate should be prepared for general anesthesia and the umbilicus evaluated. The surgeon should be prepared to perform a laparotomy in order to remove all infected tissue. The urachus should be traced to the bladder and amputated. The opening at the bladder should be closed with a double-layered Lembert or Cushing pattern.

Umbilical vessels should be identified and ligated proximal to healthy tissue and the diseased segments removed. Infection may have traveled along the umbilical veins to the liver. In this case, it is recommended that the infected tract be marsupialized to provide drainage and access for irrigation with povidone-iodine solution. Broad-spectrum antibiotics are appropriately administered when infection is present.

The neonate should be observed for evidence of urethral patency. If the owner observes urine issuing from the penis or vulva, no further treatment is indicated, but urine output should be carefully monitored following ligation to assure that urethral flow is adequate.

Catheterization should be avoided, especially through the umbilicus, since the area is always contaminated and the risk of introducing potential pathogens into the abdomen is great. Also, the risk of trauma caused by catheterization of the neonate outweighs possible benefits.

MUSCULOSKELETAL SYSTEM

Space limitation precludes detailed descriptions of all the orthopedic procedures that may be performed on camelids. Even though few procedures have been described in camelid literature, experience and discussions with colleagues make it apparent that many procedures are performed routinely, utilizing techniques described in standard surgical textbooks for horses, cattle, and dogs. The approach in this chapter will be to describe unique problems, especially to emphasize anatomic variations of SACs from other species.

Limb Amputation

INDICATIONS. Both fore- and hind limb amputations have been performed on llamas. The usual indication for such surgery is irreparable trauma to the limb, such as may be caused by shatter fractures, dog bites or other severe lacerations, inoperable tumors, nonresponsive osteomyelitis, or vascular lesions resulting in gangrene of the distal limb.

SURGERY. Limb amputation is not described in any of the current large animal surgery texts. However, an excellent illustrated description of such surgery in the dog is found in Newton and Nunamaker (20).

Insufficient numbers have been operated to establish precise recommendations of preferred sites for amputation of the camelid limbs. In general, the author recommends the midhumerus as the site for forelimb amputation and that the hind limb be amputated at the distal third or midfemur. In large animals, amputations below the carpus or tarsus usually result in trauma of the stump caused by the animal trying to step down onto the shortened limb. Little muscle mass is available to provide padding around the end of the bone if the amputation site is the radius or tibia.

POSTSURGICAL CARE. Easy access to feed and water is necessary until the animal becomes accustomed to three-legged ambulation. That llamas adapt well to amputation is indicated by the fact that one pregnant female successfully carried a fetus to term following a hind limb amputation.

COMPLICATIONS. The contralateral limb may be incapable of withstanding the additional weight and extra burden of locomotion. If so, the fetlock may overextend and the collateral ligaments of the fetlock carpus or tarsus may become weakened. Infection and wound dehiscence are also possible complications if asepsis is inadequate.

Fracture Repair

Fractures in camelids are caused by the same types of trauma reported in livestock, horses, and small animals (15). Any of the fixation techniques practiced in other domestic animals are applicable in appropriate situations in camelids. The size of llamas and alpacas places them between small animals and horses in terms of appropriate techniques. Camelids tolerate orthopedic surgery and application of various orthopedic devices well, so selection of a particular procedure should be dependent upon the bone involved and the nature of the fracture, available anesthesia, equipment and instrumentation, and the skill of the surgeon.

Although sophisticated procedures, such as compression bone plating and various pinning techniques, are valuable for many fracture repairs, they may be contraindicated in certain cases in which less sophisticated procedures are valid and effective. The Schroeder-Thomas splint has been used successfully on radial fractures. A walking bar, incorporated into a coaptation splint, may be considered for fractures below the carpus or tarsus.

Anatomic Considerations for Orthopedic Surgery

Though surgical approaches to the long limb bones are basically similar to those performed on dogs, horses, and cattle, there are slight variations (16, 18). A description of recommended approaches follows.

HUMERUS. The distal humerus should be approached from the lateral aspect of the limb, directly over the bone. The skin and fibrous sheath over the muscles should be incised. The depression between the lateral head of the triceps brachii muscle and the brachialis muscle should be palpated to incise the fascia or reflect the muscles away from the bone with blunt dissection.

The radial nerve curves diagonally around the caudal and lateral aspects of the distal third of the humerus. Prolonged pressure on this location with the animal in lateral recumbency may cause postsurgical radial paresis or paralysis.

The proximal humerus may be approached from the craniolateral aspect of the limb just cranial to the deltoid tuberosity of the humerus. The biceps brachii muscle may be reflected away from the cranial border of the humerus. If the caudal border must be exposed, it is necessary to transect the attachment of the deltoideus muscle from the deltoid tuberosity.

The major blood supply to the forelimb is the median artery, which lies on the medial aspect of the humerus but is protected from it by muscle tissue. Fractures of the humerus are less likely than femoral fractures to result in transection of major blood vessels.

RADIUS. The radius is superficial throughout its length on the medial aspect of the limb. To expose the bone, incise the skin and the heavy subcutaneous fascial sheath and reflect the extensor carpii radialis muscle from the cranial border of the radius along with the major vessels and nerves to the lower limb. The flexor carpii radialis muscle is firmly attached to the caudal border of the radius.

The medial aspect of the radius is rounded, providing a suitable surface for attaching a plate or inserting a pin. The proximal medial surface is narrow. If a plate is needed here, it must be placed on the cranial surface of the proximal radius.

METACARPUS. Both the medial and lateral aspects of the metacarpus are superficial; however, the major blood supply to the foot lies on the medial side; thus this is the approach that should be used to allow visualization of the vessels. The extensor tendons may easily be reflected out of the way. The flexor tendons, suspensory ligament, vessels, and nerves are encased in a heavy fibrous sheath, which must be incised to expose the bone. The two nutrient foramina, one for each marrow cavity, are located slightly proximal to the middle of the bone.

A large deep palmar metacarpal vein lies between the palmar aspect of the metatarsus and the suspensory ligament. When the suspensory ligament is to be transected surgically, such as to release contracture of the ligament, this vein should be isolated and reflected away from the ligament before an incision is made.

FEMUR. To expose the femur, the skin should be incised on the lateral aspect of the limb directly over the femur. The fascia lata lies immediately beneath the skin and should be incised in the same direction. The fascial sheet should be identified and incised between the biceps femoris muscle (caudal) and the vastus lateralis muscle (cranial). The biceps femoris muscle fibers run diagonally to the long axis of the limb, and those of the vastus lateralis run vertically.

The femur may be palpated at the distal end, but more proximally it is covered by the vastus intermedius muscle on the lateral and caudal borders. In order to completely expose the femur, it is necessary to sever the attachment of the vastus intermedius muscle on the lateral and cranial borders of the bone.

The sciatic nerve lies 3–5 cm caudal to the femur, well out of the way of the surgical site. The femoral artery and veins lie medial to the caudal border of the femur. Because of the close proximity of these vessels to the femur, in a fracture of the femur, they are at high risk of laceration. Exsanguination into the soft tissue and death have resulted from lacerations caused by a femoral fracture in the horse, and, presumably, this could occur in camelids.

Closure should include placement of sutures in each layer incised, especially in the fascia lata.

TIBIA. The tibia should be approached from the medial aspect. The tibia is free of muscle covering throughout its length on the medial side of the limb. Incising the skin and fascial layer will expose the bone. The cranial tibial muscle lies on the cranial border of the tibia and can be reflected out of the way. The deep digital flexor muscle is firmly attached to the caudal border of the proximal two-thirds of the tibia. This attachment must be released to completely free the tibia.

The major blood vessels and nerves to the lower hind limb lie in the fascia between the gastrocnemius muscle and the deep digital flexor muscle and thus are well out of the way.

The medial aspect of the tibia is rounded in the distal half but flattened in the proximal half, providing a suitable site for attachment of bone plates or the insertion of Kirschner/Ehmer pins.

METATARSUS. Both the medial and lateral aspects of the metatarsus are superficial and accessible for surgery. However, the major blood and nerve supply lies on the medial side, so this approach is more desirable.

Exposure may begin by incising the skin and reflecting the extensor tendons dorsally. The flexor tendons, suspensory ligament, blood vessels, and nerves of the lower limb are firmly attached to the plantar aspect of the metatarsus by a heavy fibrous sheath. The sheath must be incised to expose the bone. The major blood vessels lie on the medial side in the groove between the suspensory ligament and the deep digital flexor tendon. At the level of the junction between the middle and distal third of the metatarsus, the vessels and nerves leave the sheath and swing around to the plantar aspect of the flexor tendons, continuing distally in the space between the paired tendons, ligaments, and digits of the foot.

There appears to be only one metatarsus, as metatarsi 3 and 4 are fused. However, there are two marrow cavities, with a nutrient foramen for each, slightly dorsal to the middle of the metatarsus on the plantar aspect.

Tendon/Ligament Contraction

INDICATIONS. Trauma to a tendon or muscle may cause contracture and subsequent extension or flexure of the joint involved. The types of contraction most often encountered involve the digital flexor tendons and carpal flexors. Congenital carpal flexure has been observed in neonates with multiple birth defects. In one neonate, an intrauterine tibial fracture had apparently been caused by a severe contracture of the tarsal flexor tendon.

DIAGNOSIS. The posture of the animal is disturbed. Contraction of the carpal flexor tendons prevents proper extension of the carpus and results in a buck-kneed stance. Contraction of the digital flexor tendons may also produce a slight flexion of the carpus or act in concert with the carpal flexors to accentuate the problem.

The deep digital flexor tendon inserts on the flexor process of phalanx (P) 3. Contracture causes the fetlock to be flexed, and the llama must walk on the tips of the toes (Fig. 6.22).

The superficial digital flexor tendon inserts on the distal end of P-1 and the proximal end of P-2. Contracture increases the flexion of the fetlock, causing the pastern to become more vertical, but the llama need not walk on the tips of the toes.

Diagnosis is enhanced by palpation of the tendons under maximum flexure or extension. The degree of tautness can be felt.

In one case, the tendon of the interosseous muscle (suspensory ligament) of the hind limb developed a contracture. The stance of a llama with a contracture of the interosseous muscle is illustrated in Figure 22.54.

ANESTHESIA. General.

SURGERY. The flexor tendons of the lower limb in both fore- and hind limbs should be approached from the medial aspect. The major blood vessels lie on the medial aspect of the metacarpus and metatarsus. The flexor tendons and the suspensory ligament are encased in a heavy fibrous sheath, which must be incised to provide access to the tendons and the ligament. Blood vessels and nerves should be reflected from the surgical field.

A blunt, straight bistoury should be inserted beneath the affected tendon and the cutting edge turned outward to transect the tendon while it remains under pressure. The tendon should be transected only to the degree necessary to release the contracture and allow the limb to resume a normal position. The skin is sutured and a pressure bandage applied for 24 hours.

Angular Limb Deformity

See Chapter 23 for a discussion of this condition as a congenital defect.

INDICATIONS. This surgery should not be performed to correct a defect on a breeding animal unless there is good evidence that the condition is the result of trauma or a nutritional disorder. Excessive bowing of the limb may incapacitate an animal that otherwise could be a suitable pet or packer. To be effective, this surgery must be performed during the active growing phase, while the physis is still open. Although the distal radial physis may be open radiographically until after 2.5 years of age, surgery after 15 months of age is unlikely to be effective. The normal neonate carpus is illustrated in Figure 6.23.

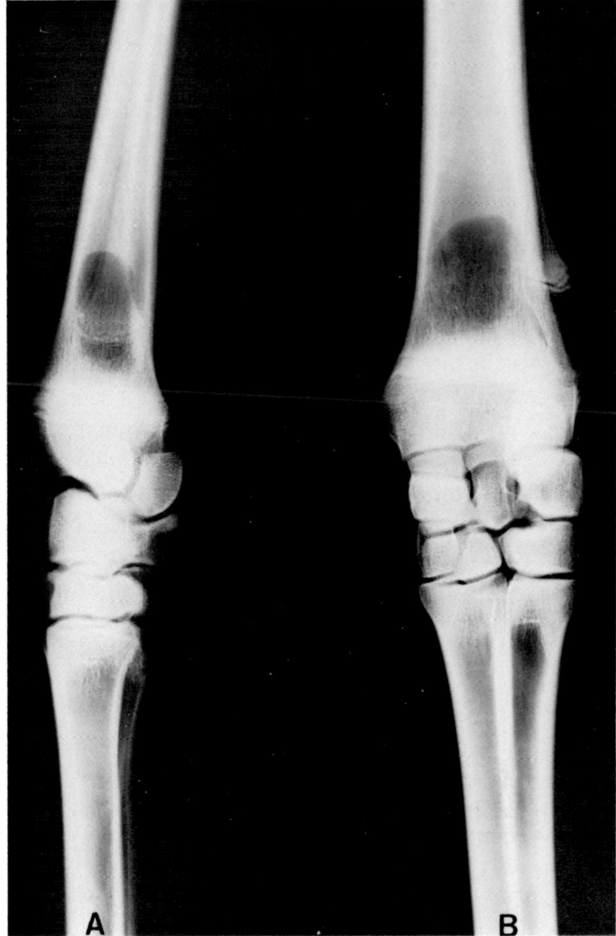

6.23 Lateral and dorsopalmar radiographs of a normal neonate llama carpus: **(A)** ulnar physis, **(B)** radial physis.

PRESURGICAL PREPARATIONS. Current radiographs should be available to aid in localization of the surgical site.

ANESTHESIA. General.

SURGERY. Two methods have been used to correct angular limb deformities. One involves the placement of cortical bone screws on either side of the physis, bridging across the physis with stainless steel wire (8). The other is periosteal stripping (1–5). Both techniques were developed in equine surgery and both have been used effectively in llamas. Each will be described.

Transphyseal Bridging

ADVANTAGES. The surgeon has control of the degree of correction. No tendons or major blood vessels are involved at the surgical site.

DISADVANTAGES. Special instruments and screws are required. A second surgery is necessary to remove the screws. Either the physis or the carpal joint may be traumatized by improper placement of the screws.

SURGERY. The physis is the most prominent palpable landmark. A 4 cm vertical incision is begun 2.5 cm dorsal to the medial physis and extended to 1.5 cm ventral to the physis. The skin and subcutaneous tissue are incised to the periosteum. The tendon of the flexor carpii radialis muscle lies immediately caudal to the surgical site and, abutting it, courses the cephalic vein. The medial collateral ligament of the carpus originates just dorsal to the physis. The incision should have penetrated the origin of the ligament parallel to its fibers. The tendon of the long digital abductor muscle crosses diagonally, cranial and ventral to the site.

The metaphyseal screw should be placed approximately 1–1.5 cm above the physeal prominence. After the hole is drilled, the depth should be checked with a depth gauge.

The required size of the cortical bone screw varies with the size of the llama. In animals less than 3 months old, the screws should be 3.5 mm in diameter and 20–22 mm long. The hole for this size screw should be drilled with a 2 mm drill and tapped with a 3.5 mm tap. Larger and older llamas require a 4.5 mm screw that is 22–24 mm long. The drill should be 3.2 mm and the tap 4.5 mm.

The epiphyseal screw is placed centrally in the epiphysis. The holes should be drilled slightly toward the physis to minimize the possibility of penetrating the carpus and add strength to the set of the screw. Proper placement of the screws should be confirmed with a dorsopalmar radiograph of the carpus. After both screws are loose-set in position, stainless steel wire (0.89 mm in diameter) is used to place a figure 8 wrap around the screws. The wires are twisted together, with the twisted tips of the wires bent to lie parallel with the strands of the wire. The screws are then tightened, and the tapered head of the screw pulls the wires taut. If the wire is not taut, growth must take up the laxity, prolonging the time necessary to straighten the leg. Proper placement of the screws is illustrated in Figures 6.24 and 6.25.

A layer of simple interrupted absorbable sutures should be placed in the subcutaneous fascia to cover the screw heads. The skin may be closed with nonabsorbable suture using a simple interrupted pattern.

POSTSURGICAL CARE. The leg(s) should be bandaged to protect the incision for 7–10 days. With severely bowed legs, the carpi are in contact while walking, which will abrade the incision site if the legs are not bandaged. A standing bandage on the lower leg will aid in keeping the carpal bandage in place. Antibiotics are not necessary.

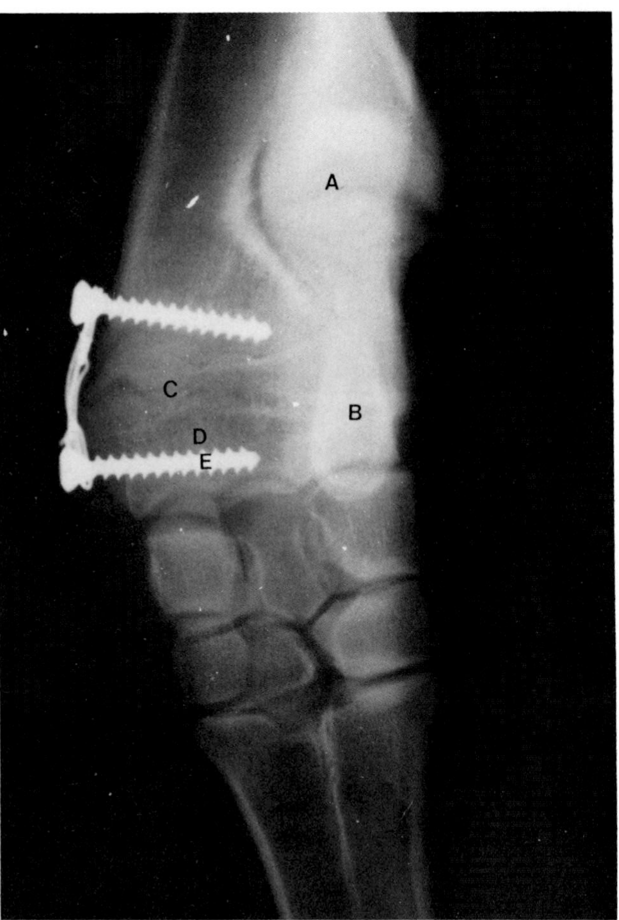

6.24 Dorsopalmar radiograph illustrating proper placement of cortical bone screws: **(A)** clubbed ulnar physis, **(B)** accessory carpal bone, **(C)** radial physis, **(D)** radial epiphysis, **(E)** cortical bone screw.

The screws should be removed when the angular limb deformity has been corrected. The time involved may be as short as 6 weeks in a 2-month-old llama or as long as 6 months in an older animal. The limb should not be allowed to overcorrect. The llama must be sedated or anesthetized to remove the screws, and aseptic techniques should be followed. A stab incision over the head of each screw will permit insertion of the hexagonal-tipped screw driver to twist out the screws. After both screws have been removed, the wires may be retrieved with a needle forceps. Each incision should be closed with simple interrupted sutures.

COMPLICATIONS. If physeal growth has halted, little or no correction will take place. If the animal is not monitored, overcorrection is possible. A seroma

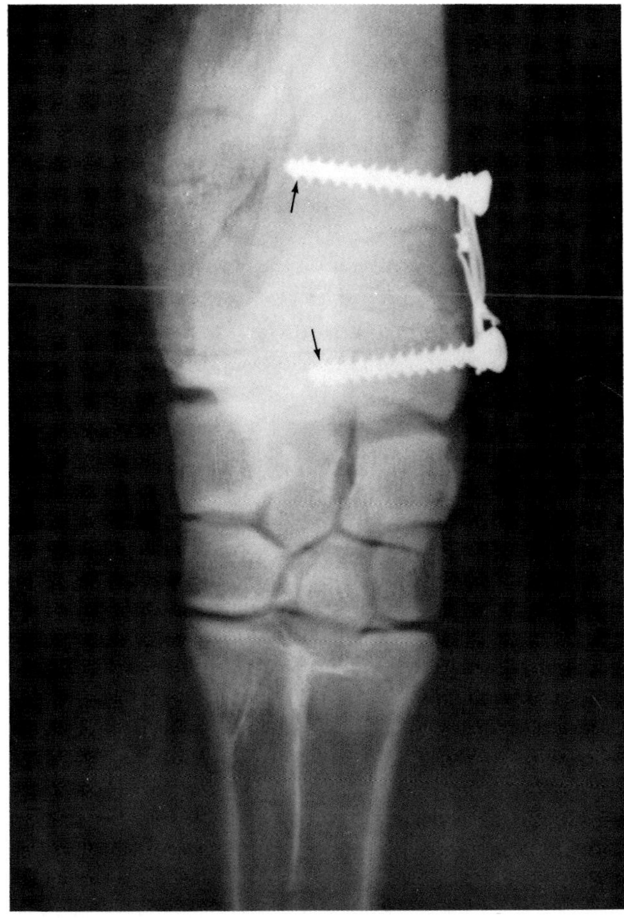

6.25 Normal divergence of cortical bone screws left in place for 30–60 days in a case of carpal valgus.

may form at the incision or the wound become infected. In either case, removal of one or two of the ventral sutures may establish drainage. The incision should not be fully opened to expose the heads of the screws.

No postsurgical pain or lameness should occur. If pain or lameness is observed, penetration of the carpal joint by the lower screw should be suspected. Epiphysitis may result if either of the screws penetrates the physis.

In one case, the owner failed to notice overcorrection (8). The tension on the wire avulsed the epiphysis into the physis and initiated an epiphysitis. The distal screw and the wire became imbedded in the inflammatory fibrous reaction, making removal of the screw extremely difficult.

Periosteal Stripping

In 1982, a new technique, called hemicircumferential transection of the periosteum and periosteal stripping, was reported for the correction of angular limb deformities in foals (2). The basic premise postulated that tension across the physis may be brought about by using the periosteum as a fibroelastic tube, uniting the proximal and distal epiphyses (2). If greater tension is exerted on one side than on the other, the growing leg will bow away from the side with the least growth. A bowed leg can be produced experimentally by performing a periosteal transection in a healthy foal (1).

This technique has been successfully applied to llamas.[2] However, the anatomy of the radius and ulna of the llama differs from that of the horse. In most but not all llamas, the distal ulnar epiphysis is fused with the radial epiphysis. The ulnar physis is approximately 3–5 cm dorsal to the radial physis. A thin section of the ulnar epiphysis wraps around the lateral radius and fuses with it. Radiographically, the radial physis appears to extend entirely across the bone; dissection has shown that this is not so.

The ulnar physis is abnormal in angular limb deformity and seems to be the structure that inhibits normal growth of the limb (Fig. 6.24).

Carpal angular limb deformity is the most common form seen in llamas and alpacas, but angulation of other joints should be evaluated to determine whether the following methods have application. If there are significant changes in the joint surfaces or of the bones in a joint, surgery may be contraindicated.

ADVANTAGES. No specialized instruments or screws are required. Surgery can be performed quickly, and a second surgery to remove screws is not necessary. There is less risk of infection with this technique because there are no bone implants.

DISADVANTAGES. There is less control over the degree of correction. To date, insufficient numbers of llamas have been operated with this technique to evaluate accurately the extent of transection or stripping that is desirable. The common and lateral digital extensor muscle tendons lie in the immediate vicinity of the surgical field.

SURGERY. The incision should be made dorsally over the prominence of the ulnar physis on the lateral aspect of the radius for a distance of 6 cm between the tendons of the common and lateral digital extensor muscles. A hemicircumferential inverted T incision is made through the periosteum approximately 1 cm dorsal to the physis. A periosteal elevator is used to strip the periosteum away from the bone, but no periosteum is actually removed.

The ulna has no weight-bearing function in the llama, and in one case, the ulna was transected with a

2. J. Paul-Murphy and E. Sharpnack, personal communication.

surgical saw following periosteal elevation. A bone chisel was used to physically separate the distal ulnar metaphysis from the radius down to the ulnar physis. The animal improved satisfactorily, but no conclusions can be drawn as to its advantages over simple transection or stripping.

The periosteum is left open. The subcutaneous fascia is closed with a simple continuous pattern using absorbable sutures. The skin may be closed with a simple interrupted or vertical mattress pattern using nonabsorbable suture or vicryl. A light bandage should be placed over the carpus and changed in 3 days. The bandage may be removed in 7–10 days.

COMPLICATIONS. The main complication is failure of adequate correction of the angulation. If this occurs, a second periosteal stripping can be performed, or cortical bone screws may be used. In severe deformities, both physeal stripping and transphyseal bridging may be necessary to achieve correction.

Choanal Atresia (7)

Choanal atresia is a congenital defect wherein there is either a membranous or osseous separation of the nasal and pharyngeal cavities at the level of the choanae. The condition may be unilateral, bilateral, partial, or complete. The paired choanae are separated by the caudal border of the vomer bone. Embryologically, the nasal cavity forms from a caudad-directed invagination of the nasal membrane and the rostrum of the embryo. A corresponding invagination moves forward from the pharyngeal pouch. The two cavities are separated by the buccopharyngeal membrane, which ultimately ruptures in normal embryologic development.

Other nasopharyngeal deformities may be associated with choanal atresia. The nasal bones may be shortened or situated abnormally close to each other, narrowing the nasal passageway. There may be total absence of the nasal cavity and nostrils.

INDICATIONS. Complete bilateral choanal atresia is a life-threatening condition. Neonate lamoids are obligate nasal breathers. They are able to breathe through the mouth with some difficulty, but when doing so they are unable to nurse. Without surgical intervention, the neonate will either starve or develop aspiration pneumonia.

It is not possible to state with assurance that choanal atresia is hereditary; however, there are indications that heredity is a factor. Therefore, surgery should not be performed on a neonate destined for breeding. Nonetheless, if the condition is fully corrected, such a neonate could become a pet or be useful for fiber production or packing.

CLINICAL SIGNS. Respiration is labored. In the characteristic breathing pattern, upon inspiration, the mouth opens slightly, air is drawn in, the lips close, and the cheeks puff out. The air in the oral pharynx is then forced around the caudal border of the elongated soft palate into the larynx and trachea. Expiration is prolonged and labored because air must again be forced around the soft palate, in reverse.

With complete choanal atresia, no air movement through the nares is possible. It is common for air entrapped in the nasopharynx to be swallowed, resulting in gastric tympanitis. The affected neonate will fail to gain weight and weaken rapidly.

DIAGNOSIS. Plain film radiography may be suggestive, and definitive diagnostic radiographs can be made by depositing 5–10 ml of a radio-dense liquid, such as renografin or barium sulfate, into the nasal cavity with a 3–5 French catheter. The llama should be placed in sternal recumbency, with the head elevated, so that the contrast medium may accumulate in the caudal nasal cavity before making radiographs.

ANESTHESIA. General anesthesia is required.

SURGERY. A tracheostomy must be performed before attempting correction of the atresia. The junction of the hard and soft palates should be palpated with an index finger, and with the other hand, a 3.5–6 cm (1/8–1/4 in.) trocar-tipped intramedullary pin is inserted into the nostril through the ventral meatus, directing the tip toward the finger within the mouth. Resistance will be felt as the tip of the pin meets the membrane. If an osseous plate is present, resistance will be strong, but the pin should be pushed through the plate. The pin may be felt in the nasopharynx through the soft palate.

A silastic tube must replace the intramedullary pin to maintain patency while healing. In one technique, a silastic tube with an inside diameter slightly larger than the pin is lubricated internally, threaded over the pin, and pushed into the nasopharynx. Then the pin is withdrawn (11).

Alternatively, the original pin is withdrawn and inserted into a silastic tube of a slightly greater diameter than the pin and reinserted within the silastic tube sheath. When the tube is positioned properly, the pin is withdrawn. In either case, the tube must be sutured to the ventromedial aspect of the nostril and cut off flush to prevent the tube from catching on objects during feeding. The process is repeated on the opposite side.

The tubes must be left in place for 3–4 weeks to allow epithelium to cover the newly created orifices. The tracheostomy must be maintained to allow breathing until the tubes can be removed.

Another approach to the obstructed choanae is via a midline trephine opening through the nasal bones directly dorsal to the choanae.[3] The choanal area is visualized through the nasal cavity on either side of the nasal septum. The choana is penetrated with a scalpel and the orifice enlarged using rongeur bone forceps.

COMPLICATIONS. The prognosis for such surgery is guarded to poor. The risk of aspiration pneumonia is high. The procedure has not been standardized. The defect is highly variable and is often accompanied by secondary defects that may complicate recovery. Even if surgery is successful, the nasal openings may be less than optimum for adequate air passage.

REFERENCES

1. Auer, J. A. 1985. Periosteal transection of the proximal phalanx in foals with angular limb deformities of the metatarsophalangeal area. J. Am. Vet. Med. Assoc. 187:496–99.

2. Auer, J. A., and Martens, R. J. 1982. Periosteal transection and periosteal stripping for correction of angular limb deformities in foals. Am. J. Vet. Res. 43:1530–35.

3. Auer, J. A., Martens, R. J. K., and Williams, E. H. 1982. Periosteal transection for correction of angular limb deformities in foals. J. Am. Vet. Med. Assoc. 181:459–66.

4. Bertone, A. L., Turner, A. S., and Park, R. D. 1985a. Periosteal transection and stripping for treatment of angular limb deformities in foals: Clinical observations. J. Am. Vet. Med. Assoc. 187:145–52.

5. Bertone, A. L., Park, R. D., and Turner, A. S. 1985b. Periosteal transection and stripping for treatment of angular limb deformities in foals: Radiographic observations. J. Am. Vet. Med. Assoc. 187:153–56.

6. Bustinza, C., and Jahuira H., F. 1985. (Frequency of genetic defects and their productivity implications in the exploitation of alpaca rearing in the department of Puno). Frecuencia de defectos geneficos y sus implicancias productivos en explataciones alpaqueras del Dpto de Puno. Alpaka 1(2):11–35.

7. Fenwick, B. W., Fowler, M. E., and Kock, M. 1982. Complete choanal atresia in a llama. J. Am. Vet. Med. Assoc. 181:1409–10.

8. Fowler, M. E. 1982. Angular limb deformities in young llamas. J. Am. Vet. Med. Assoc. 181:1338–42.

9. Getty, R. 1975. Sisson and Grossman's, The Anatomy of the Domestic Animals, vols. 1, 2, 5th ed. Philadelphia: W. B. Saunders.

10. Horney, F. D., and Wallace, C. E. 1984. Surgery of the bovine digestive tract. In P. B. Jennings, Jr., ed. 1984. Large Animal Surgery, vol. 1. Philadelphia: W. B. Saunders, pp. 493–554.

11. Kiorpes, A. L., Lindsay, W. A., and Adams, W. M. 1986. Repair of complete choanal atresia in a llama. J. Am. Vet. Med. Assoc. 189:1169–71.

12. Kock, M. 1984. Canine tooth extraction and pulpotomy in the adult male llama. J. Am. Vet. Med. Assoc. 185:1304–6.

13. Lesbre, M. F. 1903. (Anatomical research on the camelids) Recherches anatomiques sur les camelides. Arch. Mus. Hist. Nat. Lyon, vol. 8.

14. McIlwraith, C. W. 1984. Equine digestive system. In P. B. Jennings, Jr., ed. Large Animal Surgery, vol. 1. Philadelphia: W. B. Saunders, pp. 554–664.

15. Manning, J. P. 1956. Fracture of the metacarpal bones in a llama. J. Am. Vet. Med. Assoc. 129:136–37.

16. Newton, C. D., and Nunamaker, D. M., eds. 1985. Textbook of Small Animal Orthopaedics. Philadelphia: J. B. Lippincott.

17. Nickel, R., Schummer, A., and Seiferle, E. 1954. (Textbook of the Anatomy of Domestic Animals) Lehrbuch der Anatomie der Haustiere. Berlin: Paul Parey.

18. Oehme, F. W., and Prier, J. E., eds. 1974. Textbook of Large Animal Surgery. Baltimore: Williams & Wilkins.

19. Roberts, S. J. 1971. Veterinary Obstetrics and Genital Diseases, 2nd ed. Ann Arbor, Mich.: S. J. Roberts.

20. Stone, E. A. 1985. Amputation. In C. D. Newton and D. V. Nunamaker, eds. Textbook of Small Animal Orthopaedics. Philadelphia: J. B. Lippincott, pp. 577–88.

21. Sumar, K. J. 1968. (Shortened maxillary bone in alpacas or mandibular prognathism) Maxilares deprimidos en alpacas or prognatismo mandibular. Bol. Extraordinario 3:50–53.

22. Sumar, J., and Bravo, W. M. 1986. (Pelvic vasectomy in alpacas and llamas) Vasectomia pelvica en alpacas y llamas. FAO-SIDA Workshop, Lima, Peru.

23. Sumar, J., Leyva, V., and Velasco, J. 1973. (Castration in alpacas) Castracion en alpacas. Rev. Invest. Pecu. 2(1):107–8.

24. Sumar, J., Bravo, W. M., Franco, E., and Leyva, V. 1985. (Laparoscopy in llamas, alpacas and vicuñas) Laparoscopia in llamas, alpacas y vicuñas. 5th Conv. Int. Camelidos Sudam., Cuzco, Peru, p. 11.

25. Taylor, S. 1981. Male llamas—removal of "fighting teeth." 3 L llama 9:6–7.

26. Turner, A. S., and McIlwraith, C. W. 1982. Techniques in Large Animal Surgery. Philadelphia: Lea & Febiger.

3. B. Smith, personal communication.

7 Infectious Diseases

INFECTIOUS DISEASES play a prominent role in the production of llamas and alpacas (39, 50, 55, 56, 68–71, 78, 83, 103, 104). Prevention, diagnosis, and treatment are vital to the management of these animals.

VIRAL DISEASES OF CAMELIDS

The prevalence of viral diseases in camelids as a whole, and South American camelids (SACs) in particular, is unknown. Few clinically important viral diseases have been reported. Investigators have reported a few positive serologic test results, indicating exposure to viruses, but no evidence of clinical disease has been presented.

Whether or not lamoids are susceptible to a number of important viral diseases of cattle and sheep is still unknown (25). Perhaps lamoids have not been exposed to these viruses, or clinicians and researchers may not have conducted adequate virologic testing to discover them. For example, rinderpest has not been reported in SACs. Rinderpest does not occur in South America, but llamas have been experimentally challenged and found susceptible to the rinderpest virus. It is known that Old World camels are susceptible to rinderpest infection, and there is reason to believe that all members of the order Artiodactyla are susceptible to this virus, at least to some degree.

Viral diseases of cattle not known to occur in lamoids, and without known positive serology, include malignant catarrhal fever (bovine herpesvirus III), bovine leukemia (bovine leukemia virus), cowpox, pseudorabies, and bovine papilloma. Similarly, diseases of sheep that have not been reported in lamoids include ovine progressive pneumonia (ovine leukovirus), sheep or goat pox, balanoposthitis, sheep and goat papilloma, and scrapie.

Table 7.1 provides an overview of known viral diseases of camelids. Current knowledge of lamoid viral diseases is rudimentary. Comparison of SACs with camels is important to indicate possible familial susceptibility. Clinicians should be alert to recognize the presence of undiagnosed viral diseases.

Rabies

Rabies is a viral encephalitic disease endemic in many areas of North and South America. Like all other mammals, camelids are susceptible to this rhabdovirus. The virus has been studied extensively because of its zoonotic aspect and its high mortality once clinical signs appear.

EPIDEMIOLOGY. Rabies virus is primarily spread by bites from infected animals. The virus has been found in saliva and other body excretions, but it cannot penetrate the unbroken skin. Infected mouse brain suspensions have been instilled into the conjunctival sac of alpacas without producing disease (60).

Reservoir hosts vary with location. In Peru, the dog and fox are considered to be reservoir hosts (57). In tropical South America and Mexico, the vampire bat, *Desmodus rotundus,* is a serious threat to livestock production. In the United States, rabies is controlled in dogs and cats by vaccination, but wild species serve as a reservoir. The striped skunk, *Mephitis mephitis,* is the major wildlife host in the western United States. In the Southeast and along the eastern seaboard, the raccoon, *Procyon lotor,* has become a serious threat to domestic and zoo animals and humans. In the Midwest, there are foci where two species of fox, *Vulpes vulpes* and *Urocyon cinereoargenteus,* are the reservoir hosts.

In many areas of the United States and Canada, rabies is endemic in one or more reservoir hosts. Since lamoids are susceptible, they should be protected against infection by appropriate vaccination.

In one instance in Peru, 20 alpacas from a herd of 160 were bitten by a rabid dog (61); 13 died or were euthanized in extremis. The incubation period was as short as 15 days in 1 animal, 22 days in 2, 24 days in 1, and 31–34 days in 9 animals. Affected animals died 6–8 days after the development of clinical signs.

In another instance, 29 of a herd of 330 alpacas developed rabies. Dogs were implicated in this case as well. Dogs were not seen biting the alpacas, but rabid dogs were known to have been in the area and in one instance had attacked a herder. The losses occurred over a 3-month period beginning about 15 days after the suspected exposure. One neonate was involved in this outbreak. Transmission of rabies from alpaca to alpaca as a result of bites has also been reported (26). Experimental rabies has been produced (98).

CLINICAL SIGNS. Clinical signs are varied and include normal body temperature, aimless running, tremors of the head and neck, head jerking, whole body trembling, incoordination, refusal of females to permit nursing, alarm cries without cause, irritability, trampling of objects on the ground, attacks on the herder and other animals, chewing of foreign objects, excessive sexual excitement and ejaculation, and paralysis.

DIAGNOSIS. Lamoids develop Negri bodies in neurons of the hippocampus and other locations in the brain. Rodent inoculations with brain tissue are appropriate. The author is unaware of any diagnosed case of rabies in lamoids in the United States in which fluorescent rabies antibody was used as a diagnostic test and thus cannot comment on its value. Previous experience with various wild animals leads to the conclusion that no single test should form the basis of a definitive diagnosis until experience has demonstrated its accuracy and reliability.

PREVENTION. Killed rabies vaccines are appropriate for immunization of lamoids. No definitive research has been done to demonstrate that immunity has been established in lamoids by the use of these vaccines, but it would be imprudent not to attempt protection. No vaccines have been officially approved for lamoids, but Trimune (Fort Dodge) and Imrab (Pitman-Moore) have been administered to lamoids and are, at least, safe. Annual revaccination is recommended. Experience with a variety of zoo animals indicates that wild animals respond with high titers to these vaccines.

Following an outbreak of rabies in alpacas in Peru, a herd of 290 alpacas were vaccinated with a modified live virus (MLV) vaccine (26). Thirty of the alpacas (10%) developed postvaccination paralysis within 14–30 days. A MLV rabies vaccine should never be given to any animal unless it has been specifically approved for that species.

Herpesvirus

Herpesviruses are highly evolved and usually well adapted to one or more hosts. Interestingly, no herpesviruses unique to lamoids have been identified. When herpesviruses infect a nonadapted host, serious disease

Table 7.1. Viral diseases of camelids

			SACs		Camels	
Virus	Family	Disease	Clinical disease	Serologic response	Clinical disease	Serologic response
Camel pox	Poxvirus	Camel pox	0	0	++	++
Contagious ecthyma	Poxvirus	Sore mouth, orf, contagious pustular dermatitis	+	+	0	0
Rabies	Rhabdovirus	Rabies	+	+	+	+
Vesicular stomatitis	Rhabdovirus	Vesicular stomatitis	+	+	?	?
Bovine herpes type I	Herpesvirus	Infectious bovine rhinotracheitis	0	+	?	?
Equine herpes type I	Herpesvirus	Equine rhinopneumonitis	++	+	0	0
Foot-and-mouth disease	Picornavirus	Foot-and-mouth disease, aftosa	+	+	+	+
Rinderpest	Paramyxovirus	Rinderpest, cattle plague	+	+	+	+
Bluetongue	Orbivirus	Bluetongue	?	+	0	+
Bovine virus diarrhea, mucosal disease	Togavirus	Bovine virus diarrhea, mucosal disease	0	+	0	+
Rift Valley fever	Togavirus	Rift Valley fever	0	0	0	+
Influenza A	Influenza	Influenza	0	+	0	0
Influenza B	Influenza	Influenza	0	0	0	+
Parainfluenza III	Paramyxovirus	Pneumonia	0	+	0	0
Respiratory syncytial		Pneumonia	0	+	0	0
Rotavirus	Rotavirus	Virus diarrhea	0	+	0	0

or death is likely to result, which has occurred in both llamas and alpacas.

Equine herpesvirus type 1 (EHV-1) produces rhinopneumonitis and abortion in horses. The virus is endemic in most equine populations within the United States, and vaccination is routinely practiced to control the infection. In 1984, blindness was diagnosed in 21 alpacas and llamas of a herd of approximately 100 animals, which was ultimately attributed to infection with EHV-1 (38, 89, 101).

EPIDEMIOLOGY. The affected herd had been imported into the United States from Chile and had undergone the prerequisite federal quarantine at the point of origin and further quarantine at the U.S. Department of Agriculture (USDA) quarantine station in Florida. All affected animals had been kept in a large barn during a specific time period. Also housed in the barn during that time were two zebras that were sold shortly before the infection developed in the lamoids. It was not possible to subsequently trace the whereabouts of the zebras to obtain confirmation of their involvement. However, the zebras were the only possible equine exposure. The means of transmission was unknown.

CLINICAL SIGNS. Blindness, with nonresponsive dilated pupils, was the primary manifestation. Retinal degeneration and optic nerve atrophy were seen on ophthalmoscopic examination. Blindness was complete and irreversible. Four animals exhibited neurologic signs in addition to blindness. One animal died of encephalitic complications.

DIAGNOSIS. A herpesvirus, indistinguishable from EHV-1 virus, was isolated from four animals, and acute and convalescent serum titer evaluations demonstrated active infection in the blind animals. All individuals in the herd with a fourfold elevation in titer eventually developed blindness.

The lesions noted at necropsy included retinal detachment and hemorrhage, retinitis, choroiditis, vitritis, and optic nerve degeneration. The presence of intranuclear inclusion bodies, typical of herpesvirus infection, was the first clue that led to the diagnosis.

TREATMENT. Although steroids and other medications were administered, the retinal lesions were unresponsive.

PREVENTION. It is significant to note that this was an equine virus infection in an artiodactylid. With increasing production of lamoids in North America and increased opportunity for association with horses, not only this virus, but other equine virus infections, should be considered in a differential diagnosis.

Vaccines are routinely used in horses. Killed vaccines were given to exposed lamoids in the case described. The value of blanket vaccination of lamoids with equine vaccines is questionable. Before such a step is recommended, a controlled trial should be conducted to determine both the safety and efficacy of the vaccine.

Each vaccine is prepared for a specific animal. Each animal responds characteristically. Both bovine and sheep vaccines have routinely been given to lamoids, and it is more logical to use vaccines developed for ruminants than to use an equine vaccine without first exploring the ramifications of such a step.

Bluetongue

Bluetongue is an insect-transmitted viral disease caused by bluetongue virus (BTV), first described in domestic sheep but now known to affect many species of ruminants (24). There is serologic evidence that lamoids respond to BTV with the formation of antibodies, but there have been no reports of natural disease.

ETIOLOGY. BTV is classified as an arbovirus and is antigenically related to the epizootic hemorrhagic disease virus of deer. BTV exists in a multiplicity of serotypes. The degree of cross-protection against heterologous serotypes has been shown to be limited and variable.

EPIDEMIOLOGY. Small, blood-feeding gnats of the genus *Culicoides* biologically transmit BTV. After the female gnat has taken an infective blood meal, the virus replicates in the salivary glands. Ten days later, BTV may be transmitted by the gnat while taking another blood meal. The gnat may live for 28 days or more, feeding every 3–5 days. Vertical transmission has also been demonstrated in mammalian hosts.

BTV antibodies have been found in numerous species of wild animals and in alpacas (93), but there is no evidence that these animals are a reservoir for the disease in sheep. Twenty percent of the alpacas on one ranch in Peru had a positive antibody response to BTV.

BTV is probably present in most regions where sheep, cattle, and lamoids coexist. This disease should be included in a differential diagnosis.

CLINICAL SIGNS. Clinical manifestations of bluetongue vary widely according to species. In sheep, it is characterized by fever, nasal discharge, pneumonia, congestion of the lips, oral and nasal mucosa and epithelium of the tongue, necrosis of the dental pad, edema of the ears, and necrosis of skeletal and cardiac muscle. Mouth lesions may progress to shallow ulcers on the lips and gums. In a few individuals, a similar inflammatory response will occur on the coronary bands of the hoofs. Lameness is an early clinical sign in flocks of infected sheep on pasture.

Cattle may show fever, a stiff gait, drooling from the mouth, small ulcers on the oral and nasal mucous membranes and the dental pad, and/or nasal discharge. The muzzle may be hyperemic. The coronary bands may become inflamed and swollen, resulting in lameness similar to that seen with sheep. Reproductive abnormalities such as abortion, deformed calves, or unthrifty newborn calves have been associated with BTV infections in cattle. Also, many cattle apparently acquire an infection that is undetectable or not observed. Usually, cattle recover 7–10 days after clinical signs appear.

The author has seen one suspected case in a llama. A pregnant female had an episode of respiratory distress followed by an abortion. Paired serum samples taken after the abortion demonstrated a fourfold increase in BTV antibody titer.

DIAGNOSIS. Virus isolation and serologic tests are necessary for diagnosis. Gross and microscopic lesions are suggestive, but must be differentiated from vesicular diseases and rinderpest.

TREATMENT. Supportive therapy and administration of antibiotics to prevent secondary infection are recommended.

PREVENTION. Sheep are routinely vaccinated. Currently, available MLV vaccines are strain specific and have not been tested for lamoids. The use of these vaccines in lamoids, with the present state of knowledge, is not recommended.

Contagious Ecthyma

Contagious ecthyma (CE, contagious pustular dermatitis, sore mouth, orf) is a parapox viral disease primarily affecting the epidermal structures of the nose and lips of sheep and goats. Other susceptible species include musk-oxen *Ovibos moschatus;* wild sheep, *Ovis canadensis;* goats, *Oreamnos americanus;* camelids; and humans (34).

EPIDEMIOLOGY. The natural reservoir host is probably the sheep. The virus may remain viable in crusts from a lesion for longer than a year. Transmission may be by either direct contact or insect vectors.

CE is a zoonosis that produces severe ulcerating lesions on the fingers, limbs, or face of affected persons. A clinician should always wear rubber gloves while examining a suspected case. In one instance, a llama farm employee had recently returned from working on a sheep ranch in New Zealand. Although she had a finger lesion at the time, it was not recognized as CE. A month later, a number of llamas at the farm developed lesions.

CLINICAL SIGNS. In Peru, classic lesions have been seen in alpacas at 2–4 months of age (79, 80). Typical proliferative epidermal lesions at the commissures of the mouth have been seen in lamoids in North America also. The lesion may be chronic, characterized by thickening of an area of the skin of the face or the perineum. Such lesions must be differentiated from those of sarcoptic mange or ringworm.

A nursing cria may develop lesions on the lips and transmit the virus to the teats. Because of the pain associated with a lesion on the teats, the dam may prevent the cria from nursing.

In sheep and goats, CE is a self-limiting disease. In lamoids, the lesions may persist for months.

DIAGNOSIS. CE virus grows in tissue cultures, but grows poorly on the chorioallantoic membrane of chick embryos. Microscopic lesions are diagnostic in early and acute cases (40). Cytoplasmic inclusion bodies (4–8 μ) are found in swollen epidermal cells but disappear in older (6 days or more) lesions (40). Chronic lesions seen in lamoids may be difficult to diagnose.

TREATMENT. No specific treatment is recommended. Nonspecific immunostimulation with such drugs as levamisole have been attempted.

PREVENTION. MLV vaccines are routinely used in sheep and goats, but these vaccines are risky and may be unwise to use on lamoids. Faced with an outbreak of CE in a herd, a clinician would have to weigh risks against possible benefits.

Any sheep or goats kept with lamoids should be vaccinated and all traces of vaccinal lesions gone before such animals are allowed to mix with lamoids.

Foot-and-Mouth Disease

Foot-and-mouth disease (FMD, aftosa, aphthous fever, hoof and mouth disease) is a highly contagious viral disease, primarily of cattle, sheep, swine, and goats, but also affecting other artiodactylid domestic and wild animals. It is characterized by vesicular lesions and, subsequently, erosions of the epithelium of the lips, gums, soft palate, nares, muzzle, coronary bands, interdigital spaces, teats, and rumen pillar. Degenerative necrotizing lesions may have been observed in the myocardium of calves.

ETIOLOGY. FMD is caused by a virus of the picornavirus group. Seven immunologically distinct types of FMD virus (FMDV) are known. Within the seven types, over 60 subtypes have been identified over the years by complement fixation tests.

EPIDEMIOLOGY. North America is free of the disease and Canada, the United States, Mexico, Central America, and Panama have stringent regulations to prevent introduction of FMDV. FMD is of interest to the llama industry because the virus is present in most of the countries in which SACs are indigenous. Many species of artiodactylid are susceptible to FMDV, but they vary markedly as to whether or not clinical manifestations develop. Some species, e.g., the African buffalo, *Syncerus caffer,* may harbor the virus in the pharynx for 28 months, but vesicular lesions do not develop (24).

Many species of wild animals seem to be affected when an epizootic of FMD occurs in an area of Africa, but no susceptibility studies have been conducted. There are anecdotal reports, but no confirmed records, of natural infection in camels (105). Experimental infections of FMD in camels have been reported (74). In an epizootic of FMD in Ethiopia, where camels were in intimate contact with cattle, they neither developed lesions of FMDV nor produced antibodies to the strains involved (105).

During a severe epizootic of FMD in Peru approximately 15 years ago, there were reports by Peruvian regulatory veterinarians dealing with cattle that similar lesions had been seen in alpacas (49). Also in Peru, a case of FMD in alpacas was confirmed by laboratory test (type A24) in 1971 (43). A similar type isolation made in llamas in Peru that same year was not reported in the literature.

One study of lamoid susceptibility to FMDV was conducted in 1952 (49). One vicuña, 19 alpacas, and 16 llamas were exposed to FMDV by various methods, including scarification of the tongue, intradermal inoculation of the tongue, intramuscular (IM) and intravenous (IV) injection, and cohabitation with animals infected by other routes.

Animals became infected from all routes of exposure. Four animals died in the groups given IM or IV injections. The incubation period from exposure to the development of lesions was 48–72 hours. The first manifestations were vesicles on the tongue, with generalized vesicular formation occurring elsewhere within 3–4 days.

The four llamas exposed by cohabitation developed no lesions, but these same animals became infected when inoculated intramuscularly. Cattle exposed by cohabitation suffer 100% morbidity. One of the alpacas in the cohabitation experiment developed lesions in 3 days, another in 5 days, and a third in 10 days. Two other alpacas failed to develop lesions through cohabitation, but did so 20 days later when injected intramuscularly.

It was concluded from this Peruvian study that lamoids are susceptible to the virus, but less susceptible than cattle and sheep. In a study conducted at the USDA National Foreign Animal Disease Laboratory at Plum Island, New York,[1] transmission was shown to be possible from the bovine to llamas and vice versa. The virus could not be isolated from llamas after 14 days following infection. This study involved only a few animals, but indications are that the llama is not likely to be a carrier. The route of field transmission may be by respiratory aerosol, direct contact with infected animals, or exposure to contaminated feed and water.

FMDV can be inhaled in aerosol droplets by people working around infected animals. The virus lodges in the pharyngeal mucosa and may be exhaled for as long as 24 hours postexposure. Thus humans could contribute to the spread of FMD. Actual FMDV infection in humans is rare, and the disease is not considered to be a public health risk.

CLINICAL SIGNS. The incubation period varies from 3 to 5 days. In cattle, early signs include fever, depression, and anorexia. Stomatitis causes salivation, and lameness is caused by lesions on the coronary bands and interdigital spaces. Pain may cause the animal to tread, shake or kick out the feet, or lie down. Ultimately, the vesicles rupture, forming erosions, and a mucopurulent nasal discharge may develop. Pregnant cows may abort and calves die acutely. The overall mortality rate in cattle is usually less than 5%, but 50% of affected calves may die from myocardial degeneration.

Experimentally infected lamoids in Peru developed fever, up to 40°C (104°F). This was the first sign noted in all affected animals. They became totally anorectic approximately 24 hours following inoculation and chose to lie down most of the time. Vesicle locations and progress of the lesions followed patterns seen in cattle and sheep.

In the North American study, the affected llamas were depressed but had no fever. Vesicles formed on the tongue, lips, dental pad, coronets, and interdigital glands. When the vesicles ruptured, the erosion healed rapidly. Footpads became undermined.

DIAGNOSIS. The diagnosis of any suspected vesicular disease is under the control of state and federal regulatory veterinarians in the United States and comparable authorities in Canada and Mexico. Suspected cases must be reported promptly. Suspect facilities must

1. Juan Lubroth, personal communication.

be quarantined until a diagnosis is confirmed or disproved by a variety of sophisticated laboratory tests. A provisional diagnosis will be made within 24 hours of receipt of lesion material at the diagnostic laboratory. Specific vesicular diseases cannot be differentiated by clinical signs nor at necropsy.

PATHOLOGY. Vesicles, followed by erosions, may occur on the tongue, dental pads, gums, cheeks, hard and soft palates, lips, nostrils, muzzle, coronary band, the interdigital space, teats, and stomach pillars. Degenerative, necrotizing myocarditis may cause death, especially in young animals. Since lamoids are also susceptible to experimental inoculation with vesicular stomatitis virus, this disease must be considered in a differential diagnosis.

TREATMENT. There is no treatment for FMD. By law, both infected and exposed animals must be euthanized in North and Central America.

PREVENTION. Vaccines are utilized for the control of FMDV in livestock in countries in which FMD is enzootic. Vaccines are strain specific and must be prepared for a given geographic area. Vaccination is illegal in North America.

Vesicular Stomatitis

Vesicular stomatitis (VS, erosive stomatitis, pseudoaftosa) is another vesicular disease; it has a broader host range than FMD, including horses and omnivores. VS is enzootic in a number of locations in the Western Hemisphere.

VS virus is classified as a rhabdovirus. There are two major types, New Jersey and Indiana. There is no known reservoir host. It is possible that this virus primarily attacks a plant or an insect and only secondarily infects mammals.

EPIDEMIOLOGY. Definitive information on the epidemiology of VS is not complete. Epizootics occur seasonally in various geographic locations, affecting horses, cattle, swine, and deer in the United States. No natural cases of VS in lamoids have been reported. Experimentally, alpacas and llamas are susceptible to intradermal inoculation into the dorsum of the tongue, which produces localized vesicles (29). Other methods of inducing infection were unsuccessful. Attempted exposure routes included IM injection, rubbing the virus on the surface of the tongue, and cohabitation with infected animals. Only 50% of those given intradermal inoculations developed vesicles, in 48–96 hours.

Fluid taken from vesicles of lamoids was infective to susceptible cattle. Lamoids that were unaffected in the cohabitation trials were subsequently susceptible to intradermal tongue inoculation a month later.

CLINICAL SIGNS. Clinical signs of VS are indistinguishable from those of FMD. In experimental llama cases, a transient, slight elevation in temperature (0.5°C) occurred 24–48 hours after inoculation, followed by anorexia. The animals became recumbent and developed vesicles. No foot lesions were seen.

Pathology, diagnosis, and treatment are the same as for FMD.

Animals should be treated supportively.

Borna Disease

Borna (equine encephalomyelitis) is a viral disease primarily of horses and donkeys and is restricted to localities in central Europe. This disease was diagnosed in a group of lamoids that died at a zoo in Erfurt, East Germany (2, 3). The Borna virus is an arbovirus that may be transmitted by the tick *Hyalomma anatolicum.* Oral transmission in horses has also been demonstrated, and the virus has been found in saliva, urine, feces, milk, and nasal secretions.

The host range is unknown, but young horses appear to be the most susceptible, and donkeys are more resistant. Sheep and cattle have been involved in natural outbreaks. Animals may be viremic for long periods with inapparent infections. No reservoir host has been identified.

CLINICAL SIGNS. Llamas and alpacas at the Erfurt zoo exhibited anorexia and weight loss. Death occurred acutely or within 3 weeks (2). Horses developed ataxia, pharyngeal paralysis, muscle tremors, spasms, and blindness. The anorexia shown by SACs may have been neurologically induced.

DIAGNOSIS. In the outbreak at the Erfurt zoo, lamoids developed no neurologic signs, and cerebral spinal fluid and the brain were not examined in early cases of the disease. Diagnosis was confirmed by histopathologic evaluation of later cases. Histologic changes are typical of a nonsuppurative encephalomyelitis (40). Intranuclear inclusion bodies, known as Joest-Degen bodies, are diagnostic and are especially prevalent in the hippocampus.

TREATMENT AND PREVENTION. Treatment was not effective in the sick lamoids. A MLV vaccine was administered to all SACs at the Erfurt zoo in 1972 (2). A month later, an alpaca died and Borna disease was confirmed by histopathology. It is impossible to determine whether the death of this alpaca was caused by a natural infection or was vaccine induced. However, all SACs at Erfurt now receive yearly vaccination, with no outward reaction.

Rinderpest

Rinderpest is a highly contagious disease of artiodactylids characterized by fever, lymphocytopenia, erosive stomatitis, gastroenteritis, and diarrhea.

ETIOLOGY. Rinderpest is caused by a paramyxovirus closely related to the viruses that cause canine distemper and measles. Several different strains vary in virulence, but all are immunologically indistinct.

EPIDEMIOLOGY. Rinderpest has never appeared in North America and only once in South America, in Brazil in 1921. It is a devastating disease, and veterinarians dealing with such animals as camelids that may be shipped around the world need to have a basic understanding of the disease.

Natural hosts for rinderpest virus probably include all members of the order Artiodactyla. Natural rinderpest has never been reported in SACs. Limited experimental studies at the Federal Animal Disease Diagnostic Laboratory, Plum Island, have shown that llamas develop a mild febrile response, running a short clinical course, with recovery in 3–5 days.[2] Old World camels are susceptible. Primary hosts for this virus on a worldwide basis are cattle, water buffalo, and domestic swine, but no reservoir host has been determined.

Transmission of rinderpest is by direct contact. All animal discharges contain the virus, and the infection route is either via the respiratory tract or by ingestion. No carrier state of rinderpest has been established in cattle. Clinically affected animals shed the virus for 2–3 weeks if they survive.

CLINICAL SIGNS. In cattle, rinderpest is characterized by a high fever (41°C), anorexia, inflammation and necrosis of the mucous membranes, with hyperemia of buccal mucosa and development of erosions, but not vesicles or ulcerations. There is little bleeding from the erosions. Diphtheritic membranes may develop on the muzzle. Constipation precedes a severe, fetid diarrhea. Pregnant animals may abort.

The incubation period is 3–9 days. The disease course is 3–4 days in acute cases and up to 12 days in less severe cases. Animals may recover after a prolonged convalescence.

2. Juan Lubroth, personal communication.

DIAGNOSIS. Rinderpest is a reportable disease. Clinical signs may be confused with FMD or VS. Suspect cases should be reported to state and federal authorities, after which, differential diagnosis will be carried out under their direction. Isolation of the virus, animal inoculation, and serologic procedures are required for definitive diagnosis.

PATHOLOGY. Erosions and ulcerations occur throughout the digestive tract. Hemorrhage of serosal surfaces occurs with the septicemic form of the disease. Microscopically, destruction of lymphocytes and epithelial cells of the digestive tract may be seen.

TREATMENT AND PREVENTION. In North America, affected and exposed animals must be euthanized. Vaccines are used for disease control in other enzootic areas but are illegal in North America.

FUNGAL INFECTIONS

Dermatophytosis (ringworm) (96)

Various dermatophytes produce superficial infection of the epidermis in many different species of animals. Fungal dermatitis is rare in lamoids, and there are no reports of ringworm in the literature.

ETIOLOGY. Two dermatophytes have been isolated from llamas at the author's clinic. *Trichophyton verrucosum* (Fig. 7.1) is the common cause of ringworm in

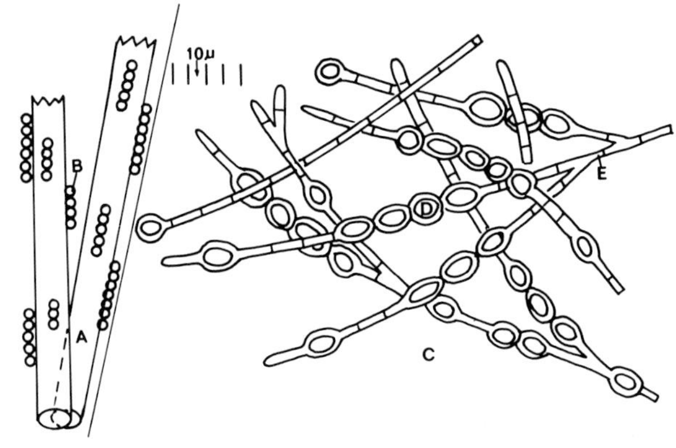

7.1 Diagrams for identification of *Trichophyton verrucosum:* **(A)** fibers, **(B)** arthroconidia on the surface of the fibers, observed on KOH preparation of skin scrapings, **(C)** growth on artificial media, **(D)** chlamydospores, **(E)** septate hyphae.

cattle and goats and more rarely in horses, donkeys, dogs, and sheep and now in llamas. Arthroconidia are seen lining the surface of hairs in potassium hydroxide (KOH) preparations of material scraped from lesions. The arthroconidia are approximately 5 μ in diameter. Colony growth on artificial media is illustrated in Figure 7.2; microscopic chains of chlamydospores are typical (Fig. 7.1).

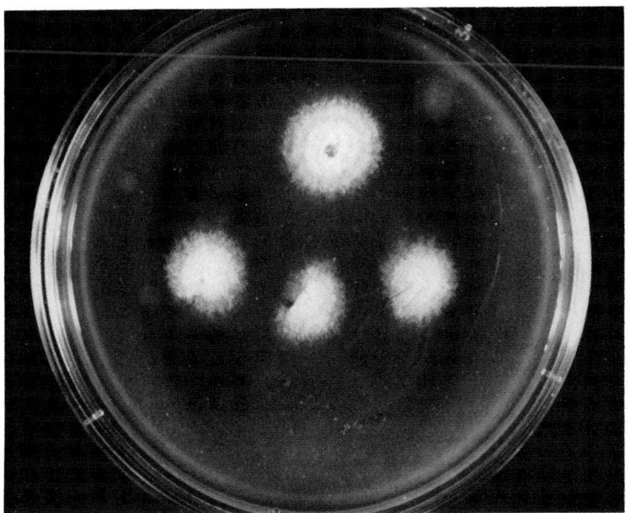

7.2 *Trichophyton verrucosum* colonies growing on Sabourad's dextrose agar.

Trichophyton mentagrophytes var *mentagrophytes* (Fig. 7.3) has also been isolated from skin lesions in llamas as well as from cats, dogs, cattle, sheep, pigs, horses, rodents, and monkeys. The organism has a ubiquitous geographic distribution. *T. mentagrophytes* var *interdigitale* is the most common organism of human athlete's foot. Arthroconidia on the surface of hairs tend to cluster. Growth on artificial media is characterized by microconidia, macroconidia, coiled hyphae, and branched, septate hyphae.

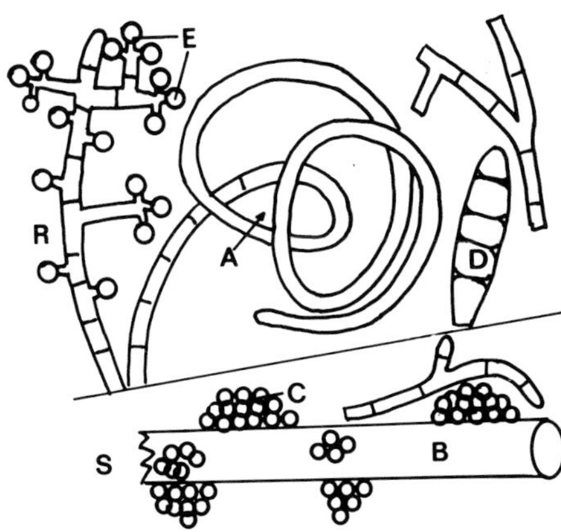

7.3 Diagrams for identification of *Trichophyton mentagrophytes:* **(A)** coiled hypha, **(B)** fiber, **(C)** arthroconidia, **(D)** macroconidia, **(E)** microconidia, **(R)** growth on artificial media, **(S)** characteristics observed on KOH preparation of skin scrapings.

CLINICAL SIGNS. In the clinical cases seen, the lesions in the llama caused by both organisms were similar to those observed in cattle, with raised, crusty, circular plaques around the poll and face. The age of the lesions was unknown in the case reported, but the plaques varied from 2 to 4 cm in diameter.

EPIDEMIOLOGY. The epidemiology of ringworm in lamoids is as yet unexplored, but direct and indirect contact are the usual modes of transmission of dermatophytes. The chlamydospores of both *T. verrucosum* and *T. mentagrophytes* may remain viable for up to 4.5 years in hair and cellular debris scraped off the animal and left attached to barn walls, fence posts, trees, feed bunks, halters, blankets, packs, brushes, and combs. Other lamoids and humans may become infected from contact with these fomites. Both organisms may be zoonotic, causing acute scalp and other areas of skin inflammatory response, with possible scarring.

PATHOLOGY. Early lesions have not been observed in lamoids, but in other species, the dermatophyte produces toxins and allergens that evoke an inflammatory response in the susceptible host, with erythema, exudation, and alopecia. The organism tends to move peripherally toward unaffected tissue, enlarging the lesion in a circular pattern. In cattle, as the lesion enlarges it becomes thicker as well as enlarging peripherally.

DIAGNOSIS. Direct microscopic examination of hair and crusts taken from the periphery of a lesion is the most rapid method of diagnosis. The material should be placed on a slide and a few drops of 10% KOH solution applied and allowed to react for 10–15 minutes, preferably accompanied with gentle heating to facilitate clearing. Fungal spores may be observed clinging to hairs when viewed microscopically at 100X, and irregular, septate hyphae may be identified.

Both *T. verrucosum* and *T. mentagrophytes* may be cultured on Sabouraud's dextrose agar. In contrast with most dermatophytes, *T. verrucosum* grows better at 37°C than at room temperature. Growth is slow, requiring 10–14 days before colonies become evident (Fig. 7.2). Chlamydospores (Figs. 7.1, 7.3) and mycelia are produced on unenriched media, but numerous microconidia and more regular mycelia grow on thiamine-enriched media (12).

A number of nonspecific and generally undiagnosed keratin-proliferative dermatoses have been seen in llamas. Any thickened lesion should be checked carefully with multiple deep skin scrapings for dermatophytes and sarcoptic mange mites (see Chap. 8).

TREATMENT. Lesions of ringworm are usually self-limiting in most species. Iodine (2% tincture) may be applied directly to a lesion daily for 2 weeks. A less caustic povidone-iodine preparation (diluted 1:4) may be equally effective. This product is used extensively to treat ringworm in livestock, horses, and dogs and has been effective in treating llamas.

Captan[3] is a fungicide for ornamental plants. It has been found to be safe and effective for the treatment of dermatophyte infections in horses, cattle, dogs, and, by inference, llamas. As a caution, captan has not been approved for use on animals intended for food. Captan may be purchased as a 50% wettable powder from nursery suppliers. The recommended dilution is 2 tablespoonfuls of the powder to 4 L (1 gal) of water. The mixture is stable for 1 week after mixing. The solution can be applied liberally to the lesion(s) and the surrounding area twice weekly for 2 weeks. The animal should not be rinsed off after application of the mixture.

Thiabendazole has antifungal action and may be applied as a 2–4% ointment to lesions of ringworm at 3-day intervals. A popular but expensive treatment for ringworm is the application of Tresaderm solution.[4]

Candidiasis

Candidiasis (candidosis, moniliasis, thrush) is a common, sporadic disease of the digestive tract caused by a yeastlike fungal infection. The disease is seen in poultry and swine and, rarely, in dogs, cats, horses, and wild animals (95). In humans, the disease causes glossitis in infants, skin infections, and vaginitis. In cattle, both mastitis and abortion have been reported. One case of gastric candidiasis has been reported in a neonatal llama in Europe (32).

ETIOLOGY. *Candida albicans* is the usual agent of infection, but other species have been isolated. *Candida* has a yeast life phase, usually encountered when the infection is on the surface of a mucous membrane, and a mycelial or pseudomycelial form that occurs when the infection becomes invasive. *Candida* is not highly pathogenic and may be isolated in the normal flora of the digestive tract. Candidiasis is probably an opportunistic infection.

EPIDEMIOLOGY. *C. albicans* is normally present on the mucous membranes of the alimentary and genital tracts of animals. The organism may be isolated from many lesions, in which it may be present as a commensal or secondary infection. The isolation of *C. albicans* should not be construed as establishing a diagnosis of candidiasis. In many species, the development of candidiasis frequently involves an immune-deficient host (neonate, chronic disease) or follows long-term antibiotic therapy. The only case that has been reported in lamoids involved a neonate llama in a European zoo (32).

Transmission may be via ingestion of contaminated food or water, but most cases are probably endogenous, the agent having been acquired during or shortly after birth.

CLINICAL SIGNS. In the single reported case, the llama was anorectic, with a yellowish diarrhea of 3 day's duration prior to death at 5 days of age. The llama had been treated for enteritis with antibiotics, fluids, and electrolyte replacement therapy.

DIAGNOSIS. Antemortem diagnosis is difficult to establish. The organism can be isolated from normal animals, and clinical signs are nonspecific. At necropsy, a mucosal scraping stained with lactophenol cotton blue, new methylene blue, Wright's, Giemsa, or a standard Gram stain may show characteristic rounded or oval budding cells (blastospores) 3–6 μ in diameter. The budding cells may be linked, forming a chain (pseudohyphae), with indentations between the buds. True mycelia may also be found.

Candida may be cultured in Sabouraud's dextrose broth or on Sabouraud's agar at either room temperature or 37°C. Standard texts describe other methods of culture for identification to species.

NECROPSY. In the clinical case reported, the walls of compartments one and two (C-1, C-2) of the stomach were thickened and edematous. A grayish-white pseudomembrane in an irregular pattern 1 to several millimeters thick was found. A whitish fluid containing necrotic debris from the pseudomembrane was found within the stomach lumen. No pseudomembrane was seen in C-3. The mucosa was hyperemic to mildly inflamed.

Microscopically, the epithelium of the mucous membrane was necrotic and invaded by masses of pseudohyphae and budding yeast cells. The invasion rarely progressed beyond the basement membrane of the

3. Orthocide Ortho-Chevron, San Francisco, CA 94120-7144.

4. Tresaderm (15 ml plastic bottle: thiabendozole 40 mg/ml, dexamethasone 1 mg/L, and neomycin 3.2 mg/ml), Merck, Sharp, and Dohm, Rahway, NJ 07065.

epithelium, and then only where deep ulceration had occurred. Yeast cells were best demonstrated in the tissue with a periodic acid-Schiff stain.

TREATMENT. No treatment has been reported for affected lamoids. Since antemortem diagnosis is difficult and the disease rare, it seems unlikely that a treatment regimen can be properly developed. However, nystatin has been recommended for intestinal infection in pigs.

PREVENTION. Prevention of candidiasis can best be accomplished by minimizing predisposing factors such as stress and prolonged antibiotic therapy. Lack of response to antibiotic therapy after 3–4 days should prompt reevaluation of the treatment regimen. Cleanliness in the management of orphan lamoids is crucial.

Aspergillosis

Aspergillosis is an opportunistic fungal infection, rare in mammals but common in birds. The disease is characterized by an inflammatory granulomatous lesion, usually of the respiratory system. The disease has been reported in a disseminated form in an alpaca (77).

ETIOLOGY. Aspergillosis is caused by *Aspergillus fumigatus* and other *Aspergillus* species. An extensive body of literature deals with *Aspergillus* sp. The hyphae are 4–6 μ in diameter and septate. Identification is dependent upon the presence of conidiophores, which are characteristic of the genus.

EPIDEMIOLOGY. *A. fumigatus* is an ubiquitous organism. Infection is rare in mammals, usually occurring when a patient is immunodepressed or has been under intense or prolonged stress. Transmission is by inhalation of fungal spores from a contaminated environment. The disease is not contagious.

CLINICAL SIGNS. The young female alpaca in which disseminated aspergillosis was diagnosed had been imported into the United States and held in quarantine for a total of 10 weeks before being examined for an apparent blindness (head tilt, intermittent circling, searching gaze, and widely dilated pupils with no pupillary light reflexes) (77). Retinal degeneration was identified by ophthalmoscopy. Further examination and laboratory evaluations failed to determine the etiology. Nonspecific steroid (30 mg prednisone daily) and amoxicillin therapy was administered for 16 days, with gradual reduction of the steroid during the last 10 days. The alpaca became anorectic and lost weight during the therapy. The day after therapy was concluded, the alpaca became moribund and died.

NECROPSY. A perforating ulcer was found in C-1, with ingesta in the greater omental sac. The lungs contained multifocal firm nodules ranging in size from pinpoint to 3–4 mm in diameter. Similar lesions were observed in the caudal pole of a kidney (77).

Microscopically, septate hyphae were identified in the lung and kidney lesions and in the necrotic retina, ciliary body, and posterior lens capsule. No hyphae were identified in sections taken from the margin of the gastric ulcer.

DIAGNOSIS. In the case described, the cause of death was probably peritonitis associated with the perforated gastric ulcer.

Typically, mycelial elements in tissue sections may be observed microscopically under 100X, using hematoxylin and eosin stains, but are more easily identified with Gomori's methenamine silver stain (77). Impression smears from suspected granulomas may be treated with KOH to clear debris from the fungal elements before staining.

Aspergillus spp. can easily be cultured on Sabouraud's dextrose agar incubated at room temperature.

TREATMENT AND PREVENTION. Treatment of aspergillosis has been unsatisfactory. As a stress-related disease, it is frequently associated with prolonged steroid or antibiotic therapy or an immune-deficient patient. Predisposing conditions must be corrected before therapy can be effective. Amphotericin B is the antibiotic of choice, but it has not been used to treat aspergillosis in lamoids.

Coccidioidomycosis

Coccidioidomycosis (San Joaquin Valley fever, valley fever) is a fungal infection primarily of the respiratory tract of humans and susceptible animals (48). It may also appear in a disseminated form or as a dermatitis.

Coccidioides immitis was first described as a protozoa, similar to coccidia, but it is actually a dimorphic fungus. Its life cycle is usually completed in the absence of animals. The literature on this organism is extensive because of human infection, but this disease is not a zoonosis.

EPIDEMIOLOGY. Coccidioidomycosis is acquired by inhalation of arthrospores from a contaminated environment. Arthrospores are the infective stage; they convert to the tissue-invasive spherules seen in animal tissues. The thick, refractile-walled spherule sporulates and becomes filled with endospores. When the spherules rupture, endospores are released, spreading the infection.

Coccidioidomycosis is an infectious disease, but is not transmitted by direct contact from animal to animal. Infection is generally considered to be restricted to specific geographic areas, but in lamoids, with extensive movement of animals from one location to another, the disease may be diagnosed in any area.

Jones[5] reported a case of coccidioidomycosis in a 1-year-old llama in 1952 (72). A number of cases have been presented to the veterinary hospital of the University of California. Dr. Ingram, in Arizona, has also dealt with cases. Whereas most other artiodactylids seem to have a low susceptibility to clinical infection with *C. immitis,* the llama, in contrast, seems to be highly susceptible. Horses frequently develop a disseminated form.

Llamas and alpacas maintained in endemic areas are at risk. The known areas in which *C. immitis* is endemic include the southern desert areas and the San Joaquin Valley of California; the southernmost parts of Utah and Nevada; most of southern Arizona, New Mexico, and southwestern and west-central Texas. The climatic conditions of these hot, arid areas of the lower Sonoran life zone are conducive to maintenance of the fungus (48).

The arid regions of northern Mexico are known to harbor *C. immitis.* In South America, endemic areas are located in northwestern Venezuela and the Gran Chaco Pampa region of Argentina and Paraguay, with possible extension into southern Bolivia. Endemic areas have also been identified in Honduras, Guatemala, and Nicaragua in Central America. Infection originating in Europe and Asia has never been authentically confirmed. It is likely that infection has been carried to the Old World by infected animals or fomites.

Disruption of the soil, such as for road building or excavation for construction, exposes the organism to winds creating dusty aerosols suitable for inhalation of the arthrospores. In California, heavy winds have transported infective dust from southern areas of the state to northern California, causing an epidemic in humans and animals in areas not normally exposed to Coccidiodes.

Transplacental infection has occurred in a llama. Previously, this was only known to occur in humans.

CLINICAL SIGNS. Clinical signs vary with the location of the lesion. One llama had a posterior paresis, with slightly impaired hind limb neural reflexes (72). A radiographic change was discernable at the level of the tenth thoracic vertebra (T-10). Although disseminated lesions were seen at necropsy in the heart, lungs, liver, and all lymph nodes, primary signs were neurologic. In other cases, respiratory signs have predominated, i.e., dyspnea and coughing.

A dermal form is characterized by nodular lesions from 1 to 3 cm in diameter or extensive raised plaques (Fig. 7.4). Lesions have been observed over most of the body surface, e.g., on the perineum, face, and limbs. Pruritus is not evident.

5. Unpublished laboratory report, California Livestock and Poultry Pathology Lab., San Gabriel, Calif., 1952. Cited in Maddy (48).

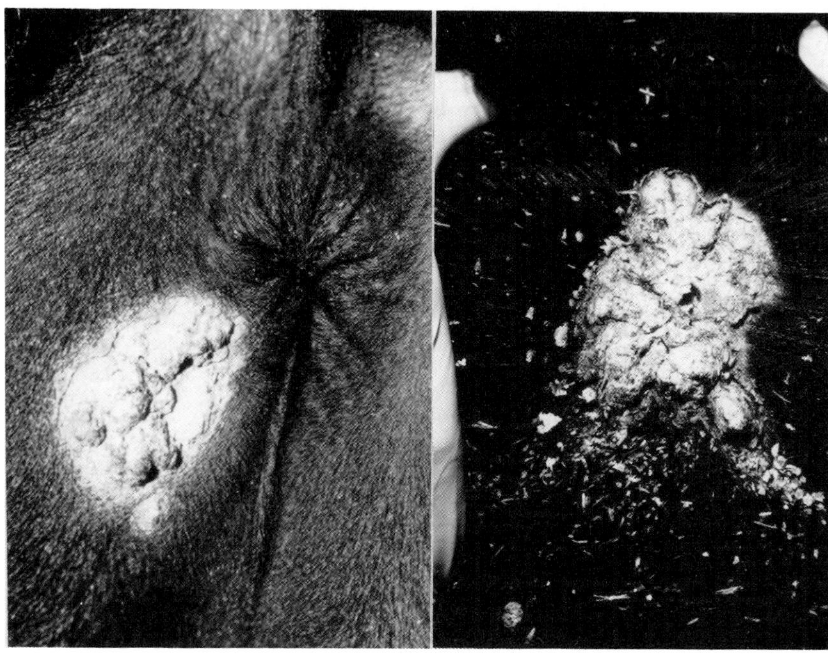

7.4 Dermal coccidioidomycosis.

PATHOLOGY. In less severe forms of coccidioidomycosis, granulomas may be restricted to the thoracic cavity, lymph nodes, and within lung tissue. These lesions may be incidental findings at necropsy. Most likely, animals in enzootic areas have inhaled the organism and developed this inapparent mild infection.

In the disseminated form, every organ or tissue of the body is a potential site for granuloma formation (Figs. 7.4–7.7). Though only a few reports have been documented in North America, granulomas affecting the pericardium, myocardium, endocardium, spleen, liver, kidney, thyroid, lungs, bone, central nervous system, visceral and peripheral lymph nodes, skin, and buccal mucosa have been seen. Lesions may appear as discrete granulomas ranging from 1 to 5 cm in diameter or coalesce in large irregularly shaped masses. The nodule is usually gray and firm. The gross lesion is nondifferentiable from those of mycobacteriosis. The microscopic lesion is characterized by granulomas or pyogranulomas, with numerous spherules present.

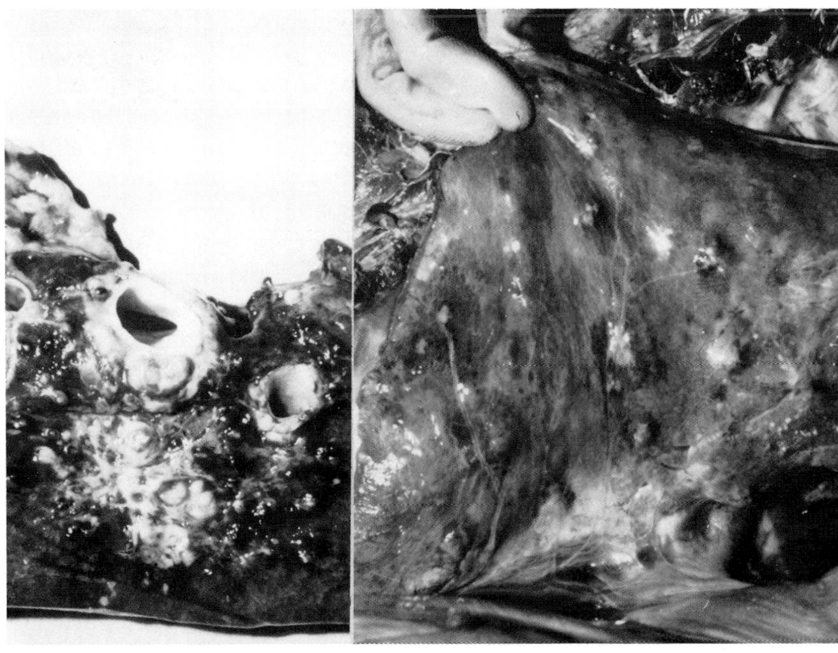

7.5 Lung granulomas caused by *C. immitis.*

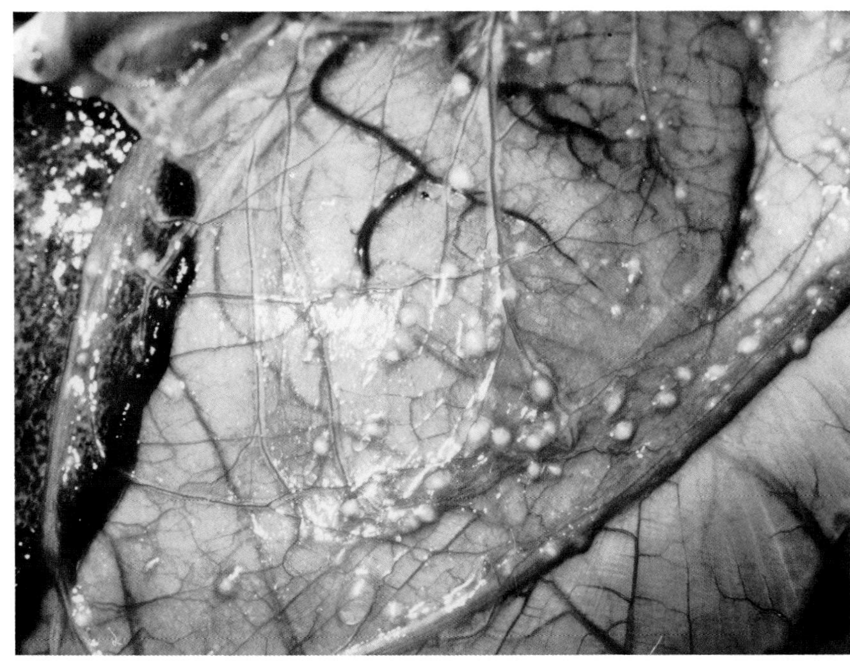

7.6 Lesions in the peritoneal cavity caused by *C. immitis.*

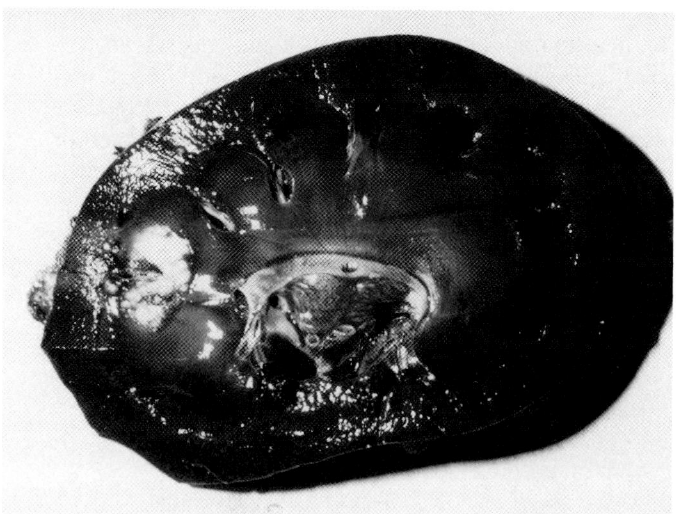

7.7 Renal granuloma caused by *C. immitis.*

DIAGNOSIS. A presumptive clinical diagnosis is difficult because of the numerous organ systems involved. If a lesion is accessible, diagnosis will be facilitated, since the organism can be readily identified by direct microscopic observation and identification of fungal spherules (10–80 μ in diameter) from respiratory secretions, pleural and peritoneal fluids, needle aspirates from abscesses and skin nodules, or biopsy samples. In the llama with posterior paresis, the cerebrospinal fluid sample collected from the lumbosacral space was normal. The granuloma at T-10 had been encapsulated, preventing development of an inflammatory response that could be detected in the cerebrospinal fluid.

The interpretation of serologic data from llamas is difficult because, as yet, insufficient numbers of individuals and herds have been tested to establish sound normal data as a basis for comparison.

The organism may be cultured on selective media such as cycloheximide-chloramphenicol agar incubated at room temperature. On artificial media, hyphae will be seen sprouting from the spherule. The hyphae are septate. Growth is rapid (3–5 days). Arthrospores develop within hyphal segments. An investigator should refer to standard texts for details of safety precautions before attempting to culture *C. immitis* because of the risk of infection from the arthrospores produced in culture.

Serologic and immunologic tests utilized in the study of coccidioidomycosis include precipitin, complement fixation, fluorescent antibody, latex particle agglutination, and agar gel diffusion precipitin tests. Some of these tests are presently being used to evaluate the status of infection in herds in endemic areas of Arizona.[6]

6. I. Ingram, Scottsdale, Ariz., personal communication.

Intradermal tests, at dilutions of 1:5, 1:10, and 1:100, have been negative in known infected animals.

Lesions within the thoracic cavity are detectable by radiography but can not be differentiated from abscesses, tumors, or other granulomatous lesions.

TREATMENT WITH AMPHOTERICIN B. On October 30, 1985, a female llama given a prepurchase physical examination was pronounced pregnant. She was losing weight according to the owner, but no other clinical signs were evident. On January 30, 1986, a biopsy obtained from a dermal lesion proved to be coccidioidomycosis. Thoracic radiographs indicated extensive granulomatous lesions in the lungs. Immunodiffusion test was positive for complement-fixing-type antibodies, and the complement fixation quantitative test was 4+ at 1:16 and 2+ at 1:32. The llama was still pregnant, with a fetus estimated to be 4 months of age.

In view of the value of the fetus, a decision was made to attempt treatment to carry the mother through pregnancy. The llama weighed 115 kg. The jugular vein was catheterized and the catheter remained in position for 6 weeks. A test dose of amphotericin B (1 mg) was given intravenously to check for adverse reactions.

The therapeutic regimen was to be 1 mg/kg amphotericin B, administered intravenously every 48 hours for 6 weeks. The regimen was begun with 34.8 mg amphotericin B mixed in 500 ml of 5% dextrose in water solution. This was administered over a 4-hour period, followed by 3 L lactated Ringer's solution containing 1.5 ml vitamin B complex solution (Bsol) and 20 mEq potassium chloride (KCl). The supplemental lactated Ringer's solution, B complex, and KCl were given to stimulate diuresis and prevent hypokalemia, a side-effect of amphotericin therapy.

The dosage of amphotericin was increased by 10 mg per treatment until the final dose of 115 mg or 1 mg/kg was reached. The llama was monitored carefully and laboratory tests (urinalysis, hemogram, and serum chemistry) performed every 3–5 days. There was no evidence of nephrotoxicity. The llama tolerated the therapy well, with anorexia appearing only during the last week of therapy.

This therapy regimen was expensive (approximately \$33/dose × 21 = \$693). After completion of therapy, the female stabilized, was discharged, and ultimately delivered a male cria on July 9, 1986. The neonate was examined carefully for evidence of coccidioidomycosis, including thoracic radiographs. Initial examinations were evaluated as normal. Approximately a month later the neonate was dyspneic. A thoracic radiograph indicated a cystic lesion in the lung; serologic tests were positive for coccidioidomycosis. The female's complement fixation titer was positive at 1:256. Euthanasia was elected, and both the neonate and the female were euthanized on September 19, 1986. Extensive diffuse lesions were found throughout the thorax and abdomen of the female. Lesions were found in the lungs of the cria also.

It was concluded that therapy was not successful in eliminating the infection from the female nor in preventing transplacental passage of the organism to the fetus.

PREVENTION. Vaccines are being developed to protect humans who must work in high-risk areas. Similar vaccines have also been used in nonhuman primates in highly endemic areas with apparent success. Vaccines for lamoids have not been evaluated, but may become important if lamoids are to be kept in endemic areas.

Mucormycosis

ETIOLOGY. There are numerous genera within the order Mucorales. The disease produced by any of these is called mucormycosis. Only one genus, *Rhizopus* sp., has been isolated from a disseminated, multisystemic infection in a llama. *Rhizopus* is a complex genus. The isolate from the llama was not speciated.

CLINICAL SIGNS. The llama was maintained in a herd used for teaching and research. The first sign of disease was bilateral facial paralysis (cranial nerve VII) that developed following an episode of struggling in a restraint chute. It was believed that the halter straps had traumatized the facial nerves. The eyelids were paralyzed at first, but in a few days the nictitating membrane failed to be pushed over the cornea, indicating an inability for the bulb to be retracted deep into the orbital socket by paralysis of the abducent (cranial nerve VI) nerve, which supplies the retractor bulbi muscle.

Ultimately, prehension and swallowing became impossible (cranial nerve IX, glossopharyngeal). The llama began to lose weight. It became apparent that multiple cranial nerves were involved, which precluded the diagnosis of trauma to superficial nerves.

The llama was anesthetized for more detailed diagnostic procedures. An endoscopic examination of the nasal cavity revealed a black membrane flecked with irregular white patches on the surface of the turbinates and the nasal mucous membrane. There was no prior nasal exudate.

DIAGNOSIS. The llama died and was necropsied. *Rhizopus* sp. was isolated from nodules (0.5–2 cm) in the lung parenchyma. The nodules were firm and black on the cut surface. Filamentous growth was present on the surface of a necrotic rhinitis, including the turbinates and cribriform plate.

The meninges on the ventral aspect of the brain were inflamed, and granulomas were present in the region of the cranial nerves, indicated by the clinical signs. The significant lesions caused by *Rhizopus* included multifocal bronchopneumonia, necrotizing rhinitis, and severe, multifocal meningioencephalitis.

Cryptococcosis

Cryptococcus sp. was isolated from a meningitis and pneumonia in a vicuña (30).

BACTERIAL DISEASES

Clostridial Diseases

The major clostridial diseases of domestic animals and humans are listed in Table 7.2. Many of these are ubiquitous and would be serious threats to livestock production if bacterin/toxoids were not available. Lamoids acquire some of these diseases.

Clostridia are Gram-positive, rod-shaped, anaerobic bacilli. All form spores that may persist in the soil for months or years. Some of these organisms may be normal flora of the digestive tract, which become pathogenic only if given access to tissue damaged as a result of deep penetrating trauma to the muscle bundles or a compromised gastrointestinal mucosa.

A few of these diseases may affect lamoid production, but the ramifications are not yet clear. For instance, *C. perfringens* type A is devastating to nursing alpacas and llamas in Peru; yet this disease has not been reported in North America.

Clostridial organisms produce potent exotoxins that are primarily responsible for the disease these agents cause. The toxins are metabolites that are produced as the organism grows in the host tissue, except for botulinum toxin, which may be ingested preformed. A given organism may produce single or multiple toxins, each with a different effect on the host. Botulinum and tetanus toxins are neurotoxic only. Most other clostridial organisms produce toxins with both local and systemic effects, including hemolysis and local tissue necrosis.

BOTULISM *C. botulinum* is distributed worldwide. One or more of the types (A–G) is probably toxic to all vertebrates. No cases have been reported in camelids, but clinical diagnosis is difficult and may have been simply overlooked. There is good reason to believe that camelids may be susceptible.

Clinical cases have not been described in camelids, but the syndrome is believed to be similar to that seen in most other mammals, consisting of a progressive paralysis of all skeletal muscles. Initially, incoordination, mus-

Table 7.2. Differential diagnosis of clostridial disease in SACs

Disease	Species	Unique clinical signs	Differential pathology	Epidemiology	Occurrence in SACs	Importance in SACs in North America
Botulism	*C. botulinum*	Flaccid muscle paralysis	None	Ingestion of toxin	?	NR
Tetanus	*C. tetani*	Tetanic muscle spasms	None	Anaerobic wound contamination	N	Mi
Blackleg	*C. chauvei*	Fever, hemorrhagic swelling and gas formation in muscles	Serosanguineous myositis with gas	Unknown in SACs	E	NR
Malignant edema	*C. septicum*	Edematous swelling around wound, no gas, sudden death	Edematous subcutaneous cellulitis	Wound infection	N	Mi
Black disease	*C. novyi* type B	Sudden death, dyspnea, ataxia	Hepatic necrosis	Spores and vegetative forms in liver of healthy animals, liver damage allows initiation	?	NR
Bacillary hemoglobinuria	*C. novyi* type D	Sudden death, hemoglobinuria, anemia	Hepatic necrosis, intravascular hemolysis	Same as above	?	NR
Type A enterotoxemia	*C. perfringens* type A	Sudden death, depression, colic, convulsions, no diarrhea	Well muscled, hemorrhages on serosae, intestine distended with fluid and gas	Not in U.S., in best conditioned neonates, 8–35 days	N	NR
Type C enterotoxemia	*C. perfringens* type C	Sudden death, severe diarrhea, distended abdomen, gas, colic, prostration, paddling	Similar to type A, with more gastrointestinal hemorrhage and enteritis, cerebral edema	In U.S., otherwise similar to type A, occurs in years with abundant grass	N	Mi
Type D enterotoxemia	*C. perfringens* type D	Sudden death, convulsions, circling, prostration, posterior paralysis, some diarrhea	Hemorrhages extensive on serosae, epicardial, endocardial, intestinal; no gas formation	Not common in neonate, usually of animal on heavy feeding schedules	N	Mi

Note: N = natural, E = experimental only, ? = not reported but suspected, M = major disease, Mi = minor disease, NR = not reported.

cle weakness, and recumbency are seen, leading finally to flaccid paralysis of all muscles, including respiratory muscles. Body temperature is not elevated. The pupils of the eyes become dilated. Salivation is decreased, and mucous membranes become cyanotic.

Diagnosis. Since *C. botulinum* may be cultured from a normal digestive tract, isolation of the organism is not diagnostic. A definitive diagnosis can be made only by the injection of filtrates of suspected feed materials or gut contents into mice or guinea pigs. Control animals are given simultaneous injections of protective doses of specific antitoxin (10).

Treatment. Once signs have developed, little can be done other than to support respiration. Antitoxins (toxin-type specific) used to treat human cases are not available for animals.

Prevention. No toxoid bacterins are available for protection of animals or humans against botulism.

TETANUS. *C. tetani* occurs worldwide as a soil saprophyte, but it can also be found in the feces of horses, humans, and cattle. Tetanus is more common in tropical regions than in cold climates. There is wide variation in the susceptibility of animal species to tetanus toxin. Horses, nonhuman primates, and swine are highly susceptible, with cattle, sheep, goats, and humans less so and dogs and cats quite resistant. The degree of susceptibility of SACs is not known. In camels, tetanus is considered to be insignificant. Two cases of tetanus in alpacas in Peru have been reported (65), one case of tetanus in a llama in Argentina (102), and one presumptive diagnosis in a llama neonate in the United States.

Tetanus develops when wounds have been contaminated with soil or feces containing *C. tetani* spores. Contaminated deep wounds with devitalized tissue are most at risk. Such wounds are poorly aerated, providing optimum conditions for growth of the anaerobic organism. It was suspected that the llama cria acquired tetanus via a navel infection.

Clinical Signs. Both of the affected alpacas in Peru had purulent rear limb wounds. Signs included prostration, muscle rigidity, dyspnea, tonic muscular contractions, joint siffness, a fixed stare, erect ears, a locked jaw, and a fever of 41.5°C (107°F) (65).

In Argentina, a llama with infected wounds on the feet was diagnosed as having tetanus. The llama remained standing in a "sawhorse" stance, with the limbs base wide. The jaw was closed and rigid, with drooling saliva, and the facial expression was wooden. There was dyspnea, erect ears, an elevated and rigid tail, and a protruding nictitating membrane (102).

Treatment. The llama was given the treatment recommended for tetanus in cattle: antibiotics were administered and the wounds were debrided and cleansed. Tetanus antitoxin was administered at a dose of 225 units/kg body weight; half was given in an IV dose and half in an IM dose (102). Anaphylactic shock is a hazard of this therapy, because tetanus antitoxin is a horse-serum product. The llama was placed in a nonstimulating environment and was tranquilized with chlorpromazine (2.2 mg/kg/6 hr).

Within a few hours, the llama began to eat, drink, and move about the stall. Medication was discontinued in 13 days, with the llama recovering fully (102).

Prevention. Tetanus toxoid vaccines are readily available. Studies have been conducted that demonstrate that llamas respond to toxoid vaccination with a rise in titer, but challenge studies have not been conducted.[7]

BLACKLEG. Blackleg (quarter evil, quarter ill, black quarter, symptomatic anthrax) is a disease of ruminants characterized by high fever, serohemorrhagic swellings, and gas formation in the heavy muscles of the body and limbs (52). The toxin is produced by *C. chauvei.* There are no reports of natural infections in SACs, but blackleg has been produced experimentally in alpacas. The alpaca seems to be more resistant than the bovine to infection (71). The disease has been reported to occur in the camel.

Blackleg is mentioned here because the disease must be differentiated from anthrax. Diagnosis is based on a positive fluorescent antibody test or isolation and identification of the organism from infected tissue.

Treatment. A recommended treatment regimen consists of antibiotic administration (penicillin, tetracycline) for 5–8 days. Clostridial toxoid vaccines contain all multiple species, including *C. chauvei,* and induce effective protection in cattle.

MALIGNANT EDEMA. Malignant edema (gas phlegmon, gas edema, bradsot, braxy) occurs worldwide in a broad host range, including domestic livestock, horses, humans, dogs, and cats (53). Wild herbivores are considered equally susceptible. Malignant edema is an economically important disease in alpacas in Peru (56), but no cases have yet been reported in lamoids in North America.

C. septicum produces the toxin that causes severe edema. It is basically a soil organism, but has been found in both spore and vegetative form in the intestines of healthy animals.

The organism invades tissue through a necrotic, deep wound that provides anaerobic conditions. Oral wounds and bruises are common entrance sites in alpacas. The organism may also gain access to body tissue from disruption of the stomach epithelium. As the organism grows, toxins are produced and clinical signs appear within 1–3 days. Two types of syndromes develop in SACs. One is the typical wound infection and edema. The other is an acute systemic disease similar to braxy of sheep. The Spanish name for this disease is "muerte súbita" (sudden death), which characterizes the primary finding. With wound infections, clinical signs include a rapidly spreading, edematous swelling in the subcutaneous tissue surrounding the wound. Little, if any, gas forms in this disease, in contrast with blackleg. Other signs include fever, rapid pulse, anorexia, depression, and weakness. *C. septicum* affects animals of all ages. Death may occur 1–2 days after signs develop.

Diagnosis, treatment, and prevention are the same as for blackleg.

CLOSTRIDIAL HEPATITIS (21). Two different diseases are caused by two different strains of *C. novyi.* Black disease is produced by *C. novyi* type B (in the United States this strain is designated *C. hemolyticum*), and bacillary hemoglobinuria (red water, icterohemoglobinuria) is produced by type D. Neither of these diseases is known to occur in camelids, but some aspects of the pathogenesis of the diseases warrant consideration.

The type B organism is a common contaminant of soils in the Western Hemisphere and may also be a normal constituent of the microflora of the digestive system of domestic livestock. Spores may be transported to the liver, where they lie dormant until conditions are suitable for vegetative growth and invasion of the hepatic parenchyma. Favorable conditions include any necrotizing or tissue-damaging insult to the liver, such as

7. J. Paul-Murphy, Davis, Calif., personal communication.

that caused by migration of immature liver flukes (*Fasciola hepatica*), chemical toxins, plant toxins, liver abscesses, or trauma (liver biopsy).

The germinating spores produce the highly necrotizing toxin, which compromises the liver further. Recognizing the likelihood that spores of *C. novyi* are present in the liver of lamoids kept with cattle and sheep, and that liver biopsy is a routine diagnostic procedure, it may be wise either to immunize SACs against *C. novyi* or administer long-acting benzathine penicillin at the time a liver biopsy is performed.

Clinical signs of black disease in cattle are those of a peracute to acute toxemia, with death occurring in many cases before signs are noticed. In subacute cases, signs include dark discoloration of the skin as a result of severe venous congestion (hence the name), severe depression, anorexia, dyspnea, ataxia, and recumbency, with death occurring within a few hours.

Bacillary hemoglobinuria is also an illness of short duration (18–36 hours). Initial signs may be similar to those of black disease, but if the animal survives for 24 hours, severe intravascular hemolysis with anemia and hemoglobinuria will develop. Death usually results from hypoxemia and respiratory depression (21).

The mortality rate for both diseases is over 90%, and treatment is of little avail because of the severe hepatic necrosis. Definitive diagnosis is based on isolation and identification of the organism in the laboratory using immunofluorescent antibody tests.

ENTEROTOXEMIA. *C. perfringens* is an anaerobic, spore-forming bacterium. Small numbers of the organism may be found in the gastrointestinal tract of healthy individuals. The organism proliferates only if the environment in the intestine deteriorates (97). The spores of *C. perfringens* are common soil inhabitants, and infections tend to recur year after year, once an area is seeded with the organism.

Five types of *C. perfringens* are known to affect animals. Collectively, the types are found worldwide, but individual types have a specific geographic distribution. There is marked variation in species susceptibility to each type. The types are designated as A, B, C, D, or E, according to the toxin produced. Lamoids are known to be susceptible to types A and C. Type D is also highly suspect. Each of the three types will be discussed separately.

Type A

Epidemiology. *C. perfringens* organisms (both spores and vegetative forms) are ingested in feed or water contaminated with infected soil or the feces of carrier animals.

Type A enterotoxemia has not occurred in North America but is the most serious disease of neonate alpacas in Peru (37, 67, 84–86, 88). Epizootics may occur during the birthing period or prolonged rainy periods or as a result of poor sanitary conditions. In different districts of Peru, mortality rates from this disease vary from 10 to 70% of alpaca crias each year. Even in carefully controlled conditions, such as prevail at La Raya Research Station, mortality from enterotoxemia varied from 1 to 56% between the years 1973 and 1979.

Death losses from type A enterotoxemia occurred in crias from 3 to 80 days of age, with over 85% of the losses occurring between 8 and 35 days. Paradoxically, crias in the best condition were most likely to be affected.

The immune status of the dam is crucial to the protection of the alpaca cria. Infant lamoids receive temporary passive immunity via the colostrum. To pass clostridial endotoxin–specific gamma globulin into the colostrum, the female must have been immunized against *C. perfringens* type A or have recovered from a natural infection. Without the protection obtained from colostrum, alpaca crias in Peru are at great risk.

Another important factor in the development of enterotoxemia is the serum protein level in the cria, especially of the globulin fraction. It is naturally low at birth (<5.2 mg/kg). With ingestion of colostrum, the protein level elevates to 5.5–6.2 mg/kg by 4 or 5 days. The globulin fraction begins to decrease, since the neonate is not yet immunologically competent and is not producing sufficient immunoglobulin G (IgG) to compensate for the diminishing of colostral IgG. The lowest level of globulin occurs between 2 and 3 weeks of age, which also corresponds to the age of highest death losses from type A enterotoxemia.

Clinical Signs. Sudden death may be the only overt manifestation. Signs, and their intensity, are dependent upon the quantity of toxin produced. Rectal temperatures may be subnormal, normal, or slightly elevated. The cria soon becomes recumbent, with the head stretched forward, eyes closed, ears directed backward, and legs stretched. Movement and vocalizations are indicative of colic. The abdomen is frequently distended, with gas tympany in the intestinal tract. The cria is anorectic and dyspneic. Diarrhea is not a sign of type A enterotoxemia but may be seen in mixed infections with *Escherichia coli* or other microorganisms. Constipation is more likely to occur in pure type A enterotoxemia.

As the disease progresses, central nervous system (CNS) disorders become apparent, indicated by convulsions and opisthotonus. Finally, the animal may become comatose and die. Death occurs too rapidly for the development of hematologic alterations.

Pathology. The carcass is usually in good muscular condition. Hyperemia and petechia of the subcutaneous tissue may be seen. Lungs are congested, and petechia of the pleural surface may occur. The bronchi contain fluid and foam, indications of pulmonary edema, and ingesta, aspirated terminally. Thoracic lymph nodes may be edematous and hemorrhagic. The thymus may be congested, with surface petechia. Variable amounts of excess serosanguineous pericardial fluid have been found. The coronary arteries are dilated, and petechia are present on the epicardium of the auricles. When the ventricles are exposed, the blood has not coagulated, as a result of thrombocytopenia.

The glandular saccule areas of the stomach are markedly congested. The intestines are typically distended with watery fluid and gas, which have a disagreeable odor. The small intestine, particularly the jejunum and ileum, is congested. The large intestine may also be congested, and Peyer's patches are prominent.

There is congestion of the renal cortices, and the capsule of the kidney peels away with difficulty. The urinary bladder is usually distended as a result of paralysis from the effects of the toxin. The brain is congested, and there is an excessive amount of cerebrospinal fluid.

Type C

Epidemiology. Type C enterotoxemia resembles type A and is included with type A as an economically important disease in Peru (66), but recently researchers have concluded that of the two, type A is much more important. No confirmed cases of type C enterotoxemia have been reported in North American lamoids, but it may have been misdiagnosed, since clinicians and pathologists base diagnoses on experience with type C enterotoxemia in lambs and calves. Not all strains of type C are infective for lamoids.

In Peru, enterotoxemia outbreaks occur in years of heavy rainfall, when grass is lush and abundant and milk production by the females is high. Types A and C affect alpacas, llamas, and vicuñas, but alpacas 10–40 days of age are more often affected. Some researchers feel that alpacas are much more susceptible to enterotoxemia than llamas.[8] Unsanitary conditions enhance the possibility of infection.

Clinical Signs. Some animals die with no clinical illness observed. Animals seen to be perfectly healthy may be moribund 4 hours later, with subnormal temperatures, 35–36°C (95 – 97°F), and subsequent death shortly thereafter. Disinterest in nursing and depression are seen early in both acute and chronic cases. In chronic cases, the temperature may be elevated, up to 40°C (104°F), and a watery diarrhea develops (62). The abdomen becomes distended, and vocalizations indicate colic. Some animals ingest great quantities of water or develop pica.

South American researchers indicate that some animals with severe diarrhea seem to recover better than those with minimal diarrhea, presumably because the toxin is flushed from the intestine by the rapid fluid expulsion (53). The morbidity rate in some herds may reach 100%, and the mortality rate may be as high as 60%.

Experience with type C enterotoxemia in North American lamoids is of a different nature. No epizootics have been reported. Incidence of the disease has been sporadic. Infection has been most frequently observed in the cria of less than 2 weeks of age that is nursing a dam with high milk production. Clinical signs are prostration, paddling (CNS involvement), and watery diarrhea. Some animals have been found dead without illness having been previously observed.

Pathology. In Peru, the lesions are essentially the same as for type A enterotoxemia (62). In North America, the usual necropsy findings are of a hemorrhagic enteritis, with blood-stained intestinal contents. The intestines are distended with gas and are intensely congested. Pulmonary interstitial edema and hydropericardium are often seen. There may be cerebral edema and neuronal degeneration in the brain (97).

Type D

Epidemiology. Type D enterotoxemia (overeating disease) has not been diagnosed in SACs in Peru. Sporadic cases have been reported in North America. Type D is a serious disease of feedlot cattle and sheep, in animals on lush pastures, or in those being overfed with grains. *C. perfringens* type D produces two major toxins, an alpha hemolytic toxin, which, in turn, aids the more damaging epsilon toxin to cause necrosis of the intestinal wall, which is then absorbed to produce similar necrotic lesions in the brain.

Clinical Signs. Type D enterotoxemia is characterized by CNS signs such as convulsions, circling, prostration with opisthotonus and paddling, posterior paralysis, and coma (10). Sudden stimuli may initiate a convulsive seizure. A slight fever, drooling, and diarrhea are other signs (97). As with most of the enterotoxemias, sudden death is common.

Pathology. Necropsy findings listed here are those seen in cattle and sheep, since the lesions in lamoids have not yet been adequately described. Petechial

8. W. Bravo, personal communication.

and ecchymotic hemorrhages may be found on any serosal surface, and both epicardial and endocardial hemorrhages are common. Excessive amounts of pericardial fluid may contain fibrin clots. Gastroenteritis is present, but there is no significant gas formation. Additional findings in animals that survive the peracute stage include intramuscular hemorrhage, pulmonary congestion and edema, edematous mesenteric lymph nodes, and focal necrosis and edema of the brain (97).

Diagnosis of Enterotoxemia. There is sufficient overlap of epidemiology, clinical signs, and pathology of the various enterotoxemias that laboratory assistance is necessary to make a definitive diagnosis. *C. perfringens* can be isolated from intestinal contents of the ileum in 100% of the affected lamoids (71). The organism may also be isolated from the blood, lungs, liver, spleen, and mesenteric lymph nodes in septicemic cases.

The isolation and identification of the organism, including the type, is carried out by standard microbiologic procedures. Ileal contents are filtered through a millipore filter. Either in vitro or in vivo techniques may be used to identify the strain. A diagnosis may also be made by identification of the toxins using immunologic procedures.

A differential diagnosis must include other diseases that cause peracute signs, severe diarrhea, and death. Failure of passive transfer of immunoglobulins to the neonate may predispose the cria not only to enterotoxemias but to other opportunistic bacterial and viral infections. Nutritional diarrheas are common in neonates, especially if they have been orphaned, and *E. coli* septicemias are not rare and may be acquired in utero. Coccidiosis is a parasitic disease that should be considered in a differential diagnosis.

Treatment. Treatment has been unrewarding in clinical cases. Administration of broad-spectrum antibiotics may arrest the growth of the organism and production of toxins, but usually severe organ damage has already occurred. Supportive treatment with fluids is indicated, but the prognosis is grave. In herd outbreaks in Peru, workers have found that chloramphenicol is most effective against type A enterotoxemia (86). In North America, herd enterotoxemias have been managed by adding chlortetracycline to the feed at a rate of 22 mg/kg feed (97).

Prevention. Feeding, sanitation, and general husbandry practices must be evaluated periodically and changed, if necessary. Toxoid administration is commonly practiced in cattle, sheep, and llamas in North America, but, in the case of llamas, studies have not been conducted to determine whether or not protection has been obtained.

The risk for development of enterotoxemia in lamoids is greatest during the first few weeks of life. Neonates have immune systems that are unable to mount an adequate response to confer protection against *Clostridium* spp. or other pathogens, even if toxoids are administered. The preferred approach is to administer toxoids to the dam approximately 2 months before parturition, with a booster at 1 month prior to parturition.

Type A toxin produced by *C. perfringens* is a poor antigen (97) and is not included in any of the multispecies clostridial preparations. Toxoids produced from type A toxins were not effective in controlling enterotoxemia in Peruvian alpacas (84, 85). Toxins other than type A, but which may be produced by type A *C. perfringens,* caused the major damage. Types A, B, C, D, and E toxins are used in typing the strain but may not be the major disease producers. Researchers are presently attempting to enlarge the toxin base for subsequent protection trials.

Tuberculosis

Tuberculosis is a chronic, bacterial, infectious disease characterized by the development of tubercles (small avascular nodules containing giant cells) in various organs of the body. Lamoids are not highly susceptible to the infection, but both natural and experimental infections have been reported (14, 59).

Four major species of acid-fast staining mycobacteria (*Mycobacterium bovis, M. tuberculosis, M. avium, M. paratuberculosis*) affect livestock, and all four have been reported in lamoids. *M. microti* has been reported in a zoo llama (76).

EPIDEMIOLOGY. Tuberculosis develops slowly. Lesions are commonly found in the respiratory and digestive systems, and excretions and secretions may be contaminated with the organism. Infection may be acquired by inhalation or ingestion.

There are rare reports of confirmed natural cases of tuberculosis in lamoids in South America, even though tuberculosis is common in cattle, sheep, and humans in the areas shared with SACs (59). In North America, *M. bovis* was isolated from eight llamas during a 5-year period at the Veterinary Services Laboratory of the USDA (100).

In 1957, 390 alpacas were tested with intradermal injections of mammalian tuberculin (59). Another 60 were injected subcutaneously to ascertain body temperature changes. None of the 450 alpacas developed positive reactions to the tuberculin. Unfortunately, the degree of exposure to tuberculosis was not mentioned in the report. However, this report is of interest, because others have reported that camelids are prone to exhibiting false positive and negative reactions to tuberculin, and these alpacas showed none.

CLINICAL SIGNS. The signs of tuberculosis vary widely, depending on the organ system involved. Since tuberculosis is a debilitating disease, emaciation is typical. Diarrhea and dyspnea accompany lesions in respective organ systems (45).

Healthy lamoids may withstand exposure to a few mycobacteria. Others may acquire a minimal infection, with the lesion healing without progressing to overt disease. Tuberculosis should be considered in the differential diagnosis of illnesses involving chronic weight loss or emaciation in lamoids.

DIAGNOSIS. Intradermal tuberculin testing with Koch's old tuberculin (OT) is the classic diagnostic test, but modern diagnostic methods include lymphocyte stimulation tests and intradermal testing with balanced, purified protein derivatives (PPD) of *M. avium* and *M. bovis.* None of these tests are infallible, but all may aid in diagnosis of tuberculosis in camelids. Tuberculin testing is considered unreliable at present.

Tuberculin testing in Bactrian camels resulted in a number of false positive reactions, both with Koch's OT and balanced bovine and avian PPD tuberculins. Lymphocyte stimulation tests in this herd were also positive, but no tubercles were observed at necropsy and no mycobacteria were isolated (42).

The author has tuberculin tested llamas during an outbreak of tuberculosis at a zoo. A significant reaction to avian PPD was observed in one llama, but a retest 1 month later was negative.

In a Peruvian experiment, alpacas were exposed to virulent organisms of *M. tuberculosis, M. bovis,* and *M. avium* by both oral and subcutaneous routes (13). Subsequently, the animals were tuberculin tested using mammalian OT intradermally. This test resulted in a mixed response, with negative reactors, suspects, and positive reactors, even to *M. avium* inoculated subcutaneously. At necropsy, localized lesions were found at the inoculation sites except for one animal given a subcutaneous inoculation of *M. tuberculosis,* in which case generalized tuberculosis developed that caused death.

A definitive diagnosis requires the culturing and speciation of the organism. It is evident that lamoids are susceptible to mycobacterial infections and that they do develop hypersensitivity responses. However, there is a problem with both false positive and negative tuberculin reactions.

Gross lesions are suggestive, but other granulomatous diseases may be confused with tuberculosis. Acid-fast staining of tissue sections is conclusive for the presence of mycobacteria but does not identify species. Tuberculosis is a reportable disease, and results of tuberculin testing must be reported to appropriate state and federal agencies in the United States. The management of a tuberculin-positive individual and its herd falls under control of these governmental agencies.

TREATMENT. Treatment is not allowed in the United States. In the past, permission has been granted to treat valuable zoo artiodactylids with isoniazid (5–10 mg/kg/day). It should be understood that isoniazid is not a mycobactericidal drug. The infection may be controlled and the tuberculin reaction suppressed, but if treatment is discontinued, the tuberculin response may reappear since the infection is still present.

PREVENTION. Vaccines are illegal in North America.

Johne's Disease

Johne's disease (paratuberculosis) is caused by an acid-fast staining bacterium, *Mycobacterium paratuberculosis.* The disease is characterized in sheep, goats, and cattle by chronic weight loss and diarrhea.

Johne's disease has been reported in a number of species of zoo artiodactylids (75), and one case has been reported in a llama from a zoo that had been maintained in a paddock with sheep (4).

Clinical signs were acute, with severe diarrhea, weakness, prostration, and death in 6 days. At necropsy, the carcass was emaciated. Lymphoid patches were prominent in the intestine, mesenteric lymph nodes were enlarged, and on cut sections areas of caseous necrosis were evident.

Histologic sections of the lymph nodes and lymphoid patches of the intestine contained numerous colonies of acid-fast-staining bacteria that were morphologically identical to *M. paratuberculosis.*

DIAGNOSIS. Antemortem diagnosis may be difficult. Body condition is not easily determined by casual observation of the lamoid because of the fluffy fiber coat. Diagnostic procedures recommended for sheep and goats should be followed.

TREATMENT AND PREVENTION. None.

Anthrax

Anthrax is an acute, septicemic disease of many species of mammals, including camelids (17). It is caused by *Bacillus anthracis,* a spore-forming, Gram-positive rod that is a constituent of the normal flora of many soil types worldwide. Spores may persist in soil for years. Infection is usually acquired by ingestion of feed or water that has been contaminated with soil containing the spores. Outbreaks are usually sporadic and may follow marked climatic changes such as heavy rainfall, flooding, or drought (41).

CLINICAL SIGNS. Cases of anthrax have been reported in SACs both in Peru and the United States. Insufficient numbers of cases have been studied to establish the incubation period in lamoids, but manifestation of the disease appears to be uniform throughout most species. The incubation period ranges from 1 to 14 days, with the more common length being 3–7 days. The first sign of anthrax is fever, as high as 42°C (108°F), but this may be missed. The general signs of total anorexia, stomach stasis, colic, hematuria, and hemorrhagic diarrhea may be more evident.

Sudden death may occur without premonitory signs being observed. If an animal survives for 24 hours, subcutaneous swellings may be seen on various parts of the body. Hemorrhagic discharges may exude from all body openings. Dyspnea indicates pulmonary involvement. Ultimately, the animal becomes severely depressed, convulsive, or comatose and may die in 1–3 days.

DIAGNOSIS. Anthrax may be confused with other diseases that cause sudden death or produce septicemia. *B. anthracis* is easily cultured from the tissues of the carcass. If anthrax is suspected, it is prudent to avoid a complete necropsy to preclude further contamination of the soil with the organism. A small quantity of blood is sufficient for the laboratory to make a direct smear or culture. A fluorescent antibody test is also available.

TREATMENT. If a rapid diagnosis is made, *B. anthracis* is susceptible to many antibacterial agents, including penicillin and tetracyclines. Therapy should be continued for 5 or more days, depending on the response.

PREVENTION. Live-spore bacterins are routinely used to protect cattle, sheep, goats, swine, and horses in endemic areas. Similar bacterins have been used in lamoids, but they should be used carefully (87). The dose of vaccine must be adjusted to the size of the animal. The live spores in the bacterin must germinate and grow in the animal's body to stimulate antibody production, but it is possible for the body's defenses to be overwhelmed and overt infection result from the bacterin.

Anthrax was diagnosed in a herd of llamas and live-spore bacterin was administered to all other animals in the herd, including the neonates. Two nursing babies died within 2 weeks following inoculation, with signs and lesions of anthrax. The infection was thought to be bacterin induced. Bacterin-induced anthrax has also been reported in foals.

The Sterne strain of anthrax bacterin[9] is currently recommended. The dose for sheep is suggested for adult SACs, and a fourth to a half dose is recommended for neonates and weanlings (41). A second dose is recommended 2–4 weeks following the first.

It is inappropriate to administer antibiotics simultaneously with the bacterin, since this will inhibit or prevent development of antibodies.

Brucellosis

Brucellosis is not a major disease of lamoids, but they have been proven to be susceptible to *Brucella melitensis* type 1 (1, 58). One significant outbreak in a herd of alpacas in Peru has been described, with classic signs of brucellosis. In the study, of 1449 alpacas tested, 20.9% had plate agglutination titers greater than 1:25. Over 25% of the 79 people caring for the animals also developed positive titers, some with active undulant fever.

B. melitensis is the primary species found in goats and sheep. It was felt that sheep were the source of infection in the Peruvian herd (1). Transmission in lamoids is assumed to be the same as in cattle, sheep, and goats, with the usual route being ingestion of feed or water that has been contaminated with the body excretions of infected individuals. The placenta and fetal fluids of infected individuals are a significant source of the organism. The organism will also be found in the milk.

Three llamas died at the London zoo a few weeks after contact with newly imported camels from Moscow (23). Serum titers for *B. melitensis* were greater than 1:1000, indicating active infection. Camels have been shown to be affected by both *B. abortus* and *B. melitensis*. Nothing is known of the susceptibility of lamoids to *B. abortus, B. ovis,* or *B. suis.*

CLINICAL SIGNS. Abortion may occur in the last third of gestation, at 9 or 10 months. Affected crias may be born dead or die shortly after birth. The extent to which brucellosis interferes with fertility in lamoids is not known. There were no reports of epididymitis or

9. Anthrax spore bacterin, Colorado Serum Co., Denver, Colo.; Anvax, JenSal Laboratories, Kansas City, Mo.; Thraxol-2, Bayvet Div., Cutter Labs., Shawnee Mission, Kan.

orchitis in the alpaca outbreak (1).

Alpacas did not develop retained placentas, as is common in cattle and sheep. This may be a result of the difference in the placental attachment (see Chap. 17).

PATHOLOGY. Mortality is nil except for fetuses. Lesions of the fetus and placenta of SACs are similar to those found in cattle specimens.

TREATMENT. *B. melitensis* is a Gram-negative coccobacillus, sensitive to many broad-spectrum antibiotics. Lamoids with positively diagnosed brucellosis should be treated for 2–3 weeks to eliminate development of the carrier state in the female. Areas in the United States that are certified brucellosis free may require euthanasia of positive reactors.

PREVENTION. Any preventive program must be integrated with the programs of regulatory authorities in a given area (see preceeding note). Strain 19 bacterin used to control brucellosis in cattle is inappropriate for lamoids because the bacterin contains MLV antigens.

Listeriosis

Listeriosis (circling disease, listerellosis, silage disease) is caused by *Listeria monocytogenes,* a Gram-positive nonspore-forming coccobacillus that has a worldwide distribution. The disease is infectious but not highly contagious, causing sporadic occurrence in a broad range of animal species, including lamoids. The herd morbidity is low, but the mortality rate of affected individuals is high, approaching 100%.

L. monocytogenes may be isolated from the intestinal tract of healthy animals and may remain dormant in the soil for years. The organisms may be saprophytic, living in a plant-soil environment, and infection may develop in domestic and wild animals or humans at any time (19). Infection does not become clinical unless resistance has been impaired by stress, concurrent disease, or pregnancy.

CLINICAL SIGNS. Lamoids develop an encephalitic syndrome, similar to that seen in cattle, with unilateral facial paralysis, circling, trembling of the head, running into objects, erect ears that may each be pointed in a different direction, salivation, depression, and a fever as high as 41.5°C (107°F) (50, 64, 99). Death occurs 2–5 days after onset of the first signs of illness. Abortion in late gestation was not described in the case in Peru, but it is a common occurrence in all other species studied.

Listeriosis was responsible for the deaths of six of the eight llamas in a German zoo (50). Other species of animals were also involved in an apparent epizootic. Because of the explosive outbreak, MLV bacterins were given to all ungulates in the zoo, including llamas, with no apparent untoward effects.

PATHOLOGY. No gross lesions have been described in lamoids. Histopathologically, miliary abscesses and perivascular cuffing, with large mononuclear cells, are especially prominent in the medulla oblongata.

TREATMENT AND PREVENTION. Treatment of clinical cases has been unsuccessful to date. Since the disease appears to be rare in lamoids, no vaccination program is recommended.

Leptospirosis

Leptospirosis is caused by various serovars of the genus *Leptospira,* a spirochete that may be visualized by use of special staining techniques. Fortunately, only a few of the more than 100 serovars of *Leptospira* cause disease in North American domestic animals (33). However, worldwide, the genus affects a broad range of hosts. There are reports of leptospirosis in lamoids (46).

EPIDEMIOLOGY. The epidemiology of the disease in lamoids is unknown but is presumably similar to that of other species. One or more primary hosts maintain each serovar as a reservoir for nonadapted species. The organism is shed to the environment from primary hosts and infected secondary hosts via the urine and can remain viable in ponds for as long as 3 months.

The infection is acquired from contaminated surface water through abrasions on the skin or through exposed mucous membranes (33). The organisms invade the liver, producing necrotic foci (leptospiremia), and secondarily affect the kidney, lung, reproductive organs, and brain.

CLINICAL SIGNS. The effects of leptospirosis are not clearly defined in lamoids. One ranch experienced an abortion epizootic. From studies considering a number of diseases, it was concluded that *L. grippotyphosa* was implicated.[10]

Leptospirosis has been diagnosed at necropsy in a zoo guanaco (35). This animal was dyspneic and refused to rise. On closer examination, the guanaco was icteric, anuric, and passed no feces. Serum creatinine was 5.5 mg/dl and the blood urea nitrogen was 80 mg/dl. These values are not markedly elevated but were significant in the overall evaluation of the case. The

10. P. Long, Corvallis, Oreg., personal communication.

guanaco died 48 hours after the first signs were observed.

Customary signs noted in cattle and sheep include fever, hemoglobinuria, icterus, anemia, encephalitis, mastitis, pulmonary congestion, orchitis, and abortion. The kidneys and reproductive organs are most often involved.

PATHOLOGY. Lesions are consistent with the signs noted. Gross lesions may be minimal but may include edema of the lungs and icterus of the fat, mucous membranes, and fascia. Histologically, there may be acute tubular and interstitial nephritis. The organisms may be observed in tissue sections if special stains are used.

DIAGNOSIS. Serologic testing, coupled with clinical signs, is the most accurate diagnostic method. Titers of over 1:100 using the microscope agglutination technique are considered significant. Acute sera and convalescent sera collected 2 weeks following the first sample are most helpful, since it is difficult to interpret a titer from a single sample.

Leptospira may be isolated from the living animal, but only during and shortly after the acute stage of the disease.

TREATMENT. *Leptospira* are susceptible to many broad-spectrum antibiotics. The success of therapy will depend on the degree of tissue and organ damage done prior to treatment. Symptomatic and supportive treatment is indicated. Renal function and urine output must be continuously monitored and fluid and electrolyte therapy adjusted accordingly.

PREVENTION. Multiple-serovar leptospiral bacterins are commercially available. These have been administered to lamoids with apparent safety and efficacy, although no experimental challenge studies have been conducted. Bacterins containing appropriate serovars for the area, as determined by diseases being diagnosed in livestock, should be used.

Necrobacillosis

ETIOLOGY AND EPIDEMIOLOGY. *Fusobacterium necrophorum* (*Sphaerophorus necrophorus*) is a Gram-negative, anaerobic bacterium. The organism has worldwide distribution and has been implicated in numerous disease processes in a broad host range of domestic and wild animals. *F. necrophorum* is not highly tissue invasive. Usually, a break in healthy epithelium or devitalized tissue is required to provide a portal for entry.

There is evidence to support the concept that *F. necrophorum* forms a symbiotic relationship with other organisms such as *Corynebacterium pyogenes,* the toxins of each enhancing the effects of the other. Multiple organisms are often isolated from necrobacillosis lesions, particularly from abscesses in the lungs or articulations.

Necrobacillosis usually occurs sporadically. If climatic and other environmental factors cause long-term stress, outbreaks of the disease may result.

CLINICAL SIGNS. Clinical signs depend on the location of the lesions, which may develop on the lips, tongue, palate, pharynx, larynx, interdigital space, sole of the foot, stomach, or mandible or maxillary bones (Fig. 7.8). Young animals are usually more at risk. Oral and pharyngeal lesions are characterized by fever, 40.5°C (107°F), anorexia, salivation, excessive drinking of water, and depression (54). Dyspnea and open-mouth breathing accompany laryngeal lesions. Oral necrobacillosis lesions produce a characteristic foul odor that emanates from the mouth and nostrils of affected individuals. Infected particles from the mouth and throat may be aspirated, causing pneumonia.

Ulcers and diphtheritic membranes may be observed in the rostral oral cavity. The pharynx and larynx can be inspected with a laryngoscope or a fiberoptic scope only after the animal has been sedated.

Lameness may result from necrotic lesions in the interdigital space and on the footpad (infectious pododermatitis) (see Chap. 10). Foot lesions are extremely resistant to therapy and, if cleared up, tend to recur with little provocation.

DIAGNOSIS. *F. necrophorum* may be isolated from lesions using standard anaerobic microbiologic methods. The necrotic lesions are characteristic, with ulcerations containing variable amounts of surface debris. Raised diphtheritic lesions are typically observed on or within the larynx and the stomach.

TREATMENT. The author has had little success in treating necrobacillosis in lamoids as well as in other species. In vitro, the organism is susceptible to many antibiotics, but the nature of the lesion precludes penetration of antibiotics.

Environmental stressors must be alleviated, which may be difficult. In a llama with infectious pododermatitis, prolonged topical therapy and systemic antibiotics resulted in healing of the pad lesions, but when the animal was returned to its original environment, the lesions recurred.

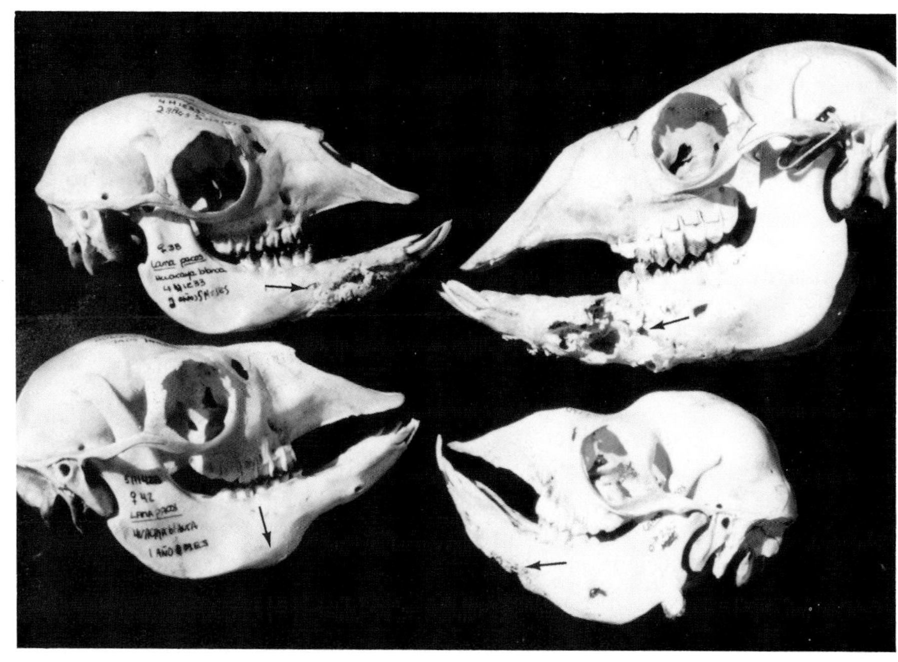

7.8 Jaws of alpacas affected with alveolar osteomyelitis, presumably caused by *Fusobacterium necrophorum.*

PREVENTION. No bacterins have been developed that will protect against this disease. Environmental stressors should be minimized.

Osteomyelitis of the Mandible

ETIOLOGY AND EPIDEMIOLOGY. Inflammatory swellings of the mandibles are seen in mammals throughout the world. Such swellings may be caused by dental anomalies or infections, tumors, trauma, or infection of the bone by osteolytic or proliferative bacteria. It has been suggested that the organisms gain access to the bone via disruptions in the mucous membranes of the mouth.

There may be regional differences in the organism responsible for the infection. In Australia, marsupials develop osteolytic lesions of both mandible and maxillary bones, and researchers there have incriminated *F. necrophorum* as the primary etiology. Marsupials in North America also suffer from mandibular lesions, but the osteitis is usually proliferative and the implicated organism is *Actinomyces* sp. Both *Actinomyces* and *Fusobacterium* should be considered in a differential diagnosis in lamoids.

Similar lesions have been observed in both domestic (15) and wild lamoids (18) (Fig. 7.8). The occurrence is sporadic and not of major economic importance.

CLINICAL SIGNS. Firm swellings along the rami of the mandible are easily observed and palpated (63). Little or no pain may be associated with palpation. General signs of anorexia, fever, and depression are usually absent. Variable degrees of soft-tissue involvement are encountered, and a fistulous tract may lead from the lesion to the ventral border of the jaw. The odor of the exudate of a dental infection or a necrobacillosis lesion is foul, but little or no odor may emanate from infections with other organisms. If swellings are in the vicinity of the teeth, the examination should investigate dental involvement (see Chap. 6). Swellings are usually unilateral, but bilateral involvement has also been observed.

DIAGNOSIS. Radiographic evaluation of the lesion is imperative to determine whether the lesion is lytic or proliferative and if the teeth are involved. Isolation and identification of the infective microorganism may be difficult, but is necessary for definitive diagnosis. Surgical extirpation and microscopic examination of the lesions may aid in the diagnosis.

TREATMENT AND PREVENTION. Therapy is entirely dependent upon the etiologic agent and the nature of the lesion and may include surgery, administration of antimicrobials, and supportive therapy. No effective preventive measures have been developed.

Streptococcosis

ETIOLOGY AND EPIDEMIOLOGY. The following species of *Streptococcus* have been isolated from alpacas in Peru and are considered to be constituents of the normal flora of mucous membranes (90): *S. pyogenes, S. faecalis, S. uberis,* and *S.* group E. Various species of *Streptococcus* have been isolated from abscesses in North American lamoids. *S. zooepidemicus* is the etiologic agent of "la fiebre de las alpaca" (alpaca fever) in Peru (5, 7, 27, 29, 60, 78, 81). This organism is also responsible for a variety of syndromes in livestock and horses worldwide. Streptococci are also responsible for diarrhea in crias (31).

CLINICAL SIGNS. Alpaca fever occurs in acute, subacute, and chronic forms. The acute and subacute forms are usually seen in young animals, resulting from ingestion of the organism. Signs include anorexia, recumbency, depression, and fever as high as 41.2°C (106.4°F). The morbidity rate in a herd is only 5–10%, but the mortality rate in those affected may be 50–100%.

The infection becomes systemic with involvement of the lungs and serosae of the thoracic and abdominal cavities, and dyspnea, colic, a tense, tender abdomen, and cessation of defecation have been described. Death may occur 4–8 days after signs are observed.

Wound, preputial, and mammary gland infections result in local, painful edema and cellulitis. Chronic forms, more commonly seen in adults, are essentially abscesses or focal infections. Abscesses may be either external or internal.

DIAGNOSIS. Diagnosis involves the correlation of signs and lesions and isolation and identification of the organism. The lesions of acute and subacute cases include significant quantities of fibrinopurulent exudation of the thoracic and abdominal cavities along with pleuritis, peritonitis, pneumonia, and petechial and ecchymotic hemorrhages of all serosal surfaces (16). Balanitis and mastitis have also been observed.

TREATMENT AND PREVENTION. Localized abscesses should be lanced and irrigated. Antibiotic therapy is not indicated, except for systemic forms. Streptococci are responsive to antibiotic therapy, but sensitivity patterns should be developed to avoid prolonged therapy with antibiotics to which the organism may be resistant.

Although mixed streptococcal bacterins are available, there is little evidence of their efficacy.

Colibacillosis

ETIOLOGY AND EPIDEMIOLOGY. *Escherichia coli* is a ubiquitous, Gram-negative, enteric bacterium. The organism may be a constituent of the normal flora of the intestinal tract, but under favorable conditions, it may become a pathogen. *E. coli* is the most common cause of uterine infection seen at the author's clinic and has been isolated in pure culture from septicemic neonates. In Peru, an atypical diarrhea of crias is felt to be a result of colibacillosis. In contrast to enterotoxemia, where the best-conditioned animals are involved, in colibacillosis the thin, undernourished animal is most likely to contract the disease. Malnourishment, as a result of decreased maternal milk production, may predispose, as does poor sanitation.

Transmission occurs via ingestion or through the umbilicus.

CLINICAL SIGNS. The most serious disease of SACs involving *E. coli* in the United States is neonatal septicemia, followed by metritis, mastitis, and abscesses. The typical signs of illness in alpaca babies are profuse diarrhea (colored whitish, yellowish, or greenish), lasting for 5–20 days, weight loss, abdominal distention, no fever, pica, and debility (53).

DIAGNOSIS. Clinical signs and lesions are not diagnostic. Isolation and identification of the organism is necessary for a confirmed diagnosis. Colibacillosis may also be seen as a secondary infection accompanying such diseases as enterotoxemia.

Lesions are consistent with the organ systems involved in the infection.

TREATMENT AND PREVENTION. Successful treatment of *E. coli* septicemias requires intensive supportive and antibiotic therapy. The aminoglycoside antibiotics are most often effective and should be begun immediately, until results of sensitivity testing are available, when more precise therapy may be instituted.

Miscellaneous and Minor Bacterial Infections

Numerous bacteria have been isolated from single cases of infection involving lamoids (36). Infection is sporadic, possibly opportunistic, and may be of no economic importance. Isolation of an organism from mucous membranes may not determine etiology (94).

For instance, *Pasteurella multicida* has been isolated from the bronchi of healthy lamoids, but this ubiquitous organism has not been reported as a pathogen in respiratory infections in lamoids, which contrasts with reports in other domestic livestock. *Staphylococcus aureus* has been isolated from lamoid infectious processes, frequently in mixed infections. Other bacterial isolates include various species of the genera *Citrobacter, Enterobacter, Pseudomonas* (30), *Campylobacter* (47), and *Proteus.*

The genus *Corynebacterium* is important in lamoid infections. *C. pyogenes* is frequently isolated from superficial abscesses in llamas and may also be a primary pathogen in endometritis, mastitis, and internal abscesses. *C. pyogenes* abscesses are thin walled and filled with thick, nonfetid exudate. (Recall that *C. pyogenes* may act synergistically with *Fusobacterium necrophorum* to facilitate necrobacillosis.)

C. equi is primarily an equine pathogen, but chronic granulomatous lymphadenitis has been reported in other species. Multiple caseous abscesses have been found in the lungs, liver, and spleen of the llama (20, 44). In Peru, *C. pseudotuberculosis* has been reported as an isolate from abscesses in alpacas (6, 7).

In a single case of keratoconjunctivitis in a llama, *Staphylococcus aureus* was isolated from the conjunctival sac, while *Moraxella liquefaciens* was isolated from the cornea (11). The clinical signs were photophobia, blepharospasms, lacrimation, conjunctivitis, miosis, and focal, unilateral corneal opacity. A 5 mm central corneal ulcer retained fluorescein stain.

The mixed infection was treated with a subconjunctival injection of benzathine penicillin (300,000 units) plus systemic administration of antibiotics and atropine. The corneal ulcer healed completely in 30 days.

Unsuccessful attempts have been made to identify mycoplasmas as agents for disease in lamoids (73). Camels may be susceptible to bovine contagious pneumonia, caused by *Mycoplasma mycoides,* but in general, mycoplasmosis is not a significant problem in camelids.

There have been no reports of naturally occurring cases of anaplasmosis as a result of *Anaplasma marginale* infection in lamoids. However, alpacas have been infected experimentally with blood from infected cattle (22, 79, 81). Anaplasma bodies were observed in the blood 29–120 days following inoculation, but the infection was subclinical, even though hemoglobin and erythrocyte levels were reduced in the affected alpacas.

Bacteroides fragilis is a large, Gram-negative, nonmotile, anaerobic rod. It is the most common anaerobe causing infections in humans (12) and recently is being increasingly isolated from animals. *B. fragilis* was isolated in pure culture from an internal abscess in a llama.[11] In the author's clinic, *Bacteroides* sp. has also been cultured along with *Fusobacterium necrophorum* from a llama with infectious pododermatitis.

PODODERMATITIS—A CASE REPORT. In April 1985, a gelding llama developed erosions and ulcerations of the footpads. A practitioner prescribed application of astringent solutions to the feet with and without bandages. In November, the llama was referred to the veterinary hospital of the University of California for evaluation and consultation.

Ulcerative lesions were present on all four footpads and interdigital spaces. The lesions were debrided and biopsied and specimens were cultured. Initial therapy consisted of soaking the feet in dilute povidone-iodine solution (1:4) for 15 minutes once daily, followed by application of a formalin solution (1:10). The feet were then bandaged.

Reports of the first biopsy supported a diagnosis of severe suppurative necrotizing pododermatitis, accompanied by periarteritis and arteriolar hypertrophy. Several colonies of bacteria grew on the original cultures, including two unspeciated Gram-negative aerobes and streptococci. Anaerobic cultures yielded *Fusobacterium necrophorum* and *Bacteroides* sp. *Bacteroides* is highly resistant to most antimicrobial therapy but has been found to be sensitive to dimetridazole (Flagyl). A 7-day course of medication with dimetridazole was initiated at a dosage rate of 7.5 mg/kg administered intravenously four times daily. Foot soaks were continued. The llama tolerated the therapy well, with the exception that salivation and drooling occurred with each treatment. The ulcers became quiescent, and epithelialization began at the periphery. The topical medication was changed to an astringent solution (white lotion, zinc sulfate, and lead subacetate), and the llama was discharged with some of the smaller lesions completely healed and the larger ones obviously healing. The owner was instructed to continue application of the white lotion and bandaging until healing was complete.

In June 1986, the llama was returned to the hospital, severe pododermatitis having recurred on all four footpads. Although IV therapy with dimetridazole had been clinically effective, the expense of the medication ($120 per day) was now prohibitive for the client, and topical medication was elected. The feet were soaked in a 5% tannic acid solution for 15 minutes, followed by application of dilute povidone-iodine solution (1:4) and pine tar under a bandage. Although the llama was docile and easily handled, the bandage changing was painful, and it was necessary to sedate the llama. Xylazine (0.04 mg/kg) and butorphanol (0.04 mg/kg) were administered intravenously. Initially, the treatment regimen was carried out daily. After a month it was conducted every other day, and at the end of a 4-month period, every third day. Healing waxed and waned, but the ulcers progressively epithelialized, and by October the llama was discharged once again.

Unfortunately, the pododermatitis recurred a third time, and in January 1987, a decision was reached to euthanize the llama. Radiographs of the severely affected feet indicated no bone involvement. At necropsy, the infection was found to be restricted to the sole and

11. Elliott, Corvallis, Oreg., personal communication.

adjacent corium of the foot and the skin and subcutaneous tissue of the interdigital space. The digital cushion was not invaded. Sections were reported as epidermal necrosis and ulceration.

Actinomyces has been mentioned in connection with osteomyelitis of the mandibles, but other species of *Actinomyces* have also been involved in soft-tissue abscessation. *Actinomyces* sp. (not *A. bovis*) was isolated from a thick-walled abscessed tract in the cheek of a llama. Repeated lancing and irrigation failed to clear up the infection. Only with radical extirpation of the entire lesion was therapy successful.

Dermatophilosis (streptothrichosis, streptotrichosis, mycotic dermatitis, lumpy wool disease) is caused by the actinomycete *Dermatophilus congolensis* (*Streptothrix congolensis*) (9). There are only anecdotal reports of the occurrence of this infection in lamoids, but the organism is known to cause a severe form of dermatitis in camels (105). The disease is characterized as an ulcerative, exudative dermatitis (9). The organism is found worldwide, but infection is more prevalent in areas of high rainfall and in tropical and subtropical climates. Administration of antibiotics, including penicillin and tetracyclines, has been highly effective in treating dermatophilosis.

For centuries, lamoids were thought to be endemically infected with syphilis, *Treponema pallidum* (92, 93). European invaders sought to discredit indigenous people and their animals, and when syphilis appeared in the Andean countries, wreaking havoc with the nonresistant indigenous people, the colonizers blamed the epidemic on the lamoids, rather than accept the responsibility for having introduced the infection themselves.

Although modern medical authorities have discounted the legend of an animal source of syphilis, it was not until 1970 that experiments proved that alpacas were not susceptible to infection with *Treponema pallidum* (91, 92).

Nocardia asteroides has been isolated from two abscesses in llamas at the author's clinic.

REFERENCES

1. Acosta, M., Ludena, H., Barreto, D., and Moro Sommo, M. 1972. (Brucellosis in alpacas) Brucelosis en alpacas. Rev. Invest. Pecu. 1 (1):37–49.

2. Altmann, D. 1975. (Most common diseases of Old-World and New-World camels) Die Wichtigsten Erkrankungen der Alt- und Neuweltkamele. Verhandlungsber. 17th Int. Symp. Erkr. Zootiere (Tunis) 17:53–60.

3. Altmann, D., Kronberger, H., Schueppel, K. F., Lippmann, R., and Altmann, I. 1976. (Enzootic meningoencephalomyelitis simplex in New-World tylopods and equines) Bornasche krankheit (meningo-encephalomyelitis Simplex enzootica equorum) bei Neuwelttylopoden und Equiden. Verhandlungsber. 18th Int. Symp. Erkr. Zootiere (Innsbruck) 18:127–32.

4. Appleby, E. C., and Head, D. K. 1954. A case of suspected Johne's disease in a llama (*L. Glama*). J. Comp. Pathol. Ther. 4:52–53.

5. Arze Borda, L. C. V. 1972. (Alpaca fever) Fiebre de alpacas. Puno Minist. Agric., Zona Agrar. 12 Divulg. 19.

6. Barsallo G., J. A., Villena, S. C., and Chavera, C. A. 1984a. (Abscesses in alpacas) Abscesos en alpacas. Sexto Congr. Peru. Microbiol. Parasitol. (Cuzco), Abstr. 113, p. 53.

7. Barsallo G., J. A., Calle, E. S., and Samame, B. H. 1984b. (Bacterial agent in a respiratory disease which causes mortality in alpacas) Agentes bacterianos en procesos respiratorios que causen mortalidad en alpacas. Sexto Congr. Peru. Microbiol. Parasitol. (Cuzco), p. 53.

8. Bautista Iturrizaga, D. 1953. (Diseases or fever of alpacas) Enfermedad o fiebre de las alpacas. Peru Inst. Nac. Biol. Andina. Rev. 4(46):27–31.

9. Berg, J. N. 1986. Dermatophilosis. In J. L. Howard, ed. 1986. Current Veterinary Therapy: Food Animal Practice, 2nd ed. Philadelphia: W. B. Saunders, p. 610.

10. Bone, J. F. 1981. Neurotoxic clostridial diseases. In J. L. Howard, ed. Current Veterinary Therapy: Food Animal Practice. Philadelphia: W. B. Saunders, pp. 680–83.

11. Brightman, A. H., McLaughlin, S. A., and Brumley, V. 1981. Keratoconjunctivitis in a llama. Vet. Med. Small Anim. Clin. 76:1776–77.

12. Carter, G. R. 1982. Essentials of Veterinary Bacteriology and Mycology. East Lansing: Michigan State Univ. Press.

13. Castagnino Rossi, D., Singer, I. N., and Hernandez Dongo, J. 1968. (Experimental tuberculosis in alpacas) Tuberculosis experimental en alpacas, *Lama pacos,* nota preliminar. Bol. Extraordinario 3:75–77.

14. Castagnino Rossi, D., Ludena, H., Huaman, D., and Ramirez, A. 1974. (Limits of infectious diseases) Linea de enfermedades infeciosas. Bol. Divulg. 15:145–47.

15. Cuba Capara, A. 1948. (Osteomyelitis of the mandible in alpacas) Osteomielitis del maxilar inferior de las alpacas. Rev. Fac. Med. Vet. (Lima) 4:25–49.

16. Cuba Capara, A., Copaira, M., and DeLa Vega, E. 1954. Comparative study of the lesions produced by "animal *Streptococcus pyogenes*" in the alpaca and the goat. Panam. Vet. Congr. Proc. 2:210.

17. Davis, J. W., Karstad, L. H., and Trainer, E. D., eds. 1981. Infectious Diseases of Wild Mammals, 2nd ed. Ames: Iowa State Univ. Press.

18. de Lamo, D. A., and Garrido, J. L. 1983. (Anomalies and dental infections and their relation with the mortality of guanacos) Anomalias e infecciones dentarias y su relacion con la mortalidad de guanacos. Gac. Vet. 45(382):783–90.

19. Dennis, S. M. 1986. Listeriosis. In J. L. Howard, ed. 1986. Current Veterinary Therapy: Food Animal Practice, 2nd ed. Philadelphia: W. B. Saunders, p. 562–65.

20. Elissalde, G. S., and Renshaw, H. W. 1980. *Corynebacterium equi:* An interhost review with emphasis on the foal. Comp. Immunol. Microbiol. Infect. Dis. 3:433–45.

21. Erwin, B. G. 1981. Clostridial hepatitis. In J. L. Howard, ed. Current Veterinary Therapy: Food Animal Practice. Philadelphia: W. B. Saunders, pp. 690–94.

22. Fernandez, L., Lora, C. A., and Marble, D. 1967. (Experimental infection of alpacas with *Anaplasma marginale*) Infeccion experimental de alpacas con *Anaplasma marginale*. Rev. Cent. Nac. Patol. Anim. 7(11):2–8.

23. Fiennes, R. N. T. -W. 1965. An outbreak of brucellosis in camels, llamas, and ibex in the London Zoo. Verhandlungsber. 7th Int. Symp. Erkr. Zootiere (Zuerich) 7:153–58.

24. Fowler, M. E. 1985. Livestock diseases caused by wild mammals. In S. M. Gaafar, ed. Parasites, Pests, and Predators. Amsterdam: Elsevier, pp. 509–35.

25. ______. 1986. Camelids. In M. E. Fowler, ed. Zoo and Wild Animal Medicine, 2nd ed. Philadelphia: W. B. Saunders, pp 969–81.

26. Franco, E. 1968. (An outbreak of rabies in alpacas on a ranch in the Department of Puno) Brote de rabia en alpacas de una hacienda del Departamento de Puno. Bol. Extraordinario 3:59–60.

27. Gallegos Loza, M. 1964. (An outbreak of fever of streptococcosis in alpacas) Sobre un brote de fiebre de alpacas o estreptococosis. Asoc. Med. Vet. Peru Bol. Inf. 40.

28. ______. 1970. (Fever in alpacas) Fiebre de alpacas. Primera Conv. Camelidos Sudam., Peru. pp. 104–5.

29. Gomez, U. D. 1964. (Tests on the sensitivity of South American camelids to vesicular stomatitis) Ensayos sobre receptividad de los auquenidos a la estomatitis vesicular. An. Segunda Congr. Vet. Zootec. (Lima), pp. 403–6.

30. Griner, L. A. 1983. Camelidae. In L. A. Griner, ed. Pathology of Zoo Animals. San Diego: Zool. Soc. San Diego, pp. 501–5.

31. Guerra, L. A. 1964. (Pathologic studies of the diplostreptococci of South American camelids and its differentiation with infant diarrhea of baby alpacas) Estudio patologica de la diploestreptococia de los auquenidos y su diferenciacion con la disenteria de las crias de alpacas. An. Segundo Congr. Nac. Vet. Zootec. (Lima), p. 110.

32. Hajsig, M., Naglio, T., Hajsig, D., and Herceg, M. 1985. Systemic mycoses in domestic and wild ruminants. I. Candidiosis of forestomachs in the lamb, calf, kid and newborn llama. Vet. Arh. 55(2): 53–58.

33. Hanson, L. E. 1986. Leptospirosis. In J. E. Howard, ed. Current Veterinary Therapy: Food Animal Practice, 2nd ed. Philadelphia: W. B. Saunders, pp. 594–96.

34. Hartung, J. 1980. (Contagious ecthyma of sheep, cases in man, dog, alpaca and camel) Lippengrind des Schafes. Tieraerztl. Prax. 8(4):435–38.

35. Hodgin, C., Schillhorn van Venn, T. W., Fayer, R., and Richter, N. 1984. Leptospirosis and coccidial infection in guanaco. J. Am. Vet. Med. Assoc. 185:1442–44.

36. Hoffman, R. K., Otte, K. C., Ponce, C. F., and Rios, M. A. 1983. (Diseases of vicuña) Enfermedades de la vicuña. El Manejo de la Vicuña Silvestre, vol. 1. Weisbaden: Eschbom, pp. 97–123.

37. Huaman, D., Ramirez, A., and Samame, H. 1981. (Production of the toxins of three strains of *C. perfringens* type A isolated from alpacas) Produccion de alfa toxina de 3 cepas de *Clostridium perfringens* Tipo A aisladas de alpacas. Resumenes 5th Congr. Peru. Microbiol. Parasitol. (Arequipa), p. 56.

38. Jenkins, D. 1985. Alpacas and llamas are susceptible to an equine disease. Llamas 30(Nov.–Dec.):15–16.

39. Jessup, D. E., and Lance, W. R. 1982. What veterinarians should know about South American camelids. Calif. Vet. 36(11):12–19.

40. Jubb, K. V. F., and Kennedy, P. C. 1970. Pathology of Domestic Animals, vol. 2, 2nd ed. New York: Academic Press, p. 595.

41. Kaufmann, A. F. 1986. Anthrax. In J. L. Howard, ed. Current Veterinary Therapy: Food Animal Practice, 2nd ed. Philadelphia: W. B. Saunders, pp. 566–67.

42. Kennedy, S., and Bush, M. 1978. Evaluation of tuberculin testing and lymphocyte transformation in Bactrian camels. In R. J. Montali, ed. Mycobacterial Infections of Zoo Animals. Washington, D.C.: Smithsonian Inst. Press, pp. 139–43.

43. Konigshofer, H. O., ed. 1971. Foot and Mouth Disease in Peru. Animal Health Yearbook. FAO-WHO-OIE, p. 178.

44. Leite, R. C., Negrelli Filho, H., and Langenegger, C. H. 1975. (*Corynebacterium equi* infection in a llama) Infeccao por *Corynebacterium equi* em lhama (*Lama glama*). Pesqui. Agropecu. Bras. Ser. Vet. 10(8):57–59.

45. Lucet, A. 1909. (Pulmonary tuberculosis of the llama) Tuberculose pulmon chez *Lama glama*. Rev. Vet. 66:129.

46. Ludena, J., and Vargus, A. 1982. (Leptospirosis in alpacas) Leptospirosis en alpacas. Adv. Vet. 2(2):27–28.

47. Luechtefeld, N. W., Cambre, R. C., and Wang, W. L. L. 1981. *Campylobacter fetus-jejuni* in zoo animals. Abstr. 81st Annu. Meet. Am. Soc. Microbiol. 81:296.

48. Maddy, K. T. 1960. Coccidioidomycosis. In C. A. Brandley and E. L. Jungherr, eds. Advances in Veterinary Sciences, vol. 6. New York: Academic Press, pp. 251–86.

49. Mancini, A. 1952. (Tests on susceptibility of South American camelids to foot-and-mouth disease) Ensayos sobre la receptividad de los auquenidos a la fiebre aftosa. Bol. Inst. Nac. Antiaftoso (Lima) 1(3):127–46.

50. Mayer, H., and Gehring, H. 1975. (Listeriosis in llama) Listeriose bei lamas. Verhandlungsber. 17th Int. Symp. Erkr. Zootiere (Tunis) 17:307–12.

51. Morgan, C. O. 1981a. Blackleg. In J. L. Howard, ed. Current Veterinary Therapy: Food Animal Practice. Philadelphia: W. B. Saunders, pp. 684–87.

52. ______. 1981b. Malignant edema and braxy. In J. L. Howard, ed. Current Veterinary Therapy: Food Animal Practice. Philadelphia: W. B. Saunders, pp. 688–89.

53. Moro Sommo, M. 1955a. (Bacillary diarrhea in young alpacas) Diarrea bacilar de las crias de alpaca o diarrea de las crias de alpaca. Fac. Med. Vet. Bol. (Lima) 2:1–35.

54. ______. 1955b. (Report on the study of disease of young alpacas) Informe sobre el estudio de las enfermedades de las crias de alpaca. Fac. Med. Vet. Bol. (Lima) 6(26):23–24.

55. ______. 1955c. (Report on the study of disease of young alpacas) Informe sobre el estudio de las enfermedades

de las crias de alpaca. Fac. Med. Vet. Bol. Vet. Zootec. (Lima) 7(17):30–33.

56. ______. 1956. (Contributions to the study of the diseases of the auquenidos) Contribucion al estudio de las enfermedadas de los auquenidos. Rev. Fac. Med. Vet. (Lima) 7(11):15–177.

57. ______. 1957a. (Rabies in alpacas) Rabia en alpacas. Rev. Fac. Med. Vet. (Lima) 12:15–39.

58. ______. 1957b. (Preliminary investigation of brucellosis in alpacas) Investigacion preliminar de la brucelosis en alpacas. Rev. Fac. Med. Vet. (Lima) 12:130–34.

59. ______. 1957c. (Preliminary investigation of tuberculosis in alpacas) Investigacion preliminar de la tuberculose en alpacas. Rev. Fac. Med. Vet. (Lima) 12:135–37.

60. ______. 1958–59a. (Alpaca fever or streptococcosis) Fiebre de las alpacas o estreptococosis. Rev. Fac. Med. Vet. (Lima) 13–14:7–25.

61. ______. 1958–59b. (On an outbreak of rabies in alpacas) Sobre un brote de rabia en alpacas. Rev. Fac. Med. Vet. (Lima) 13–14:35–40.

62. ______. 1960. (Enterotoxemia of young alpacas) Enterotoxemia o diarrea bacilar de las crias de alpacas. An. Primer Congr. Nac. Med. Vet. (Lima), pp. 1–29.

63. ______. 1961–62a. (Infectious diseases of alpacas. I. Necrobacillosis) Enfermedades infecciosas de las alpacas. I. Necrobacilosis. Rev. Fac. Med. Vet. (Lima) 16–17:138–53.

64. ______. 1961–62b. (Infectious diseases of alpacas. II. Listeriosis) Enfermedades infecciosas de las alpacas. II. Listeriosis. Rev. Fac. Med. Vet. (Lima) 16–17:154–59.

65. ______. 1961–62c. (Infectious diseases of alpacas. III. Tetanus) Enfermedades infecciosas de las alpacas. III. Tetanos. Rev. Fac. Med. Vet. (Lima) 16–17:160–62.

66. ______. 1963-66. (Infectious diseases of alpacas. IV. Enterotoxemia *C. welchii* type C) Enfermedades infecciosas de las alpacas. IV. Enterotoxemia diarrea bacilar por *Clostridium welchii* tipo C. Rev. Fac. Med. Vet. (Lima) 18–20:74–84.

67. ______. 1963. (Infectious diseases of alpacas. V. Enterotoxemia produced by *C. welchii*) Infermedades infecciosas de las alpacas. V. Enterotoxemia o diarrea bacilar producida por *Clostridium welchii,* tipo A. Rev. Fac. Med. Vet. (Lima) 18(20):85–87.

68. ______. 1964. (Infectious diseases of alpacas) Enfermedadas infecciosas de las alpacas. Rev. Univ. Nac. Tec. Altiplano (Puno) 1(1):9–21.

69. ______. 1968a. Diseases of the Auchenidae. Panam. Health Org. Publ. 182:158–64.

70. ______. 1968b. (Diseases of South American camelids) Enfermedades de los auquenidos. Bol. Extraordinario 3:61–74.

71. Moro Sommo, M., and Guerrero, C. 1971. (The alpaca, infectious and parasitic diseases) La alpaca: Enfermedades infecciosas y parasitarias. Bol. Divulg. 8:1–64.

72. Muir, S., and Pappagionis, D. 1982. Coccidioidomycosis in the llama: Case report and epidemiologic survey. J. Am. Vet. Med. Assoc. 181:1334–37.

73. Noe, N., and Moro Sommo, M. 1967. (Isolation of mycoplasma of domestic animals) Aislamiento de micoplasma de animales domesticos. Rev. Fac. Med. Vet. (Lima) 21:77–83.

74. Nasser, M., Moussa, A. A., Metwallz, M. A., and Saleh, R. E. S. 1980. Secretion and persistence of foot-and-mouth disease virus in faeces of experimentally infected camels and ram. J. Egypt Vet. Med. 40(4):5–13.

75. Pallaske. 1965. (Generalized paratuberculosis in an antelope and a llama) Verallgemeinern Paratuberculose bei die Antelopen und bei die Lama. Zentralbl. Allg. Pathol. Anat. 107:95.

76. Pattyn, S. R., Antoine-Portaels, F., Kageruka, P., and Gigase, P. 1970. *Mycobacterium microti* infection in a zoo llama, *Lama vicugna.* Acta Zool. Pathol. Antverpiensia 51:17–24.

77. Pickett, J. P., Moore, C. P., Beehler, B. A., Gendron-Fitzpatrick, A., and Dubielzig, R. R. 1985. Bilateral chorioretinitis secondary to disseminated aspergillosis in an alpaca. J. Am. Vet. Med. Assoc. 187:1241–43.

78. Preston Smith, H. 1935. (Diseases of the alpaca) La enfermedades de las alpacas. Granja Model. Puno Bol. 9:14–30.

79. ______. 1940. (The camelids of Peru, ecthyma of alpacas) Los camello Peruanos, auquenidos, alpacas ectima. Minist. Agric. Bol. (Lima).

80. ______. 1947. (Ecthyma of animals of Peru, contagious pustular dermatitis) Ectima de los animales del Peru, dermatitis pustular contagiosa. Ganaderia (Peru) 1(1):27–32.

81. ______. 1950. (Diseases of the alpaca) Enfermedades del alpaca. Rev. Inst. Nac. Biol. Anim. Peru 1:10–12.

82. ______. 1951. (Fever of alpacas) Fiebre de las alpacas. An. Congr. Panam. Med. Vet. (Lima).

83. ______. 1953. (Fever of alpacas) Fiebre de las alpacas. Rev. Peru Inst. Nac. Biol. Andina 3(4):91–95.

84. Ramirez, A., and Huaman, D. 1980–81. (Evaluation of enterotoxemia vaccination in infant alpacas) Evaluacion de la enterotoxemia en crias de alpacas vacunados. Resumenes Proyectos Invest. Realizados (Lima) 3:48–49.

85. Ramirez, A., Lauerman, L., Huaman, D., and Vargas, A. 1983. (Preliminary induction of enterotoxemia type A [*Clostridium perfringens*] in alpacas) Induccion preliminar de la enterotoxemia A *Clostridium perfringens* tipo A en alpaca. Resumenes Proyectos Invest. Realizados (Lima) 3:48–49.

86. Ramirez, A., Ludena, H., and Acosta, M. 1983. (Mortality in alpacas of the livestock center at La Raya-Puno for 7 years) Mortalidad en alpacas del centro pecuario La Raya-Puno en siete años. Resumenes Proyectos Invest. Realizados (Lima) 3:47–48.

87. Rath, E. 1950a. (The anthrax vaccine immunizes the alpaca against the so-called fever or septicemia of alpaca) La vacuna de carbunclo sintomatico immaniza a las alpacas contra la i llamada "fiebre o septicemia de las alpacas." Copias Mecanografiadas.

88. ______. 1950b. (Symptoms and anatomic pathologic charts of the diseases of livestock in the Department of Puno) Sintomas y cuadros anatomo-patologicos de las enfermedades de ganado en el Departamento de Puno. Rev. Agrop. Peru 1(2):68–70.

89. Rebhun, W. C., Jenkins, D. H., Riis, R. C., Dill, S. G., Dubovi, E. J., and Torres, A. 1988. An epizootic of blindness and encephalitis associated with a herpesvirus indisti-

guishable from equine herpesvirus I in a herd of alpacas and llamas. J. Am. Vet. Med. Assoc. 192(7):953–56.

90. Rios, M., Ramirez, A., Ellis, R., and Barsallo, J. 1985. (Presence of streptococcus in alpacas in relation to factors of management) Presencia de streptococcus en alpacas en relacion a factores de manajo. Proc. Int. Camelidos Sudam, Cuzco, Peru, p. 40.

91. Rivera, G. H. 1970a. (Investigations of syphilis in alpacas) Investigacion de sifilis en alpacas, *Lama pacos.* Tesis, Fac. Med. Vet. Univ. Nac. Mayor San Marcos (Lima), pp. 1–25.

92. ______. 1970b. (Investigation of syphilis in alpacas) Investigacion de sifilis en alpacas, *Lama pacos.* Bol. Extraordinario 4:105–115.

93. Rivera, H., Madewell, B. R., and Ameqhino, E. 1987. Serologic survey of viral antibodies in the Peruvian alpaca, *Lama pacos.* Am. J. Vet. Res. 48(2):189–91.

94. Rodriguez, H., and Mimbela, M. 1983. (Microbiology of nasal and buccal secretions in alpacas) Microbiologia de secrecion nasal y bucal en alpacas. Resumenes Proyectos Invest. Realizados (1980–81) (Lima) 3:4.

95. Saez, H., and Rinjard, J. 1975. (Animal candidiasis in a captive wild animal environment) La candidose animale en milieu sauvage captif. Bull. Soc. Fr. Mycol. Med. 4(2):131–34.

96. Scott, D. W. 1988. Large Animal Dermatology. Philadelphia: W. B. Saunders.

97. Smith, D. H. 1981. Enterotoxemia. In J. L. Howard, ed. Current Veterinary Therapy: Food Animal Practice. Philadelphia: W. B. Saunders, pp. 695–97.

98. Tamayo, M. O. 1905. (Experimental rabies in llama) La rabia experimental en la llama. Cron. Med. 22:269–72.

99. Tapia Cano, F. 1965. (Investigations of *Listeria* in the medulla oblongata in apparently normal alpacas) Investigacion de *Listeria monocytogenes* en la medula oblongata de alpacas aparentemente normales. B. S. tesis, Fac. Med. Vet. Univ. Nac. Mayor San Marcos (Lima), pp. 1–45.

100. Thoen, C. O., Richards, W. D., and Jamagin, J. L. 1977. Mycobacteria isolated from exotic animals. J. Am. Vet. Med. Assoc. 170:987–90.

101. Torres, A., Dubovi, E. J., Rebhun, W. C., and King, J. M. 1985. Isolation of a herpesvirus associated with an outbreak of blindness and encephalitis in a herd of alpacas and llamas. Abstr. 66th Conf. Res. Workers Anim. Dis.

102. Toucedo, G. A. 1965. (Infection with *C. tetani* in a llama) Infeccion a *Clostridium tetani* en una llama. Gac. Vet. (Argentina) 27(13):432–36.

103. Urbain, A., et al. 1944. (Relationship between registered births and deaths at the Vincennes Zoo for the year 1943) Rapport sur la mortalite et la natalite enregistres au Parc Zoologique du Bois de Vincennes en 1943. Bull. Mus. Nat. Hist. (Paris) 16:56.

104. ______. 1949. (Relationship between registered births and mortality at the Vincennes Zoo) Rapport sur la mortalite et la natalite enregistres au Parc Zoologique du Bois de Vincennes. Bull. Mus. Nat. Hist. (Paris) 21:178–93.

105. Wilson, R. T. 1984. The Camel. Burnt Mill, Harlow, England: Longman Group, p. 120.

8 Parasites

THIS CHAPTER is not meant to be a definitive discussion of all the ramifications of the parasites of camelids; however, sufficient information will be discussed to allow general identification, provide the life cycle, if known, and aid in the management of parasitism in South American camelids (SACs).

The classification of parasites is in constant flux. Therefore, a recent reliable author should be selected as a source for taxonomy. In this book, the classifications of Levine for nematodes (56) and protozoa (57) are followed. For other parasites, Soulsby (70) and Georgi (22) are the sources. Taxonomy is not of great importance to the clinician except to know that closely related species tend to share similar life cycles, which aids in more effective management planning. For instance, if a particular parasite is known to be a trichostrongylid, plans to control the parasitism can be based on knowledge of the probable life cycle and susceptibility to certain anthelmintics.

A classification of parasitic genera reported to affect camelids follows:

PHYLUM ARTHROPODA

Class Insecta
- Order Mallophaga—biting lice
  - *Damalinia breviceps*
- Order Siphunculata [Anoplura]—sucking lice
  - Family Linognathidae
    - *Microthoracius cameli*
    - *M. praelongiceps*
    - *M. mazzai*
- Order Siphonaptera—fleas
  - *Vermipsylla* sp.
- Order Diptera—flies
  - Suborder Nematocera
    - Family Culicidae—mosquitoes, miscellaneous genera
    - Family Simuliidae—black fly
  - Suborder Brachycera
    - Family Tabanidae
      - *Tabanus* sp.—horse fly, deer fly
  - Suborder Cyclorrhapha
    - Family Muscidae
      - *Musca domestica*—house fly
      - *Musca autumnalis*—face fly
      - *Stomoxys calcitrans*—biting stable fly
    - Family Calliphoridae—blow flies
      - *Calliphora* sp.—blue blow fly
      - *Cochliomyia hominivorax*—primary screw worm
      - *Phaenicaia* sp.—green blow fly
      - *Phormia* sp.—black blow fly
    - Family Oestridae—Bot flies
      - *Oestrus ovis*—sheep nasal bot
      - *Cephenemyia* sp.—deer nasal bot
      - *Cephalopsis titillator*

Class Arachnida
- Order Acarina
  - Suborder Metastigmata—ticks
    - Family Argasidae—soft-bodied ticks
      - *Otobius megnini*—spinose ear tick
    - Family Ixodidiae—hard-bodied ticks, various genera
  - Suborder Mesostigmata—mites
    - Family Sarcoptidae
      - *Sarcoptes scabiei*
    - Family Psoroptidae
      - *Psoroptes ovis*
      - *Chorioptes bovis*

PHYLUM PROTOZOA

Subphylum Sarcomastigophora—flagellates
- *Trypanosoma* sp.
- *Trichomonas* sp.
- *Giardia* sp.

Subphylum Apicomplexa (Sporozoa)
- *Eimeria lamae*
- *E. alpacae*
- *E. punoensis*
- *E. macusaniensis*
- *Sarcocystis* sp.
- *Toxoplasma gondii*

PHYLUM PLATYHELMINTHES (Flat worms)

Class Trematoda—flukes
- Order Digenea
  - *Fasciola hepatica*
  - *Fasciola gigantica*
  - *Eurytrema pancreaticum*
  - *Dicrocoelium dendriticum*

Class Eucestoda—tapeworms
- Family Taeniidae
  - *Echinococcus granulosus*

Family Anoplocephalidae
Moniezia expansa
Thysaniezia sp.

PHYLUM NEMATOHELMINTHES
Class Secernentea (Phasmida)
Order Strongylida
Superfamily Trichostrongyloidea
Trichostrongylus axei
Trichostrongylus sp.
Ostertagia ostertagi
Ostertagia sp.
Marshallagia (Ostertagia) marshalli
Camelostrongylus mentulatus
Graphinema aucheniae
Haemonchus contortus
Haemonchus sp.
Lamanema chavezi
Spiculopteragia peruvianus
Nematodirus lamae
Nematodirus battus
Cooperia sp.
Dictyocaulus viviparus
Dictyocaulus filaria
Superfamily Metastrongyloidea
Family Protostrongylidae
Parelaphostrongylus tenuis
Superfamily Strongyloidea
Family Strongyloidae
Oesophagostomum sp.
Chabertia ovina
Superfamily Ancylostomatoidea (hookworms)
Family Ancylostomatidae
Bunostomum sp.
Order Spirurida
Superfamily Thelaziodea
Family Thelaziidae
Thelazia californiensis
Thelazia sp.
Superfamily Spiruroidae
Gongylonema sp.
Class Adenophorea (Aphasmidia)
Order Enoplida
Superfamily Trichuroidea
Trichuris ovis
Capillaria sp.

The identification to species of the gastrointestinal (GI) parasites of SACs in North America has never been reported. Thus it is not known whether the species found in SACs are the same as those found in cattle, sheep, and goats or if they are different species from the same genera (23). Though important from an epidemiologic standpoint, information will not be available until a classic taxonomist of parasites takes an interest in SACs.

The parasites of herd or flock importance in South America have been studied intensively. Those of lesser importance are rarely investigated. The lack of reported instances of parasitism from major taxonomic groups may only reflect a failure to observe, identify, or report. As yet, only 75 species of parasites have been reported to cause clinical disease in camelids. SACs share no nematode genera with equids, and there are no reports of ascarids in SACs.

EXTERNAL PARASITES

Lice

IDENTIFICATION. Lice are wingless insects that live a complete life cycle on a single host (70). They are generally host specific, i.e., lice found on livestock and pets will not spread to camelids, nor will camelid lice transfer to other species (49, 81). Both biting, *Damalinia breviceps,* and sucking, *Microthoracius minor,* lice and *M. mazzai, M. praelongiceps,* and *M. cameli* (Fig. 8.1) have been identified on camelids (8, 15, 19).

Biting lice vary in size from 0.5 × 1.2 to 1.5 × 4 mm. They may be white or light tan. People with average vision can see these lice without magnification, but a hand lens (10X) assists the observer. Unless recently groomed, a camelid fleece contains detritis, which may be confused with lice. Lice move when disrupted by parting of the fiber and will be found near the surface of the skin. Biting lice have a blunted head. This characteristic can usually be seen without magnification, but precise identification would require microscopic evaluation.

Sucking lice of SACs are approximately two-thirds the size of biting lice. Sucking lice are more sedentary than biting lice and thus are more difficult to see. They have elongated mouth parts, but these are so small that microscopic identification is necessary.

LIFE CYCLE. The life cycle of lice is simple (Fig. 8.2). Adult lice copulate and the female deposits fertilized eggs (nits) on fibers and cements them in place. The eggs hatch within 1–3 weeks and tiny replicas of adult lice emerge. As the louse matures it undergoes two or three molts, but in each case it is growth, not a change of body structure. The maturation phase lasts 1–2 weeks. The entire life cycle may be completed in as little as 2–5 weeks. Adults live for 15–40 days.

EPIDEMIOLOGY. Lice may complete the life cycle on a single animal. There is no free-living stage. Transmission from one camelid to another is by close body contact, as may occur with maternal care of infants, during breeding, or between individuals when they lie down touching each other. Transmission can also occur by the use of communal grooming equipment such as combs, brushes, and carding combs or by group use of

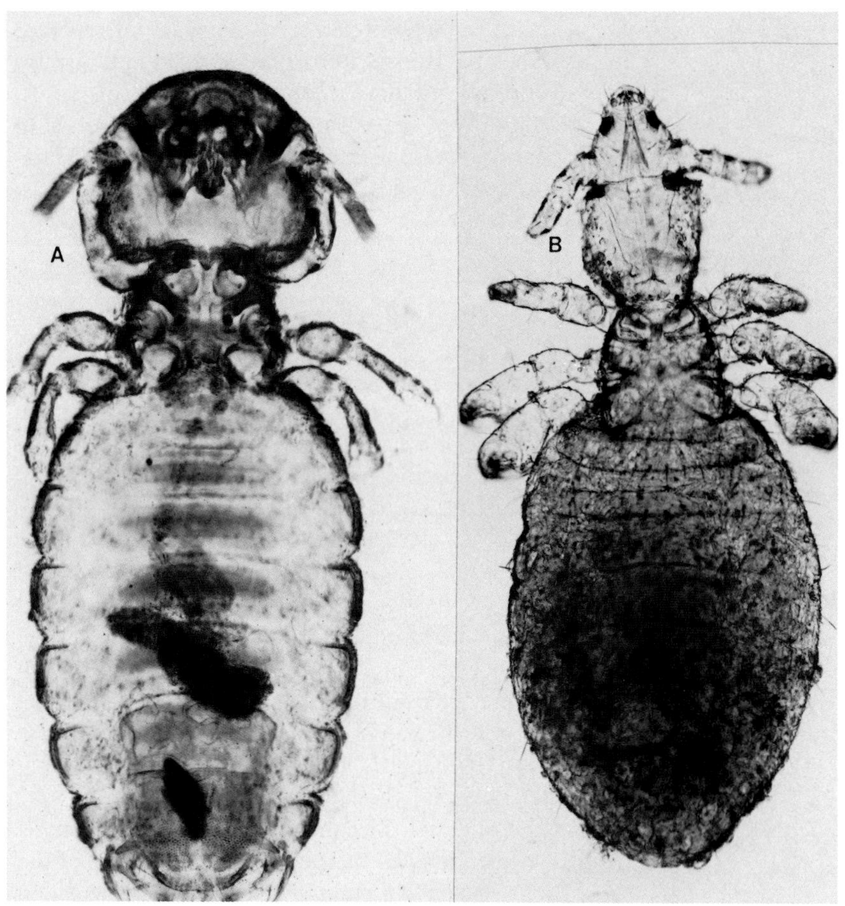

8.1 Lamoid lice: **(A)** biting louse, *Damalinia breviceps,* **(B)** sucking louse, *Microthoracius cameli.*

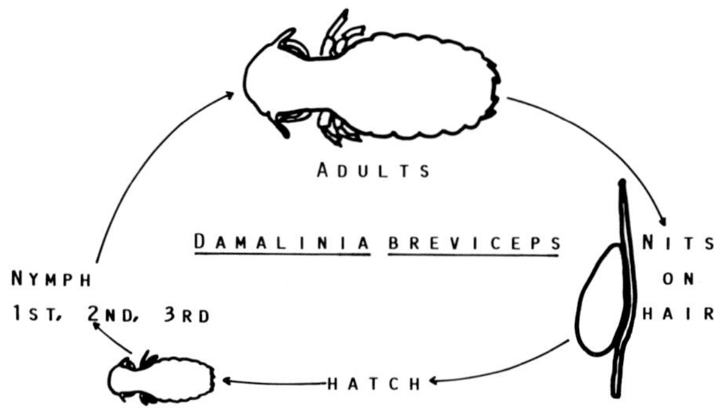

8.2 Life cycle of a louse.

blankets, scratching posts, dust bath areas, narrow doorjambs, and feed bunks.

Populations of lice tend to build up during the colder months of the year. Perhaps the long fiber provides a warmer environment conducive to reproductive success. Although the cycle may be completed in as little as 2–5 weeks, it may be extended many months by arrested development in the nit stage, or a few lice may lie dormant until environmental conditions become conducive to rapid development of a population.

CLINICAL SIGNS. The syndromes of the two types of lice are different.

Biting Lice. The fiber coat lacks luster and has a ragged appearance. Heavy infestation results in matting and loss of fibers. The llama may bite at itself or rub against fences, trees, shrubs, poles, or buildings. In one case, the animal rubbed raw a spot over the dorsal spine of the vertebra. The egg cases (nits) may be observed attached to the fibers.

The areas of the body most likely to be infested are around the base of the tail, along either side of the vertebral column, on the side of the neck, and along the sides of the body. To search for lice, part the fibers down to the skin, use a bright light, and observe for movement of the tiny specks. If no lice are seen, change locations and repeat the procedure.

Sucking Lice. Of the two types of lice, sucking lice are more pathogenic. In addition to the signs noted for biting lice, sucking lice may cause anemia since they extract blood and tissue fluid from the host. Anemic llamas are more susceptible to cold stress and secondary infections.

Sucking lice prefer sites around the flanks, head, neck, and withers. The lice will be found clinging to the fibers close to the skin or actually imbedded in the skin taking a blood meal.

TREATMENT. Lice may be destroyed by direct contact with numerous insecticides, including pyrethrins, chlorinated hydrocarbons, carbamates, and organic phosphates (Tables 8.1, 8.2). The problem is to

Table 8.1. Pesticides registered for use on livestock and horses

Pesticide	Formulation	Beef cattle	Dairy cows	Sheep, goats	Horses
1. Calcium polysulfide (sulfur)	EC, WP, S, D	*	*	*	*
2. Carbaryl (Sevin)	WP, D				*
3. Chlorpyrifos (Dursban)	SO	*			
4. Coumaphos (CoRal)	EC, WP, PO, S, D	*	*	*	*
5. Crotoxyphos (Ciodrin)	EC, S	*	*	*	*
6. Diazinon	EC			NL	
7. Dichlorvos (Vapona)	EC, S	*	*	*	*
8. Dioxathion (Co-Nav)	EC	*		NL	*
9. Famphur (Warbex)	SO, D	*	NL		
10. Fenthion (Tiguvon)	PO, SO	*	NL		
11. Fenvalerate (Ectrin)	ET, S	*	*		
12. Ivermectin[a] (Eqvalen for horses, Ivomec for cattle)	IM, SC	*	*		*
13. Lindane (Gamma BHC)	EC, WP, S, D	*		NL	*
14. Malathion	EC, WP, S, D	*	*	NL	*
15. Methoprene (Altosid)	F	*	*		
16. Methoxychlor (Marlate)	EC, WP, D	*	*	NL	*
17. Naled (Dibrom)	EC				*
18. Nicotine sulfate (Blackleaf 40)[c]	EC				
19. Permethrin (Atroban, Ectiban, Permectrin)	ET, ETT, S	*	*		
20. Phosmet (Prolate)	EC, PO	*	NL		
21. Pyrethrins, plus piperonyl butoxide	S	*	*	*	*
22. Ronnel (Korlan)	ASC, SM, G		*		*
23. Stirofos (Rabon)	EC, WP, F, D	*	*		
24. Toxaphene[b]	EC	*			*
25. Trichlorfon (Neguvon)	SO	*	NL		

Source: Extension Veterinary Medicine, Univ. of Calif., Davis. Used by permission.

Note: EC = emulsifiable concentrate; WP = wettable powder; S = usually in dilute, ready-to-use form; D = dust; SO = spot-on (high concentrate, low dose); PO = pour-on (low concentrate, low dose); ET = ear tag; IM = intramuscular injection; SC = subcutaneous injection; F = feed mixtures or medicated salt blocks; ETT = ear tag tape; ASC = aerosol spray can; SM = smear; G = granules; NL = use only on nonlactating animals.

*Registered for use in that species.

[a]Prescription drug only by a veterinarian.

[b]Registered only for use in scabies mite control on beef animals.

[c]Registered but no longer used.

Table 8.2. Registered pesticides for external parasite control on livestock and horses

Parasite	Beef and nonlactating dairy cattle	Lactating dairy cows	Sheep and goats	Horses
Blow flies (in wounds)	4, 13, 22	4, 13, 22	4(NL), 13(NL), 22(G)	13, 14, 22
Face fly	4, 5, 7–9, 11–16, 19, 20, 21, 23, 24	4, 5, 6, 11, 14, 16, 19, 21, 23		4, 5, 7, 8, 14, 16, 21, 23
Horn fly	4, 5, 7–9, 11–16, 19, 20, 21, 23, 24	4, 5, 7, 11, 15, 19, 21		
Horse fly	19, 20	19, 20	4, 13(NL)	2, 4, 5, 6, 8, 14, 16, 21, 23, 24
House and stable flies	5, 7, 19, 21, 23	5, 7, 19, 21, 23		2, 4, 5, 6, 8, 14, 16, 21
Heel fly	3, 4, 9, 10, 12, 20, 25			
Mosquitoes, black flies, and gnats	5, 7, 21	21	21	21
Lice and sheep ked	3–5, 7–10, 13, 14, 16, 19, 20, 23, 24	4, 5, 7, 19, 21, 23	4(NL), 5, 6(NL), 7, 8, 13(NL), 14(NL), 16(NL), 19, 24(NL)	4, 5, 7, 8, 14, 24
Ticks—body	3–5, 7, 8, 13, 14, 19, 20, 23, 24	5, 7, 19	1, 3(NL), 14(NL), 19, 24(NL)	4, 5, 7, 8, 14, 19, 24
—ear	4, 5, 11, 13, 19, 22	4, 5, 11,19	13(NL)	4, 13, 22
Mites	1, 13, 19, 20, 24	1, 19	1, 3(NL), 13(NL), 14(NL)	1, 24

Source: Extension Veterinary Medicine, Univ. of Calif., Davis. Used by permission.

Note: Numbers correspond to drugs in Table 8.1; NL = use only on nonlactating goats; G = use only on goats.

establish contact with the lice. Dusts and sprays applied superficially will not reach them. Drenching sprays or dips are not practical for temperate climates, especially since the problem is more pronounced in the winter.

Ivermectin is not effective against biting lice but has excellent activity against sucking lice at a dose of 0.2 mg/kg body weight administered subcutaneously. It should be noted that although ivermectin has not been approved by the Federal Drug Administration (FDA) for use in llamas, it has been used extensively as a general anthelmintic in llamas and has proven to be safe and effective. This should be discussed with a client before this drug is administered.

The author has had poor results from the use of "pour on" organic phosphate insecticides for biting lice, but others recommend its usage. The most effective product in the author's experience is a 50% wettable powder of methoxychlor (Marlate, obtainable at orchard and garden supply companies). The powder can be dispensed from a large shaker-top container like those used for salt in food establishments. The fibers should be parted down the topline and the powder shaken next to the skin. Manipulating the wool will aid in distributing the powder. More powder should be applied 2–3 inches to the side, parting the fibers as before. This process should be continued until all of the problem areas have been covered. It is a laborious process but is an effective method during cold winter months. Carbaryl powder is also effective but is likely to be more expensive than methoxychlor.

Fleas

IDENTIFICATION. Fleas are wingless insects with laterally compressed bodies (70). They vary in size from 1.5 to 4 mm. Fleas are not host specific, thus several different types may be found on camelids. No specific reports of flea infestations have appeared in the literature on SACs, but the genus *Vermispsylla* contains a number of species that infest camels. Llama owners have described flea infestation to the author.

LIFE CYCLE. Adult fleas copulate and the female lays approximately 20 eggs at a time in detritis on the host or in dust/dirt in the llama's environment. Larvae hatch in 2–16 days and feed on dried blood, feces, or other organic matter. The larval stage is completed in 7–10 days and the insect enters the pupal stage, which may last for 10–17 days or remain dormant for months. The adult emerges from the pupal case to seek a suitable host.

EPIDEMIOLOGY. Fleas may be transmitted from one llama to another by close body contact. Fleas are active and may jump prodigious distances. Contamination of the environment with flea eggs and pupae enables infestation to be acquired by simply walking through any area previously exposed to animals with fleas. The life span of an individual flea may be over 1 year. During this time the female may lay as many as 400 eggs.

Fleas are notorious vectors for infectious and parasitic diseases; however, no such instances have been documented in SACs.

CLINICAL SIGNS. Adult fleas consume only blood and may cause anemia. In massive infestations, exsanguination from fleas may be fatal. While biting the host, fleas deposit saliva, which may stimulate an allergic response varying from mild irritation to marked pruritus, hyperemia, swelling, and dermatitis.

TREATMENT. Same as for lice.

Mosquitoes

IDENTIFICATION. Mosquitoes are slender-bodied, long-legged, winged insects with spherical heads and a long slender proboscis, which is used to cannulate capillaries to ingest blood meals from the host (70). The numerous species differ in habitat preference but have no significant host specificity. Camelids in mosquito territory will be bitten.

LIFE CYCLE (70). The gravid female lays eggs in water. The eggs hatch in less than a week to become air-breathing larvae. Larvae undergo four molts over a period of 2 weeks, progressing to the pupal stage that lasts 2–7 days. The adult emerges from the puparium and must dry itself before being able to fly off in 24 hours. The entire cycle requires approximately a month, less in warm moist habitats.

EPIDEMIOLOGY. Since mosquitoes fly, they can easily reach hosts. They do not remain on the host but, rather, light, ingest a blood meal, and leave. A swarm of mosquitoes can be annoying and may stimulate a bite response similar to that of fleas. Like fleas, mosquitoes are vectors for numerous infectious diseases, serving as the intermediate host for some and as mechanical vectors for others.

CLINICAL SIGNS. Mosquito bites, even in large numbers, will not likely cause anemia. Individual bites may be pruritic, hyperemic, and swollen.

TREATMENT. Reducing mosquito numbers requires management of the environment (decreasing breeding habitat, insecticide treatment). Mosquito repellents used in humans are effective for a short period and are recommended for those who pack with llamas.

Black Flies (buffalo gnats)

IDENTIFICATION. Simulid flies are closely related to mosquitoes but have a short, piercing proboscis and a hump over the thorax. The legs are not as long as those of mosquitoes.

LIFE CYCLE (70). The female black fly lays eggs only in running water, either on the surface or on submerged stones, twigs, or vegetation. The eggs may remain in the water for months, overwintering in this state, or hatch in a few days. Larvae are mobile, with the lopping type of ambulation typical of an "inch worm." Larvae molt six times before entering the pupal stage, which floats near the surface so that a special respiratory tube can take in the necessary air. Adults emerge from the puparium and may swarm in dense clouds if the population is large.

EPIDEMIOLOGY. Black flies are found throughout the world but are concentrated in warmer climates (70). Flies are active in the morning and evening. They do not live on the hosts but take blood meals from them.

CLINICAL SIGNS. Swarms of black flies are annoying to the animals and may inhibit feeding. The bites may simulate those from mosquitos in sensitive animals.

TREATMENT. Same as for mosquitoes.

Tabanids (horse flies, deer flies)

IDENTIFICATION. Tabanids are medium to large flies with powerful wings and large eyes.

LIFE CYCLE (70). Females lay eggs in damp soil or decaying organic matter. The eggs are glued in masses near a water source so that when the larvae, hatching in about 1 week, will fall into the water to continue maturation. The larvae and subsequent pupae may burrow into the mud at the bottom of a pond or stream and overwinter there. Adults emerge from the puparium and soon require a blood meal to complete the life cycle, which requires a minimum of 4 months or may extend to the next season.

EPIDEMIOLOGY. Tabanids are diurnal and are especially active on hot, bright, humid days. Only the females take blood meals every 3 or 4 days. The bite from a tabanid is painful. Tabanids may be responsible for transmission of parasites and infectious agents, but this has not been documented for SACs. Tabanids are an important intermediate host for *Trypanosoma evansii,* the cause of surra in camels and other artiodactylids in Africa and Asia. There is circumstantial evidence of *T. evansii* infection in South America, with a potential for infection in SACs.

CLINICAL SIGNS. The large mouth parts may pierce capillaries, which continue to flow after the tabanid has departed, attracting other nonbiting flies. Sensitive individuals may develop erythema and swelling at the bite site. The flies may annoy the animal.

TREATMENT. No treatment or prevention is available other than swatting the fly if observed near or on the animal.

Miscellaneous Flies

IDENTIFICATION. Llamas and other camelids are plagued with the same types of flies that afflict domestic livestock. The house fly, *Musca domestica,* has four dark stripes on the thorax and yellow spots on the side of the abdomen and is approximately 7 mm long (59).

The face fly, *Musca autumnalis,* is slightly larger than the house fly and lacks the yellow color on the abdomen.

The biting stable fly, *Stomoxys calcitrans,* is also annoying to llamas. It is the same size as the house fly but has a long, stiff proboscis and gray-brown spots on the abdomen.

Other species of flies may annoy or afflict llamas. The species that are present will depend on the environment.

LIFE CYCLE (70)

House Fly. The female lays eggs on manure or decaying organic matter. The larvae hatch in less than 24 hours, then grow and molt twice in a few days to become third-stage larvae, which move to a drier area and pupate. The adults emerge in 2–3 weeks, climb to the surface, and spread their wings to dry. Adults live for 6–8 weeks, during which time the female will lay 2000 eggs. The entire cycle takes 3–5 weeks.

Face Fly. The life cycle is similar to that of the house fly (Fig. 8.3), except that the female lays eggs in fresh cattle feces, where hatching, larvation, and pupation occur. Hence, face flies will be a problem only where camelids are housed contiguous to cattle (70).

Biting Stable Fly. The life cycle is similar to those of the house and face flies. Eggs are laid in decaying organic matter or manure. Both sexes suck blood and feed once or twice daily.

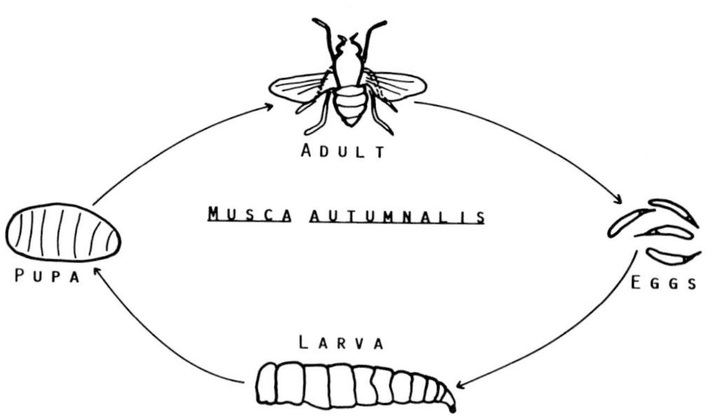

8.3 Life cycle of a fly.

EPIDEMIOLOGY. House flies are found both inside and outside of barns and sheds. Face flies usually do not enter buildings, so llamas may gain respite by going inside; however, face flies may enter buildings to escape cold weather. They may overwinter as adults, becoming active on days of unseasonably warm weather. All flies are more active on warm days than on cool and cease activity at dark.

CLINICAL SIGNS. Flies are annoying to the llama. Biting flies may cause additional irritation. Flies are particularly irritating if there is excessive lacrimal secretion. They may exacerbate the problem until conjunctivitis is produced.

MANAGEMENT. Fly control is a never-ending challenge to any animal enterprise. All the methods employed by livestock raisers have application with camelid enterprises. A visor of cloth or leather strips, similar to those used on horses, may be employed to keep the flies from the eyes.

Blow Flies

IDENTIFICATION. Many species of flies deposit eggs in fresh or necrotic wounds of animals. Camelids are equally susceptible to the attacks of these flies. Some examples of blow flies follow (59).

The blue blow fly, *Calliphora* sp., is up to 11 mm in length. The thorax is dull colored and the abdomen is blue-green. The green blow fly, *Phaenicaia* sp., is approximately 7 mm long, with green to bronze coloration of the thorax and abdomen. The black blow fly, *Phormia* sp., is approximately 8 mm long and is bluish-black. The primary screw worm, *Cochliomia hominivorax,* is a special problem because it will invade healthy tissue.

LIFE CYCLE. The female screw worm lays eggs (200) in a fresh wound. The eggs hatch in 24 hours and the larvae feed on flesh, invading contiguous tissue. The matured larvae leave the wound in 7 days to pupate. Adults emerge in from 1 to several weeks. The entire life cycle may be completed in as little as 2.5 weeks or continue for several. The primary screw worm could be considered an obligatory parasite.

The facultative parasitic calliphorids have a similar life cycle but do not invade fresh wounds. They are attached to suppurating or necrotic wounds or areas solid with feces and urine. The neonatal umbilicus is a favored site. Downer animals may develop decubitus on soiled areas and be subject to attacks.

EPIDEMIOLOGY. Primary screw worms have been eradicated from the United States but may be present in other areas of the New World. The other flies are ubiquitous.

CLINICAL SIGNS. Larvae will be seen crawling and feeding in the wound.

TREATMENT. The wound should be cleaned and debrided to remove necrotic tissue. Fiber should be clipped to allow proper drainage of the wound and exposure to the air. Larvae may be removed mechanically or killed by the instillation of insecticides into the wound. Since the vehicle used to solubilize the insecticide may be irritating to the tissue and will be absorbed into the system much more readily than through healthy skin, only as much fluid as is absolutely necessary to destroy the larvae should be applied. Chloroform, ether, and hydrogen peroxide will also cause the larvae to retreat from crevices and cavities. Once larvae are destroyed, the wound should be properly treated and dressed. The wound should be monitored to remove missed larvae or deal with reinvasion. Ivermectin is also effective.

Bot Flies

IDENTIFICATION. Only three species of bot flies have been reported from camelids: the sheep and goat nasal bot, *Oestrus ovis;* various species of the deer nasopharyngeal bot fly, *Cephenemyia* sp.; and the camel bot, *Cephalopsis titillator.* The first two species are important for SAC owners and will be discussed separately.

Oestrus ovis

Identification. The adult fly averages 12 mm in length, about the size of a small honeybee. Soulsby describes the fly as having a dark gray color with tiny black spots that are especially prominent on the thorax. First instar larvae are whitish, translucent, and less than 2 mm long. As the larvae mature, dark transverse bands develop on the dorsal aspect of the segments. Mature larvae are approximately 3 cm long, with a long, tapering anterior end and a flat posterior end. There are two black stigmal plates on the posterior surface (Fig. 8.4), black oral hooks on the anterior end, and rows of small spines on the dorsal surface.

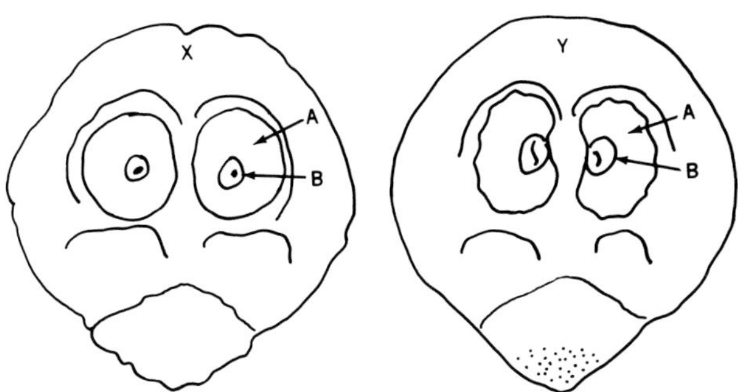

8.4 Third instar larvae: (X) *Oestrus ovis,* (Y) *Cephenemyia* sp. (A) peritreme, (B) button, posterior view.

Life Cycle (20). The fly deposits larvae around the nostrils of the llama. The flies cause considerable annoyance to the animal, and it may take evasive action by pressing the muzzle close to the ground or against other animals. The larvae instinctively crawl upward into the nasal cavity. Larvae may stay in the turbinate area or crawl into a sinus. The cycle in the llama has not been defined as to the location or length of time necessary to complete maturation, if, indeed, the larvae reach maturity in this species. In sheep, the first instar progresses to the second in from 2 weeks to as much as 9 months. The second instar matures in 25 days or more. Mature larvae crawl out of the nasal cavity, fall to the ground, and pupate for 3–6 weeks in warm weather or remain viable in the pupal stage for months if protected from freezing.

Epidemiology. The fly is active during the day but spends most of its time resting in cracks or crevices. In temperate climates, the fly is active in all but winter months, and in warm climates throughout the year. This fly is a serious parasite in sheep and goats in many areas. It has been only circumstantially identified from a camelid. Proper identification should be pursued on any nasal larvae found in a camelid, since the more common larva found has been the deer bot.

Clinical Signs. The syndrome seen in llamas has not been reported in the literature. Affected llamas exhibit signs similar to those seen in sheep, with nasal exudation, sneezing, and head shaking prominent. Visualization of the larvae with endoscopic examination would be fortuitous since the larvae are usually in the sinuses.

Treatment. Ivermectin therapy, at doses of 0.2 mg/kg, has been successful.

Cephenemyia sp. (deer nasopharyngeal bot, throat bot, deer nasal bot)

Identification. The adult fly superficially resembles a small bumblebee and is approximately 14 mm in length (20). First instar larvae are approximately 1 mm long and may molt up to 3 mm. Second instar larvae vary in length from 3 to 13 mm. Third instar larvae vary from 12 to 40 mm. The puparium is 16–20 mm long. Third instar larvae of all species are similar, making it difficult to identify the species. First instar larvae are most easily identified but are rarely seen or recovered.

A third instar larva removed from the nasopharynx of a llama had the following characteristics: cream color, 2.5 cm long, and approximately 0.7 cm in diameter (Fig. 8.5). The peritremes (stigmal plates) were crescent shaped, with the outer margins slightly sinuous. The button was on the inner margins (Fig. 8.4). In contrast, the peritremes of the third instar *Oestrus ovis* larva are circular with a central button (Fig. 8.4) (20).

Life Cycle (Fig. 8.6). Primary hosts for *Cephenemyia* sp. are cervids. Whether the cycle is completed in llamas is unknown. In deer, the adult fly lives for 2–3 weeks without feeding. Larvipositing by the female is carried out by spraying larvae into the nostrils of the host. Larvipositing evokes a behavioral response in deer. The head is jerked back, and sneezing and snoring ensue, accompanied by head shaking. Older animals may lower the head, pressing the nose against the ground. A few animals will run a few yards immediately following a strike (20).

The larvae may remain for a time in the nasal passageways but ultimately migrate to the nasopharynx, where they take up residence in the retropharyngeal pouches found in cervids, and develop to the second and third instar. At maturity, the third instar larvae migrate or are sneezed out through the nostril, fall to the ground, pupate, and after 16–31 days emerge as adult flies.

Epidemiology. A number of llamas have been infested with the deer nasopharyngeal bot (20). Camelids cohabiting pastures with deer are at risk. Various species of flies of this genus can be found in any area of North America where there are cervids. The llama is an

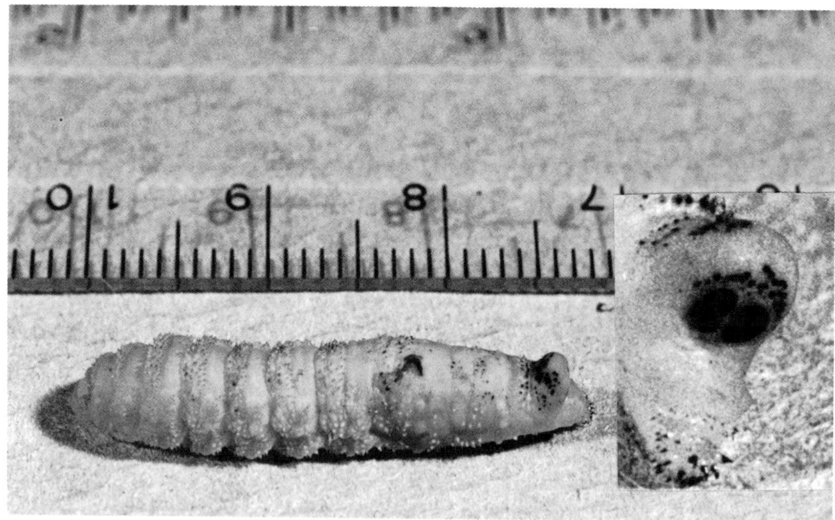

8.5 Third instar larva of *Cephenemyia* sp.

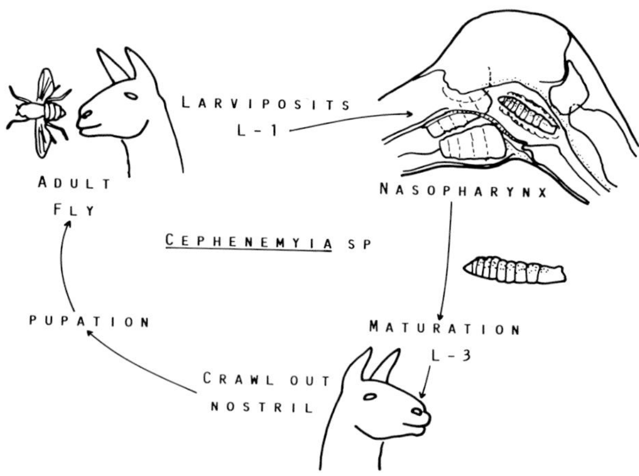

8.6 Life cycle of *Cephenemyia* sp.

aberrant host for this parasite, and it is not known whether or not the cycle is completed in the llama.

Clinical Signs. In deer, the oral hooks and spines of the larvae irritate the mucosa of the nasopharynx, inducing secretion of a viscous mucoid exudate that apparently provides nourishment for the larvae. Affected deer may have a nasal exudation and sneeze periodically.

In llamas, being an aberrant host, there is a more significant host reaction, with the development of a granulomatous swelling in the nasopharynx and nasal cavity. None of the affected llamas have died, and no biopsies have been taken to establish the histologic picture of this mass. However, the larvae can be seen embedded in the surface of the mass with endoscopic examination.

Prominent signs in the llama are sneezing and coughing, with or without a nasal discharge. The lesion is in the nasopharynx, and any exudation may be swallowed, not pushed out through the nasal cavity. Owners have reported that the llama is short of breath or fails to keep up with others on the trail. Though the llama is an obligate nasal breather, if the lesion becomes too obstructive, the llama will be forced to mouth breathe, with all its debilitating effects (see Chap. 22). Audible breathing will also be heard. There is usually no febrile response or changes in the hemogram. This is significant in differential diagnosis to rule out respiratory infectious diseases.

Diagnosis. The characteristic clinical syndrome, observed in a llama in an area harboring deer, would be primary evidence. The lesions and perhaps the larvae may be seen via endoscopic examination in an anesthetized individual. The mass appears as a radio-dense area in a radiograph (Fig. 8.7). A final diagnosis may be made on the basis of response to treatment.

Treatment. Although too few cases have been seen and treated to be conclusive, there is evidence that ivermectin is effective at 0.2 mg/kg given subcutaneously, although in two llamas, live larvae were seen after treatment and the dose was increased to 0.4 mg/kg.

Ticks

IDENTIFICATION. There are two major groups of ticks: hard-bodied ticks (family Ixodidae) and soft-bodied ticks (family Argasidae). There are numerous genera of hard-bodied ticks. Although no reports in the literature list the species found in SACs, it is likely that those that are not host specific will be identified according to the locality inhabited by SACs (16). Tick paralysis (discussed later) has been reported in a llama as a result of hard-bodied tick attachment.

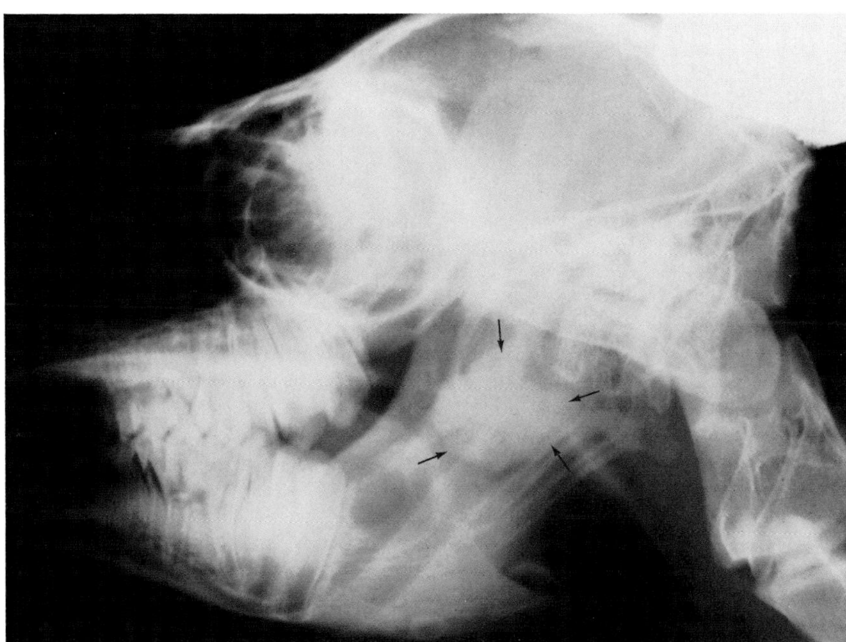

8.7 Lateral radiograph of the head of a llama with a *Cephenemyia* granuloma in the nasal pharynx.

The only soft-bodied tick that has caused a problem in llamas is the spinose ear tick, *Otobius megnini*. The adult tick, which is not parasitic, is about 8 mm long and has a constriction at the middle, giving it a fiddle shape (70). The larvae are pear shaped to spherical and about 2–3 mm long. The nymph, which is the primary parasitic stage, molts twice and when engorged will measure 7–10 mm in length.

LIFE CYCLE

Spinose Ear Tick. Adult ticks do not feed and may live for 6 months in cracks and crevices of barns, sheds, and fences or under feed bunks or stones (Fig. 8.8). The female may oviposit 500–600 eggs in the previously mentioned areas during her lifetime. The eggs hatch to six-legged larvae, ready to attach to a host in 10 days. The larvae migrate to the ear canals and begin to feed on lymph. Larvae survive only 2–4 months without a suitable host (70).

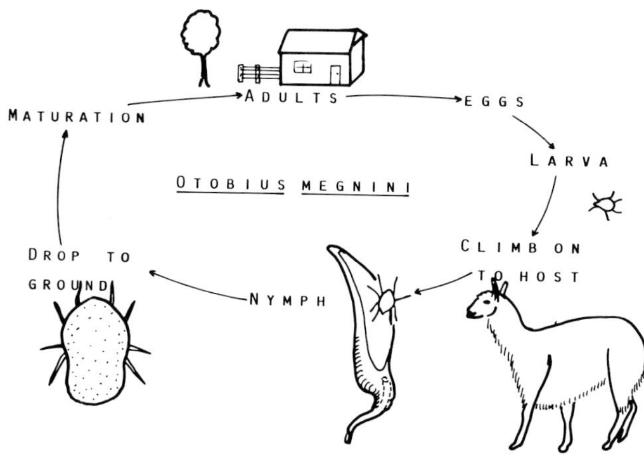

8.8 Life cycle of *Otobius megnini*.

The eight-legged nymphs molt twice within the ear canal, remaining on a single host for 1–7 months, feeding on blood. The mature nymph climbs out of the ear canal, drops to the ground, and molts to the adult stage. Usually only one mating cycle is completed each year.

Hard-bodied Ticks. Some species complete the entire cycle utilizing a single host species; others require two hosts; and a few, three separate hosts for each of the life stages. The female oviposits only once, producing thousands of eggs. Larvae feed only once, and there is only one nymph stage, taking only a single feeding. Hard-bodied ticks are more likely to be encountered in open grassland or shrubby areas rather than near sheds and barns, as is the case with soft-bodied ticks.

EPIDEMIOLOGY. Spinose ear ticks are a problem in llamas and alpacas in localized pockets in the western United States. Animals kept entirely on pasture or open range will be less likely to encounter the ticks because the preferred habitat of ticks is around buildings, sheds, wooden fences, and rough-barked trees, e.g., *Eucalyptus* sp.

Hard-bodied tick infestation is a problem in much of the West, especially with llamas used for packing into wilderness areas.

CLINICAL SIGNS. The two prime signs of spinose ear tick infestation are head shaking and exudation from the external ear canal. Further examination should reveal the nymphs within the ear canal. Anemia may result in young llamas with heavy infestations.

TREATMENT. Ivermectin (0.2 mg/kg) administered subcutaneously is effective for both the larvae and nymphs of the spinose ear tick. The individual ear canal may be physically cleaned with standard techniques and an insecticide solution instilled into the ear canal. The problem is to prevent reinfestation. There is little hope of eradicating the tick from an environment wherein the adults hide in crevices and under objects difficult to reach with sprays. Periodic inspection and treatment is necessary to prevent a buildup of infestation.

TICK PARALYSIS

Epidemiology. Tick paralysis has been recognized for over 50 years, and 43 species in 10 different genera of ticks have been incriminated (17). Usually only female hard-bodied ticks produce toxin, which is localized in the saliva and is injected into the host when the tick ingests a blood meal. No information is available as to why a given tick produces the toxin.

The neurotoxin from *Dermacentor* sp., in the United States, interferes with acetylcholine liberation at the neuromuscular endings, causing a lower motor neuron paresis. The bite from a single tick is sufficient to kill an animal if the tick is not removed.

Based on work in other species, there is variable host susceptibility. There may also be seasonal or annual variability, since there have been reports of epidemics of paralysis in some years and none in other years.

Clinical Signs. Tick paralysis has been diagnosed in the llama (48). A 1-year-old male llama was observed as normal on one day and the following day was totally paralyzed. A diffuse lower motor neuron disease was suspected. *Dermacentor* sp. ticks were found.

The llama was sprayed with a pyrethrin insecticide and ivermectin (0.2 mg/kg) was administered parenterally. Muscle tone reappeared within 12 hours and the llama was standing in 36 hours.

An affected llama would probably follow a similar progressive course as noted in other species. Signs may not develop for 5–7 days after the tick begins to feed. Paresis and paralysis are progressive, beginning in the rear quarters and moving cranially. Ataxia develops, followed by a loss of all motor function. Pain perception remains, according to human victims.

The signs may progress rapidly over a few hours or more slowly over a period of 24–48 hours. Paralysis ascends to the forelimbs, neck, head, and face. In early stages, the victim is bright and alert, able to eat and drink, but as the paralysis ascends, difficulty in chewing and swallowing develops. The cause of death is respiratory arrest from involvement of the respiratory centers of the brain.

Treatment. No drug can counter the effects of the neurotoxin. The cure is to remove the tick from the animal. The difficulty lies in finding a tick on an unshorn llama or alpaca. Since only one tick may be sufficient to cause the paralysis, finding it is crucial. In one tragic death in a human infant, the tick was located within the vulva.

Removal of the tick may reverse the signs in 2–12 hours. Assuming inability to find the offending tick, a standard insecticide dip may be employed. Amatraz (Mitaban, UpJohn, Kalamazoo, Mich.) may be applied as a dip in a concentration of 250 ppm of the active drug (10.6 ml bottle/2 gal water).

If dyspnea and respiratory arrest occur, the patient must be intubated and maintained on artificial respiration until the effects of the neurotoxin wear off.

Mites

Three types of mange mites have been reported from camelids: sarcoptic, psoroptic, and chorioptic. Of these, the one causing sarcoptic mange is the most common and troublesome. The true identify of the mite must be established in order to institute proper therapy and determine whether or not the case must be reported to regulatory authorities. Psoroptic mange (scab) is a reportable disease in the United States, and all forms of mange are reportable in certain states.

TRANSMISSION. Direct contact is usually necessary for a new animal to acquire any of the mange mites. However, objects such as clothing, bedding, and grooming tools may serve as mechanical vectors. Dust bathing areas are also a source. Mites may survive off the host on epithelial debris for a limited time. Adults are able to survive off the host for a maximum of 30 days. Eggs will hatch in 4–10 days. Larvae must feed within 10 days or die.

Sweatman has shown that *Psoroptes* sp. and *Chorioptes bovis* are not host specific, and cross transfers are theoretically possible (71, 72, 84). Sarcoptic mites are still thought to be host specific. No cases of zoonosis from lamoid sarcoptic mange have been reported, but it has been reported from camels in Australia.

DIAGNOSIS. Any of the mange mites can be seen (but not identified) at 30X with either a dissecting or a compound microscope. At 100X, the mite will fill the field of view, and most of the identifying characteristics can be seen; however, the segmentation of the pedicel attached to the suckers in *Psoroptes* sp. can be clearly seen only at 400X.

Scrapings for mange mite identification should be taken at the periphery of a lesion. When scraping lesions, it is necessary to penetrate deep enough to draw blood. The debris should be scraped into a glass tube or plastic container, placed on a slide, bathed with 10–15% potassium hydroxide solution warmed to boiling, and examined for mites.

TREATMENT. Psoroptic and chorioptic manges respond readily to insecticide dusts, sprays, and dips, since the mite lives on the surface of the skin. Sarcoptic mange is more difficult to treat topically, but ivermectin (0.2 mg/kg) given subcutaneously has proven to be highly effective (51).

SARCOPTIC MANGE MITE (7, 11, 21, 50, 61, 66, 68, 83)

Identification. *Sarcoptes scabiei* is morphologically identical in all animals. The identifying characteristics of the mite are a globose or round body with short legs (13). The caudad two pairs of legs do not extend beyond the margin of the body. There are bell-shaped suckers (caruncles) on the long, nonsegmented stalks (pedicels) on the tarsi of all the legs in the male but only on the anterior two pairs in the female mite. The male has no adanal suckers (copulatory discs). The capitulum (head or false head) is broad (Fig. 8.9). The maximum size of the female mite is about 0.5 mm and of the male, 0.3 mm.

Life Cycle (70). The entire life cycle is completed in the skin of the llama (Fig. 8.10). Adult male and female mites copulate on the surface of the skin. The fertilized female burrows into the skin, depositing eggs behind her as she tunnels along. The eggs hatch in 3–8 days. Larvae migrate to the skin surface and mature through the nymph stage to become adults in 4–6 days. The entire life cycle is completed in 7–14 days. Males and unfertilized females may also burrow or may follow the tunnels of the fertile female.

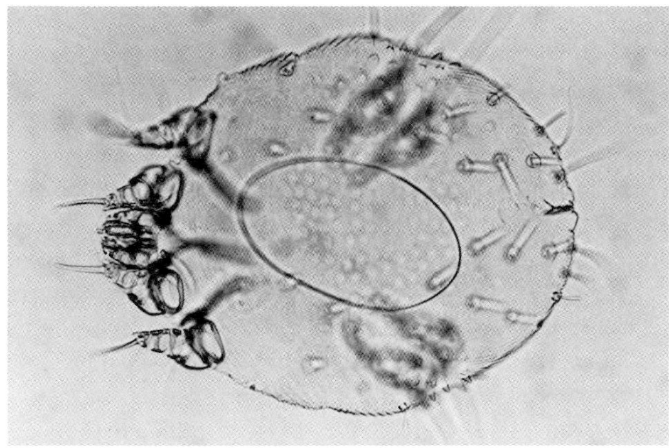

8.9 Gravid *Sarcoptes scabiei.*

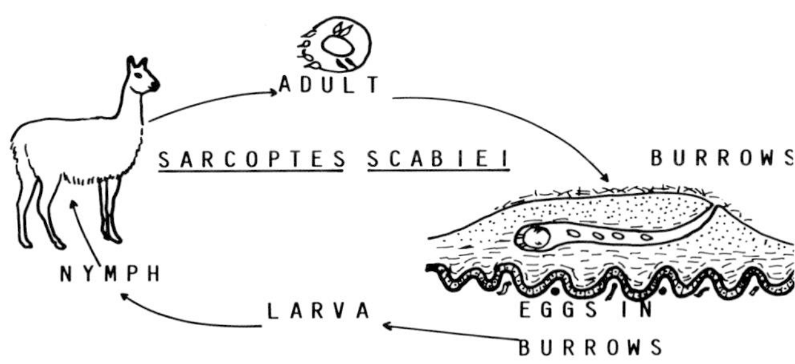

8.10 Life cycle of *Sarcoptes scabiei.*

Clinical Signs. The burrowing mite causes hyperemia, papules, and pustules, which become encrusted (83). The skin becomes thickened in affected areas and loses its vitality, thus becoming susceptible to secondary bacterial infection, with subsequent exudation. Pruritus is common. Lesions are usually found on the limbs (between the toes), medial thighs, ventral abdomen, chest, axilla, and perineum of the female and prepuce of the male. This distribution is similar to that seen with chorioptic mange, but the thickening of the skin is the differential characteristic of sarcoptic mange. In severe cases of infestation, the entire head, body, and limbs may be involved (Figs. 8.11–8.13) (53).

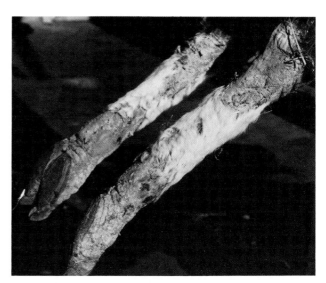

8.11 Limb lesions of sarcoptic mange.

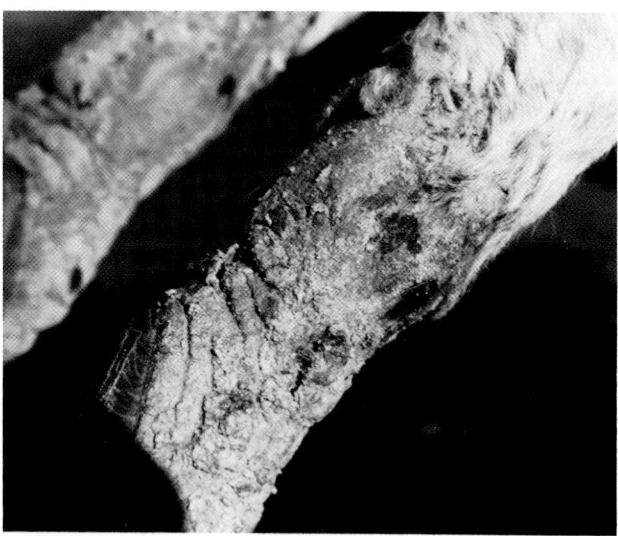

8.12 Close-up of sarcoptic mange.

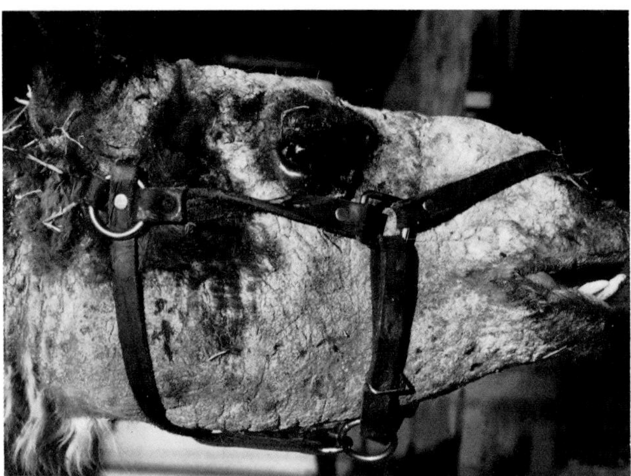

8.13 Severe sarcoptic mange of the head.

PSOROPTIC MANGE MITE

Identification (45, 70, 72). The body of *Psoroptes* sp. is more oval shaped than that of *Sarcoptes scabiei,* and the legs are longer, projecting beyond the margin of the body (Fig. 8.14). The pedicels of the tarsal suckers are long and composed of three segments (Fig. 8.15). In the female mite, the third set of legs end in bristles instead of suckers (Fig. 8.16). In the male mite, all legs have suckers, and the fourth set of legs (caudal set) are much shorter than the third. The male mite also has a pair of adanal suckers. The posterior margin of the abdomen of the male is bilobed, and the capitulum is elongated (Fig. 8.14). The maximum size of the male mite is 0.7 mm, that of the female about 0.8 mm.

Life Cycle. The entire cycle is completed on the host. Eggs are deposited on the skin at the periphery of the lesions and hatch in 1–3 days if the eggs remain in

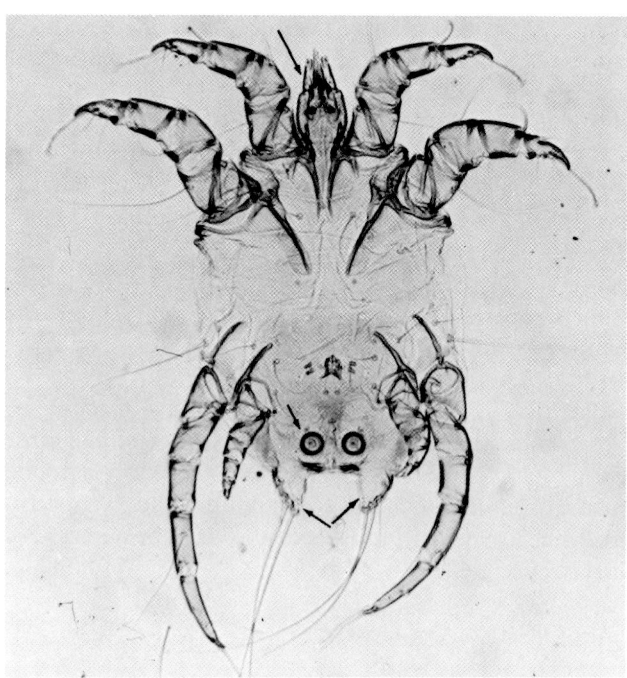

8.14 Male *Psoroptes* sp. mite. Note elongated capitulum, adanal suckers, and bilobed abdomen.

contact with the skin. If separated from the skin by crusts, hatching becomes delayed until 4–5 days, and if detached from the body along with wool, the eggs will either hatch in 10 days or die. The larval stage lasts for 2–3 days, during which time feeding occurs. The nymphal stage lasts from 3 to 4 days. Adults copulate soon after maturation. A female mite lives for 30–40 days, laying about five eggs daily. The cycle may be as short as 10 days but is usually about 3 weeks.

Clinical Signs. The mouth parts of the mites penetrate the epidermis to suck lymph and in so doing stimulate a local inflammatory reaction that exudes serum. The serum coagulates to form crusts (hence the name "scab"). The dermatitis produced causes pruritus and fiber loss. Psoroptic mites prefer the heavily fibered areas of the body. When fibers are pulled, rubbed, or fall out, the mites move to the margins of the lesion. This habit should be kept in mind when scrapings are collected to check for the presence of the mites.

Lesions are usually located around the shoulder and along the back, sides, and tail head. An early lesion or one at the margin of an established infestation consists of small papules about 5 mm in diameter. The papules are yellowish and have a moist surface. A mite is likely to be found in the center of a papule. Within 4–5 days, the serum will exude, congeal, and form the crusts characteristic of scab. Although dermatitis is produced, the skin does not become thickened to the extent observed in sarcoptic mange.

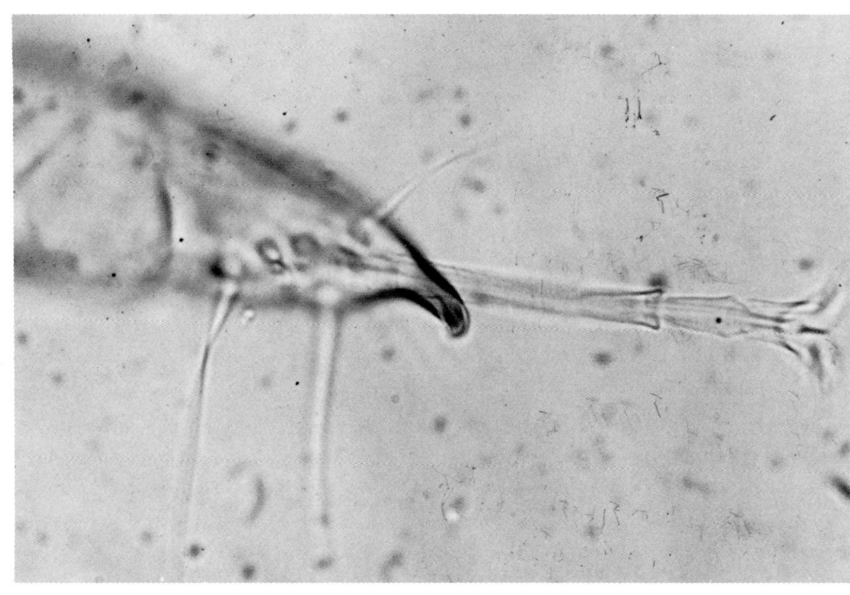

8.15 High-power magnification (400X) of the segmented tarsal pedicel of the tarsal suckers of *Psoroptes* sp.

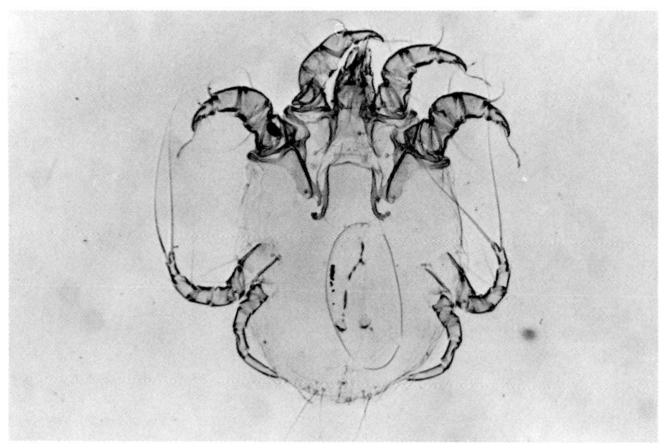

8.16 Gravid female *Psoroptes* sp. mite.

Epidemiology. Little is known about the seasonality of psoroptic mange in llamas, but in sheep, it is most active during the fall and winter. Psoroptic mange is a reportable disease in the United States. No cases have been reported from camelids in the United States, but it has been reported in SACs in South America (45).

CHORIOPTIC MANGE MITE (71, 84)

Identification. *Chorioptes bovis* closely resembles *Psoroptes* sp. except that the tarsal suckers are on short, unsegmented pedicels. The capitulum is shorter and blunter than that of *Psoroptes* sp. (Fig. 8.17). Female chorioptic mites are approximately 0.4 mm long, and males, 0.35 mm (Fig. 8.18); larvae are 0.2 mm.

Clinical Signs. Chorioptic mites feed on epidermal debris on the skin surface. These mites have short chelicerae adapted for chewing in contrast with the penetrating cheliceae of psoroptic mites. In some cases diagnosed by the author, the lesions were found on the ventrum of the tail, around the anus and vulva (Fig. 8.19), and extending ventrally on the inner sides of both hind legs to the ventral abdomen (Fig. 8.20). The lesions extended laterally up to more heavily fibered areas. Lesions were also present in the axilla, again involving lightly fibered areas. Other sites included the tips and inner surfaces of the ears and between the digits, extending up to the fetlock. The basic lesion of chorioptic mange is similar to that of psoroptic mange. The skin is hyperemic and covered with incrustations 0.5–1.5 cm in diameter (Fig. 8.21). The pathogenesis of the lesion is unknown.

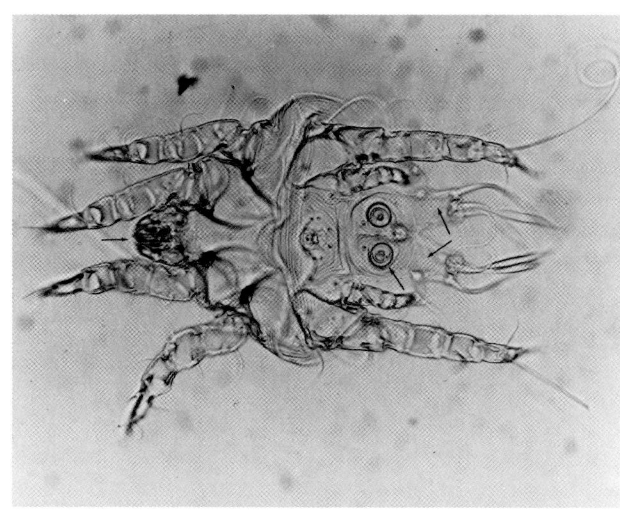

8.17 Male *Chorioptes bovis* mite from a llama. Note the broad, shortened capitulum, adanal suckers, and bilobed abdomen.

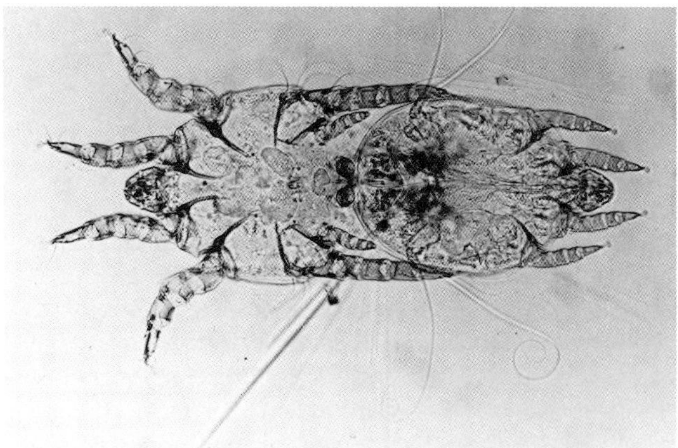

8.18 Copulating adult male (left) and nymphal female *Chorioptes bovis* mites.

Epidemiology. Chorioptic mange is supposedly more ubiquitous and less debilitating to the host than the other two manges. Chorioptic mange is rarely reported in llamas, but the author has diagnosed cases and it has been reported in South Africa (84) and by Sweatman (71).

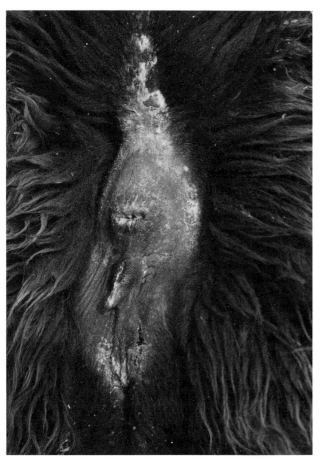

8.19 Chorioptic mange on the perineal area of a llama.

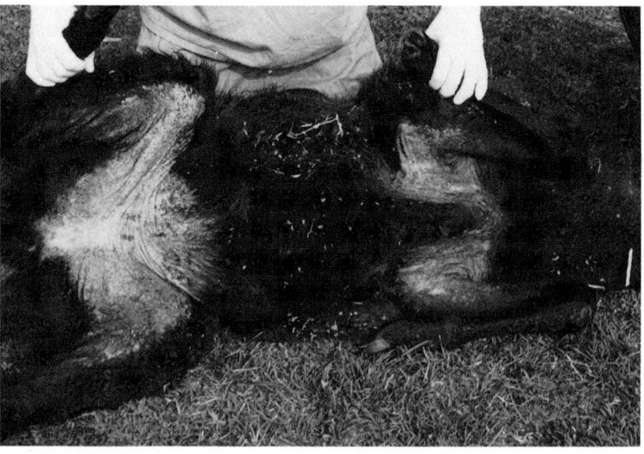

8.20 Chorioptic mange on the ventrum of a llama.

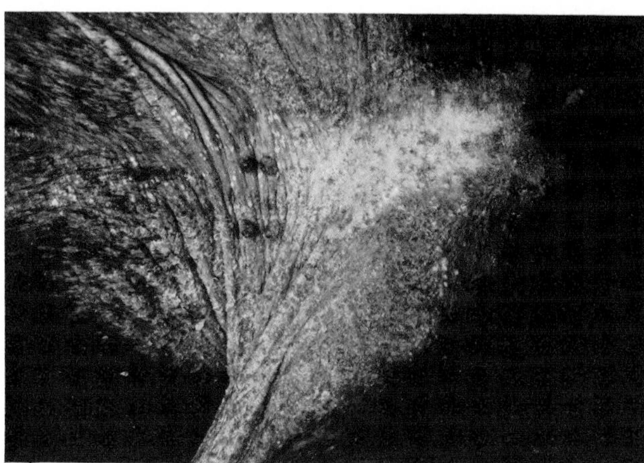

8.21 Encrustations typical of both psoroptic and chorioptic mange.

INTERNAL PARASITES

Protozoa (60)

TRYPANOSOMIASIS (SURRA)

Identification. Old World camels are highly susceptible to infection by a number of species of *Trypanosoma* sp. Camels are not commonly used in the region called the Tsetse Belt. Illness and death caused by *T. brucei,* causing nagana, may be the key factor of their absence from the area. *T. evansi* is the major trypanosome affecting camels, causing a disease called surra (18). Surra is an Indian word meaning "rotten." *T. evansi* may have some significance in SACs for reasons to be enumerated.

Trypanosome species are similar, and species identification may be impossible without animal inoculation and other sophisticated diagnostic procedures. They have a leaflike shape, with a single flagellum attached to the cell by a undulating membrane (70).

Life Cycle. *T. evansi* does not require a period of maturation in an insect vector and thus has a noncyclic transmission. Any biting or blood-sucking insect or tick may serve as a vector. Flies of the genera *Tabanus* and *Stomoxys* are commonly implicated. Mechanical transmission by contaminated hypodermic needles is also possible.

Epidemiology. The geographic distribution of *T. evansi* is extensive, occurring in North Africa, Asia Minor, the U.S.S.R., Pakistan, Afghanistan, India, Burma, Malaya, Indochina, South China, Indonesia, and the Philippines (18). It has also been reported from Central and South America, though trypanosomiasis has not been reported in SACs in these areas, despite the presence of the organism. However, trypanosomes have been isolated from llamas imported into the United States from Chile.[1]

Clinical Signs. Acute surra is characterized by fever, depression, weakness, and edema. The presence of pulmonary edema may contribute to the development of secondary pneumonia. Females may abort, and the milk of lactating females may become caseous. Large numbers of trypanosomes are seen in peripheral blood samples. Death may occur within a few weeks.

Chronic surra is characterized by intermittent episodes of fever, anemia, pendant edema, and emaciation. Between episodes of fever, the parasite may be absent from peripheral blood vessels. A camel may live for 3 or 4 years, depending on the care provided.

1. G. F. Ferris, USDA, Plum Island, N.Y. 1985, personal communication.

TOXOPLASMOSIS. *Toxoplasma gondii* is a ubiquitous protozoan parasite. Overt disease has not been described in SACs, but serum titers have been reported, and it is likely that the disease will be reported in time (64). Much has been written on this parasitic disease, and the reader is referred to recent reports.

COCCIDIOSIS (26, 27, 32, 33, 35, 37, 38, 74)

Identification. Coccidia tend to be host specific. A few species of the genus *Eimeria* have been described from SACs (Table 8.3) (27). Eimerian oocysts are frequently encountered on routine fecal flotations, and cases of coccidiosis have been reported, but none of the North American coccidia have been identified. Coccidia identified from camels are listed in Table 8.4.

Life Cycle. The life cycle of coccidia includes both sexual and asexual phases (Fig. 8.22). The asexual cycle is called schizogony or merogony. Sporulated oocysts are ingested by the animal and pass along the digestive tract to the small intestine. The oocyst frees sporozoites, which invade the epithelial cells. The sporozoite changes shape and becomes a trophozoite, which, in

Table 8.3. Coccidia of llamoids

Species	Size of oocyst (μm)	Shape of oocyst	Micropyle
Eimeria alpacae	22–26 × 18–21	Ellipsoidal	+
E. lamae	30–40 × 21–30	Ovoid to ellipsoidal	+
E. macusaniensis	81–107 × 61–80	Ovoid	+
E. punoensis	17–22 × 14–18	Ellipsoidal or oval	+
E. peruviana	28–37 × 18–22	Ovoid	–

Source: Soulsby 1982.

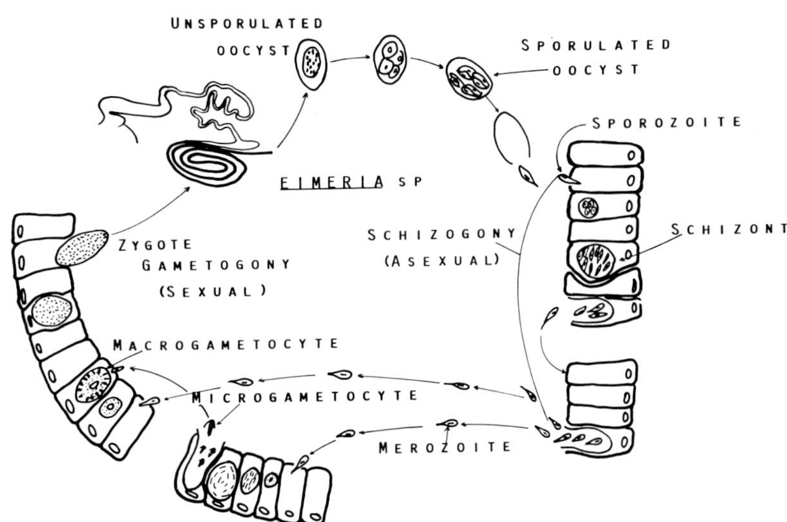

8.22 Life cycle of *Eimeria* sp.

Table 8.4. Coccidia of camels

Species	Size of oocyst (μm)	Shape of oocyst	Micropyle	Sporulation time (days)
Eimeria bactriani	32 × 25–27	Spherical-ellipsoidal	+	10
E. cameli	81–100 × 63–94	Truncate	+	10–15
E. dromedarii	22–33 × 20–25			15–17
E. pellerdyi	23.2 × 12.6			5

Source: Soulsby 1982.

turn, grows larger and forms a schizont (merzont). Within the schizont, merozoites form and ultimately rupture the cell and escape to infect other cells. This process may be repeated two or three times.

The sexual cycle is called gametogony. The merozoites produced by the last schizogony cycle infect a cell and develop into either male (microgametocyte) or female (macrogametocyte) gamonts. The male gamont fertilizes the female gamont while it is still in the cell, producing a zygote. The zygote matures to become an oocyst, which ruptures from the host cell and is shed in the feces. The oocyst sporulates in 1–2 days to become infective.

Epidemiology. Coccidial infections are generally self-limiting because asexual reproduction is repeated only two or three times (70). Unless reinfection takes place, only one cycle of development can occur, but in a contaminated environment, reinfection is the rule and heavy buildups can occur that may kill the host. The concept is important to the clinician, who must manage coccidiosis.

Ruminant livestock have a definite immune response to infection with coccidia. Whether or not this occurs in lamoids is unknown. It is not uncommon to see eimerial oocysts on fecal flotation, but coccidiosis is uncommon in lamoids in North America. It is a serious problem of recently weaned llamas and alpacas in Peru.

Clinical Signs. Coccidia invade the epithelial mucosa of the small intestine, causing enteritis and diarrhea. The diarrhea may be mild catarrhal or, more serious, hemorrhagic.

Treatment. Numerous coccidiostats are used in ruminants. Their use in lamoids in North America has not been reported. Monensin should not be used in lamoids until testing is carried out, since there is species sensitivity to this drug. Horses have been killed by feeding from the same feed bunks as cattle being given medicated feed.

SARCOCYSTIASIS

Identification. *Sarcocystis* sp. has an interesting two-host life cycle. *Sarcocystis* sp. is a genus of coccidia, closely related to the *Eimeria*. The primary host is a carnivore, in which gametogony, fertilization, and sporulation occur. Lamoids serve as an intermediate host in which only schizogony and encystment occur. Two species have been reported from the lamoid. *Sarcocystis aucheniae* has been reported from Bolivia and Peru (43) in the llama and alpaca and *Sarcocystis tilopoidi* from the guanaco in Argentina (63).

Life Cycle. Life cycles for lamoid sarcocysts have not been established (31). Whether dog, fox, cat, or human serves as the primary host is unknown. In general, the carnivore ingests the muscle of the herbivorous intermediate host (Fig. 8.23). Zoites are released in the intestine and invade the epithelial cells. Gametogony is completed in the wall of the intestine of the carnivore up to and including the sporulated oocysts. This cycle differs from the eimerian cycle, in which nonsporulated oocysts must undergo sporulation outside the primary host.

The lamoid ingests the sporocyst; sporozoites are released in the intestine and invade vascular endothelial cells. One or more asexual cycles are completed in these cells before the merozoites enter muscle cells and form sarcocysts.

Epidemiology. Sarcocysts have been encountered as a secondary finding at necropsy in North American llamas, but no cases of clinical disease have been described. In Peru, it has been reported that in certain areas, over 50% of the lamoids over 3 years of age are infected with sarcocysts.[2] Meat is downgraded as a result of the infection.

A carnivore or omnivore must serve as the definitive host, passing the sporulated oocysts with the feces. The lamoid serves as the obligatory intermediate host.

Clinical Signs. Little or no damage is done to the definitive host. No signs may be noted in light infections. In high numbers, the schizogonous cycles in endothelial cells may produce acute febrile disease, resulting in abortion and death. Sarcocysts may cause mild myositis with myalgia and interference with muscle function.

2. W. Bravo, 1986, personal communication.

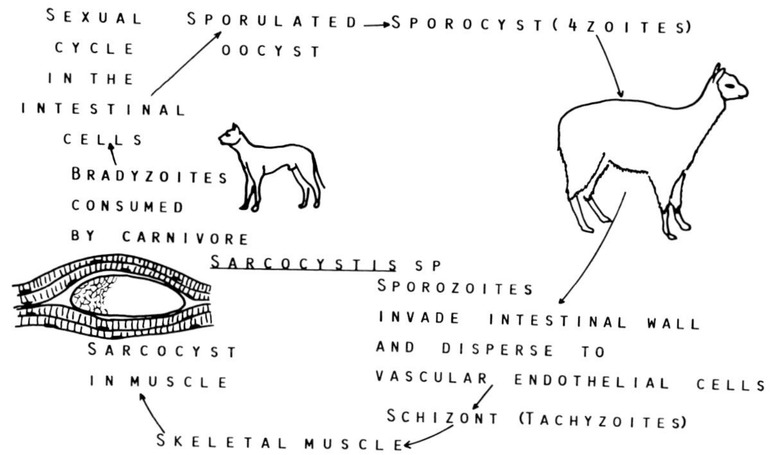

8.23 Life cycle of *Sarcocystis* sp.

Treatment. No treatment is available. Prevention requires disruption of the life cycle from the carnivore host.

FASCIOLIASIS (*Fasciola hepatica, F. gigantea*)

Identification. The common liver fluke, *Fasciola hepatica,* is locally ubiquitous and found throughout tropical and temperate regions of the world. This fluke is leaf shaped (Fig. 8.24) and reaches a maximum size of 30 × 13 mm.

Life Cycle (70). Adult flukes live in the bile ducts (Fig. 8.24). Eggs are discharged into the bile duct, carried to the intestine, and excreted in the feces. The eggs must fall into water for maturation to the ciliated miracidium stage to take place. This takes 10–12 days. The miracidium bores into one of many species of snail. *Lymnaea truncatula* is one of the more common intermediate hosts, but other species of *Lymnaea* may also act as hosts. While in the snail, the miracidium loses its cilia and matures to become a sporocyst, then a redia, and finally a cercaria. This phase requires 4.5–7 weeks.

The cercaria leaves the snail and is free swimming for a few minutes to 2 hours, attaches to a plant just below surface level, loses its tail, and becomes a metacercaria, which is the infective stage for the llama. The metacercaria are ingested, and immature flukes (marita) are released into the duodenum; they penetrate the wall of the intestine, enter the peritoneal cavity, and migrate to the liver. By 3–7 days after infection, the majority of the young flukes will have reached the liver, where they penetrate the capsule. Following this, a migratory period of some 5–6 weeks in the liver parenchyma occurs before the flukes enter the bile duct and mature.

The prepatent period is about 8 weeks, but development may be retarded, delaying maturity another 2 months. Adult flukes may live for 9 months or longer.

6-8 WEEK OLD IMMATURES AND ADULT FLUKES IN BILE DUCT
IMMATURE FLUKES IN PARENCHYMA
PERITONEUM
FASCIOLA HEPATICA
EGG
INTO WATER
MIRACIDIUM
SMALL INTESTINE
METACERCARIA ON PLANT
SNAIL
CERCARIA LEAVES SNAIL

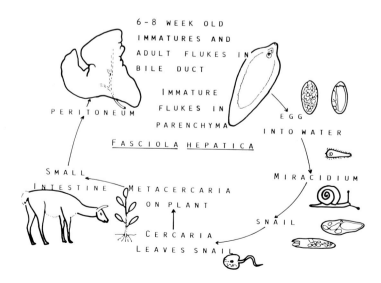

8.24 Life cycle of *Fasciola hepatica.*

Epidemiology (70). The completion of the fluke life cycle is dependent upon the presence of snail intermediate hosts, which, in turn, are dependent upon an aquatic environment. The eggs will not develop at temperatures below 10°C, and there is a direct correlation of development time with temperature (at 13°C, 60 days; at 15°C, 40 days; and at 26°C, 12 days).

Some snail hosts are capable of estivation for as long as 13 months under certain circumstances, e.g., during drought conditions. The infection may be maintained while the snail is buried in the dried mud.

Metacercaria can persist for a few days to a few weeks while encysted on the plant. Some of the cysts may fall to the bottom of the water and be stirred up and ingested when an animal walks into the water to graze or drink. The cyst may survive for as long as 8 months on moist hay, but the usual drying process will shorten life to a few weeks (70).

Liver fluke infection in lamoids has been reported from South America (3, 8, 47, 75) and occurs in localized problem areas in the western and southern United States. If flukes are endemic in local cattle and sheep, and llamas or alpacas inhabit similar swampy, poorly drained pastures, it is reasonable to assume that the lamoids will have a fluke problem also.

Clinical Signs. Both acute and chronic forms of fascioliasis are seen. The acute form is seen with overwhelming infections that produce signs of hepatic insufficiency similar to those caused by other agents (see Chap. 13). The chronic form is more often seen. Chronic stasis of the bile, caused by flukes obstructing the ducts, produces a hepatic fibrosis, which ultimately causes an elevation of intrahepatic blood pressure. A hyperplastic cholangitis, which allows leakage of plasma protein, causing hypoproteinemia, also occurs. Adult flukes suck blood, causing intrabiliary hemorrhage, which results in anemia.

The affected llama will become anorectic. Mucous membranes may be pale, and pendant edema may be seen. The fiber becomes dry and brittle, with "breaks" associated with intense periods of the disease. Depression and emaciation will follow anorexia. Either diarrhea or constipation may be seen.

Treatment. Many different drugs have been used to treat fluke infestation. Currently, the only recommended drug in the United States is Clorsulon (Curatrem) at a dose of 7 mg/kg body weight. This is given per os, twice at 45- to 60-day intervals.

The unhealthy, fluke-infested liver may be susceptible to secondary bacterial infection from clostridial organisms or enterics. One disease of concern to livestock people is Black's disease, caused by *Clostridium novyi.* Vaccination with a multiple-antigen clostridial toxoid may prevent complications from this disease.

Tapeworms

HYDATID DISEASE

Identification. Hydatid disease, caused by *Echinococcus granulosus,* is worldwide in distribution. The adult tapeworm resides in the intestine of a carnivore, with dogs, foxes, coyotes, and wolves all potential definitive hosts. This is a small tapeworm, 2–7 mm long, consisting of only three or four proglottids, which usually disintegrate in the intestine, so only eggs are seen in the feces (67, 75).

Life Cycle (70). The feces of the carnivore contaminate the feed of the lamoid (Fig. 8.25). The eggs are immediately infective to any of many ungulate in-

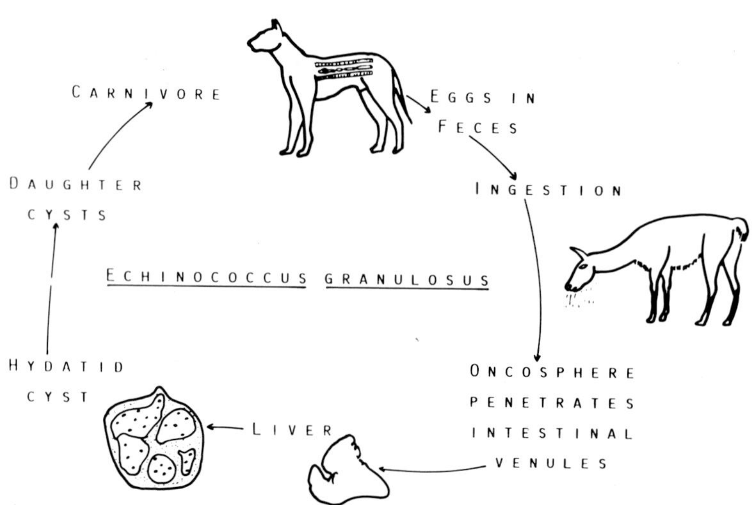

8.25 Life cycle of *Echinococcus granulosus.*

termediate hosts, the lamoid being one. The eggs hatch in the intestine, releasing oncospheres, which penetrate the intestinal venules or lymphatics and migrate to the organ of predilection for the species (liver, lung).

The hydatid cyst (metacestode) develops slowly over several months (2, 70), reaching a diameter of 8–10 cm. The inner membrane of the cyst or bladder is composed of germinal epithelium and is surrounded by fluid enclosed in a capsule of inflammatory cells. Brood capsules, each with its own scolex, may develop within the outer capsule. Some of the brood capsules rupture, releasing scolices into the fluid ("hydatid sand"). The fluid is infective if the outer capsule is ruptured.

The hydatid cyst is consumed by the carnivore when it scavenges a carcass or is fed offal. The protoscolices are released in the intestine, evaginate, and penetrate between the villi into the crypts of Lieberkuhn, developing to maturity in about 47 days (70). Dogs may maintain an infection for 2 years.

Epidemiology. Only one species of *E. granulosus* has been identified, but in the field, apparently, various strains or cycles exist between a particular species and a certain carnivore (sheep/dog, cattle/dog, camel/dog, wallaby/dingo [Australia], deer/coyote [California], moose/wolf). The cycle in lamoids in South America is lamoid/dog or lamoid/fox.

Clinical Signs. The adult tapeworm is usually harmless to the carnivore, and, except under unusual circumstances, a mild infestation in a herbivore will produce no clinical signs. The cysts usually develop in the liver or lungs, but in humans and other hosts, they may develop in the brain or heart as well. In any case, malfunction of any organ will occur if large numbers of cysts develop or if one develops in a vital area. If the outer wall of a brood cyst ruptures, metastasis may occur, with numerous new cysts developing as a result.

Treatment. No treatment can destroy the hydatid cyst in the intermediate host. Cysts can be removed surgically after the cyst has been injected with formalin to obviate accidental rupture of the cyst and subsequent contamination of the surgical site. Prevention consists of ridding the carnivore of the tapeworm. This may be successful in a controlled situation involving a pet dog cycle but is not possible in sylvatic cycles or areas where feral dogs roam.

MONIEZIASIS

Identification. *Moniezia expansa* has been recovered from lamoids in the United States, and *M. expansa* and *M. benedeni* are significant problems in some areas of South America (8). Adult tapeworms have been found in the small intestine of lamoids. An intact tapeworm may reach 600 cm in length and be 1.6 cm wide. The scolex is 0.36–0.8 mm and has prominent suckers and no hooks (70).

Life Cycle. Mature proglottids separate from the rest of the tapeworm and, along with the contained eggs, are passed with the feces. Cysticercoid development occurs in oribatid mites, which are a true intermediate host. Infective stages develop in approximately 4 months.

Lamoids acquire the infection by consuming forage contaminated with the mites. Further maturation to the adult tapeworm in the small intestine takes 37–40 days.

Epidemiology. *Moniezia* occurs worldwide but is usually not a major disease-producing parasite. Heavy infestations could obviously impair nutrition and cause debility or even intestinal obstruction. There may be a seasonality of infestation in temperate climates because of the overwintering of the oribatid mites. Neonate lamoids begin to nibble on grass early in life and could acquire an infestation and be passing proglottids by the age of 6 weeks (70).

Clinical Signs. Diarrhea and unthriftiness may accompany heavy infestations.

Treatment. Praziquantel (Droncit) at a dose of 2.5–10 mg/kg given orally or as an injection is probably effective. Fenbendazole at 10–15 mg/kg is effective in cattle and sheep and may be effective in lamoids.

THYSANIEZIASIS. Tapeworms of *Thysaniezia* sp. have been reported in llamas. Little is known about the life cycle or epidemiology. Adult tapeworms of the genus have been found in the small intestine of sheep, goats, and cattle. Little or no clinical significance seems to be associated with this parasite.

Taenia helicometra, T. hidatigena

Infections with larval stages of these two *Taenia* sp. have been reported in alpacas and vicuñas in South America (8).

Nematode Parasites

Nematodes are the most numerous and most detrimental of the lamoid parasites (76, 77). The taxonomic outline at the beginning of this chapter lists all the nematodes that have been reported from lamoids. Most of these parasites are located in the GI tract. Many aspects of GI parasitism are similar, regardless of which species of parasite is involved (28, 55, 58). The following introductory remarks will obviate the need to repeat the same information for each species.

PATHOGENESIS. Most GI parasites produce a protein-losing gastroenteropathy. In severe cases, hypoalbuminemia may develop. Enteritis will induce changes in the secretory status of the gut.

Appetite and utilization of the feed consumed is reduced, depriving the body of vital nutrients. Absorption of calcium and phosphorus is depressed, causing, in turn, arrested skeletal development in the young animal. Selenium uptake is also retarded. Young animals are at greatest risk when affected by parasitism because no resistance has been developed to the invading organisms.

CLINICAL SIGNS. There are peracute, acute, and chronic forms of most parasitisms. Death may be caused by overwhelming invasion of an organ or system, but usually parasitism results only in debilitation in varying degrees. Over a period of time, the body loses the ability to resist minor infectious agents, and a secondary infection may take the animal's life. Some degree of unthriftiness usually accompanies parasitism. The fiber coat may lack luster.

Emaciation may be seen in longstanding cases, a result of inappetence, leading to complete anorexia, combined with poor food utilization. Inappetence and poor food utilization also inhibit growth and maturation of parasitized young animals. Diarrhea is the most prominent sign of enteritis, but it is important to recognize that diarrhea need not always be present in parasitism, especially when larvae invade such tissues as the liver or lungs.

Anemia may be seen in heavy infestations, even with parasites that are not blood suckers. The cutting mouth parts used for attachment may result in leakage of plasma and cells from capillaries.

In adult animals, production and quality of fiber and milk will be depressed. Thus a baby may be doubly jeopardized, both by its own parasite load and lack of nourishment as a result of the effect of parasitism on the mother.

DIAGNOSIS. The presence of one or more of the signs noted above should direct attention to a differential diagnosis, including parasitism. Unless adult parasites have already been seen in the feces, some type of fecal examination should be conducted to begin the process of diagnosis. Reference to standard texts will provide an explanation of the methodology for fecal examinations (22, 70).

Table 8.5 lists sizes of male and female adult parasites, larvae, and eggs and location of the internal para-

Table 8.5. Internal parasites of llamas

		Size (mm)				Anatomic location			
Scientific name	Common name	Adult male	Adult female	Larva (μm)	Egg (μm)	Adult	Immature	Intermediate host	Prepatent period (days)
Fasciola hepatica	Liver fluke	13–30			130–150 × 63–90	Bile ducts	Small intestine, peritoneum, liver	Snail, *Lymnaea* sp.	56
Echinococcus granulosus	Hydatid	2–7			32–36 × 25–30	Intestine of carnivores	Lungs, liver	SAC (primary host is dog)	
Moniezia expansa	Tapeworm	600 cm × 1.6 cm wide			56–67	Small intestine	Small intestine	Oribatid mite	37–40
Thysaniezia sp.	Tapeworm	200 cm × 1.2 cm wide				Small intestine	Small intestine	?	
Trichostrongylus colubriformis	Stomach worm	4–5.5	5–7	620–790	79–101 × 39–47	Stomach, small intestine		None	20
Ostertagia ostertagi	Medium brown stomach worm	6.5–7.5	8.3–9.2	L-3 797–910	80–85 × 40–45	C-3		None	21
Ostertagia (Marshallagia) marshalli	Stomach worm	10–13	12–20		178–217 × 78–100	C-3, duodenum		None	
Camelostrongylus mentulatus	Stomach worm	6.5–7.5	8.3–9.2		75–85 × 40–50	C-3		None	

Table 8.5. (*continued*)

Scientific name	Common name	Size (mm) Adult male	Adult female	Larva (μm)	Egg (μm)	Anatomic location Adult	Immature	Intermediate host	Prepatent period (days)
Bunostomum sp.	Hookworm	12–17	19–26	500–678	79–97 × 47–50	Small intestine		None	30–56
Skrjabinema ovis	Pinworm	2.3–3.7 × 110–180 μm	5–10 × 350–500 μm		47–63 × 27–36	Colon, rectum	Small intestine	None	17–25
Parelaphostrongylus tenuis	Meningeal worm		39–91	348		Central nervous system (may never mature in llama)	Small intestine, spinal cord		90
Thelazia californiensis	Eye worm	17 (11–19.5)				Conjunctival sac, lacrimal duct	Conjunctival sac, lacrimal duct	*Musca autumnalis,* face fly	
Gongylonema sp.	Cattle gullet worm	30–62 × 150–300 μm	80–145 × 300–500 μm		50–70 × 25–37	Esophagus, C-3	?	Beetles	?
Trichuris sp.	Whipworm	50–80	35–70		70–80 × 30–42	Cecum, large intestine	Small intestine	None	28–35
Capillaria sp.		8–13	12–20		45–50 × 22–25	Small intestine		None	
Eimeria sp. *Sarcocystis* sp.	Coccidia Sarcocyst					Small intestine Muscle			
Toxoplasma gondii	Toxoplasma				(oocysts) 11–14 × 9–11	Sexual cycle in cats	Multiple organs	SAC	2–7 in cats
Haemonchus contortus	Large stomach worm	10–20	18–30	650–750	70–85 × 41–48	C-3	C-1	None	15
Cooperia mcmasteri		4.5–5.4	5.8–6.2	780		Small intestine		None	14–21
Nematodirus	Thread-necked strongyle	10–15	15–23	922–1120	175–260 × 106–110	Lumen of small intestine	Mucosa of small intestine	None	15
Graphinema aucheniae	Stomach worm	5.5–7.8	9–12		80–90 × 40–45	C-3		None	
Lamenema chavezi		10–13	14–18		150–170 × 70–80	Small intestine	Liver	None	
Spiculopteragia peruvianus	Stomach worm	6.7–7.7	8.4–10.3		81–95 × 45–49	C-3		None	
Dictyocaulus viviparus	Lung worm	40–55	60–80	L-1 300–360	82–88 × 33–38	Bronchi	Small intestine, mesenteric lymph node, thoracic duct	None	30
Oesophagostomum columbianium	Nodular worm	12–16.5	15–21.5	771–923	73–89 × 34–45	Small intestine, large intestine		None	41
Chabertia ovina	Strongyle	13–14	17–20	710–789	90–105 × 50–55	Large intestine	Small intestine	None	49

sites in the body (14). Table 8.6 lists external parasites. Figures 8.26–8.29 illustrate the eggs for identification when recovered from the feces. Identification in this situation will be possible only to the genus level and maybe only to the family. However, this will usually suffice to indicate methods of management and therapy.

A direct smear is used as a quick preliminary procedure to determine the presence of nematode eggs, but it is even more important for detecting motile protozoan parasites such as giardia or trichomonas. The feces must be freshly passed so that the parasites are still alive and moving.

Various types of differential centrifugation or flotation are used to identify eggs, which are separated by the specific gravity unique to each parasite. Likewise, various counting procedures allow estimation of the parasite burden. Interpretation of these counts should be done by experienced persons.

Special methods, such as a Baerman apparatus, are required for detection of parasites that pass larvae in

Table 8.6. External parasites of South American camelids

		Size (mm)			Anatomic location	
Scientific name	Common name	Adult	Larva	Pupa	Adult	Immature
Culex, Anopheles, Aedes	Mosquitos				Fiberless areas of head, neck, limb	Water
Vermipsylla sp., others	Fleas	1.5–4	<6	4 × 2	Same	Soil
Tabanus sp.	Horse fly Deer fly				Same	Same
Musca domestica	Housefly	6.5–7.5	10–12		Around eyes, ears, nostrils	Feces, organic debris
Musca autumnalis	Face fly	Slightly larger than housefly			Same	Cattle feces
Stomoxys calcitrans	Stable fly	11			Same	Same
Calliphoridae (various sp.)	Blow flies	8			Free-living flies	Infected and necrotic wounds
Oestrus ovis	Sheep botfly	12	L-1 = 2 L-3 = 30		Same	Nasal cavity, sinuses
Cephenemyia sp.	Deer nasobot fly	14	L-1 = 1–3		Same	Naso-pharynx
Otobius megnini	Spinose ear tick	8	2–3	Nymph 7–10	Around farm and ranch structures	External ear canal
Ixodidae (various sp.)	Hard ticks				Attached to body	Depends on species
Sarcoptes scabiei	Sarcoptic mange mite	0.3–0.5			In tunnels in epidermis	Same
Psoroptes bovis	Psoroptic mange mite	0.7–0.8			At periphery of scab	Same
Chorioptes ovis	Chorioptic mange mite	0.35–0.4	0.2		Same	Same

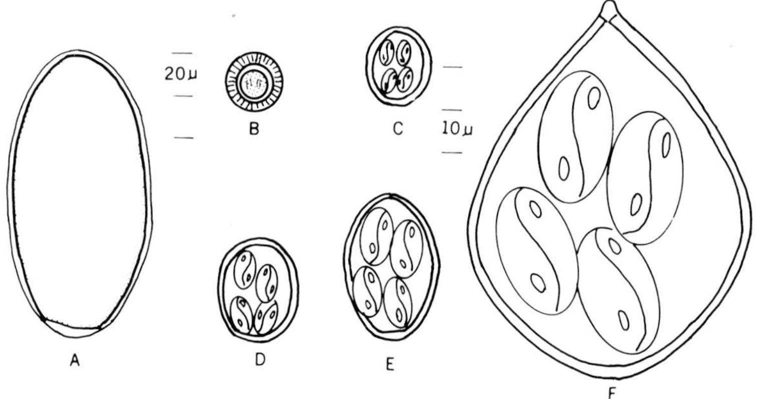

8.26 Miscellaneous parasite ova of lamoids: **(A)** *Fasciola hepatica,* **(B)** *Echinococcus* sp., **(C)** *Eimeria punoensis,* **(D)** *Eimeria alpaca,* **(E)** *Eimeria lamae,* **(F)** *Eimeria macusaniensis.* (*Eimeria* scale = 10 μ, others = 20 μ.)

the feces instead of eggs (*Dictyocaulus* sp.). A final diagnostic tool is response to treatment. The clinician may choose to treat on the basis of suspicion and previous experience.

MANAGEMENT AND TREATMENT. The basic principles involved in the management and treatment of parasitism are identification of parasite(s), at least to genus, and review of the life cycle. The same management procedures may be used as have been outlined for similar parasitism in ruminants. The nutritional status of the herd should be evaluated and appropriate changes made.

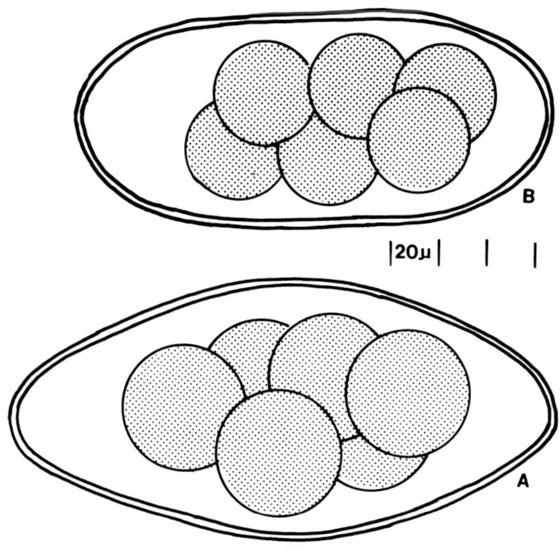

8.27 Nematode ova from lamoids: **(A)** *Nematodirus* sp., **(B)** *Ostertagia (Marshallagia) marshalli.*

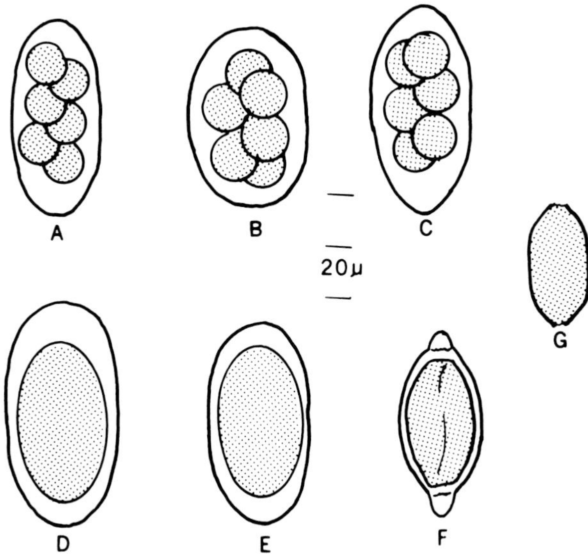

8.28 Nematode ova from lamoids: **(A)** *Cooperia* sp., **(B)** *Haemonchus contorta,* **(C)** *Oesophagostomum columbianum,* **(D)** *Trichostrongylus* sp., **(E)** *Ostertagia ostertagi,* **(F)** *Trichuris ovis,* **(G)** *Capillaria* sp.

Numerous anthelmintics are safe and effective against GI nematodes in ruminants (Table 8.7) (1, 10, 11, 29, 41, 46, 65, 74, 78, 79, 80, 82). All of these have been used in camelids, but the pharmacodynamics of anthelmintics in camelids is unknown. Until such information is available, the clinician should use ruminant doses and dosing intervals.

As in the case in ruminants, local populations of parasites in camelids may develop resistance to an anthelmintic or class of anthelmintics. For instance, the failure of ivermectin to control previously sensitive parasites has been reported to the author by practitioner colleagues.

Both internal and external parasites may be treated or repelled by a wide variety of therapeutic agents. Tables 8.1 and 8.2 list drugs approved for use on livestock and horses. None of these have been tested for efficacy or safety in lamoids. In clinical practice, the preparations recommended for cattle, sheep, and goats are customarily used. Concentrations recommended for sheep are lower than those for cattle. The concentration for sheep should be selected if choice is provided.

In addition, when an animal is suffering from severe dermatitis associated with external parasitism, chemicals are more likely to be absorbed through the damaged skin, which may lead to the development of toxicosis. It is suggested that such animals be treated in stages.

A final management recommendation is that fecal samples be monitored semiannually to evaluate the ef-

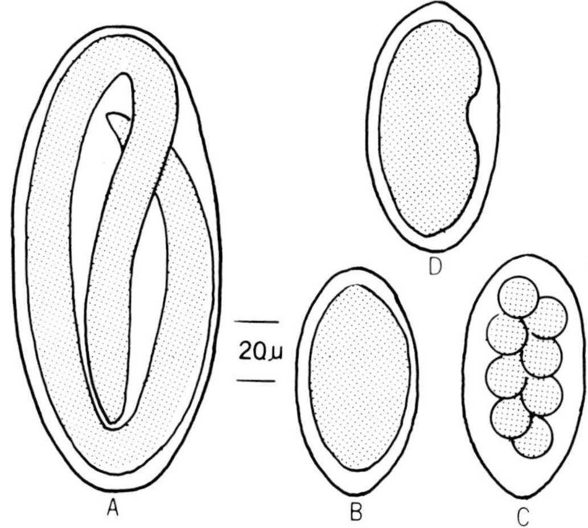

8.29 Nematode ova of South American parasites: **(A)** *Lamanema chavezi,* **(B)** *Camelostrongylus mentulatus,* **(C)** *Graphinema aucheniae,* **(D)** *Spiculopteragia peruvianus.*

Table 8.7. Anthelmintics used in lamoids

Generic name	Commercial name(s)	Company[a]	Route of administration	Dose (mg/kg)
Fenbendazole	Panacur	B	Oral suspension, paste	10–15
Ivermectin	Ivomec	G	Oral, subcutaneous	0.2
Levamisole	Ripercol-L,	A	Intramuscular	5–8
	Levasole,	F	Oral	
	Tramisole	A	Oral	
Mebendazole	Telmin	F	Oral	22
Pyrantel pamoate	Strongid	E	Oral	18
Thiabendazole	Equizole, Omnizole, Thibenzole	D	Oral	66
Praziquantel	Droncit	C	Oral	5
Clorsuon	Curatrem	D	Oral	7

[a]A = American Cyanamid (Ripercol), One Cyanamid Place, Wayne, NJ 07470; B = American Hoechst (Panacur) National Lab Corp., Somerville, NJ 08876; C = Haver-Lockhart Labs, Box 390, Shawnee, KS 66201; D = MSD Agvet. Division Merck & Co., P.O. Box 2000, Rahway, NJ 07065; E = Pfizer, Inc., Animal Health Div., 235 East 42nd Street, NY, NY 10017; F = Pitman-Moore Inc. (Levasol, Telmin), P.O. Box 344, Washington Crossing, NJ 08560; G = Upjohn Co. (Ivermectin), 7000 Portage Rd., Kalamazoo, MI 49001.

fectiveness of chemotherapy. The examination should coincide with known exacerbation of parasite loads for the area.

Trichostrongylus sp., *T. axei* (8, 9, 52), *T. vitrinus* (52), *T. colubriformis* (8, 52), *T. longispicularis* (30)

Life Cycle (70). A generalized life cycle for *Trichostrongylus* sp. is as follows (Fig. 8.30). The female produces eggs containing embryos in the morula stage. The eggs are passed in the feces, and the morula mature to become first-stage (L-1) larvae within the egg case. Under ideal conditions, hatching occurs in 1–2 days. The free-living L-1 larvae feed on microorganisms in the feces and molt to L-2 and again to L-3, which is the infective stage, taking 4–6 days.

L-3 larvae migrate out of the feces in about 1 week and climb onto vegetation. The life cycle is direct, and the lamoid ingests grass containing L-3 larvae, which mature through L-4 and L-5 to become adults in the third compartment (C-3) of the stomach or the intestine. The prepatent period is about 20 days.

Epidemiology. The length of time necessary for maturation of free-living larvae is dependent upon climate, season, and temperature. Some larvae will survive a mild winter in protected areas. Drought and desiccation are detrimental to the survival of most larvae, but some species have evolved in such environments and have developed adaptations for survival.

The clinician faced with a trichostrongyle problem in a group of lamoids should review one of the standard texts on the subject in ruminants and apply the same principles.

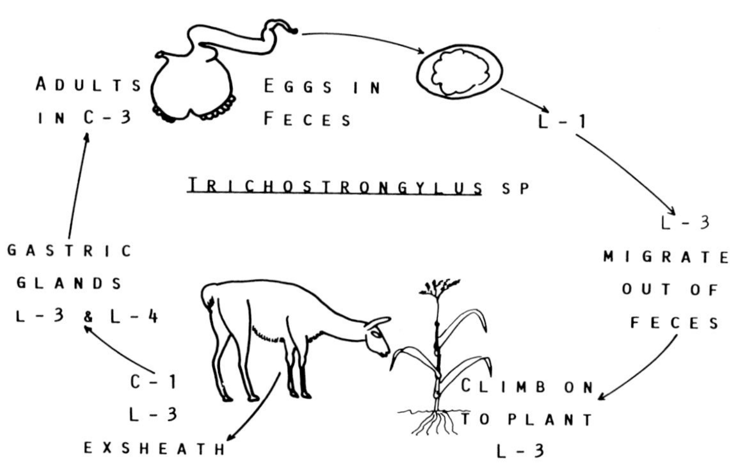

8.30 Life cycle of *Trichostrongylus* sp.

Ostertagia ostertagi (8, 42, 52), *O. circumcincta* (8, 42), *O. lyrata* (8, 30)

Life Cycle. There are two phases or types of cycles in this species (Fig. 8.31). Type I is typical of a trichostrongyle life cycle, with larvae maturing to the adult without passing through a developmental arrest stage. Type II involves developmental arrest in the mucosa of the stomach. Larvae become arrested in early fall and begin development again in winter in northern temperate regions. In southern temperate regions with dry summers and winter rainfall, arrest occurs in late winter and spring, and development begins again in late summer and fall. Larvae in the glands of the wall of the stomach stimulate formation of grayish-white nodules (Fig. 8.31). Maturation of previously arrested larvae can cause a buildup of pathogenic adults with heavy egg levels in the feces and gastritis caused by the adults.

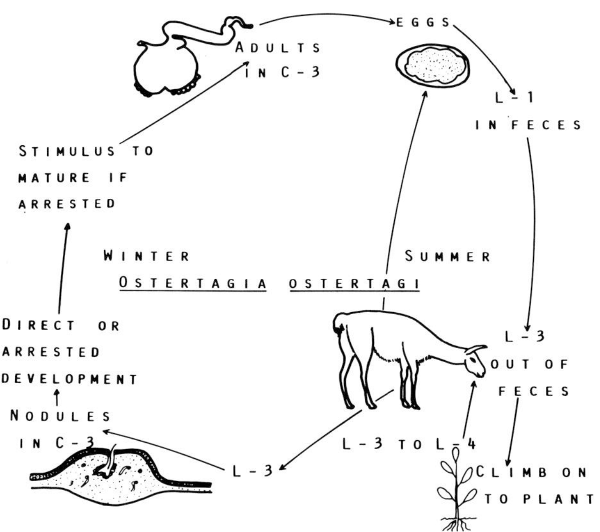

8.31 Life cycle of *Ostertagia ostertagi.*

Epidemiology. The life cycle of *O. ostertagi* may vary according to the climate and species affected, i.e., cattle, sheep, or SACs. The cycle described for cattle in a given area may not be the cycle that will occur in cattle in another area and is even less likely to be the cycle followed in llamas in yet a third area or another country. Until information has been obtained by detailed studies, however, reliance must be placed upon information that is known of ruminants of a given area.

Marshallagia (Ostertagia) marshalli (8, 42)

Life Cycle. This species has been shifted back and forth from its own generic status to that of a species of *Ostertagia.* It is closely related to *Osteragia* and has a similar life cycle. When ingested, the larvae penetrate into the gastric mucosa of C-3 and produce a nodule that is 2–4 mm in diameter. Instead of one larva per nodule, as in ostertagiosis, each nodule contains two or three larvae that will mature in 15–18 days. The prepatent period is up to 3 weeks, but there may be arrested development in this species also. The eggs of this parasite are large and frequently confused with that of *Nematodirus* sp. (see Fig. 8.30 and Table 8.5).

Epidemiology. *Marshallagia* has a limited distribution, but pockets of infection are located in the western United States. It has been seen in llama herds in northern California.

Camelostrongylus mentulatus (8, 42, 54)

This is another species that is closely related to *Ostertagia.* It is a common stomach (C-3) parasite of camels in the Middle East, but it is also found in Australia, South America, and the United States (54). The life cycle and epidemiologic patterns are similar to those of *Ostertagia.*

Graphinema aucheniae (9, 27)

This trichostrongyle has been reported only from South America. Adult parasites are found in C-3. The life cycle and epidemiology are similar to those of other trichostrongyles.

Haemonchus contortus (9, 30, 52)

Life Cycle. This parasite is similar to other trichostrongyles in the preparasitic stage. Infective larvae are present 4–6 days after the eggs have been passed in the feces. Eggs in the prehatch stage are more resistant to freezing and desiccation than the larvae, but all stages of the eggs and larvae can tolerate some degree of desiccation and low temperature.

Once the infective larvae have been ingested, they may enter an arrested-development stage resembling that of *Ostertagia.* The nodules in C-3 are not so pronounced as in ostertagiosis. Redevelopment begins when environmental conditions suitable for preservation of the eggs and larvae in the free-living state occur.

Epidemiology. In ruminants there is a breed-associated resistance to infection with *H. contortus.* Whether or not lamoids may be resistant is unknown. Other species of *Haemonchus* may have slightly different cycles and be adapted to either hot and dry climates or moist and cool climates. Infection in ruminants may stimulate an immune response. Conversely, animals that are stressed have lowered immunity, and infection and disease may be more debilitating.

A preparturient relaxing of immunity that may be accompanied by a buildup of the parasite load in a lamoid has been reported by Soulsby (70). Any period of stress ought to be monitored for the possibility of parasitism override.

Clinical Signs. *H. contortus* differs from other trichostrongyles in that it is a blood sucker. The trauma to the mucosa produced by these parasites also allows seepage of blood into the lumen of the intestine. The amount of blood loss caused by each nematode has been calculated to be 0.05 ml/day (70). Blood may appear in the feces 6–12 days following infection.

In addition to erythrocyte loss, there is a significant loss of plasma protein through such seepage. Some compensation for the protein loss may be achieved by increased albumin synthesis, but ultimately, protein reserves will become depleted and hypoalbuminemia will develop.

There are hyperacute, acute, and chronic forms of haemonchosis. The chronic form is the more important in lamoids, with affected animals being unthrifty, weak, and emaciated. The fecal egg count cannot be used as a gauge of the severity of the disease. Neither can the degree of anemia or hypoproteinemia, since the animal may have the capacity to compensate for the loss of cells and plasma as described above (70).

Lamanema chavezi (5, 36, 39, 40, 44, 69)

Identification. This nematode is one of the more important parasites of lamoids in the Andes. Fortunately, no instances of parasitism outside of South America have been reported, but lamoids being imported from South America should be carefully examined. The description of this parasite is based only on the adult male, larvae, and eggs (Table 8.5) (5, 36).

Life Cycle. The life cycle of *L. chavezi* is not well understood (Fig. 8.32). The adults are found in the small intestine rather than in C-3. The stages, up to ingestion of infected larvae, are probably similar to those of other trichostrongyles. Ingested larvae penetrate the intestinal wall and migrate to the liver and lungs. It is in the liver that the most serious damage occurs. Ultimately, maturation is completed with migration back to the small intestine via the trachea.

Epidemiology. This is a serious parasite of recently weaned lamoids. In one study, 4-month-old alpacas were given 200,000 larvae. In 20 days some of the alpacas were dying.

Clinical Signs. Massive infections cause hepatic and respiratory failure from involvement of the liver and lungs.

Pathology. The migration of the larvae through the wall of the intestine produces a catarrhal, hemorrhagic enteritis, with areas of necrosis of the mucosa. In acute cases, with recent migrations, the liver is congested, with multiple foci of coagulative necrosis, petechial hemorrhage, and punctate abscessation. There are also areas of congestion in the lungs.

Following maturation and remigration of the larvae, the liver lesions will become fibrotic and may calcify. These residual foci have been seen on adult alpacas slaughtered for meat.

Spiculopteragia peruvianus (9, 30)

Identification. The trichostrongyle nematode is found in C-3 of llamas, alpacas, and vicuñas on the Altiplano, near Lake Titicaca, in Peru. Little is known about the biology of this parasite other than its description (Table 8.5). It was mistaken for other trichostrongyles for a long time (30).

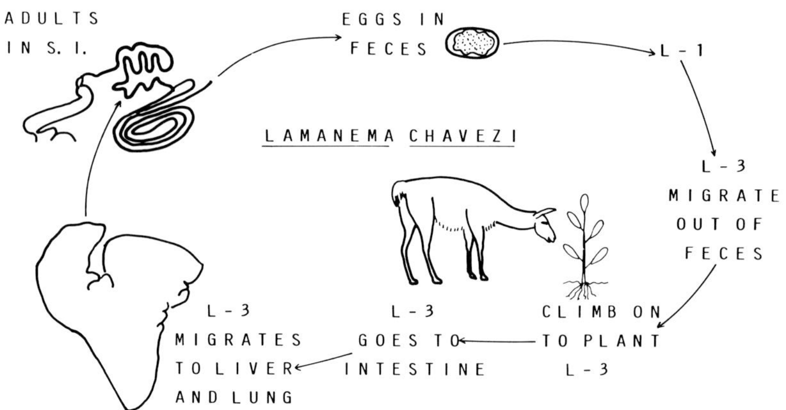

8.32 Life cycle of *Lamanema chavezi*.

Nematodirus lamae (5), *N. battus* (52), *N. spathiger* (8, 52), *N. filicollis* (9, 52), *N. lanceolatus* (52), *Nematodirus* sp. (3, 28)

Life Cycle (70). Adult nematodes are located in the small intestine. Eggs are passed in the feces and undergo slow development, over 2 or 3 months, to the L-3 larvae. If eggs at this stage are ingested in late summer, the larvae are infective, but this is not the normal route of exposure. Rather, the larvated eggs usually overwinter, and cold temperatures are required to ultimately induce the eggs to hatch and release the larvae. In the spring, when soil temperatures begin to rise, the mobile larvae climb onto herbage and are ingested (70).

Following ingestion, infective L-3 larvae penetrate the intestinal mucosa, where they molt to L-4 and L-5. L-5 larvae leave the mucosa and become adults in the lumen of the small intestine. The prepatent period is 15 days under optimum circumstances. Adult parasites live for only a few weeks.

Epidemiology. Since the larvated eggs overwinter, an infection in a given year is dependent upon contamination of a pasture the previous year. The major disease problem is in young animals with no prior exposure to the parasite, because animals develop some degree of resistance to the parasite over a period of time. A few older juveniles and adults harbor some parasites and contribute to contamination of the pastures, but overt disease is usually not seen in adults.

The degree of severity of the problem will be dependent upon the timing of the birth of the baby and the hatching of the eggs to free the infective larvae. Once freed, larvae live for only a few weeks.

Clinical Signs. Most of the damage occurs as the larvae embed in the intestinal mucosa, causing enteritis with its characteristic syndrome.

Cooperia zurnabada (C. mcmasteri) (9, 25), *C. oncophora* (8, 24, 52)

Cooperids are small trichostrongyles living in the small intestine of ruminants and camelids throughout the world. The life cycle and epidemiology are similar to those of *Trichostrongylus* sp. The infective larvae are able to survive on pastures 9–26 weeks and even overwinter. There may be an arrested-development stage in the wall of the intestine (70). Peruvian workers believe that *C. zurnabada* and *C. mcmasteri* are separate species, based on size differences (25).

Dictyocaulus filaria (34, 37), *D. viviparus*, *Dictyocaulus* sp. (12)

Identification. These lungworms are included in the superfamily Trichostrongyloidea because the life cycle is direct. See Table 8.5 for measurements (12, 34).

Life Cycle (70). Adult parasites live in the lumen of the bronchial tree (Fig. 8.33). The female lays a larvated egg, which is coughed up and swallowed. Hatching usually occurs during passage through the digestive tract. The free-living larvae, unlike other trichostrongyles, live on stored nutrients rather than on microorganisms. The larvae develop from L-1 to the infective L-3 in 5 days or more. Larvae then climb onto herbage and are ingested. The larvae penetrate the wall of the small intestine and migrate to the mesenteric lymph nodes and thence, via the blood vessels or lymphatics, to the lungs. About 4 weeks are required for maturation of L-5 to the adult nematode. The prepatent period is 4–5 weeks.

Epidemiology. The larvae require a moist environment, so are not a problem in hot, dry regions. Infective larvae can overwinter, but the more serious problem seems to arise in the fall, after a summer buildup of infection. The larvae are not usually evident on a standard fecal flotation. A Baerman apparatus is necessary to evaluate feces for lungworm larvae. It is also important to remember that clinical disease may be seen before larvae appear in the feces. The larvae developing in the lungs produce a marked catarrhal bronchitis.

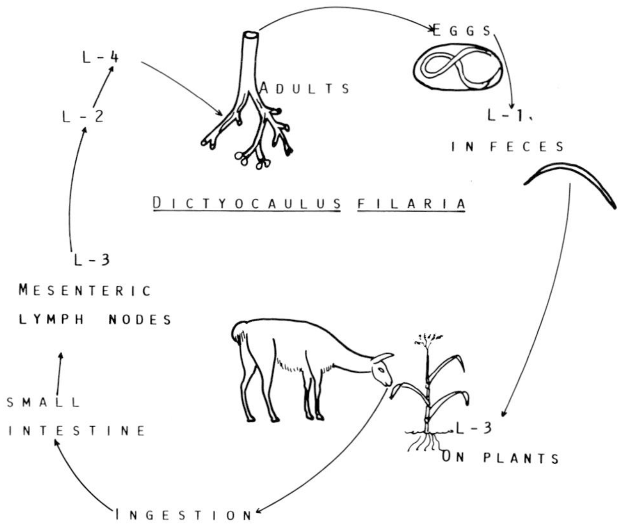

8.33 Life cycle of *Dictyocaulus filaria.*

Clinical Signs. The cardinal signs are cough, dyspnea, and nasal exudate. Not all of the signs need to be present at the same time. The body temperature is normal unless a secondary pneumonia develops.

Oesophagostomum sp. (3), *O. venulosum* (9, 52)

Identification. The nodular worm, *O. venulosum* is a strongyloid nematode found in the small and large intestines of camels and ruminants. None of the parasites found in SACs have been identified as to species. A similar strongyloid, found in sheep, is *Chabertia ovina,* which has also been reported in camels and in the vicuña in South America (9). See Table 8.5 for measurements.

Life Cycle (70). The life cycle of lamoid oesophagostomums has not been established. Based on *O. columbianum* or *O. venulosum,* it should be as follows. The thin-walled eggs are passed in the feces and require 6–7 days to reach the infective larval stage. The larvae climb onto herbage, are ingested, and exsheath in the small intestine. Larvae penetrate the wall of the intestine according to species predilection and may or may not produce nodules. L-4 and L-5 maturation takes place in the wall of the intestine; then the larvae migrate back to the lumen, and the adults take up residence in the large intestine. The prepatent period of *O. columbianum* is 41 days, and 28–31 days for *O. venulosum. O. venulosum* has less tendency to form nodules and thus is less pathogenic.

Epidemiology. Nothing is known about this parasitism in SACs.

Bunostomum sp.

Identification. *Bunostomum* sp. is a hookworm that is found only rarely in SACs and then only in warm tropical climates. See Table 8.5 for measurements.

Life Cycle (70). The life cycle is direct (Fig. 8.34). Adults are attached to the mucosa of the small intestine and are blood suckers. The eggs require a few days after passage in the feces before infective larvae are produced. These larvae may enter the body via the mouth or through the skin. If via the skin, the larvae migrate to the lung via the venous or lymphatic vessels and mature to L-3. These are coughed up and swallowed. L-4 larvae migrate to the intestine. The prepatent period is 30–56 days.

Epidemiology. Infective larvae are subject to desiccation, so this parasite is a problem only where there is permanent moisture or high humidity. There is no encystment in the muscles, nor is there transmammary migration as occurs in ancylostomiasis.

Skrjabinema ovis (52)

Identification. This parasite is the sheep pinworm. It has been reported in the guanaco in Argentina. The males are 2.3–3.7 mm long and 110–180 μm wide, making them wider than most other GI nematodes (56). The eggs are slightly flattened on one side and are 47–63 × 27–36 μm.

Life Cycle. The life cycle is direct. The adults live in the rectum, but the female traverses the anal sphincter to deposit eggs around the anus at night (56).

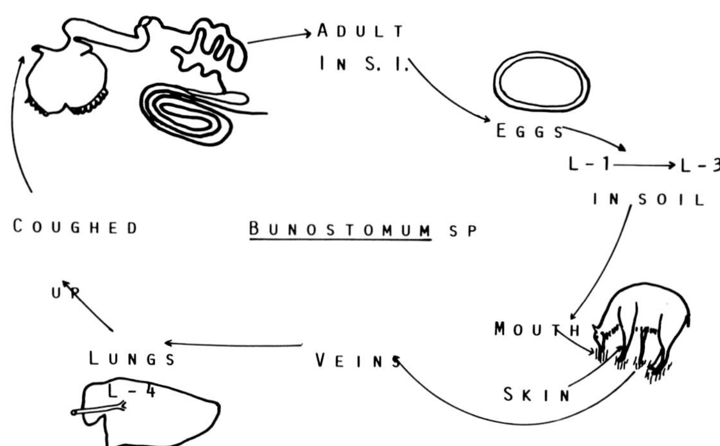

8.34 Life cycle of *Bunostomum* sp.

Infective larvae develop within the eggs. The eggs drop off and contaminate feed and water. When ingested, eggs hatch in the small intestine and the larvae migrate to the large intestine where they become mature worms in 17–25 days.

Epidemiology. The parasite probably does little harm to the host. Nothing is known about environmental requirements for persistence of the eggs (56).

Clinical Signs. Possible anal pruritis. Eggs will not usually be seen in a fecal flotation. Scotch tape applied to the anus and then applied to a glass slide is the customary diagnostic technique.

Parelaphostrongylus tenuis

Identification. The meningeal worm, *Parelaphostrongylus tenuis* (*Pneumonstrongylus tenuis*), is in the Protostrongylidae family. The white-tailed deer, *Odocoileus virginianus,* is the primary host for this parasite. See Table 8.5 for measurements (4, 6, 13).

Life Cycle (13). The life cycle in the deer will be described first (Fig. 8.35). It is not known whether the cycle is completed in the llama. Adult nematodes are located in the veins and sinuses of the dura mater of the brain. The eggs are deposited there and may or may not hatch. Eggs and larvae pass via the blood vessels to the lungs, and L-1 larvae break out into the alveoli. The larvae are then coughed up, swallowed, and passed in the feces. The larvae are picked up by terrestrial snails and slugs, *Deroceras graciles, D. reticulatum, D. laeve, Cionella lubrica, Arion circumscriptus, Zonitoides nitidus,* or *Z. arboreus.*

Development continues within the snail for 3–4 weeks. The snail or slug is then ingested by the deer. Larvae are released in the stomach, penetrate the wall of the peritoneal cavity, and migrate to the spinal cord, usually via the spinal nerves, within 10 days. The larvae mature in the dorsal horns of the gray matter for 20–30 days. The adults then move to the spinal subdural space and migrate to the brain. They move into their ultimate location by penetrating the dura mater and passing into the venous sinuses. The prepatent period is 82–91 days (70).

Epidemiology. The llama is an aberrant host for this parasite. A number of instances of affected llamas have been reported (4, 6, 62). The white-tailed deer has a broad distribution in the southern, eastern, and northern United States. The parasite is uniformly found wherever deer are found. Llamas cohabiting in pastures with white-tailed deer are at risk. It should be mentioned that other ungulate species may also be aberrant hosts for this parasite, e.g., moose, *Alces alces;* wapiti, *Cervus canadensis;* caribou, *Rangifer tarandus;* black-tailed deer, *Odocoileus hemionus;* red deer, *Cervus elaphus;* and sheep and goats.

Clinical Signs. The parasite is well adapted to the primary host, in which little or no clinical disease develops. In aberrant hosts, such as the llama, migration of the larvae in the spinal cord produces neurologic deficits commensurate with the location of the larvae, including lameness, ataxia, stiffness, circling, blindness,

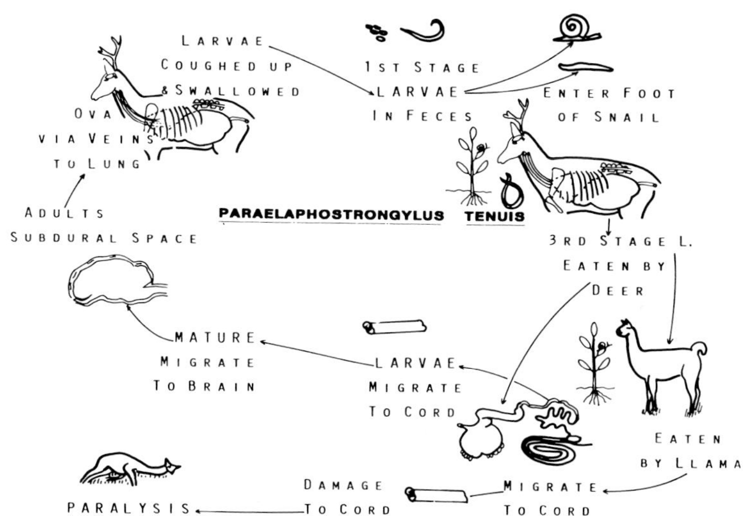

8.35 Life cycle of *Parelaphostrongylus tenuis.*

hypermetria, paraplegia, paralysis, and abnormal positions of the head (4, 6).

Treatment. Ivermectin is effective against the stages prior to entering the spinal cord. Ivermectin does not readily penetrate the blood-brain barrier. A few management procedures may be of help in protecting valuable llamas from this parasite. A deer-proof fence could exclude white-tailed deer from the llama pastures. A molluscicide could be used to destroy the snails and slugs that serve as intermediate hosts, and monthly treatment with ivermectin could be used during the spring, summer, and fall.

Diagnosis. No definitive antemortem diagnosis is possible. There may or may not be a peripheral eosinophilia and, likewise, the cerebrospinal fluid may or may not provide significant information.

Thelazia californiensis, Thelazia sp.

Identification (70). The eyeworm, *T. californiensis,* is a spirurid nematode found in the conjunctival sac of deer, elk, cattle, sheep, dogs, cats, foxes, rabbits, llamas, and humans. See Table 8.5 for measurements.

Larvated ova are found in the lacrimal secretions (Fig. 8.36). Muscoid flies, such as the face fly (*Musca autumnalis*), ingest the ova or larvae. L-2 larvae migrate to the fly's ovarian follicles and mature to L-3 in 15–30 days. L-3 larvae migrate from the follicles to the labia of the fly, and infective larvae are deposited in another eye when the fly feeds on lacrimal secretions. Maturation to the adult nematode takes 16–20 days, the prepatent period.

Epidemiology. The life cycle also describes the epidemiology. The parasite is locally common and is transmitted only during the fly season.

Clinical Signs. Excessive lacrimation may be the only sign noted. Nematodes may be seen on the surface of the cornea or in the conjunctival sac. They may lodge beneath the nictitating membrane or be found in the nasolacrimal duct. With large numbers, a mild conjunctivitis may develop.

Treatment. The parasites can be mechanically removed under sedation with a local anesthetic. Diethylcarbamazine in a concentration of 2 mg/L may be instilled into the conjunctival sac. Ivermectin drops may be instilled into the conjunctival sac also.

Gongylonema sp.

Identification. *G. pulchrum* has been reported from alpacas in Peru (8). This is a spirurid nematode. *G. pulchrum* has a broad host distribution and is called the "cattle gullet worm." No speciation was done on the specimens collected from the alpacas.

Male *G. pulchrum* are 30–62 mm long and 150–300 μm wide; females are 80–145 mm long and 300–500 μm wide. The eggs are 50–70 × 25–37 μm (56).

Life cycle. The life cycle requires an intermediate host. The adults are embedded in the mucosa or submucosa of the esophagus and stomach. Eggs are passed in the feces and ingested by beetles. The eggs hatch and mature to infective larvae in about 4 weeks (56). The lamoid must then ingest the beetle to complete the cycle. The migration route of the larvae to the esophagus is not known.

Epidemiology. Unknown, other than that beetles serve as intermediate hosts.

Clinical Signs. These parasites are nonpathogenic to cattle, and no reports of signs or pathology in lamoids have been published.

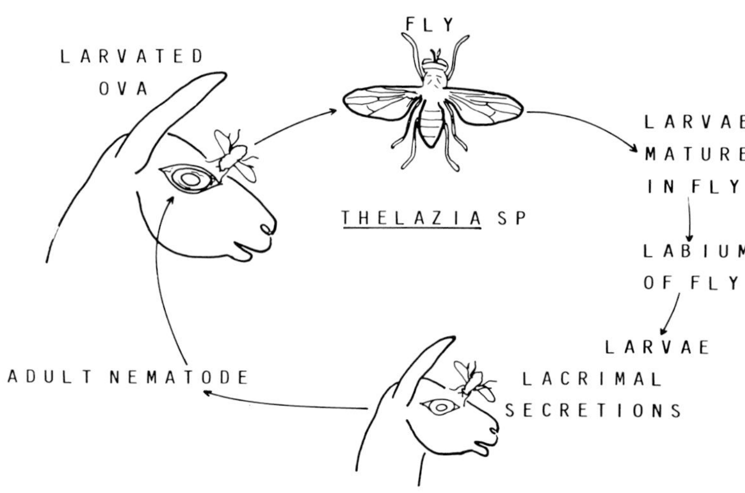

8.36 Life cycle of *Thelazia californiensis.*

Trichuris sp. (3, 8), *T. ovis* (8, 9, 25, 52)

Identification. Whipworms, *Trichuris* sp., are significant parasites of camelids and are resistant to treatment. They are characterized by a long, slender anterior and a thicker posterior segment. See Table 8.5 for measurements. The eggs are doubly operculated and thus are easy to identify, but they must be differentiated from those of *Capillaria* sp. Adult parasites are found in the cecum and large intestine. Trichurids identified from camels include *T. globulosa, T. cameli,* and *T. skrjabini* (70).

Life Cycle. Trichurids found in lamoids have not been speciated, so the precise life cycle is not known. However, trichurids all have a similar cycle, which is direct. Eggs are passed in the feces, requiring about 3 weeks to become infective. The infective eggs are ingested by the lamoid. The larvae hatch and penetrate the wall of the anterior small intestine. Maturation proceeds for 2–10 days, and the larvae migrate to the cecum and large intestine and become adults (70). The prepatent period for *T. ovis* is 7–9 weeks.

Epidemiology. The persistence of infective eggs in the environment makes management of this parasitism difficult.

Clinical Signs. These nematodes tunnel into the intestinal mucosa with the slender anterior ends. They traumatize vessels, causing hemorrhage, which is ingested by the parasites, producing a catarrhal enteritis. The syndrome is similar to that of haemonchiasis.

Capillaria sp. (8, 9, 52)

Identification. Capillarids are closely related to *Trichuris* but lack the slender and thick variation of the body. Little is known about the species found in SACs, but eggs identified in the laboratory are presumed to be identical to species found in ruminants.

Life Cycle. Not known.

Epidemiology. Not known.

REFERENCES

1. Aguilar G., A. C. 1970. (Anthelmintic effectivity of pyrantel tartrate in alpacas) Efectividad antihelmintica del tartrato de purantel en alpaca. Bol. Extraordinario 4:96–99.

2. Alvarez, I. 1972. (Fertility of hydatid cysts in bovine, sheep and alpaca in Peru) Fertilidad quistes hidaticos en vacunos, ovinos y alpacas en Puno. Tesis, Med. Vet. Puno, Univ. Nac. Tec. Altiplano.

3. Arnao, M., Gonzales, E., and Arbaiza, E. 1949. (Parasitism in alpacas) Paristos en *Lama glama pacos* o alpaca. Rev. Fac. Med. Vet. (Lima) 4:64–65.

4. Baumgaertner, W., Zajac, A., Hull, B. L., Andrews, F., and Garry, F. 1985. Parelaphostrongylosis in llamas. J. Am. Vet. Med. Assoc. 187:1243–45.

5. Becklund, W. W. 1963. Nematodes: Trichostrongylidae from the alpaca (*Lama pacos*) and the vicuña (*Vicugna vicugna*) in Peru. J. Parasitol. 49:1023–27.

6. Brown, T. T., Jr., Jordon, H. E., and Demorest, C. N. 1978. Cerebrospinal parelaphostrongylosis in llamas. J. Wildl. Dis. 14(4):441–44.

7. Castro, J. 1974. (*Sarcocystis auchenicae* in llamas) Sarcocystic auchenlae en llamas, *Lama glama.* Rev. Invest. Pecu. 4(1):91–92.

8. Chavez Garcia, C. E., and Guerrero Dias, C. A. 1960. (Identification of ecto and endoparasites by the Department of Parasitology, School of Veterinary Medicine) Ecto y endoparasitos identificados en el departamento de Parasitologia de la Facultad de Medicina Veterinaria. Rev. Fac. Med. Vet. (Lima) 15:48–68.

9. Chavez Garcia, C. E., Guerrero, D., Alva, J., and Guerrero, R. J. 1967. (Gastrointestinal parasitism in alpacas) El parasitismo gastrointestinal en alpacas. Rev. Fac. Med. Vet. (Lima) 21:9–19.

10. Chavez Garcia, C. E., Guerrero, D., Vallenas P., A., and Ochoa, B. J. 1961. (Inhibition [erythrocyte] of cholinesterase activity by the action of organic phosphate compounds in alpacas) Inhibicion de la actividad colinsterasica eritrocitica por accion de un compuesto fosforado organico en alpacas. Rev. Fac. Med. Vet. (Lima) 16(17):69–78.

11. Chu-vela, J., and Guerrero Diaz, C. A. 1973. (Evaluation of methods of treatment of sarcoptic mange in alpacas) Evaluacion de metodos en el tratamiento de la sarna de alpacas. Rev. Invest. Pecu. 2(1):23–28.

12. Cordonrena, N. 1968. (Dictyocaulosis in alpacas in the zone of Macusani in the department of Puno) Dictocaulosis en alpacas de la zona de Macusani Depto. de Puno. Bol. Extraordinario 3:56–58.

13. Davis, J. W., and Anderson, R. C., eds. 1971. Parasitic Diseases of Wild Mammals. Ames: Iowa State Univ. Press, pp. 10, 38.

14. Durette-Desset, M. C. 1978. (New morphologic data on the trichostrongyloid nematodes of the collections of the USA National Museum). Bull. Mus. Nat. Hist. Nat. Zool. 352:135–48. French.

15. Ferris, G. F. 1951. The Sucking Lice. San Francisco: Pacific Coast Entomological Society, p. 301.

16. Filippova, N. A., and Panova, I. V. 1978. (*Anomalohimalya iotozkyi,* a new species of ixodid ticks from Peter I Ridge (Ixodoidea, Ixodidae). Parazitologiya 12(5):391–99. Russian.

17. Fowler, M. E. 1985. Tick paralysis. Calif. Vet. 39 (2):25–26.

18. ______. 1986a. Camelids. In Zoo and Wild Animal Medicine, 2nd ed. Philadelphia: W. B. Saunders, pp. 969–81.

19. ______. 1986b. Lice in llamas. Avian Exot. Pract. 3(1):22–25.

20. Fowler, M. E., and Paul-Murphy, J. 1985. *Cephenemyia* sp. infestation in the llama. Calif. Vet. 39:10–12.

21. Gehring, H. 1981. (Sarcoptes in llama and alpaca) Sarkoptersraeude bei Lamas und Alpakas. Verhandlungsber. 23rd Int. Symp. Erkr. Zootier 23:257–60.

22. Georgi, J. R. 1985. Parasitology for Veterinarians, 4th ed. Philadelphia: W. B. Saunders.

23. Gonzalez-Mungaburu, L., Sarmiento, L., and Arnao, M. 1951. (List of parasites identified in domestic animals and their geographic distribution in Peru) Lista de parasitos identificados en los animales domesticos y su distribucion geografica en el Peru. Lima Congr. Panam. Med. Vet. An.

24. Guerrero Diaz, C. A. 1960. (Helminths in vicuñas) Helmintos en vicuñas (*Vicugna vicugna*). Rev. Fac. Med. Vet. (Lima) 15:103–5.

25. ______. 1961–62. (*Cooperia mcmasteri* in alpacas and vicuña) *Cooperia mcmasteri* en alpacas y vicuña. Rev. Fac. Med. Vet. (Lima) 16–17:131–37.

26. ______. 1967a. Coccidia of the alpaca, *Lama pacos*. J. Protozool. 144:616–25.

27. ______. 1967b. (New species of parasites in alpacas) Nuevas especies de parasitos identificados en alpacas. Bol. Extraordinario 2:68.

28. Guerrero Diaz, C. A., and Alva, M. J. 1968. (Some aspects of the epidemiology of gastrointestinal nematodes of alpacas) Algunos aspectos epidemiologicos de la gastroenteritis verminosa en las alpacas. Bol. Extraordinario 3:54–55.

29. Guerrero Diaz, C. A., and Chavez Garcia, C. E. 1961–62. (Anthelmintic effectivity of O,O,dimethyl,2,2,2 trichloro-1-hydroryethyl phosphate in alpacas) Efectividad anthelmintica del O,O-dimetil-2,2,2-tricloro-1-hidroxietilfosfonat (Neguvon). Rev. Fac. Med. Vet. (Lima) 16–17:104–8.

30. ______. 1967. (Helminths recorded for the first time in alpacas, *Lama pacos,* with a description of *Spiculopteragia peruvianus* New species) *Vicugna vicugna, Ostertagia lyrata, Trichostrongylus longispicularis, Lama glama, Haemonchus contortus, Camelostrongylus mentulatus* New Records Host. Bol. Chileno Parasitol. 22(4):147–50.

31. Guerrero Diaz, C. A., and Hernandez, J. 1967. (Life cycle of sarcocystis) Cirlo evolutivo del sarcosystis. Bol. Extraordinario 2:70–71.

32. Guerrero Diaz, C. A., Hernandez, J., and Alva M., J. 1967a. (Coccidiosis in alpacas) Coccidiosis en alpacas. Bol. Extraordinario 2:66–67.

33. ______. 1967b. (Coccidiosis in alpacas) Coccidiosis en alpacas. Rev. Fac. Med. Vet. (Lima) 21:59–68.

34. Guerrero Diaz, C. A., Bazalar, H., and Tabacchi, L. 1970. (Experimental infection of an alpaca with *Dictyocaulus filaria* from sheep) Infeccion experimental de una alpaca con *Dictyocaulus filaria* de ovine. Bol. Extraordinario 4:74–78.

35. Guerrero Diaz, C. A., Alva M., J., Bazalar, H., and Tabacchi, L. 1970a. (Experimental infection of alpacas with *Eimeria*) Infeccion experimental de alpacas con *Eimeria lamae*. Bol. Extraordinario 4:79–83.

36. Guerrero Diaz, C. A., Alva M., J., and Vega, I. 1970b. (Preliminary note about the infection of *Lamanema chavezi* in alpacas) Nota preliminar sobre la infeccion experimental de *Lamanema chavezi* en alpacas *Lama pacos*. Bol. Extraordinario 4:71–73.

37. Guerrero Diaz, C. A., Alva M., J., Legui, G., and Bazalar, H. 1970c. (Prevalence of coccidia in alpacas) Prevalencia de coccidias en alpacas *Lama pacos*. Bol. Extraordinario 4:84–90.

38. Guerrero Diaz, C. A., Hernandez, J., Bazalar, H., and Alva M., J. 1971. *Eimeria macusaniensis* of the alpaca. J. Protozool. 18:163–65.

39. Guerrero Diaz, C. A., Alva M., J., and Rojas, M. 1973a. (Anthelmintic activity of L-tetramisole against experimental infections of *Lamanema chavezi* in alpaca) Actividad anthelimintica del L-tetramisole contra infecciones experimentales de *Lamanema chavezi* en alpacas (*Lama pacos*). Rev. Invest. Pecu. 2(2):141–44.

40. Guerrero Diaz, C. A., Alva M., J., Vega, I., Hernandez, J., and Rojas, M. 1973b. (Biological and pathological features of *Lamenema chavezi* in alpacas) Algunos aspectos biolgoicos del *Lamanema chavezi* en alpacas, *Lama pacos*. Rev. Invest. Pecu. 2(1):29–42.

41. Guerrero Diaz, C. A., Rojas, M., and Vargas, J. 1974a. (The activity of L-tetramisole against natural infections of nematodes in alpacas) Actividad del L-tetramisole contra infecciones naturales de nematodes en alpacas. Rev. Invest. Pecu. 3(1):9–14.

42. Guerrero Diaz, C. A., Alva M., J., Rojas, M., and Bazalar, H. 1974b. (Limits of parasite diseases) Linea de enfermedades parasitaris. Bol. Divulg. 15:139–44.

43. Guerrero Diaz, C. A., Hernandez, J., and Alva M., J. 1976. (Sarcocystis in alpaca) Sarcocystis en alpaca. Rev. Fac. Med. Vet. (Lima) 21:69–76.

44. Guerrero Diaz, C. A., Rojas, M., and Alva M., J. 1981. *Lamanema chavezi,* an enterohepatic nematode of South American camelidae and its control using levamisole. Rev. Latinoam. Microbiol. 23(2):121–23.

45. Guerrero La Rosa, G. V. 1962. (Psoroptic mange in alpacas) Sarna psoroptica en alpacas) J. Microsc. Parasit. Ann. Trujillo (Peru) 13–14.

46. Guerrero La Rosa, J., and Chavez Garcia, C. E. 1963–66. (Anthelmintic evaluation of thiabendazole in alpacas) Evaluacion antihelmintica del 2-(4 Thiazolill) Benzimidazole (Thibenzole) en alpacas. Rev. Fac. Med. Vet. (Lima) 1820:203–17.

47. Hernandez, J., and Condorena, N. 1967. (*Fasciola hepatica* in the liver of alpacas) *Fasciola hepatica* en highado de alpaca. Rev. Fac. Med. Vet. (Lima) 21:138–39.

48. Hook, J. 1983. Tick paralysis. 3 L Llama 17:22.

49. Hopkins, G. H. E. 1949. The host associations of the lice of mammals. Proc. Zool. Soc. Lond. 119:387–604.

50. Kraft, H. 1956. (Observations of sarcoptic mange in camelids) Betrachtungen zur Sarcoptesraeude der Cameliden. Berl, Munch. Tieraerztl. Wochenschr. 69:365–66.

51. Kress, P. J. 1983. Use of ivermectin for treatment of scabies in llamas. Llama World 1(3):18–19.

52. Larrieu, E., Bigatti, R., Lakovich, R., Eddi, C., Bonacci, E., Gomez, E., Niec, R., and Oparto, N. 1982. (Contributions to the study of gastrointestinal parasitism in guanacos and llamas) Conribucion al estudio del parasitismo gastrointestinal en guanacos (*Lama guanicoe*) y llamas (*Lama glama*). Gac. Vet. (Buenos Aires) (374):958–60.

53. LaValley, W. 1983. Mites—one person's battle. 3 L Llama 18:26.

54. Led, J. E., and Boero, J. J. 1972. (*Camelostrongylus*

mentulatus: First report from the Republic of Argentina and of a new host, *Lama glama*) *Camelostrongylus mentulatus:* Primera cita para la Republica Argentina y su nuevo huesped, *Lama glama.* Gac. Vet. 34:187–90.

55. Leguia, G., and Bendezu, P. 1974. (Field observations on the epizootiology of helminth gastroenteritis in alpacas (*Lama pacos*) of Sierra de Pasco) Observaciones de campo sobre la epidemiologia de la gastro-enteritis verminosa en alpacas (*Lama pacos*) de Cerro de Pasco. Rev. Invest. Pecu. (1):3–7.

56. Levine, N. D. 1980. Nematode Parasites of Domestic Animals and of Man, 2nd ed. Minneapolis: Burgess.

57. ______. 1985. Veterinary Protozoology. Ames: Iowa State Univ. Press.

58. Lim, Y. J., and Lee, W. C. 1977. (Epidemiological study on infestation rates of parasites in zoo animals). Korean J. Vet. Res. 17(1):17–26. Korean.

59. Loomis, E. C. 1982. Common External Parasites and Pests of Livestock and Poultry in California. Univ. Calif. (Davis) Ext. Bull.

60. Lubinsky, G. 1964. Ophryoscolecidae of a guanaco from the Winnipeg zoo. Can. J. Zool. 42:159.

61. Mellanby, K. 1946–47. Sarcoptic mange in the alpaca. Trans. R. Soc. Trop. Med. Hyg. 40:359.

62. Murtaugh, T. 1983. *Parelaphostrongylus tenuis* in a llama. Llama World 1(3):19.

63. Quiroga, D. A., Lombardero, O. J., and Zorilla, R. 1969. *Sarcocystis tilopodi,* new species in the guanaco, *Lama guanacoe* in Argentina. Gac. Vet. (Buenos Aires) 31:67–70.

64. Riemann, H. P., Behymer, D. E., Fowler, M. E., Schulz, T., Lock, A., Orthoefer, J. G., Silverman, S., and Franti, C. E. 1974. Prevalence of antibodies to *Toxoplasma gondii* in captive exotic mammals. J. Am. Vet. Med. Assoc. 165:798–800.

65. Rojas, M., and Guerrero Diaz, C. A. 1970. (Anthelmintic evaluation of Maretin 80 μ in alpacas) Evaluacion antihelmintica del Maretin 80 en alpacas, *Lama pacos.* Bol. Extraordinario 4:91–95.

66. Rusch, K. 1965. (Sarcoptic mange in SAC) Sarkoptesraude be den Aucheniden. Vet. Med. Nachr. 4:294–98.

67. Santivanez, M. J., and Cuba, C. A. 1949. (Hydatid cysts in alpaca) Quiste hidatico en *Lama glama pacos* o alpaca. Rev. Fac. Med. Vet. (Lima) 4:22–26.

68. Sharpnack, E. 1982. Sarcoptic mange in llamas. Llama World 1(1):18.

69. Sillau, H., Llerena, L., Esquere, J., Rojas, M., and Alva M., J. 1973. (Hepatic function in alpaca babies experimentally affected with *Lamanema chavezi*) Pruebas funcionales hepaticas en crias de alpaca nomales y in fectadas experimentalmentee con *Lamanema chavezi.* Rev. Invest. Pecu. 2(1):102–5.

70. Soulsby, E. J. L. 1982. Helminths, Arthropods and Protozoans of Domesticated Animals, 7th ed. Philadelphia: Lea & Febiger.

71. Sweatman, G. K. 1957. Life history, nonspecificity, and revision of the genus *Chorioptes,* a parasitic mite of herbivores. Can. J. Zool. 35:641–89.

72. ______. 1958. On the life history and validity of the species *Psoroptes,* a genus of mange mites. Can. J. Zool. 36:905–29.

73. Teng-K., -E., and Huang, C. -A. 1981. *Anomalohimalaya cricetuli,* new species from China. Acta Entomol. Sin. 24(1):99–102. Chinese.

74. Tilc, K., and Hanuskova, Z. 1976. Dynamics of coccidioses and helminthiases in Siberian ibexes and other ruminants in a zoo and the respective control measures. Acta Vet. Brno 45(1):133–40.

75. Ueno, H., Arandia, C. R., Morales, L. G., and Medina, M. G. 1975. Fascioliasis of livestock and snail host for fasciola in the Altiplano region of Bolivia. Natl. Inst. Anim. Health Q. 15(2):61–67.

76. Unger, H. 1976. (Camels) Kamele. In H. G. Kloes and E. M. Lang, eds. Zootierkrankheiten. Berlin: Paul Parey, pp. 187–94.

77. ______. 1982. Camelidae. In H. G. Kloes and E. M. Lang, eds. Handbook of Zoo Medicine. New York: Van Nostrand Reinhold, pp. 223–32.

78. Vallenas P., A., and Ochoa B., J. 1961–62. (Erythrocyte cholinesterase activity in the normal blood of alpacas) Actividad colinesterasia eritrocitica en la saugre normal de alpacas. Rev. Fac. Med. Vet. (Lima) 16–17:57–68.

79. Vallenas P., A., Ochoa B., J., Chavez G., C., and Guerrero Diaz, C. A. 1960. (Anthelmintic dosage in alpacas) Dosificacion anthelmintica en alpacos. Rev. Fac. Med. Vet. (Lima) 15:31–40.

80. Vallenas P., A., Ochoa B., J., and Guerrero Diaz, C. A. 1961–62. (Inhibition of erythrocyte cholinesterase activity by organic phosphate compounds in alpacas) Inhibicion de la actividad colinesterasia eritrocitica por accionde un compuesto fosforado organico en alpacas. Rev. Fac. Med. Vet. (Lima) 16–17:69–78.

81. Vanzolini, P. E., and Guimares, L. R. 1955. South American land mammals and their lice (llama). Evolution 9:345–47.

82. Vargas, J., Guerrero Diaz, C. A., and Rojas, M. 1972. (Field trials of levamisole against nematodes in alpacas) Pruebas de campo controladas del levamisole contra nematodes de alpacas. Rev. Invest. Pecu. 1(2):137–44.

83. Wagenaar, G. 1964. (*Sarcoptes scabiei* in a llama). Tijdschr. Diergeneeskd. 89(9):623–24. Dutch.

84. Young, E. 1966. Chorioptic mange in the alpaca. J. S. Afr. Vet. Med. Assoc. 37:474–75.

9 Multisystem Disorders

THIS CHAPTER deals with noninfectious and nonparasitic disorders affecting multiple organ systems.

NEOPLASIA

There is only one reference to a tumor in the lamoid literature. Perhaps this is a reflection of lack of attention to individual animal health until recently. The basic premise is that if a determined search were made through a sufficient population of lamoids, neoplasia would be noted in all organ systems (7, 9). The more thorough the necropsy, the more likely is the detection of a lesion. Many necropsies of lamoids are conducted by persons without specialized training in pathology. Therefore, many subtle lesions may go unnoticed, hence unreported. This is especially true of neoplasia that may be incidental to the actual cause of death.

The etiology of neoplasia in lamoids is unknown, as it is for most tumors of domestic and wild animals.

Lymphosarcoma in a Llama: A Case Report (8)

The patient was a 4-year-old breeding male llama, kept with approximately 30 other llamas. Clinical signs included self-imposed isolation from the herd, anorexia, emaciation, weakness, stumbling gait, stomach atony, and dyspnea. Thoracic radiographs indicated pleural effusion. Cytologic examination of the sterile serosanguineous fluid from the pleural space demonstrated large numbers of immature, pleomorphic, nondifferentiated lymphoid-type cells. Similar cells were observed from a bone marrow aspiration.

The llama was euthanized and necropsied. A large lymphoma (10 × 15 × 20 cm) was found in the region of the pancreas, duodenum, and adjacent loops of colon (Fig. 9.1). The liver was infiltrated. There was fibrinous pleuritis, with lymphomas on the parietal pleural surfaces, within the lung, and in mediastinal lymph nodes (Fig. 9.2). Both external and internal lymph nodes were enlarged. A nodule was found in a kidney. The microscopic lesions were similar to those observed in other domestic animals with lymphosarcoma. The primary nidus was not determined.

Other tumors have been observed in llamas and re-

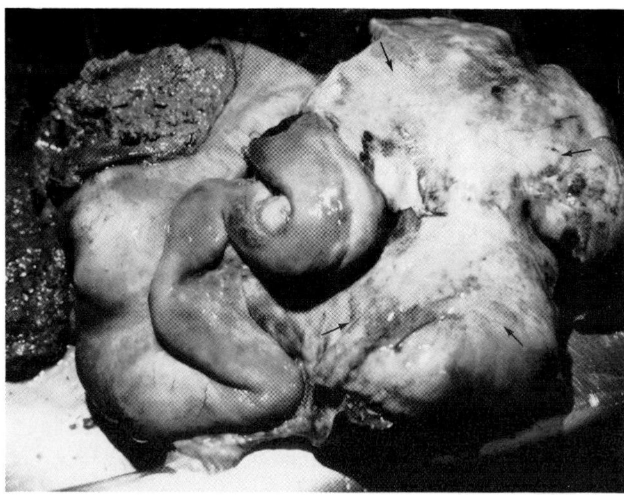

9.1 Lymphosarcoma of abdominal organs.

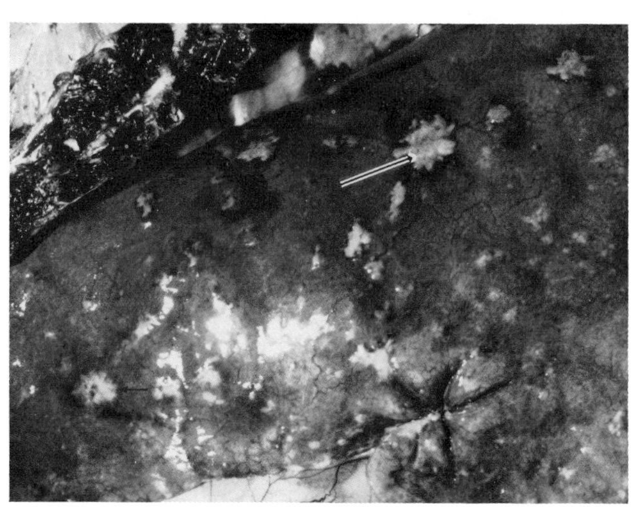

9.2 Lymphosarcoma of the lungs.

ported by clinicians at seminars and conferences. Those known to the author include carcinoma of the uterus, carcinoma of the intestinal tract, and basal cell carcinoma of the urinary bladder.

STRESS

Definition of Terms

"Stress" is the cumulative response of an animal to interaction with its environment via receptors (5, 13). Stress is an adaptive phenomenon. All responses are primarily directed at coping with environmental change. Each reaction to a stressor has adaptive significance. Intense or prolonged stimulation induces detrimental responses that may be fatal in the llama.

A "stressor" (stress-producing factor) is any stimulus that elicits a nonspecific response when perceived by an animal. A listing of some of the potential stressors acting on lamoids may direct attention to consideration of these important factors. Somatic stressors (stimulation of the physical senses) include temperature changes; strange sights, sounds, touches, or odors; stretching of muscles during restraint procedures; close confinement; thirst; and hunger.

Psychological stressors include anxiety, fright, terror, anger, rage, and frustration. Closely allied are behavioral stressors, including overcrowding, lack of social contact, hierarchial upsets, unfamiliar surroundings, trailer transport, and lack of habitual foods. Medical stressors include toxins, parasites, infectious agents, burns, malnutrition, drugs, and anesthetics.

A "specific response" is the appropriate response (of a llama) for the stimulated receptor. For instance, when cold receptors are stimulated, the body experiences a sensation of coolness. Various somatic and behavioral changes occur that conserve heat and stimulate increased heat production. The llama is adjusting to a new situation (homeostatic accommodation) (Fig. 9.3).

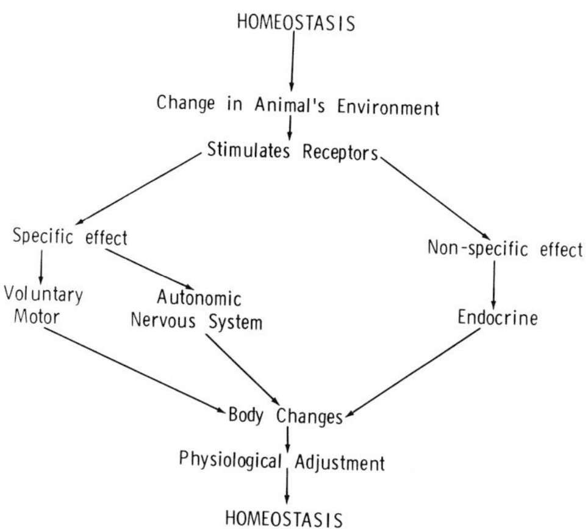

9.3 Homeostatic mechanisms.

In addition to specific responses to individual stimuli, the body reacts with "nonspecific responses" to stressors. When a cold receptor is stimulated, an impulse also acts upon the hypothalamic adenohypophyseal adrenal pathway (HAAP). As the animal attempts to adapt to the temperature change, numerous nerve pathways respond, biochemical and endocrine systems react, and subtle changes occur in the body. Similar changes may be produced in response to fright, malnutrition, restraint procedures, frustration, surgery, infections, or social incompatibilities. Nonspecific effects may not be immediately identifiable.

Basic Concepts

The animal is stimulated by stressors (environmental changes) via receptors. The nervous system analyzes and processes impulses from receptors and feeds responses back through various components of the nervous system to effector organs, producing either a specific or nonspecific reaction or both. Responses to the stimulation of a receptor may follow one of three pathways: voluntary motor, adrenal medulla, or HAAP (Fig. 9.4).

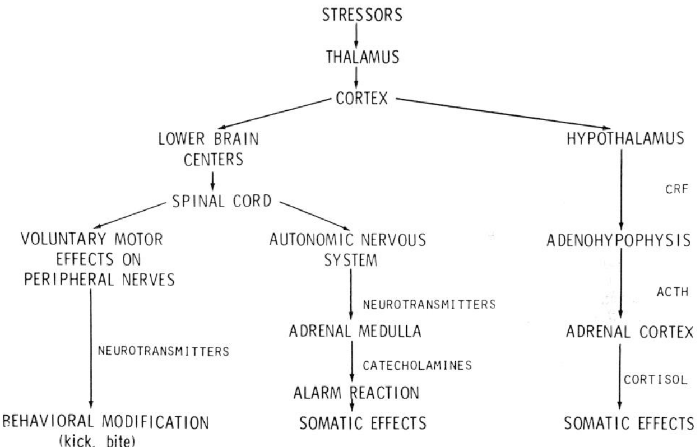

9.4 Stress pathways.

The voluntary motor pathway processes specific responses as described previously. The adrenal medullary response is via the sympathetic nervous system, producing the flight or fight reaction or, as described by Selye (13), the alarm reaction (Fig. 9.5, Table 9.1). It is important to note that both of these pathways also result in stimulation of the neuroendocrine system (HAAP) (Fig. 9.6).

Continuous adrenal cortex stimulation and excessive production of cortisol elicit many adverse metabolic responses. Psychological as well as physical changes occur. The clinical syndromes of adrenocortical stimulation have been identified in some species (human, dog, horse, laboratory animals). Nothing is known about the effects

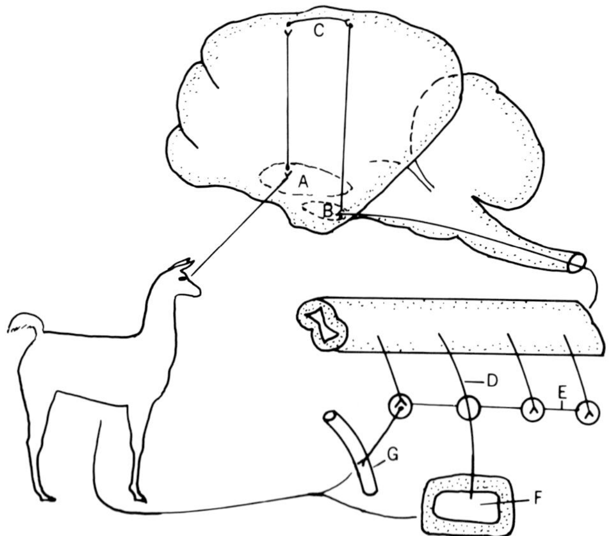

9.5 Neuroendocrine pathways of the alarm response: (A) thalamus, (B) hypothalamus, (C) neocortex, (D) preganglionic fiber of the sympathetic nerves, (E) sympathetic trunk, (F) adrenal medulla–producing catecholamines, (G) postganglionic fiber of sympathetic nerves.

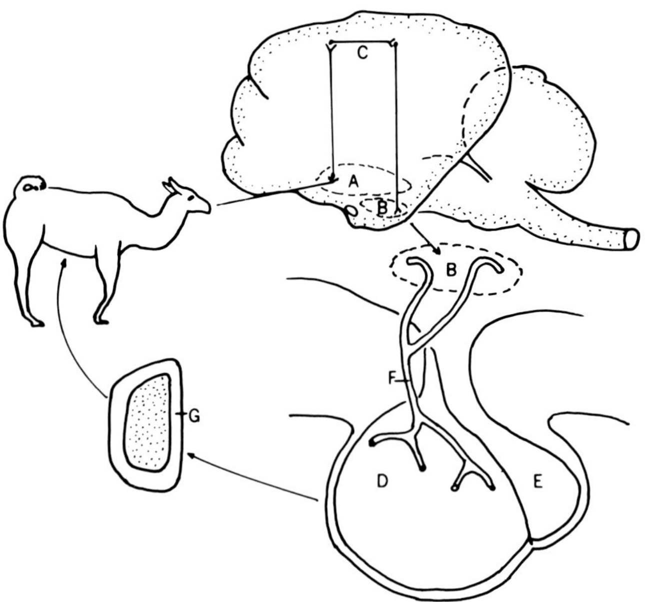

9.6 Hypothalamic adenohypophyseal adrenal pathway: (A) thalamus, (B) hypothalamus, (C) neocortex, (D) adenohypophysis, (E) neurohypophysis, (F) hypothalamic adenohypophyseal portal vein, (G) adrenal cortex–producing cortisol.

of hypercorticism in lamoids. However, the basic biologic effects of cortisol should be understood. Cortisol stimulates protein catabolism. It is also glycolytic, gluconeogenic, lipolytic, antiinflammatory, and antiimmunologic. All these actions have a bearing on the well-being of a llama.

Interference with DNA synthesis causes atrophy of lymphoid tissue throughout the body. Cell-mediated immune responses are diminished. A neutrophilia, eosinopenia, and lymphopenia are produced. Leukocytosis and an absolute lymphopenia and eosinopenia are the characteristics of a stress hemogram of a lamoid because of the preponderance of neutrophils in the leukocyte series.

Gastric and intestinal ulcers are common in llamas. No etiologic agent has been identified. Stress ulceration of the gastrointestinal system is a well-known syndrome in humans, rats, and marine mammals. Whether stress is a factor in llama ulcers is unknown, but one should be mindful of the basic effect of cortisol on the digestive system. Most of the studies have been performed on humans and laboratory animals, and as there may be significant species differences, direct extrapolation is unwise. The pathogenesis of gastric stress ulcers in humans and marine mammals is multifactorial. Hypercortisolism causes hypersecretion of acid and digestive enzymes. A duodenal reflux introduces substances from the duodenum into the stomach (lysolecithin) that reduce the effectiveness of the mucous membrane barrier. A third factor is vasoconstriction of the vasculature of the stomach, which in turn causes local hypoxia and a deficiency of adenosine triphosphate. These also contribute to the reduction of the mucous membrane barrier. Whether these factors are operating in the llama is unknown, but should be considered.

Table 9.1. Clinical signs of the alarm response

Vasoconstriction	Bronchodilation
skin and intestine	Piloerection
Vasodilation	Mydriasis
muscles and heart	Coagulation time ↓
Blood glucose ↑	Pain threshold ↑
Metabolic rate ↑	Blood pressure ↑
Muscle fasciculation	Secretions ↓
Alertness ↑	

Ulcers also occur in compartment 1 of the lamoid stomach (no gastric enzymes or acid production) and the colon. A different mechanism is the likely explanation of the pathogenesis of ulcers in these locations.

Catecholamines (epinephrine) contribute to the production of gastric secretions, so stimuli mediated via the sympathetic nervous system (fear, anxiety, frustration, anger) may have a potential effect on ulcerogenesis.

Hemorrhagic gastroenteritis and ulceration are sequelae to severe trauma (head injuries, burns, multiple fractures, spinal surgery) in humans, dogs, and other mammals (13). A juvenile alpaca with a congenital cervical vertebrae defect developed hemorrhagic gastroenteritis 24 hours following an extensive myelographic examination.

The lesions produced by harmful stress are difficult to document. Pathologists often negate a diagnosis of death caused by stress. Many of the effects of stress are functional, leaving no definitive physical lesion to mark their presence. Nonetheless, it is known that tissues and organs are weakened by prolonged insult, lowering resistance to disease. Classic lesions are lymphoid tissue atrophy, adrenal cortical hyperplasia, gastrointestinal ulceration, lymphopenia, and eosinopenia. Though the actual cause of death may be pneumonia, parasitism, or starvation, stress may have paved the way for development of these terminal ailments (5).

Conclusions

Veterinarians providing health care for lamoids should consider stress as a contributory factor to specific diseases. Husbandry practices should be evaluated and correction of those that may be harmful advised. Lamoids are social animals. Isolation for therapy or recuperation may be counterproductive. Malnutrition is a stressor, as are repeated restraint episodes. More detailed information about stress may be obtained in the references (5, 6, 13).

THERMAL STRESS

Physiology of Thermoregulation and Water Balance (1–4)

Lamoids are especially adapted for dealing with a cool environment, but they have been introduced to a wide variety of habitats in North America and other countries and have demonstrated a general adaptability. The fiber coat has a high insulation value, preventing heat loss and inhibiting radiant heat loss or gain. The ventral regions of the body are sparsely covered with hair, providing a thermal window for dissipation of heat. The rectal temperature of adult lamoids ranges from 37.5 to 38.6°C (99.5–101.5°F). Neonate temperatures range from 37.2 to 38.9°C (99.0–102°F) (3, 6).

Behavioral activities that aid lamoids in thermoregulation include seeking shade, orientation to minimize radiant heat gain when lying in direct sunlight, recumbency when in sunlight to cover the thermal window, standing in a stream or pond for cooling, standing over a sprinkler or allowing sprinklers to shower them for cooling.

Lamoids have epitrichial sweat glands, probably distributed over much of the body but especially numerous on the relatively fiberless areas of the ventrum (1). In a study of evaporative water loss in the llama, there was no detectable loss when the llama was maintained at 20–25°C (68–77°F) (11). When the ambient temperature was raised to 40°C (104°F), vapor loss became evident and gradually increased to 100–240 g/m^2/body surface/hr (1). Intravenous (IV) injection of epinephrine caused an increased loss of water vapor similar to that caused by exposure to high ambient temperatures.

Only one water balance study has been made in the llama, in which the llama was compared with the goat (11). Water turnover rates were calculated under conditions of ad libitum water intake with adequate feed intake, water deprivation and adequate feed, and reduced feed intake with ad libitum water intake. Nondesert-adapted species usually lower feed intake when water is restricted. The llama continued to ingest feed when water was restricted, thus making oxidative water available to cope with potential dehydration. Both the llama and goat were able to increase the osmolarity of urine under conditions of feed and water restriction, indicating an ability to conserve moisture by diminishing renal excretion (11).

The energy metabolism of a llama under restricted food intake lowers from 61 kcal/kg$^{.75}$/24 hr to 52 kcals/kg$^{.75}$ (12). This is associated with a concomitant decrease in water requirements.

In a study of guanacos, it was determined that this wild lamoid can deal with heat stress and dehydration, but to a lesser degree and with different mechanisms than the camel (10). Water was withheld from a female guanaco for 5 days, while feed was supplied ad libitum. A 14.8% loss of body weight resulted. Body temperature remained within a normal range.

Water was withheld from a male guanaco for 4 days, with an ambient temperature of up to 28°C (84°F). A 23.4% loss of body weight occurred, but there was no elevation in body temperature (10). At the conclusion of the foregoing period, the male was subjected to an ambient temperature of 45°C (113°F) for 6 hours. Even with heat stress added to the marked dehydration, body temperature elevated less than 1°C (1.8°F). The heart rate of the heat- and water-stressed guanaco was not elevated, in contrast to the response of domestic animals and humans, who exhibit a significant increase in heart rate under such stress (10).

The packed cell volume (PCV) of the 23.4% dehydrated guanaco increased from 30.6 to 43.6% and the hemoglobin (Hb) from 13.9 to 18.9 g/dl. This indicated an approximate 40% reduction in blood plasma (10). The camel has only a 2.3% reduction in blood plasma during severe dehydration and thus is better adapted to endure dehydration without ill effects.

The respiratory rate was not elevated above normal when guanacos were heat stressed, but when the animals were dehydrated and then subjected to heat stress, the respiratory rate increased two- or threefold. This may be explained as follows. Since there is no body temperature elevation in undehydrated but heat-stressed guanacos, thermal balance must be accomplished by dermal evaporative cooling. In the dehydrated guanaco, there is a reduction in plasma volume and a diminished ability to sweat; when heat stress is added, hyperpnea provides an alternative to dermal evaporative cooling.

Guanacos, like camels and donkeys, are able to correct severe dehydration quickly when offered water. A 23.4% dehydrated guanaco was able to drink 9 L water in 8 minutes, restoring 66% of the deficit (10).

The dromedary camel is one of the most well adapted to hot arid climates. Contrary to popular opinion, the camel does not store water any more than any other species, yet it need not drink water for days. The camel is able to tolerate extreme dehydration and has been known to safely lose body water equal to 40% of its body weight. Such a water loss would be lethal in any other animal. In the camel, plasma volume is maintained at the expense of tissue fluid, thus circulation is not impaired. The small oval erythrocyte of the camel continues to circulate despite increased blood viscosity.

Even after severe dehydration, the camel is able to drink sufficient water at one session to make up the deficit. This amount of water would cause severe osmotic problems in humans or other animals. In the camel, water is absorbed from the stomach and intestines slowly, allowing equilibrium to be established. The erythrocytes are able to avoid osmotic problems by swelling to 240% of their initial volume without rupturing. In other species, erythrocytes can swell to only 150% (6). Lamoids share some of these characteristics with camels.

The camel is able to endure a diurnal fluctuation of body temperature, from 36.5 to 42°C (97.7–107.6°F) (6). The body acts as a heat sink during the heat of the day, thus conserving vital water that would otherwise be lost through evaporative cooling. During the cool night of the desert, excess body heat is dissipated by conduction.

The kidney of the camel is capable of concentrating urine markedly to diminish water loss. The urine becomes as thick as syrup, and salt content may be increased to twice the concentration of salt in sea water. Water is extracted from the fecal pellets to such a degree that they can be used for fuel immediately upon voiding. All these unique physiologic characteristics must be considered when evaluating clinical signs in a diseased camel.

Clinical Conditions

HYPERTHERMIA (HEAT EXHAUSTION, HEAT STROKE, SUN STROKE, HEAT STRESS) (6). The conditions that predispose to the development of hyperthermia in lamoids include prolonged, high ambient temperatures; high humidity; excessive muscular activity (fighting, restraint procedures, trekking); intense metabolic activity (eating); lack of air movement; dehydration; lack of salt; fever; and forced, prolonged recumbency.

It was stated previously that the guanaco can tolerate heat stress without becoming hyperthermic. Perhaps the llama and other South American camelid species can as well; however, some individual llamas are prone to develop hyperthermia. It is common for llamas to develop mild afternoon hyperthermia, up to 41°C (106°F), when prevented from actions that promote cooling (seeking shade, wetting the ventrum of the body).

Temperatures in enclosed vehicles and trailers parked in the sun quickly rise to 49–54°C (120–154°F). These temperatures are lethal in a short time. Reduced cardiac efficiency is a contributing factor that may be brought about by malnutrition, lack of exercise, infection, or congenital cardiac anomalies.

Trauma (extensive contusions, fractures, lacerations) causes the release of pyrogens as products of tissue destruction. This reaction also takes place following surgery, and a slight elevation in body temperature may be expected (5).

Signs. It is difficult to differentiate between the signs of hyperthermia and dehydration. As already noted, the guanaco shows different signs of heat stress if dehydrated. An elevated rectal temperature is the objective sign of hyperthermia. Prolonged body temperatures of 41–43.3°C (106–110°F) are debilitating and may be lethal. Body temperatures at or above 45°C (113°F) are critical, and death will ensue if the body is not immediately cooled.

An increased heart rate, commonly seen in hyperthermic temperature–adapted species, is not a reliable sign in lamoids. There is an increased respiratory rate, but only if dehydration accompanies hyperthermia (one previous study suggested no increased respiratory rate if not dehydrated). Open-mouth breathing is an indication of heat stress. However, males may stand with their mouths open for a period following a fighting bout. This is a behavioral stance and is not necessarily an indication of hyperthermia, although fighting may lead to hyperthermia.

Sweating is difficult to evaluate in lamoids because of the heavy fiber coat, but sweating may be seen in the early stages of hyperthermia on the ventrum of the body. With dehydration there is a loss of plasma, and sweating will cease. Salivation may be seen. If body temperatures of 42–43°C (107.6–109.4°F) persist for hours, the pulse weakens and the animal becomes restless, depressed, and uncoordinated. Cerebral hypoxia from the increased metabolic rate in the face of impaired circulation results in neuronal degeneration with convulsions, collapse, and death ensuing.

Other metabolic and pathologic changes associated with hyperthermia include metabolic acidosis, hypercalcemia, myoglobinuria, hemoglobinuria, disseminated

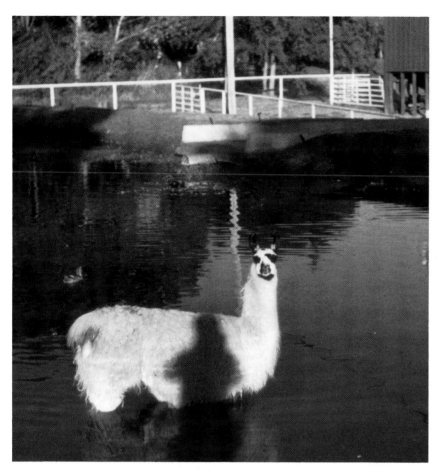

9.7 Llama cooling itself in a pond.

intravascular coagulation, hemolytic anemia, and renal shut down. Hyperthermia is characterized by peripheral vasodilatation in an attempt to cool the blood. This results in a relative hypovolemia (6).

Hyperthermia produces signs similar to those of septicemia, high fevers, and other convulsive syndromes, which should be considered in differential diagnosis. Hypoxic damage to parenchymal organs may result in a later illness such as pneumonia or nephrosis. The animal should be monitored for several days following a known hyperthermic episode.

Necropsy. The lesions of hyperthermia are nonspecific. Petechia and ecchymoses may be seen on serosal surfaces. Autolysis is extremely rapid in hyperthermia, with tissue destruction beginning prior to the animal's death and proceeding at a rapid rate after death. Coliform bacteria invade the liver and kidney antemortem. Carcasses moved to a refrigerator within minutes of death may yet be decomposed in 2 hours.

Therapy. The body temperature may be lowered by the use of cool water sprayed on the underside of the body and between the legs. Water flowing over the skin is more effective than a single dousing. A cold water enema is effective, but ability to monitor the rectal temperature is lost. Crushed ice may be packed between the legs and on the ventral abdomen. Air fanned over the crushed ice is helpful. If available, oxygen should be administered via a mask or with a tube inserted into the nostril. If dehydration or shock is also suspected, cold lactated Ringer's solution should be administered intravenously. Sodium bicarbonate should be given to counteract metabolic acidosis. Action must be taken quickly to avoid brain damage. The client should be advised on a course of action to follow until it is possible to reach the animal.

Males that are mildly hyperthermic for a few weeks may become temporarily infertile. This has not been studied, but it is an opinion of some breeders that males do not impregnate females during hot months in certain areas of the country.

Prevention. A plentiful water supply should be provided. If an animal is moved to a new enclosure, make certain that it will drink from the container provided. Novices packing with llamas have been concerned because their animals did not drink at streams or lakes along the trail. This is normal behavior for some llamas, though others may drink at each opportunity.

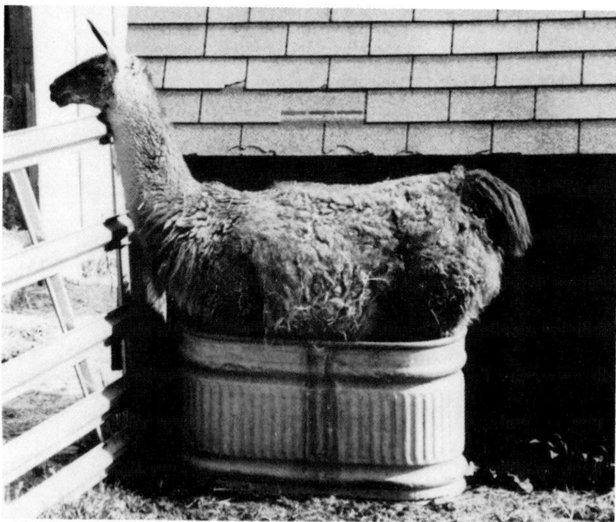

9.8 Llama cooling itself in a water tank.

Shade should be made available, especially during the afternoon. Even with shade available, some llamas choose to lie in direct sunlight on a hot day. They may lie on grassy or moist areas of the enclosure, making contact with the thermal window, and orient themselves to minimize exposure to the sun. The fiber coat insulates the skin from heat as well as retaining heat. Llamas have been observed standing under irrigation sprinklers during the hottest periods of the day or on top of a sprinkler to bathe the underside. Llamas have been seen standing or sitting in the water of ponds or streams during particularly hot weather (Fig. 9.7). When no other water was available, they have climbed into drinking tanks (Fig. 9.8). A few owners have constructed special air-conditioned stalls for the hot weather.

Restraint procedures should be avoided on warm days. Clients should be advised against heavy work for packers during the afternoons on hot days. Concentrates and high-protein forages should be avoided, since llamas excrete excessive nitrogen byproducts via the urine, thus increasing fluid requirements.

North American llama owners resist shearing their animals because it takes months for the fiber coat to grow back and make them presentable. Total shearing does not automatically allow the llama to thermoregulate better; in fact, it is undesirable to closely shear a llama at the approach of the hot season. Partial shearing of a heavily wooled animal, leaving 8–10 cm (3–4 in.) of fiber, is an appropriate course of action for the hyperthermia-prone llama, especially if it is dark colored.

HYPOTHERMIA

Predisposing Factors. Although lamoids are adapted to the cool temperatures of their native lands, temperatures there do not reach the extremes found in North America, where winter nighttime temperatures may dip to minus 40°C (−40°F). When combined with wind chill, the effective temperature may be minus 73°C (−100°F). Without shelter, llamas will have difficulty coping with such severe cold.

Neonates are particularly susceptible to hypothermia because they have poorly developed thermoregulation mechanisms and a higher metabolic rate. Their relatively greater proportion of skin surface allows for rapid dissipation of heat. Neonates lack a shivering reflex. Even adult llamas under anesthesia or in shock are prime candidates for hypothermia if in a cold ambient environment.

Insufficient food intake reduces metabolic heat production. Restricted muscular activity prevents heat generation. A poor fiber coat has less insulation capacity and contributes to heat loss. Any or all of these factors predispose llamas to hypothermia.

Signs. Clinical thermometers record body temperatures only to as low as 33.3°C (92°F). With more sensitive thermometers, temperatures as low as 29.4°C (85°F) have been recorded in living llamas (5). Other signs include depression progressing to coma. In contrast to hyperthermia, the hypothermic llama may live for hours.

A decrease in body temperature is accompanied by a decrease in cardiac output, heart rate, blood pressure, and glomerular filtration rate. Blood viscosity and hematocrit levels increase. Signs noted with temperatures below 30°C (86°F) include slow and shallow breathing, metabolic acidosis, "sludging" in the microcirculation, ventricular arrhythmias leading to fibrillation, and coagulation disorders (5).

Therapy. Total body immersion in warm water 40.5–45.5°C (105–114°F) is the fastest way to warm an animal. Total body immersion is impossible with an adult llama but possible with a neonate. Running the fingers through the fiber coat will keep warm water flowing over the skin. If the whole body cannot be immersed, warm water should be applied to the legs and the legs massaged.

A warm-water enema is highly effective, but the ability to monitor the body temperature is temporarily lost. A hair dryer may be helpful in warming a neonate. Covering the animal with blankets will help conserve heat, but if the temperature is below 32.3°C (90°F), metabolic heat production is proportionately reduced, and endogenous rewarming is slowed.

IV infusions of warm saline are effective. Surgical exposure of a suitable vein may be necessary to effect IV administration because of the vasoconstriction. Circulating water–type heating pads are effective in preventing hypothermia in neonates during surgery and in treating accidental hypothermia, but electric heating pads have caused skin burns and sloughs. Hypothermic and shock patients normally suffer from skin vasoconstriction and exhibit a reduced ability to carry heat away from the skin. Be cautious when applying heat directly to the skin (5). Measure the temperature between the skin and the pad and keep it below 42°C.

Hot water bottles may be used to raise the ambient air temperature in a small enclosed area. Plastic milk cartons or plastic bags may be substituted for hot water bottles. The air surrounding the patient may be warmed with infrared heat lamps, forced-air driers, or electric floor heaters.

Prevention. Shelter from wind and rain should be provided. Lamoid fiber is quite resistant to moisture penetration, but wet face, ears, and limbs may allow significant heat loss. Deep straw bedding may minimize heat loss from the thermal window in extremely cold climates. A shelter should be small enough to be warmed by a group of animals huddling together. A box stall may be made smaller by blocking with bales of hay or straw. Insulated and heated barns may be required in particularly harsh, cold climates.

High-quality feed should be provided, including concentrates if the animals are used to eating them. Water must be available. Llamas are not likely to break through ice and are reluctant to drink sufficient amounts of icy water. A stock tank heating unit may be required.

For birthing in cold weather, a maternity stall with provisions for supplemental heat should be available.

Llamas generally lie down when being transported. If trailering in cold weather, the trailer floor should be deeply bedded with straw to avoid hypothermia from lying on a cold or freezing surface.

FROSTBITE. Hypothermia causes peripheral vasoconstriction to conserve energy to maintain the core body temperature. Intense or prolonged skin vasoconstriction of exposed structures may result in ischemic necrosis and gangrene. The ears are the primary site of gangrene in llamas. Neonates are most frequently affected.

Signs. The skin of the ear becomes devitalized. A sharp line of demarcation will separate the healthy tissue from the necrotic tip. The skin and the cartilage become hardened and leathery, then slough (Fig. 9.9).

Frostbite must be differentiated from congenital shortening of the pinna. Frostbite usually produces a squared tip rather than the tapered tip of the congenitally shortened ear.

Therapy. Once freezing has occurred, no treatment will halt the process. The necrotic tissue may be amputated, but it is not necessary or advisable, because more of the ear may be saved by nature than by the surgeon. Antibiotic therapy may be indicated for 5–8 days to prevent tetanus in animals not otherwise immunized against it.

Prevention. All the factors mentioned for prevention of hypothermia are appropriate.

DEHYDRATION

The mammalian body is composed of 60–80% water. High percentages of body fat decrease the percentage of water (5). Desert-adapted animals, such as certain species of antelope and rodents, have developed methods of

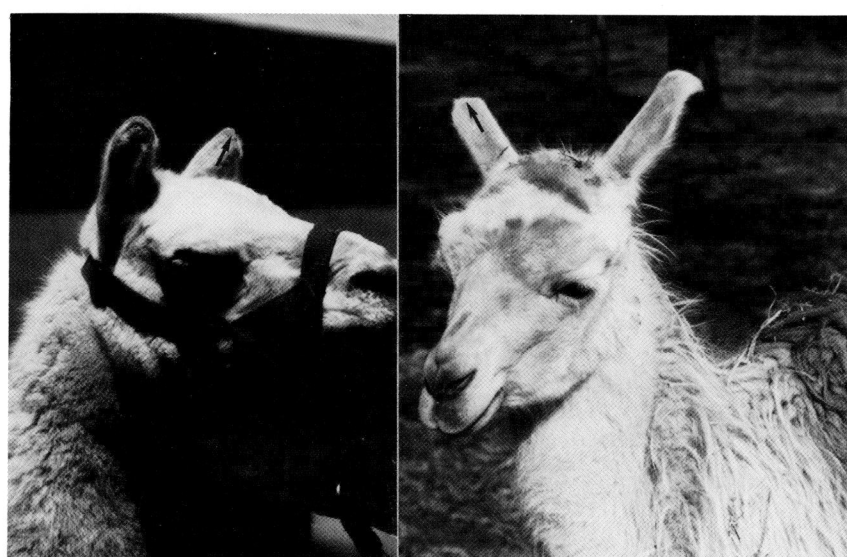

9.9 Frostbitten ears.

water conservation similar to those previously described for the camel. Mammals adapted to temperate climates require water in amounts of approximately 40 ml/kg/ body weight daily to maintain normal water balance in a basal metabolic state. Exact water requirements are based on metabolic weight rather than actual body weight. The basal amount is equivalent to fluid lost in urine and feces and through insensible evaporation via skin and lungs. The actual amount required is increased by activity and a rise in ambient temperature. As already described in the section on the physiology of heat stress and dehydration, lamoids are able to tolerate degrees of dehydration that would be fatal to humans or other temperate climate–adapted species. Water requirements of lamoids are listed as ml/kg (12). See Chapter 2 for more details.

Etiology

Dehydration is usually caused by water deprivation brought about by failure of a newly acquired animal to recognize the water source, a frozen water source, failure to use automatic waterers, failure to provide sufficient water during hot weather, overheating, prolonged muscle exertion, severe diarrhea, hemorrhage, or loss of fluid resulting from burns (5).

Signs

In one study, a guanaco experienced a 23.4% weight loss from 4 days of water deprivation, yet exhibited no clinical signs (10). He continued to eat and had no circulatory deficits. There was hemoconcentration, with the PCV elevating from 30.6 to 43.6%. It is important to note that the normal PCV is lower in lamoids than in other domestic animals, and though a 43.6% PCV would cause no alarm in other species, a rise of that magnitude represents a plasma volume loss of as much as 40%. The hemoglobin level in the blood elevated from 13.9 to 18.9 g/dl. The respiratory rate may increase in dehydrated lamoids, especially if under heat stress, because of the loss of plasma volume and the inability to sweat or thermoregulate.

No studies have been conducted to determine the ultimate clinical signs of severe dehydration for lamoids. However, expected signs would include weakness, loss of skin elasticity, sunken eyes, lowered blood pressure in the early stages of nonadaptive dehydration, and, as severity increases, circulatory failure with signs of shock and coma. The kidneys may be damaged, resulting in uremia and acidosis. Animals recovering from severe dehydration may succumb later to the secondary effects of renal failure.

Therapy

Body fluids must be replaced. Lamoids are able to rapidly restore a deficit by oral fluids without causing the osmotic upsets seen in temperate climate–adapted species. Gastric intubation may be necessary to relieve moribund animals. Fluid is readily absorbed from the colon, so enemas are effective in rehydration (5). IV administration of physiologic saline may be life saving in severe dehydration. Surgical exposure of a vein is often necessary because of low blood pressure.

It is common to underestimate the volume of fluid necessary to rehydrate an animal. A 150 kg llama with 10% dehydration would require 15 L fluid to make up the deficit. With 20% dehydration, 30 L (8 gal) are required.

Prevention

Attention to all the factors discussed in the section on etiology will prevent dehydration. Special attention must be given to the llama with persistent vomiting (rhododendron poisoning) or severe diarrhea. Electrolyte imbalances must also be alleviated.

REFERENCES

1. Allen, T. E., and Bligh, J. 1969. A comparative study of the temporal patterns of cutaneous water vapour loss from some domesticated mammals with epitrichial sweat glands. Comp. Biochem. Physiol. 31:347–63.

2. Baumann, I., Bligh, J., and Vallenas P., A. 1975. Temperature regulation in the alpaca, *Lama pacos*—thermoregulatory consequences and inconsequences of injections of nonadrenaline, 5-hydroxytryptamine, carbamyl choline and prostaglandin E, into the lateral cerebral ventricle. Comp. Biochem. Physiol. [C] 50:105–9.

3. Bligh, J., Baumann, I., Sumar, J., and Pocco, F. 1975. Studies of body temperature patterns in South American camelidae. Comp. Biochem. Physiol. [A] 50:701–8.

4. Engelhardt, W. von, Becker, G., Engelhardt, W., Hauffe, R., Hinderer, S., Rübsamen, K., and Schneider, W. 1975. Energy, water and urea metabolism in the llama. In Tracer Studies on Non-Protein Nitrogen for Ruminants. Vienna, Austria: International Atomic Energy Agency, pp. 111–22.

5. Fowler, M. E. 1978. Restraint and Handling of Wild and Domestic Animals. Ames: Iowa State Univ. Press.

6. ______. 1985. Thermal stress in llamas. 3L Llama (27) May/June:17–20.

7. ______. 1987. Neoplasia in nondomestic animals. In G. H. Theilen and B. R. Madewell, eds. Veterinary Cancer Medicine, 2nd ed. Philadelphia: Lea & Febiger, pp. 649–62.

8. Fowler, M. E., Gillespie, D., and Harkema, J. 1985. Lymphosarcoma in a llama. J. Am. Vet. Med. Assoc. 187:1245–46.

9. Moulton, J. E., ed. 1978. Tumors in Domestic Animals, 2nd ed. Berkeley: Univ. of California Press.

10. Rosenmann, M., and Morrison, P. 1963. Physiological response to heat and dehydration in the guanaco. Physiol. Zool. 63:45–51.

11. Rübsamen, K., and Engelhardt, W. von. 1975. Water metabolism in the llama. Comp. Biochem. Physiol. [A] 52:595–98.

12. Schneider, W., Hauffe, R., and Engelhardt, W. von. 1974. (Energy and urea metabolism) Energie und Stickstoffumsatz beim Lama. In K. H. Menke, ed. Energy Metabolism of Farm Animals. Hohenheim, West Germany: Univ. Hohenheim Dokumentationsstelle.

13. Selye, H. 1976. Stress in Health and Disease. London: Butterworth.

10 Integumentary System

THE INTEGUMENTARY SYSTEM consists of the skin, hair (fiber), mammary gland, adnexal glands (sebaceous, sweat, scent), and toenails.

SKIN

The functions of the skin are manifold (25). Primarily, the skin serves as a protective barrier between the body and the external environment and is an important organ for homeostasis, preventing excessive water loss and invasion of the body by pathogenic microorganisms. The flexibility and elasticity of the skin allow motion and provide shape and form. The skin also plays a vital role in thermoregulation and sensory perception.

The skin contains both sebaceous and sweat glands, which serve a secretory function. Melanin provides the variety of colors found in lamoids. Precursors for vitamin D_3 synthesis in the skin are acted upon by solar ultraviolet light to produce the vitamin that is later converted to 1,25 dihydroxycholecalciferol, the active hormone, via metabolism in the liver and kidney. Special appendages of the skin include hair and nails.

The skin of lamoids is thick and nonpliable. Scent glands are located in the interdigital space and the medial and lateral metatarsal regions. Callosities form over the sternum, carpus, and stifle in response to recumbency patterns. The anatomy of the skin of llamas and alpaca is similar, and both will be considered as an entity.

Anatomic studies of lamoid skin are few in number (6, 10) and are confined to limited areas of the body surface. Detailed, complete studies are needed, because the skin of camelids is unique among domestic animals, and few dermatopathologists understand the anatomy of normal skin, complicating evaluation of pathologic states.

The layers of the skin are illustrated diagrammatically in Figure 10.1. The epidermis consists of four layers, rather than the five described in other animals. The stratum corneum (horny layer) is a thin layer of anuclear remnants of flattened, fully keratinized cells pushed up from basal layers. The stratum granulosum (granular layer) is a single layer of cells in some areas and discontinuous in others. The nuclei are pycnotic, and most of the cytoplasm has been replaced with keratin.

The stratum spinosum (prickle layer) is reduced in lamoids but is composed of daughter cells of the basal layer. These cells are viable and nucleated and actively synthesize keratin (25). The stratum basale (basal layer) is the deepest layer of the epidermis and consists of a single layer of cuboidal or columnar cells, most of which are keratinocytes with a few melanocytes.

Melanocytes contain melanin pigment in pseudopods distributed between epidermal cells of the skin and hair. Skin color is determined by the number, size, arrangement, and dispersion of melanin granules. In chronic dermatitis, there may be overproduction of melanin, which causes darkening of the skin. Conversely, depigmentation may result from trauma, burns, or infection of the skin. Albinism occurs in lamoids as it does in all species.

The *dermis* (corium) of lamoids is thick (up to 1 cm in the cervical region of a mature male) and consists of a superficial layer composed of loose connective tissue interdigitating with undulations in the epidermis and the deep dermis, which is composed of dense fibrous tissue (6). The dermis contains hair follicles, blood and lymph vessels, nerves, and sebaceous and sweat glands (21). The middermis of lamoids is characterized by a proliferation of blood vessels, in contrast to other domestic animals. Vessel walls are hyalinized. This normal histologic picture is frequently misinterpreted as an abnormal vascular proliferation by the pathologist. There is variation in the thickness of the epidermal layers in various areas of the body. Also, the degree of vascularity and mononuclear infiltration may vary.

The *hypodermis* (subcutis) is composed of loose connective tissue, which attaches the skin to the underlying bones or muscles. Some sweat glands extend into the hypodermis.

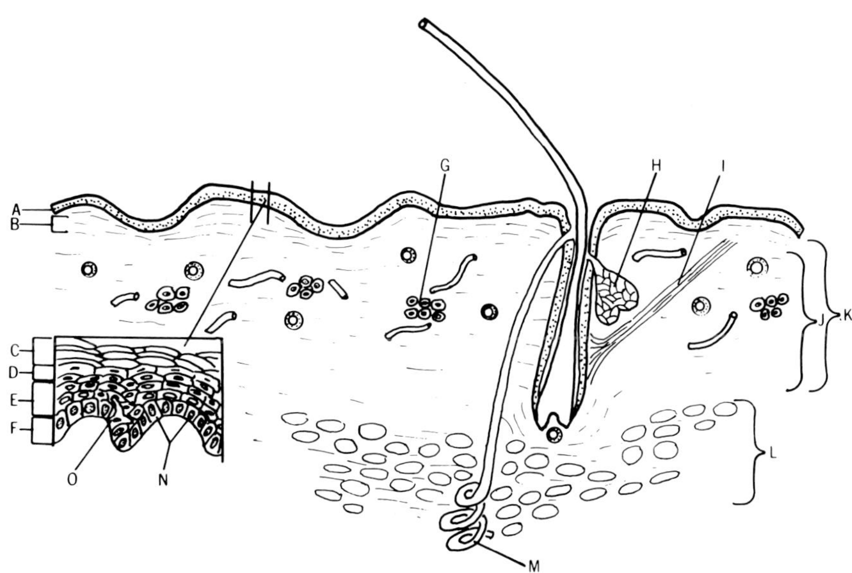

10.1 Schematic diagram of lamoid skin: **(A)** epidermis, **(B)** superficial layer of dermis, **(C)** stratum corneum, **(D)** stratum granulosum, **(E)** stratum spinosum, **(F)** stratum basale, **(G)** mononuclear infiltrate, **(H)** sebaceous gland, **(I)** arrector pili muscle, **(J)** mid- and deep dermis, **(K)** dermis, **(L)** hypodermis, **(M)** apocrine sweat gland, **(N)** keratinocytes, **(O)** melanocyte.

HAIR (FIBER COAT, WOOL)

(12, 13, 19, 20, 24, 28, 31, 38)

Wool is the fine, soft, wavy hair forming the fleece of sheep characterized by its property of felting, made possible by overlapping of minute surface scales (1, 4). Technically, the term "wool" should be restricted to the fiber from sheep. Although wool is commonly used to designate lamoid hair in North America, in South America the term used is alpaca or llama fiber, but hair will be used in this chapter. Table 10.1 lists the characteristics of camelid and other domestic animal wool and hair. Table 10.2 defines terms used to describe hair.

The hair coat of a llama consists of two types of hairs, the coarse guard hairs and a finer undercoat. The coat of most alpacas consists of only undercoat hairs.

Table 10.1. Wool and hair characteristics

	Diameter (μ)	Cross section of hair shape	Medulla	Shed
Sheep				
Merino (fine wool)	10–30	Circular to oval	Rare in fibers	None
Lincoln (coarse wool)	30–50		<35 μ	
Kemp fibers, guard hair	>70	Dumbbell (bilobed)	Heavy	Annual
Angora goat				
Mohair		Circular	Rare	
Kids	10–30			
2 years	20–50			
4 years	50–60			
Down goat				
Cashmere		Circular		Annual
Kashmir, Pashu	14–17			
Camel				
Bactrian	5–40		Interrupted	Annual
Dromedary	20–50			
Llama				
Undercoat	(26)	Circular to elliptical	Most are medullated	Partial
(woollike crimped)	10–40			
Outer coat	(70)			
(straight hairs)	40–150		Strongly	
Alpaca	(22)			
Huacayo	16–40	Smooth margin, staple crimped	Strongly	
	(23)			
Suri	16–35	Crenated margin	Strongly	
Vicuña	(13–14)	Circular to elliptical	Fibers less than 18 rare	
	10–30			
Guanaco	18–24	Circular to elliptical	Strongly	
Horse hair	(150)			

Note: Numbers in parentheses denote averages.

Table 10.2. Definition of terms used to describe hair, wool, and camelid fibers

Cotting—The entanglement of fibers into an irreversible matt.
Crimp—The natural curl or wave in a wool fiber.
Felting—Producing a compact, irreversibly entangled structure when subjected to friction in a soluble medium.
Fiber—The hair of animals other than sheep.
Fleece—The wool that covers a sheep or similar animal. The quantity of wool cut from a sheep at one time.
Kemp—Kemp fibers, guard hairs are coarse, relatively flattened fibers with a long tapering tip. They are found in llamas and in the coarse wool breeds of sheep. They are periodically shed.
Luster—Silver luster from finest merino wool, silk luster in medium to long wool, and glass luster in mohair and other goat fibers.
Staple—(1) Locks or tufts of wool shorn from a sheep. (2) Natural fibers or cut lengths from filaments, also called staple length.
Suint—That part of the new fleece that is soluble in cold water. The dried residue of the sweat glands.
Wool—The fine, soft, curly hair forming the fleece of the sheep characterized by this property of felting due to the overlapping of minute surface scales.
Wool wax—The fatty product obtained from wool. Also known as wool fat or wool grease. Purified form known as lanolin. Produced by the sebaceous glands.

Llama guard hairs comprise approximately 20% of the fleece and are 10–150 μ in diameter (35). Guard hairs must be removed from the fleece prior to spinning and garment manufacture.

In Peru, alpacas are sheared approximately every 12–18 months, the time required for regrowth (5). This fact should be kept in mind when contemplating clipping the coat from an area for diagnostic or therapeutic purposes. In North America, llamas and alpacas are rarely sheared; rather, the fiber is harvested by brushing. Llamas have only a partial annual shed. Wild lamoids and camels shed annually.

The density of the hairs vary with the location on the skin, with the thickest coat over the back and sides of the animal (2).

Hair follicles are tubular invaginations of the epidermis into the dermis. In lamoids, there are two types: simple follicles containing a single coarse hair and complex follicles containing multiple, fine hairs (2, 34). Both sebaceous and sweat glands empty into the hair follicles (6).

The fine hairs of the undercoat of llamas and alpacas have three distinct layers: the medulla, cortex, and cuticle (7). In contrast to sheep, lamoid hairs are strongly medullated, except for most of the guard hairs. The cortex is circular to elliptic in cross section. The cuticular layer is evident within the follicle but becomes flattened as the hair emerges.

Crimp is the natural curl or wave in a hair. The crimp and scaled cuticle of sheep wool hairs provide excellent binding of the hairs as they are spun into yarn. The crimp also provides resiliency, the garment conforming to changing shapes as it is worn. There are two breeds of alpaca. The huacaya (see Fig. 1.5) has a shorter fleece coat with moderate crimping of the hairs, while the suri breed (see Fig. 1.6) has a longer fleece with no crimping of the hairs. A pure alpaca hair garment does not resume its original shape if stretched. Special procedures must be used to spin alpaca hair, and frequently a percentage of fine sheep wool is mixed with it to ease spinning and knitting and improve garment usage. Llama hair is coarse and has no crimp. Garments made from llama hair have a harsher feeling than those made from alpaca hair.

A cottage industry for making llama hair garments has developed in North America, while in South America, llama hair is handled locally by the indigenous people and used to make blankets, ropes, bags (corresponding to burlap or jute bags) called costales, and inexpensive garments. Indigenous people say that llama hair sweaters are warmer than those made from alpaca hair but recognize that llama hair is harsher and may cause the skin to itch.

Fine garments are made from pure alpaca hair or alpaca hair mixed with fine sheep wool or synthetic fibers. The bulk of alpaca hair is sold to companies that sort, grade, clean, and spin it into yarn. The yarn is shipped to England, where special procedures have been developed to produce fabric and garments that are then shipped back to South America.

Hair Quality

Hair quality may be modified by such environmental factors as day length, temperature, elevation, and general nutrition, but the dominant factor in determining quality is heredity.

Hair Loss

It is often difficult to establish the etiology of patchy or generalized loss of hair in llamas. Certain specific diseases, such as mange, cause alopecia, but pediculosis does not, unless the animal rubs the hair from such locations as over the spinous processes of the vertebrae. Alopecia may also occur at other sites of excessive wear, such as alongside the neck of animals fed in a slatted manger. Mention has already been made of alopecia over the bridge of the nose and on the inside of the pinnae.

Large patches of hair may be lost with no apparent inciting cause. There may be no evidence of an inflammatory response of the skin, yet when the skin surface is examined carefully it will be noted that the hairs have broken off. This is likely similar to a condition called "wool break" in sheep. The term "break" may be used to describe the actual breaking of the hair as a result of excessive thinning or the visible line on a fleece caused by the thinning of the diameter of the hairs. Studies have not been conducted to establish breaking as a phenomenon occurring in llamas and alpacas, but it is reasonable to assume that it does.

To explain this phenomenon, it is necessary to understand that such a change in the diameter of the hair can occur only in animals that have a long growth cycle (anogen) (sheep, llamas, alpacas). Wild sheep and most other domestic animals shed wool and hair annually and the fleece grows back to a genetically predetermined length. While in anogen, various nutritional, metabolic, and environmental factors may influence the development of the hair while it is still in the follicle.

Sheep wool grown during the winter is finer (the hairs are thinner in diameter) than that grown in summer. Studies have shown that this is not a result of cold weather but rather a response to the shorter day length. Poor general nutrition may also cause thinning. If both the foregoing are combined, the hairs may become fragile and break easily.

Sheep that have been stressed by illness or fever develop a break line in the hair that is growing in the follicle during that time. The entire fleece may be lost in 1 or 2 weeks. Thinning of the hairs can be produced by the administration of cortisol parenterally, indicating that any stressor may cause thinning of the hair and a potential break.

Lack of any essential nutrient in the diet may contribute to the production of hairs that are uneven and fragile. A deficiency of dietary copper will weaken wool hairs. Since molybdenum has an inhibitory effect on copper metabolism, animals fed forage grown in areas known to have high concentrations of molybdenum may develop a copper deficiency. Low-protein diets, especially if deficient in sulfur-containing amino acids such as cysteine, will result in thinning of the hairs.

Thyroid hormone stimulates growth (both length and diameter) of hair. Estrogens tend to promote finer hairs and testosterone, coarser ones.

In sheep, specific bacterial and fungal diseases of wool cause the hairs to deteriorate. Such diseases have not been identified in lamoids.

MAMMARY GLAND

There are four nipples on the mammary gland of both Old and New World camelids. There may also be supernumerary teats, either cranial or caudal to the normal teats, some of which may connect with glandular tissue. Each nipple has two streak canals that enter into separate teat and gland cisterns (Figs. 10.2, 10.3). Variable numbers and sizes of milk ducts collect milk from the gland and empty into the gland cistern.

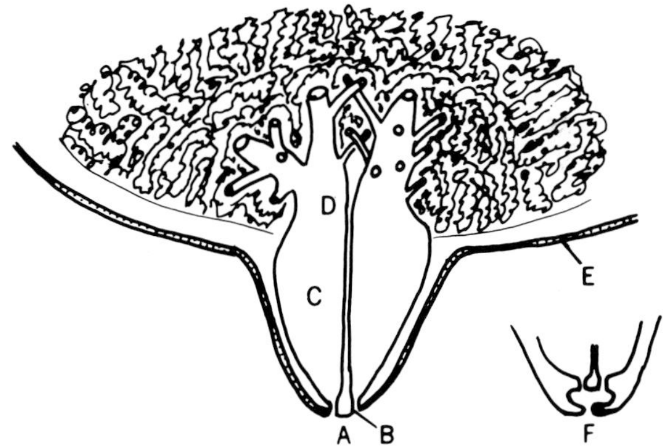

10.2 Diagram of a camelid teat and collecting system: **(A)** streak canals opening on tip of teat, **(B)** streak canal, **(C)** teat cistern, **(D)** mammary gland cistern, **(E)** skin, **(F)** alternate morphology: streak canals emptying into a sinus with a single external orifice.

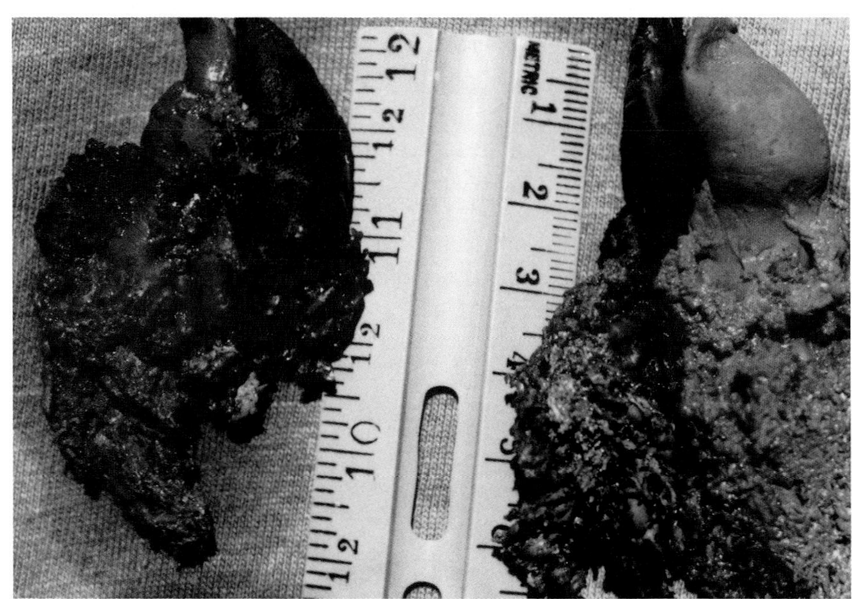

10.3 Latex cast of mammary gland–collecting system.

Although the glands and milk ducts draining into a single teat overlap and interdigitate with one another, they are separate and distinct, with no anastomosis as determined by evaluation of latex cast preparations (Fig. 10.3). Thus, in effect, there are eight mammary glands. Double teats have been identified (Fig. 10.4).

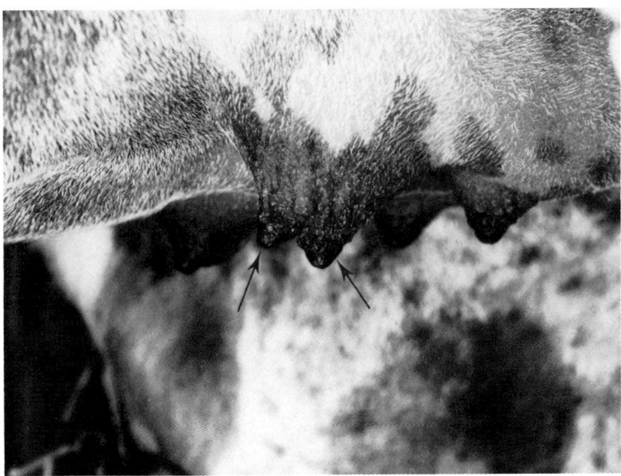

10.4 Double teat in a llama.

The streak canals are short (2 mm) and so small that conventional tubes used to instill antibiotics into the udder of a cow or sheep are too large for lamoids. A 1 mm (3.5 French) catheter is about the maximum usable size. The streak canals may exit the teat on the conical surface of the tip of the teat, or both canals may exit into a sinus at the tip of the teat, giving the erroneous impression that there is only one orifice (Fig. 10.2). The teat and gland cistern are not separated. The combined cistern is approximately 2.5 cm long and 1 cm in diameter.

The glands are compound tubuloalveolar glands similar to those of cattle. The right and left halves of the mammary gland are separated by an incomplete suspensory ligament of the udder. The front and rear quarters cannot be visually or surgically separated, but there is no connection between the collecting system of the two quarters. The udder of the camel is similar, except that there are two or three teat ducts with independent teat cisterns leading to the gland cistern (32).

The recognition that there are eight separate glands is important clinically in the management of mastitis. If infusion of antibiotics into the gland is prescribed as a treatment for mastitis, it is crucial that the appropriate gland be infused.

Hand milking a llama is a challenging task because of the short teat. At best, a thumb and one or two fingers are all that can be used. Even then, some llamas have such short teats that they are difficult to grasp. The cria may fail to grasp such short teats as well. This is particularly true if there is edema of the udder at the time of parturition.

One or more supernumerary teats may connect with glandular tissue, and milk may be obtained from these, or such teats may lack patency. Supernumerary teats may be much smaller or the same size as normal teats, and the cria may be frustrated if it grasps a blind teat to no avail.

The total weight of the udder in a nonpregnant mature female is approximately 250 g. Udder enlargement may begin approximately 2 months before parturition, especially in a primiparous female. The udder of a fully lactating female is relatively small, weighing only 450 g, and may appear empty all the time if nursed properly. As in all species of mammals, a genetic component determines mammary gland size and milk production. Breeding female llamas and alpacas have not been evaluated on the basis of milk production, nor is any information available on evaluation of the udder.

Milk composition is variable, and different values have been reported in the literature. Some values are based on a few individual samples. Values were based on thousands of reports for other domestic animals. Some values are averages of numerous reports from the literature. Precise values for the milk of lamoids (Table 10.3) may be somewhat unreliable, since they are based on limited data. However, trends are noticeable. For more detailed information on other species, the following references are provided (3, 8, 14, 15, 16).

Alpaca and llama milk is similar and may be considered together. Determination of alpaca milk composition is incomplete (17, 22, 23, 26, 27), and llama values are based on reports from just a few animals (36, 37). Moro describes alpaca milk as having a white porcelain color and an odor similar to that of cows milk. Alpaca milk has a sweetish taste and is more viscid than cows milk. The fat content varies from 0.7 up to 5.7% during the course of a lactation period, but with marked variation from day to day (23). Alpaca milk is more acidic than cows milk, having a pH of 6.4–6.8. The volume of milk production ranges from 40 to 1200 ml per day, but most animals produce less than 320 ml.

Consult Table 10.3, for composition values for camelids and other species. Numerous factors affect the composition of milk, including genetic predisposition, nutrition, stage of lactation, age of the female, season, ambient temperature, and presence of chronic infection of the glands.

It may be of interest to compare the milk of lamoids with that of their Old World cousins. Camel milk is used extensively for human food. The Koran speaks of God answering the prayers of the desert people by giving them the she camel that they may drink her milk. Camels are uniquely adapted to subsistence on harsh, dry desert herbage and intermittent supplies of drinking water while continuing to produce milk that is suitable for camel calves and human infants alike. Mammals adapted to a temperate climate cease to lactate when subjected to drought and dehydration. Not so the camel (40, 41).

The normal composition of camel milk is similar to that of lamoid milk (Table 10.3). Milk yields of camels vary from 3.5 to 14 kg per day, with lactation yields (9–18 months) totaling 1000–4000 kg. Camel milk has a sweet, sharp taste and sometimes is salty. Milk taste and odor are modified by plant ingestion and other environmental conditions. Camel milk is rich in vitamin C, three times higher than cows milk and 1.5 times higher than human milk. It is an important source of vitamin C for humans in a vitamin-impoverished environment. The fat droplets in camel milk are small and will not rise to the top of standing milk (40, 41).

Cattle, sheep, and goats produce milk with a higher than normal percentage of total solids when water is scarce. Such milk is contraindicated for the health of nursing young. The camel, on the other hand, produces milk with 4.5% fat and 84% water when provided with optimal water, but when chronically dehydrated, the fat content drops to 2% and the water content elevates to 90%. Such milk admirably serves the needs of camel calves and humans alike as a source of both moisture and nourishment.

The secretion of dilute milk by a hot desert–adapted camel is explained on the basis of the effect of the pituitary antidiuretic hormone on secretion of water by the mammary gland (the mammary gland is a modified sweat gland). Camels have minimal sweat glands otherwise, which is one of the many physiologic adaptations that aid camels in dealing with high temperatures and dehydration (40, 41).

OTHER SKIN GLANDS

Adnexal Glands

In lamoids, sebaceous (holocrine) glands are associated with each hair follicle, but the production of sebum (wool wax, wool fat, wool grease, lanolin) is low in comparison to that of sheep. Sebum is a mixture of waxes, cholesterol, and cholesterol esters that, when mixed with sweat, coat the skin and wool hairs to enhance water repellency, inhibit microorganism penetration, and inhibit dehydration via the skin.

Clippers used to shear sheep are naturally lubricated with wool wax as shearing proceeds. The lack of wool wax in lamoids causes rapid overheating of sheep clipper heads. Clippers used to shear llamas and alpacas must be dipped alternately into oil and water for cooling. The blades oscillate at a rate of approximately 300 per minute in contrast to sheep clippers that oscillate at about 1000 per minute.

Sweat (apocrine) glands are generally found widely distributed over the surface of the skin but are more dense on the ventrum, which is sparsely covered with hair (thermal window). The sweat glands are poorly developed in llamas and alpacas and consist of simple, tubular, or unilobular glands in contrast with sheep, which have multilobular glands (6).

Metatarsal Glands

Lamoids have unique, oval-shaped, hairless patches on both the medial and lateral surfaces of the

Table 10.3. Composition of llama milk compared with other species of livestock

Type of milk and species	Water	Fat	Protein	Lactose	Ash	Caloric density
	(%)	(%)	(%)	(%)	(%)	*(Kcal/ml)*
Colostrum (first milk)						
Llama	74.0	0.95	16.50	7.75	0.8	0.659 NE
Mare	73.5	1.52	8.83	16.3	0.32	0.95 NE
Cow	70.0	3.04	17.00	9.25	1.0	0.955 NE
Ewe (sheep)	58.8	17.7	20.1	2.2	1.0	2.123 NE
Doe (goat)	73.5	6.0	12.0	7.5	1.0	1.254 NE
Transition milk, 3 days postbirth, llama	87.4	2.87	5.23	3.7	0.8	0.668 GE
Mature milk						
Llama	86.2	5.66	4.25	3.34	0.8	0.813 GE
Mare	89.0	1.6	2.7	6.1	0.6	0.496 GE
Cow	87.3	3.6	3.3	4.9	0.8	0.652 GE
Doe	87.0	4.0	3.3	4.7	1.0	0.680 GE
Ewe	81.0	7.9	6.2	4.0	0.9	1.119 GE
Artificial milk formula						
Foal-lac, diluted 1:45	54.0	2.8	3.9	10.1	0.1	0.807 GE
Land-O-Lakes Lamb Milk, replacer, diluted 1:6	85.0	4.0	5.0	4.3	1.0	0.782 GE

Note: Data on llama from L. W. Johnson, personal communication; NE = net energy; GE = gross energy.

metatarsal regions of the rear limbs (Fig. 10.5) (33). Associated with the patches are multilobulated holocrine glands, with ducts emptying on the surface. The dermis is markedly papillated, corresponding to invagination into the epidermis. The function of these glands is probably the excretion of alarm pheromones, perceived as "burned popcorn" odor to humans. The glandular secretion solidifies upon excretion into a leathery sheet on the surface of the skin that can be peeled off. Some references describe these structures as chestnuts, but, histologically, they are not comparable to the chestnuts of horses (9, 30, 33).

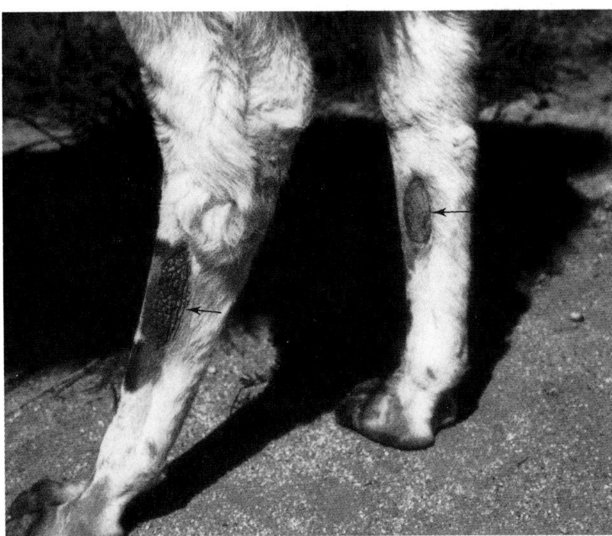

10.5 Metatarsal scent glands of the llama.

Interdigital Gland

Interdigital glands are found on all four feet. The structure and specific function of these glands is unknown, but they are probably associated with individual and group identification.

FOOT

The camelid foot is unique, with two digits on each foot. The plantar surface is covered with a soft, cornified layer of epithelium similar to that of the bulb of the heel in sheep and goats (Fig. 10.6). This is called the slipper. In lamoids, there is a separate slipper for each digit, while in the camel, a single slipper covers the entire bearing surface. Deep to the slipper is a layer of dense connective tissue, the corium, containing blood vessels and nerves.

Camelids are modified digitagrades, with phalanx two (P-2) and P-3 lying horizontally within the foot and

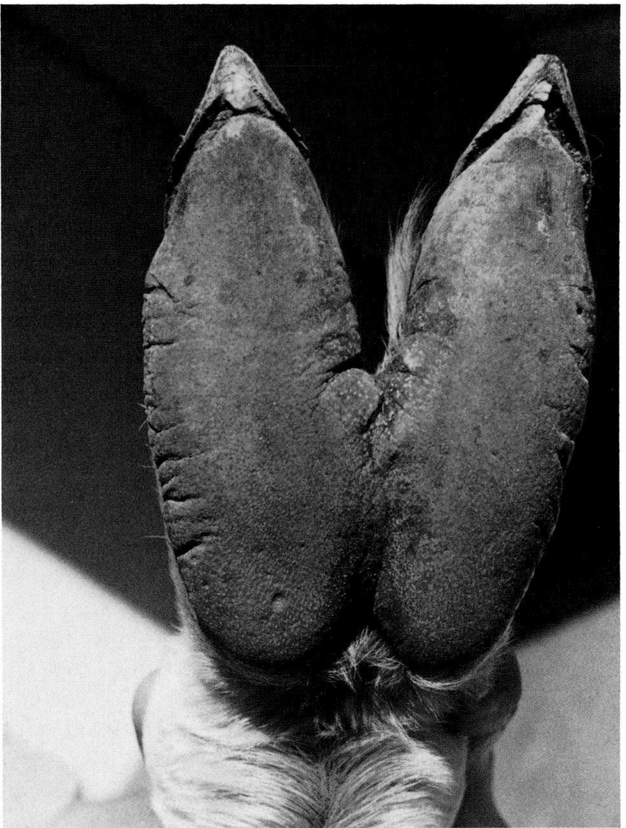

10.6 Bottom view of llama foot.

P-1 upright at approximately 45 degrees (Figs. 10.7–10.10). A small, nonweight-bearing nail, similar to a human nail, is located at the extremity of each digit and closely attached to P-3 via the corium (11) (Fig. 10.7). Primary nail growth occurs at the coronary band.

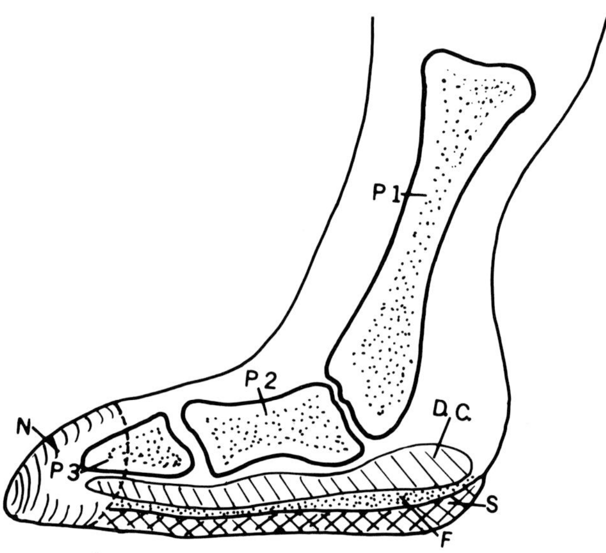

10.7 Diagram of lamoid foot and pastern: (N) toenail, (DC) digital cushion, (F) sole corium, (S) sole (slipper).

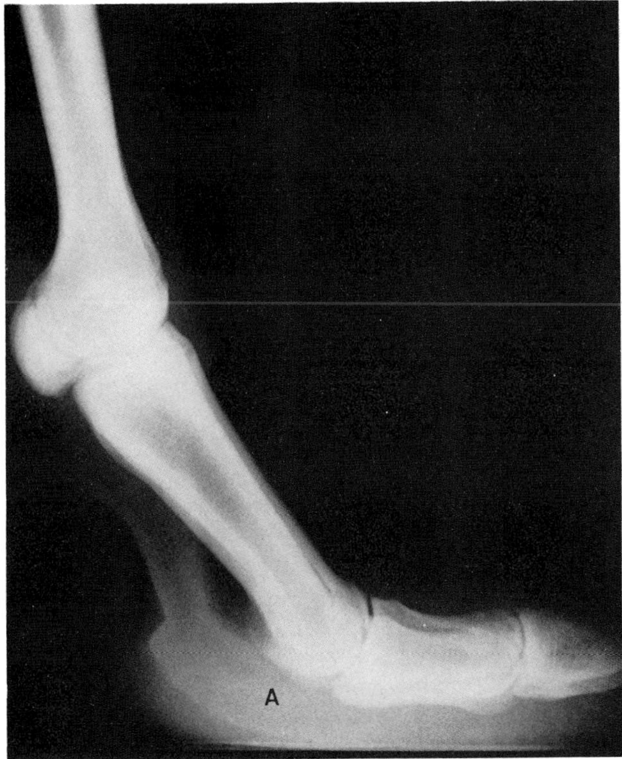

10.8 Lateral radiograph of the foot, pastern, and fetlock of a llama: **(A)** digital cushion.

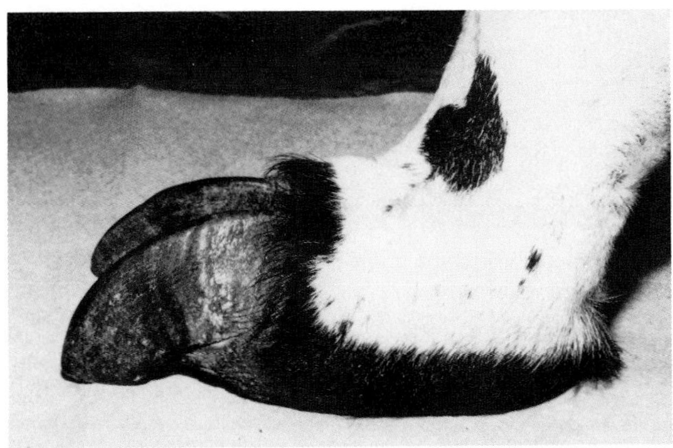

10.9 Normal llama foot, lateral view.

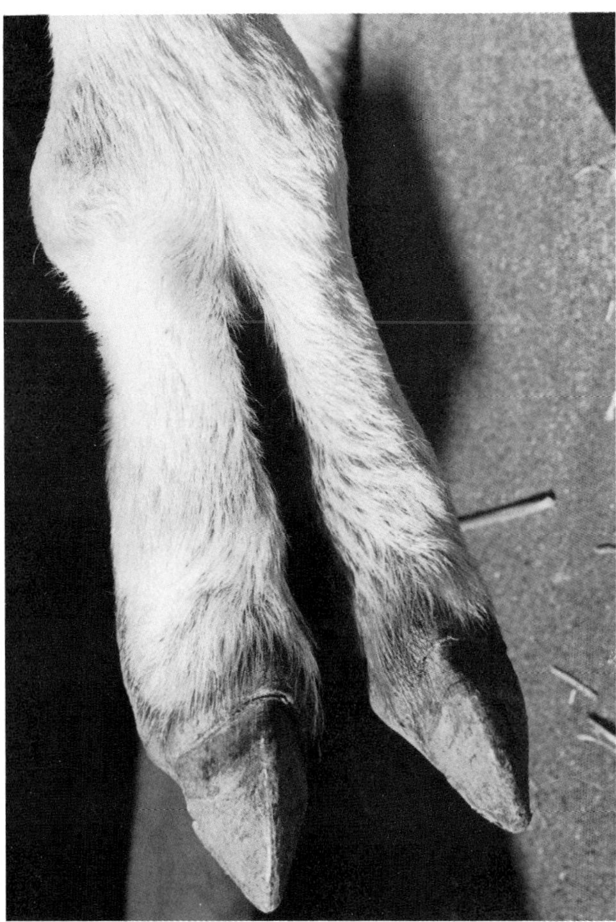

10.10 Normal llama foot, dorsal view.

The suborder name for camelids is Tylopoda, meaning padded foot, so named because of the digital cushion interspersed between the slipper, corium, and P-2 and P-3. The digital cushion consists of a poorly vascularized meshwork of collagenous and elastic fibers with interspersed masses of fat and, occasionally, cartilage tissue, all encased in a fibrous sheath (Fig. 10.11) (11).

DISEASES OF THE INTEGUMENT

Definition of Terms

The dermatopathologist uses special terminology to describe lesions of the integument. Following are definitions of a few terms, from Muller (25), that have relevance to the discussion of integumental diseases in lamoids.

Acanthosis is diffuse hypertrophy of the prickle cell layer of the epidermis. *Acantholysis* is loss of cohesion between epidermal cells. *Hypergranulosis* is increased thickness of the stratum granulosum. *Hyperplasia* is increased thickness of the noncornified epidermis. *Hyperkeratosis* is increased thickness of the stratum corneum. In normal skin of most species, the epidermal renewal time is 13–22 days. With inflammation, the renewal time may be reduced to 3–5 days, resulting in thickening (stacking) or excessive scaling. *Parakeratosis* is abnormal retention of keratinocyte nuclei in the stratum corneum.

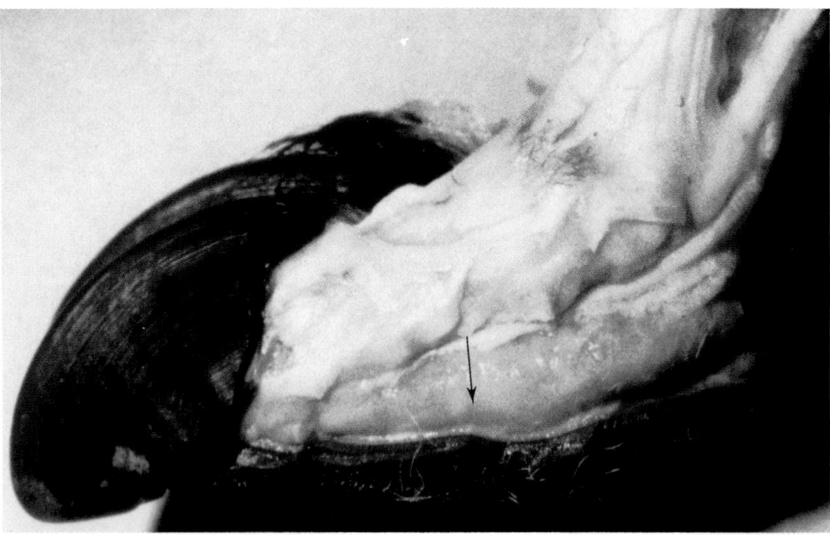

10.11 Digital cushion, lateral view.

Traumatic Lesions of the Skin

Lacerations, contusions, abrasions, and puncture wounds of the skin occur in lamoids as they do in other animals. The management of such injuries is similar to that used for livestock and companion animals. Llamas and alpacas should have been immunized against tetanus. If an individual has not been immunized, whether or not tetanus antitoxins should be administered may be controversial. Only two bonafide cases of tetanus in lamoids have been reported, and one of these was produced experimentally. Apparently, lamoids are much less susceptible to the organism than horses. Since tetanus antitoxin is prepared in horse serum, there is a risk of anaphylaxis when antitoxin is administered to animals other than the horse. Even if there is no immediate reaction, the lamoid may become sensitized to horse serum, and if such a product is administered in the future, anaphylaxis is a possibility. It is recommended that tetanus antitoxin not be used; rather, tetanus toxoid and benzathine penicillin should be administered at 3-day intervals until the wound heals.

Parasitic diseases of the skin include mange (sarcoptic, chorioptic, psoroptic, demodectic), pediculosis (*Damalinia* sp., *Microthoracius* sp.), and myiasis (see Chap. 8). The few infectious diseases of the skin include staphylococcal folliculitis, dermatophytosis, contagious ecthyma, and coccidioidomycosis (see Chap. 7).

Photosensitization may occur with hepatopathy (Figs. 10.12, 10.13).

Many lamoid dermatoses are undiagnosed as to etiology. Specific etiologies are suspected, but critical studies have not been conducted (Figs. 10.14–10.16). Alopecia and chronic dermatitis over the bridge of the nose of dark-skinned llamas and alpacas frequently occur (Fig. 10.17). Dermal plaques are frequently seen on the surface of the pinnae.

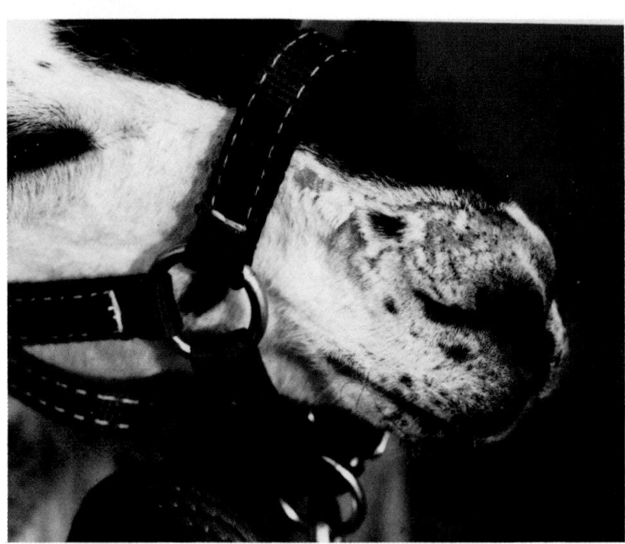

10.12 Photosensitization of the muzzle associated with fascioliasis.

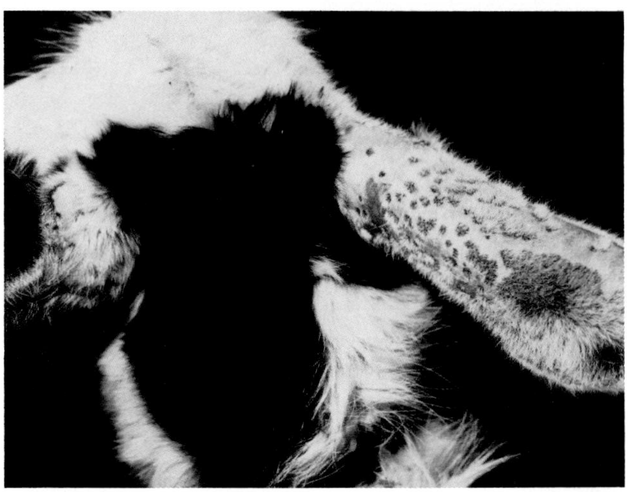

10.13 Photosensitization of the ears.

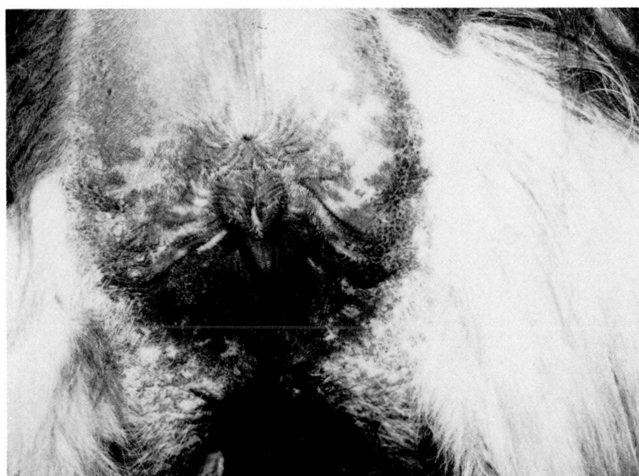

10.14 Acute nonspecific perineal dermatitis.

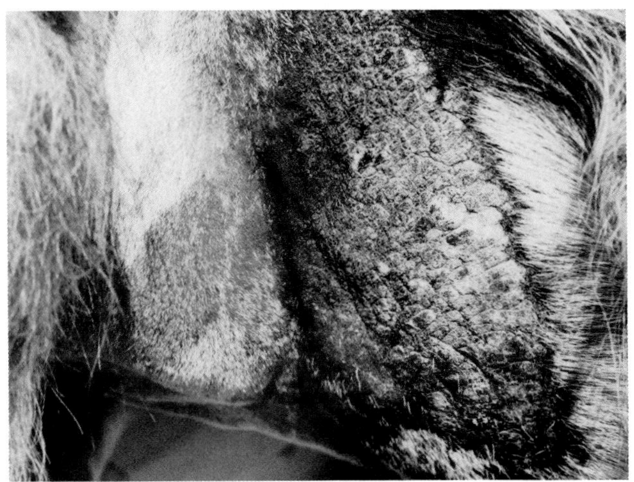

10.15 Acute nonspecific dermatitis.

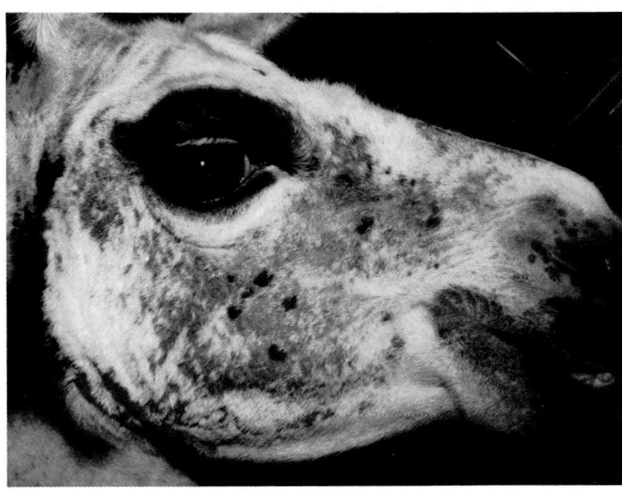

10.16 Acute facial zinc-responsive dermatitis.

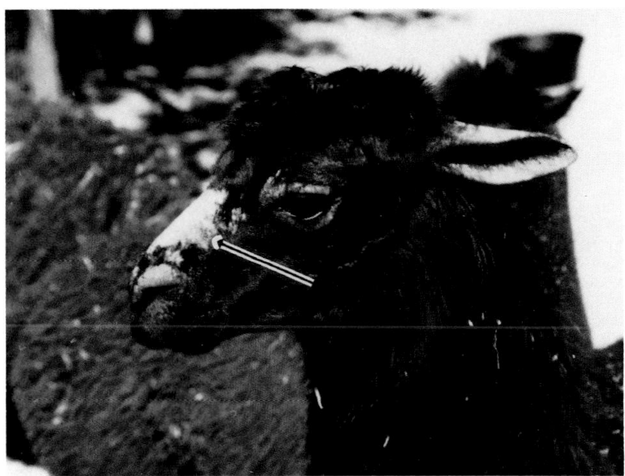

10.17 "Dark nose" dermatitis in an alpaca.

Zinc-responsive Dermatosis

Nonspecific dermatoses of llamas are often treated empirically by adding supplemental zinc to the diet. Colleagues report variable success as a result of this treatment, possibly because a precise diagnosis has not been made, and all dermatoses are treated alike.

Zinc-deficiency dermatosis has been described in swine, sheep, goats, and laboratory animals. Parakeratosis is a prominent feature of the disease in swine and laboratory animals but not in sheep and goats. In llamas, the lesions described at conferences have been hyperkeratosis with variable perivascular infiltrates of lymphocytes, plasma cells, macrophages, and eosinophils.

The clinical syndrome is characterized by nonpruritic alopecia, dermal thickening, scaling, and hyperpigmentation involving the face, ventral abdomen, medial thorax, and thighs (29). Black llamas may have a predilection for the disease. A tentative diagnosis may be made by finding serum zinc levels of less than 0.6 μg/dl and evaluation of a biopsy.

Zinc deficiency may be the result of an absolute dietary deficiency, poor absorption from the intestine, or the binding of zinc with calcium in the intestinal tract. Zinc is a required trace element. Pharmacologically, it is an immune system modulator and has some antiinflammatory effects also.

Zinc-responsive dermatoses are treated by supplying zinc sulfate in the diet at a dosage rate of 1 g/day. Improvement requires at least 30 days of supplementation.

Foot Diseases of Lamoids

Overgrowth of the toenail is the most common disorder of the lamoid foot (Figs. 10.18–10.22). The cause may be insufficient wear or congenital curling of the

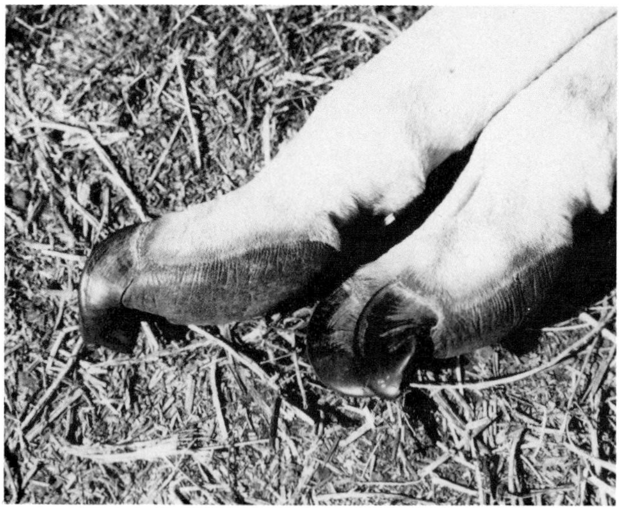

10.18 Elongated toenails on a llama.

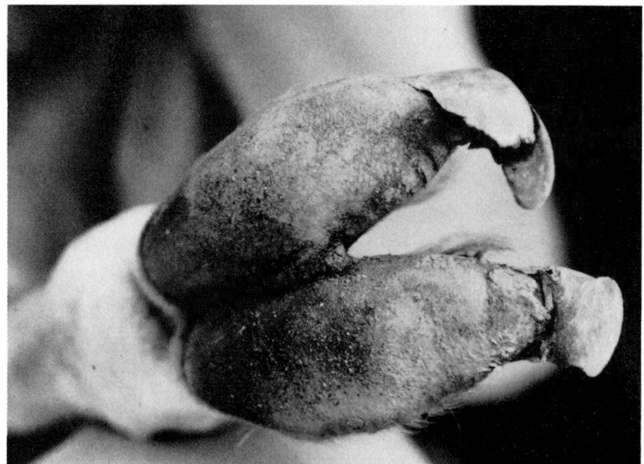

10.19 Elongated toenails on a llama.

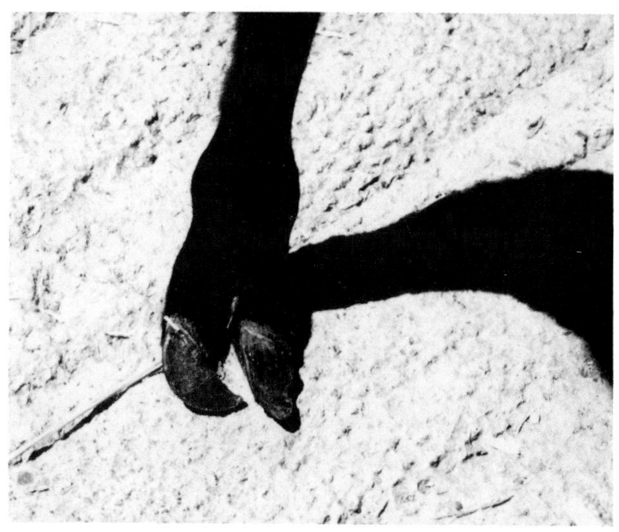

10.20 Elongated toenails, both curved to one side.

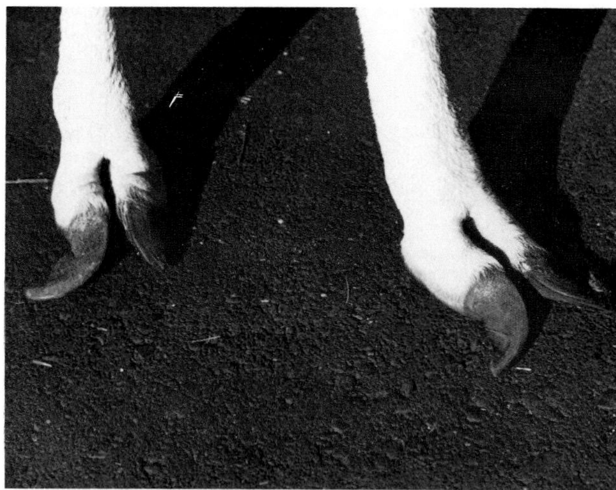

10.21 Elongated toenails, both curved outward.

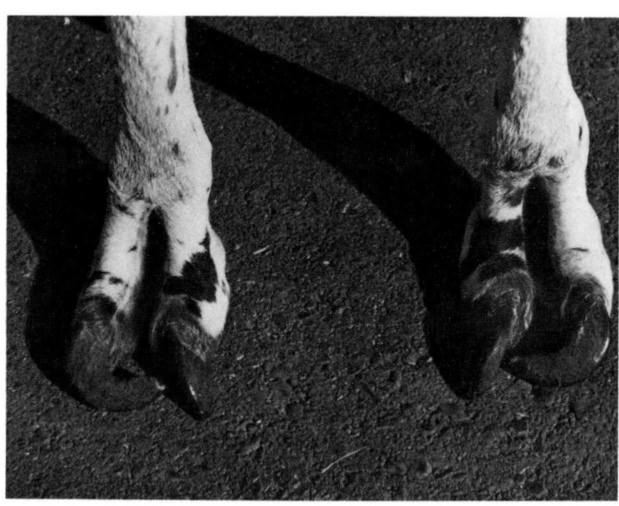

10.22 Elongated toenails, both curved inward.

toenail, in which the nail is pushed out of position for normal wear. The toenails should be trimmed as needed, using Burdizzo sheep hoof trimmers, pruning shears, or equine hoof nippers (Figs. 10.23, 10.24).

The toenail of a llama may be avulsed from the digit (Figs. 10.25, 10.26). The nailbed must be protected by a light bandage until the nail regrows, usually within 2 months.

Onychia is inflammation of the corium beneath the nail. Paronychia involves the tissue at the margins of the nail (11). Both conditions may occur in lamoids as a result of contusion or laceration of the nail. Neglected toenail trimming may allow infection to migrate dorsally under the nail. Drainage should be established and treatment continued with local disinfectant medications.

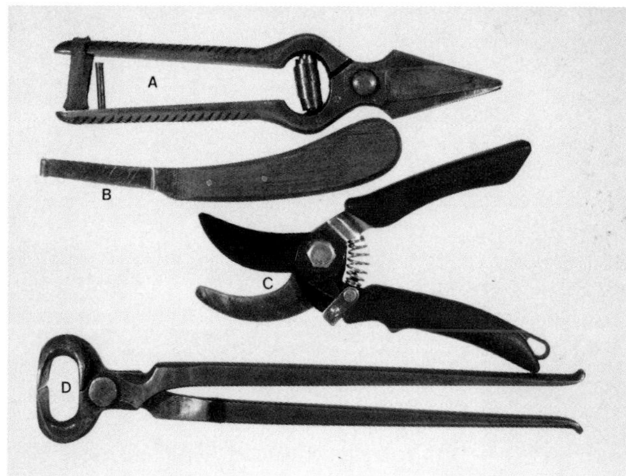

10.23 Hoof trimming tools: **(A)** Burdizzo sheep nail trimmer, **(B)** hoof knife, **(C)** pruning shears, **(D)** equine hoof nipper.

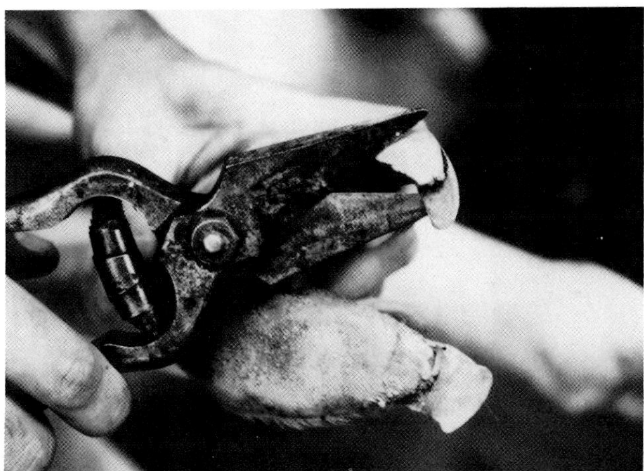

10.24 Trimming llama toenail with Burdizzo hoof trimmer.

The footpads are subject to laceration, contusion, foreign body penetration, erosion, and ulceration. Subfootpad abscessation may result in complete undermining of the pad. To repair this ailment, the detached slipper must be removed and the sensitive underlying tissue protected by bandaging until recornification takes place.

Infectious pododermatitis occurs in llamas (Figs. 10.27, 10.28). In South America, it is felt that *Fusobacterium necrophorum* is the primary etiologic agent, but a variety of anaerobic organisms have been isolated from pad ulcerations in North America. *Bacteroides* sp. is particularly difficult to eradicate since it is resistant to most antibiotics (see Chap. 7).

Povidone-iodine, diluted 1:4, is excellent for disinfection underneath a bandage. Another antimicrobial medication, copper naphthenolate (Kopertox, Ayerst Labs, New York), can be sprayed onto the exposed surface. It will adhere readily. A light bandage aids in keeping the medication from wearing away.

Mastitis

Mastitis is not common in llamas, but when it does occur, prompt attention is necessary to avoid loss of function in one or more quarters or even death (18). Lamoid mastitis occurs in the same forms as seen in dairy cattle, namely, subclinical, chronic, acute, and peracute.

PREDISPOSING FACTORS. In lamoids the udder is not pendulous and the teats are relatively short, so trauma is minimized. Nonetheless, trauma (laceration,

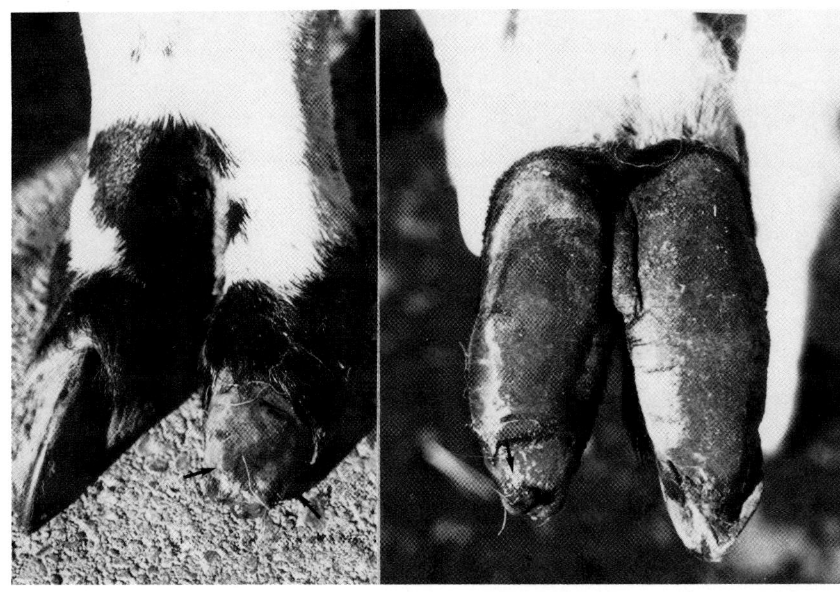

10.25 Avulsed toenail of a llama.

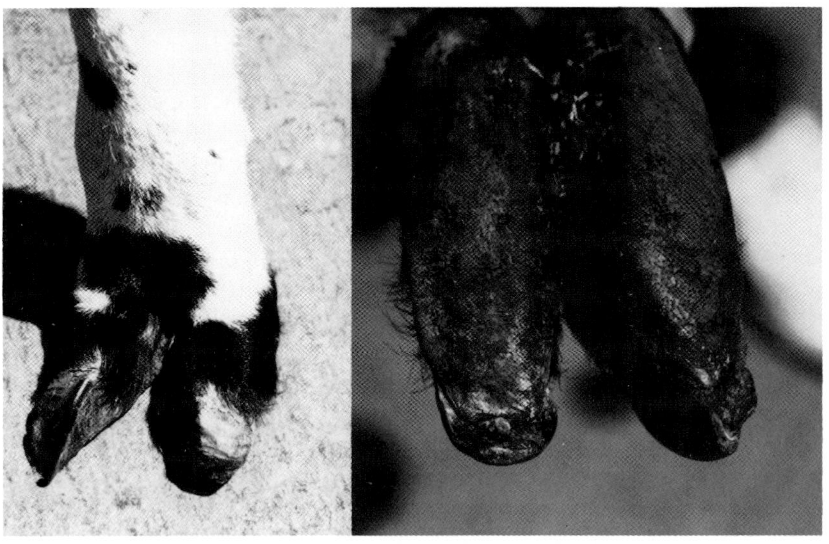

10.26 Healed avulsed toenail of a llama.

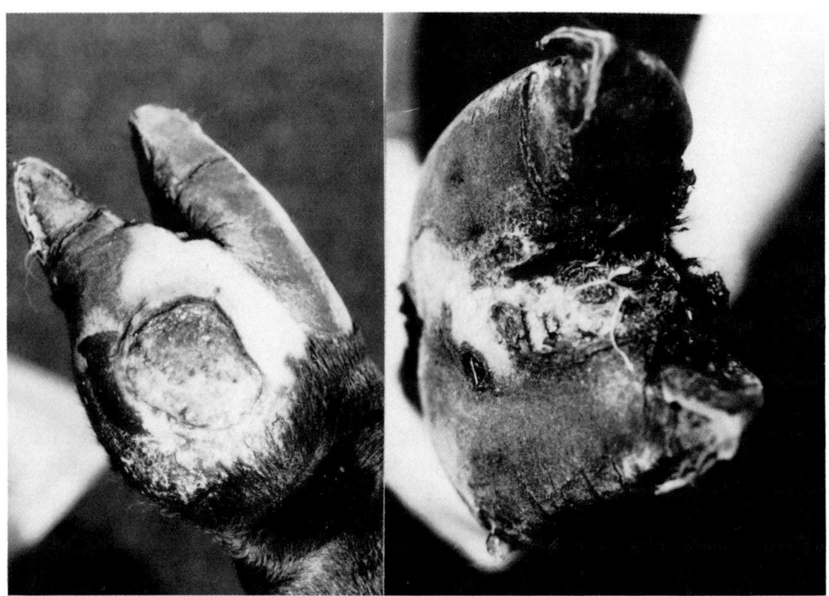

10.27 Infectious pododermatitis.

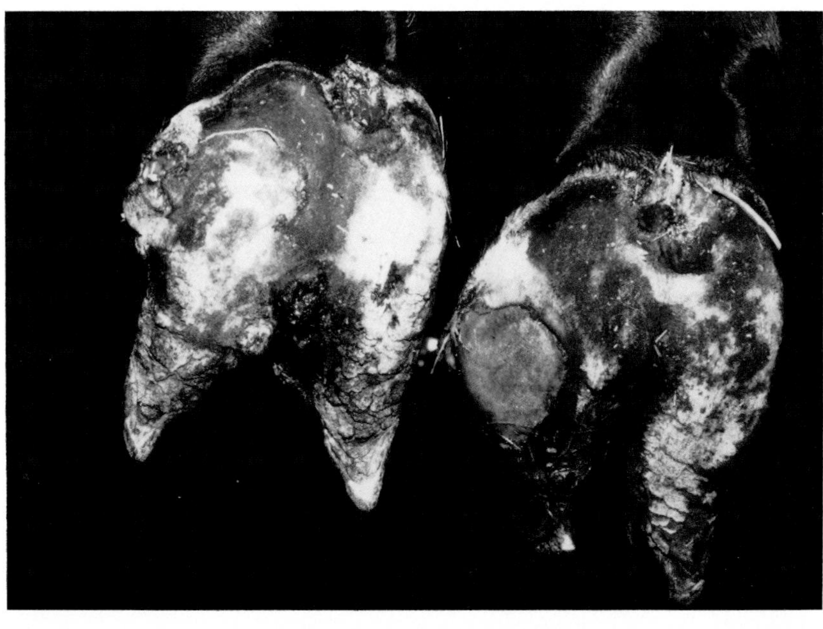

10.28 Infectious pododermatitis.

contusion, abrasion) of the glands and teats is possible if a female attempts to jump a fence or is mauled by dogs. Trauma to the tip of the teat may weaken the sphincter of the streak canal, which in the normal state tends to prevent access to the gland of pathogenic bacteria. Even though the location of the udder minimizes exposure to filth, when the female is recumbent, if there is no access to dry, clean areas, she may be forced to lie down in mud.

Milk is an excellent medium for bacteria, and any condition that allows milk to stagnate within the gland fosters growth of any organism that may have gained temporary entrance (39). Failure of the cria to nurse, blockage of a streak canal with a waxy plug, pre- and postparturient udder edema, and stricture of the streak canal are factors that may cause stagnation.

ETIOLOGY. There are no reports on specific bacteria that cause mastitis in lamoids. It might be anticipated that all of the organisms causing mastitis in cattle could do likewise in lamoids, because those organisms have been isolated from other disease conditions in lamoids. An exception is that no mycoplasmas have been isolated from diseased lamoids. Isolates from peracute lamoid mastitis have included *Escherichia coli, Klebsiella pneumoniae,* and *Aerobacter enterobactum,* which are the same organisms causing peracute mastitis in cows.

CLINICAL SIGNS. Subclinical mastitis can be detected only by culturing for an organism in the milk or testing the milk with one of the mastitis tests such as the California mastitis test (CMT). Indurated areas may be palpable within a gland, but there are no systemic signs and the gland is not swollen or hot. Chronic mastitis results in periodic changes in the quality of the milk.

Acute mastitis is usually seen just before or within a few days after parturition and is characterized by heat, swelling, hardness of the affected gland, and evident pain on palpation (Fig. 10.29). The secretion may be watery, hemorrhagic, thickened, stringy, or odorous. The female may refuse to allow the cria to nurse because of the pain, or the cria may refuse to nurse because of the unpalatable secretion. The cria may also develop gastroenteritis or septicemia from ingestion of the pathogen. The female may be anorectic and have a low-grade fever.

Peracute mastitis may have all of the signs of acute mastitis (Fig. 10.30) plus severe depression and toxemia, even leading to gangrene (Fig. 10.31), septicemia, and death. Peracute mastitis is usually seen within a few days of parturition.

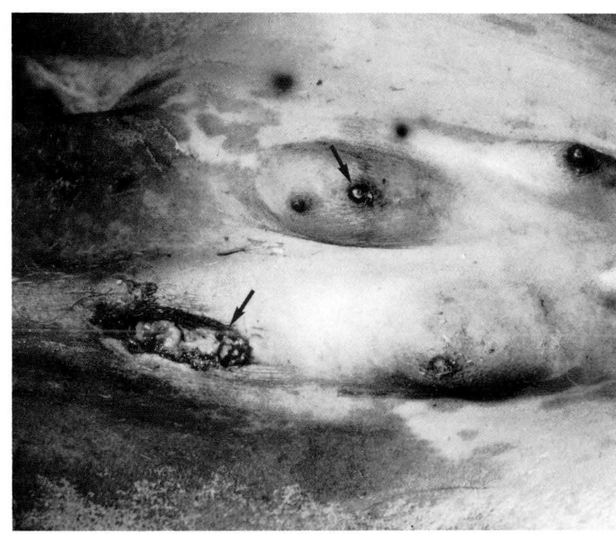

10.29 Acute mastitis with abscessation.

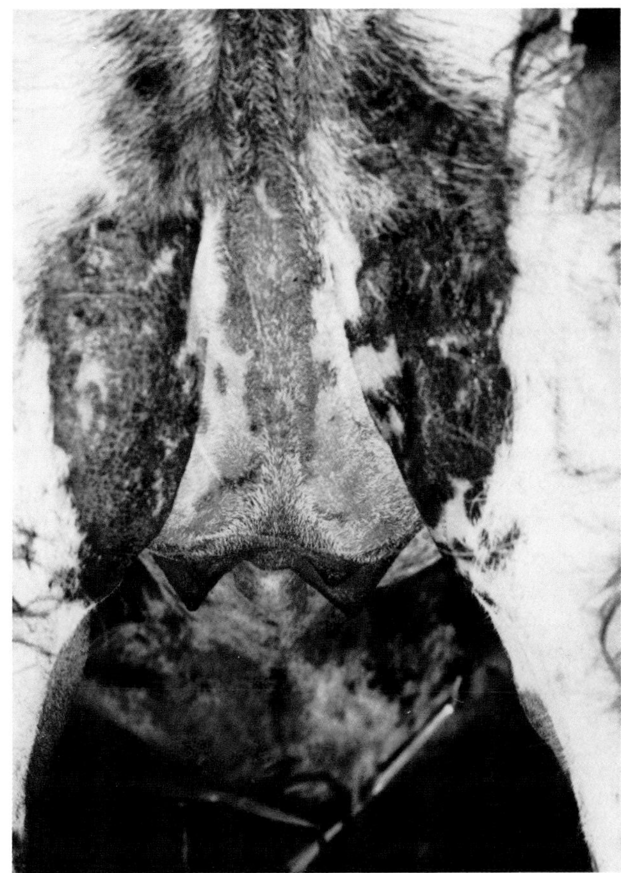

10.30 Acute mastitis and dermatitis caused by *E. coli* infection.

DIAGNOSIS. The diagnosis is based on a thorough physical examination; evaluation of the secretion for consistency, color viscosity, presence of debris, and sediment; culture and sensitivity; and evaluation with

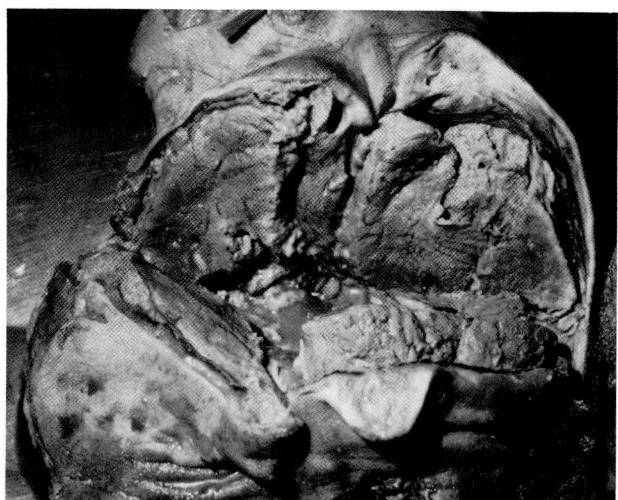

10.31 Necrotic mastitis caused by *E. coli* infection.

the CMT. All quarters should be examined, not just the obviously affected gland. Ultrasonography may be used to locate walled-off abscesses.

Pre- and postparturient edema occurs in lamoids and must be differentiated from mastitis. Edema is symmetric and uniformly distributed over the gland. The swelling is not hot or painful, and the secretion quality is not altered. Edema may cause swelling of the teats, which may mechanically interfere with the cria's ability to grasp the teat in its mouth. Massage and manual milking may be necessary to reduce the swelling. Colostrum should be saved and offered to the cria via a bottle or by tube feeding. Continued engorgement of the gland may be predisposing toward mastitis.

THERAPY. The objectives of treatment are to save the life of the female, restore the function of the gland, and improve milk quality (39). These objectives are achieved by removing the cause of the mastitis, providing systemic support, locally infusing the glands with antimicrobial agents, and promoting the healing of the damaged tissue.

The veterinarian must be fully aware of the anatomy of the camelid mammary gland, with a noncommunicating double gland associated with each teat. If local infusion is selected, both streak canals must be cannulated simultaneously to ensure treatment of the affected portion. The streak canals are tiny, and 1 mm (3.5 French) tomcat catheters are required. The streak canal is easily traumatized. Do not attempt to infuse with bovine teat cannulae or commercial infusion tubes.

Peracute and possible acute mastitis cases require parenteral administration of antibiotics along with local infusion. In both instances, the selection of an antibiotic should be based on culture and sensitivity. The toxemia should be treated aggressively with steroids and intravenous fluids. The exudate should be removed from the gland three to five times daily. Alternate hot and cold packs and gentle massage will facilitate removal of the exudate.

Following is the protocol used for successful treatment of a case of peracute mastitis. The left rear quarter became hot and swollen. Milk production in that quarter ceased and was replaced by a hemorrhagic fluid containing clots of debris. The secretion was CMT positive throughout the treatment period. A culture and sensitivity was conducted, yielding *E. coli* and *Klebsiella* sp., with sensitivities to gentamicin, trimethoprim sulfas, and third-generation cephalosporins.

Gentamicin (1 mg/kg) was administered intramuscularly three times daily for 10 days. The unaffected quarters were stripped every 4 hours. The affected quarter was infused with a solution of polymyxin B (250,000 units diluted in 40 ml sterile saline) at 8:00 A.M. and 8:00 P.M.; 20 ml were infused simultaneously into each streak canal, using tomcat catheters. The medication was left in the quarter for 4–6 hours, following which the affected quarter was stripped every 2 hours day and night. Infusion therapy was continued for 10 days.

At completion of the treatment, gland secretion had returned to milk of normal appearances, with a weak CMT positive reaction. Heat and swelling had disappeared.

In acute and peracute cases, it is imperative that the cria be temporarily orphaned as a protection to itself and to minimize painful manipulation of the affected gland and teat.

PREVENTION. Careful attention to the nursing behavior of the cria and observation and palpation of the udder will allow early detection of problems. A weak or premature cria will not remove sufficient milk to prevent stagnation. The female should be milked regularly until the cria is strong enough to nurse unassisted. The cria generally removes milk from all four teats at each nursing episode. A single swollen teat should be investigated.

REFERENCES

1. Appleyard, H. M., and Wildman, A. B. 1967. The structure and identification of animal fibers. Rev. Zootec. Numero Spec. 14–16:43–46.

2. Arana Benavides, L. R. 1972. (Distribution of follicular density in the skin of alpaca in relation to fiber diameter) Distribucion de la densidad folicular en la piel de alpaca y en su relacion con el diametro de fibra. Tesis, Ing. Zoot. Lima, Univ. Nac. Agraria.

3. Ben Shaul, D. M. 1971. The composition of the milk of wild animals. Int. Zoo Yearb. (4):333–42.

4. Bergen, W. von. 1963. The Wool Handbook, 3rd ed. New York, London: John Wiley and Sons.

5. Beytia Copello, J. 1949. (Health and animal production in the exploitation of wool in Puno) Sanidad y produccion animal en las explotaciones lanares de Puno. Tesis, Fac. Med. Vet. Univ. Nac. Mayor San Marcos (Lima), pp. 1–113.

6. Ciprian R., C., Chanbilla F., V., and Bustinza C., V. 1985. (Histology of the skin of the alpaca and llama) Histologia de la peil de alpaca y llama. Projecto—Piel alpaca. Univ. Nac. Altiplano (Puno), pp. 42–62.

7. Clement, J.-L., Hagege, R., Le Pareaux, A., and Carteaud, J.-P. 1981. Ultra-structural study of the medulla of mammalian hair. Scanning Electron Microsc. (3):377–82.

8. Davies, D. T., Holt, C., and Christie, W. W. 1983. The composition of milk. In T. B. Mepham, ed. Biochemistry of Lactation. Netherlands: Elsevier, pp. 71–117.

9. Disselhorst, R. 1926. (Chestnuts on the limbs of alpaca) Castanas en los miembros de lama huanachos. Anat. Anz. Jena 61:206–7.

10. Everts, W. 1973. Comparative functional-anatomical study of the skin of several South American mammals. Z. Wiss. Zool. 185(3):319–60.

11. Fowler, M. E. 1980. Hoof, claw and nail problems in nondomestic animals. J. Am. Vet. Med. Assoc. 177:885–93.

12. Gillespie, J. M., and Broad, A. 1972. Ultra-high-sulphur proteins in the hairs of the Artiodactyla. Aust. J. Biol. Sci. 25(1):139–45.

13. Hausman, L. A. 1944. Applied microscopy of the hair (camel, vicuña). Sci. Mon. (New York) 59:195–202.

14. Jenness, R. 1974. Composition of milk. In B. L. Larson and V. R. Smith, eds. Lactation, vol. 3. New York: Academic Press, pp. 3–96.

15. ______. 1980. Composition and characteristics of goat milk. Rev. 1968–1979 Int. Symp.: Dairy Goats.

16. Jenness, R., and Sloan, R. E. 1970. The composition of milks of various species: A review. Dairy Sci. Abstr. 32(10):599–612.

17. Jimenez O., R. 1970. (Studies on some aspects of alpaca milk) Estudio de algunos aspectos sobre la leche de alpaca. Bol. Extraordinario 4:60–70.

18. Kress, P. J., and Torrey, S. 1983. Mastitis in llamas: Diagnosis, treatment, prevention. Llama World 1(3):21.

19. Langley, K. D., and Kennedy, T. A., Jr. 1981. The identification of specialty fibers (mohair, cashmere, camel hair, alpaca, and angora rabbit). Text. Res. J. 51(11):703–9.

20. Mauersberger, H. R., ed. 1947. Matthew's Textile Fibers, 5th ed. New York: John Wiley and Sons, pp. 637–50.

21. Montalvo, C., and Cevallos, E. 1973. (Mycopolysaccharides in the apocrine or epitrichial sweat glands of the alpaca) Mucopolisacarides en la glandula sudoripara apocrina o epitrica de la alpaca (*Lama pacos*). Rev. Invest. Pecu. 2(2):137–40.

22. Moro Sommo, M. 1956. (A brief summary of the result of studies during the present year (1956) on the diseases and milk of the alpaca) Breve resumen de los estudios realizados en el presente ano sobre las enfermedades y la leche de alpaca. Ganaderia (Lima) 14(15):98–99.

23. ______. 1957. (Contributions to the study of the milk of alpacas) Contribucion al estudio de la leche de las alpacas. Rev. Fac. Med. Vet. (Lima) 7(11):117–41.

24. Morrison, P. 1966. Insulative flexibility in the guanaco. J. Mammal. 47:18–23.

25. Muller, G. H., Kirk, R. W., and Scott, D. W. 1983. Small Animal Dermatology, 3rd ed. Philadelphia: W. B. Saunders.

26. Ochoa, R. J. 1970. (Study of some aspects of alpaca milk) Estudio de algunos aspectos sobre la leche de alpaca. Bol. Extraordinario 4:60–70.

27. Ramirez, A., Zegarra, A., Ogi, A., Sumar, J., and Valdivia, R. 1983. (Physical and chemical characteristics of llama milk) Caracteristicas fisico-quimicas de la leche de la llama. Resumenes Proyectos Invest. Readizados (1980–81) (Lima) 3:46–47.

28. Riera, S. 1969. (Growth rate and the fineness of the wool of the llama) Ritmo del crecimiento y finura del pelo de la llama. Bol. Exp. Estac. Exp. Ganad. Patacamaya, La Paz, Bolivia No. 39.

29. Rosychuk, R. A. W. 1987. The llama integumentary system in health and disease. Proc. Llama Med. Workshop Vet. Fort Collins, Colo.

30. Roux, J. S. 1947. Chestnuts, knothead. Zoonooz 20(6):3–4.

31. Russell, K. P. 1977. The specialty animal fibres. Textiles 6(1):8–12.

32. Saleh, M. S., Mobarak, A. M., and Fouad, S. M. 1971. Radiological, anatomical and histological studies of the mammary gland of the one humped camel, *Camelus dromedarius*. I. The teat. Zentralbl. Veterinaermed. [A] 18:347–52.

33. Schuntermann, E. 1925. (Chestnutlike formations of the members of *Lama huanachus*) Ueber kastnaienartgie Bildungen an den Gliedmasson von *Lama huanachus*. Anat. Anz. 60:87–93.

34. Tapia C., M. 1969. (Preliminary follicle study of the skin of alpaca, variety suri) Estudio preliminar folicular de la piel de alpaca de la vaeiedad Suri. Tesis, Ing. Zootech. Univ. Nac. Agraria (Lima).

35. Torrey, S. 1978. Llama wool characteristics. Llama Newsl. 2:1–4.

36. Toyoda, M., Yamauchi, K., and Tsugo, T. 1970a. Comparative studies on the fatty-acid composition of milks of various animals (cow, sow, tapir, human, llama). Nippon Nogei Kagaku Kaishi 44(10):484–87.

37. ______. 1970b. Comparative studies on caseins of several different animals by polyacrylamide gel electrophoresis. Nippon Nogei Kagaku Kaishi 44(11):505–11.

38. Verscheure, S. H., and Garcia, D. G. 1980. (Guanaco, *Lama guanicoe,* as a renewable natural resource. I. Some wool metric characteristics) El guanaco, *Lama guanicoe,* como recurso natural renovable. I. Algunas caractericas lanimetricas de sus fibras. Adv. Prod. Anim. 5(1):15–22.

39. Winker, J. K. 1986. Mastitis. In J. L. Howard, ed. 1986. Current Veterinary Therapy: Food Animal Practice, 2nd ed. Philadelphia: W. B. Saunders, pp. 765–71.

40. Yagil, R. 1982. Camels and camel milk. FAO Anim. Prod. Health Pap. 26, pp. 14–16.

41. ______. 1985. The desert camel, comparative physiological adaptation. In Comparative Animal Nutrition V. Basel: Karger, pp. 107–20.

11 Musculoskeletal System

ANATOMY

No text describes the anatomy of the musculoskeletal system of lamoids. There are some theses on the subject (5, 16, 17, 23) and a few references in the periodic literature (1–3, 6–11, 13–15, 18, 20–22, 24). Only those aspects of anatomy that are unique to lamoids and clinically important will be discussed here. Figure 11.1 is a diagrammatic representation of the skeletal system of a lamoid. The anatomy of certain sections of the musculoskeletal system has been described in other chapters, such as Surgery, Chapter 6. Anatomy of the head has been described in the discussions of disorders of the teeth and congenital disorders of the head. The anatomy of the limbs is discussed in the section dealing with orthopedic surgery of the long bones, presented in Chapter 6.

RADIOGRAPHY

Vertebrae

CERVICAL. Lamoids have a highly mobile neck covered by thick skin (up to 1 cm). The seven cervical vertebrae are elongated and from C-3 caudad, a ventral projection of the cranial segment of the transverse process forms an inverted U osseous channel on the ventrum of the neck (Figs. 11.2, 11.3). The channel protects the vital structures of the neck from accidental laceration during intermale aggressive bouts. Figures 11.4–11.6 are of cervical vertebrae.

More pronounced ventral projections (2.5 cm) are seen on C-4 and C-5. There are ventral projections on both the cranial and caudal segments of the transverse processes of C-6. This vertebra is easily recognized on a

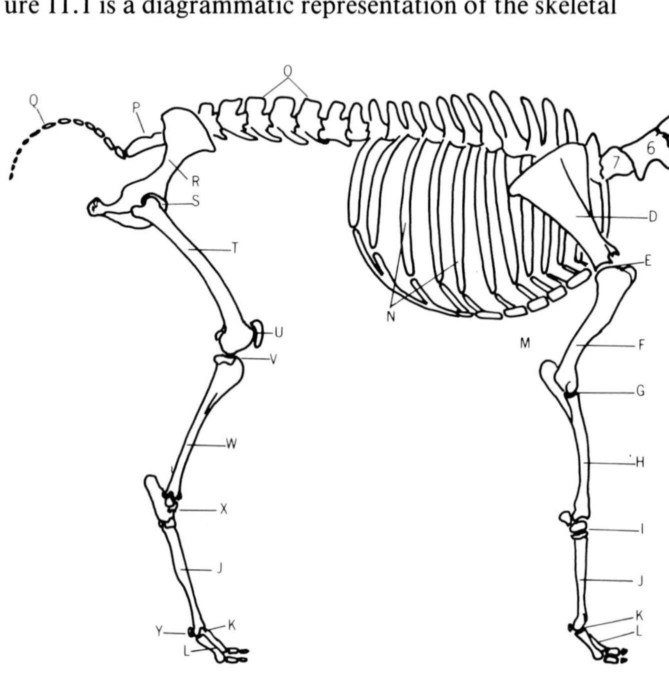

11.1 Diagram of llama skeleton. (**A**) orbit, (**B**) mandible, (**C**) cervical vertebrae, (**D**) scapula, (**E**) shoulder, (**F**) humerus, (**G**) elbow, (**H**) radius, (**I**) carpus, (**J**) metacarpus, (**K**) fetlock, (**L**) pastern, (**M**) sternebrae, (**N**) ribs, (**O**) vertebrae, (**P**) sacrum, (**Q**) coccygeal vertebrae, (**R**) ilium, (**S**) hip, (**T**) femur, (**U**) patella, (**V**) stifle, (**W**) tibia, (**X**) hock (tarsus), (**Y**) sesamoid.

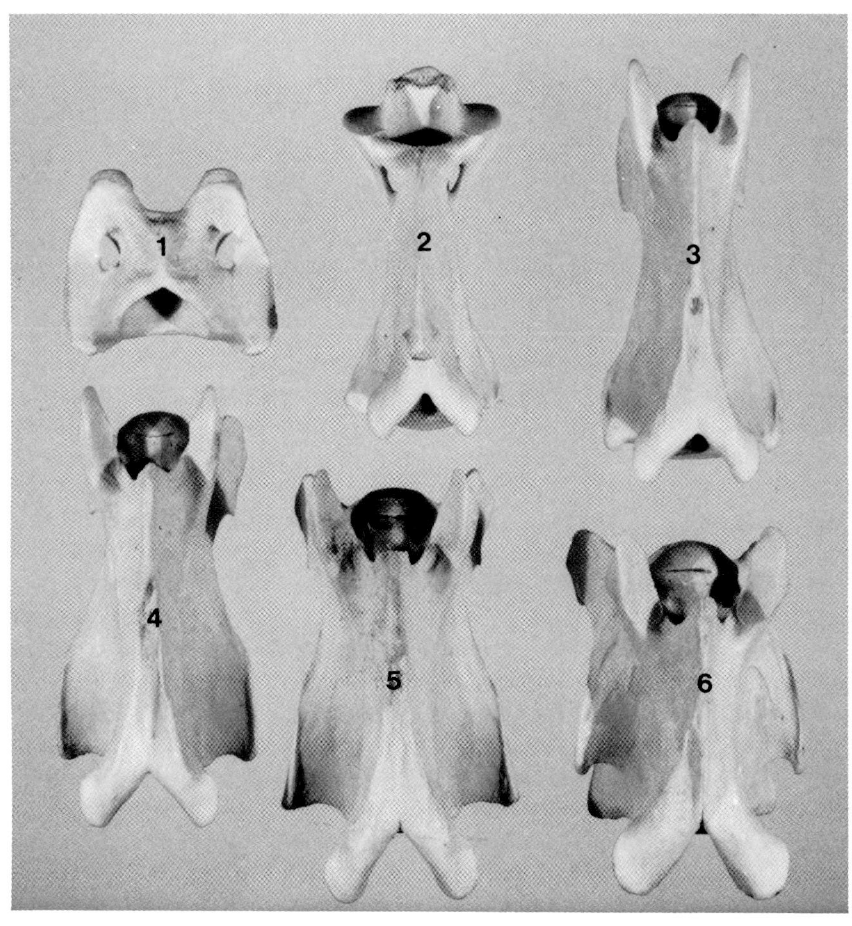

11.2 Llama cervical vertebrae (C-1 to C-6), dorsal view.

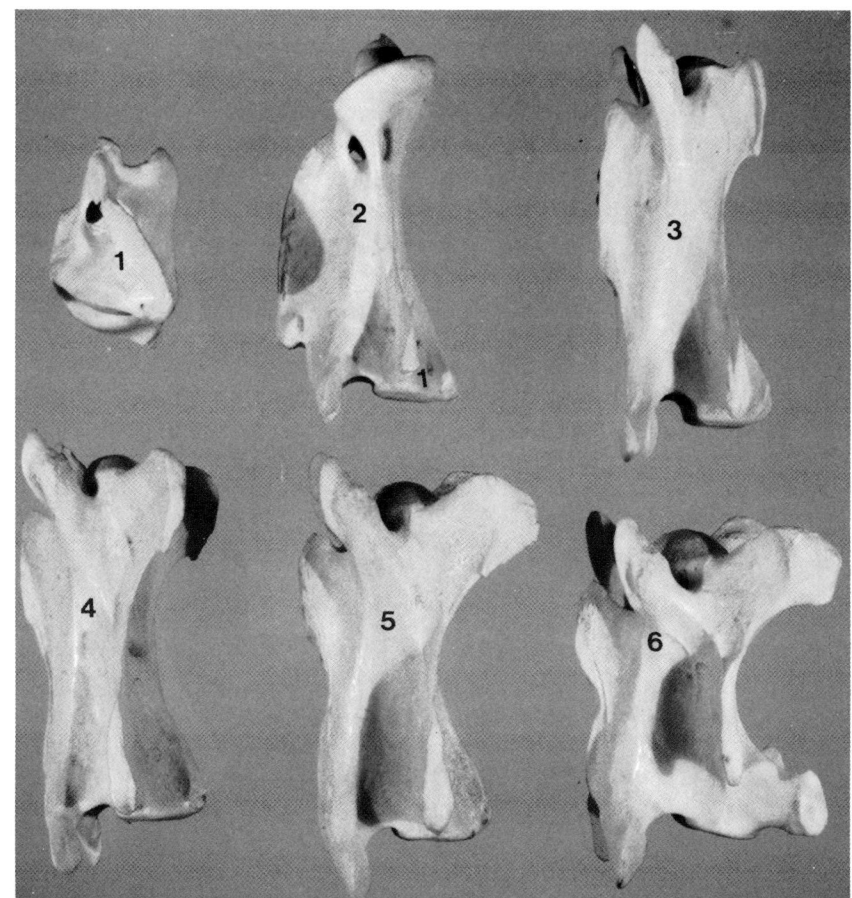

11.3 Llama cervical vertebrae (C-1 to C-6), right lateral view.

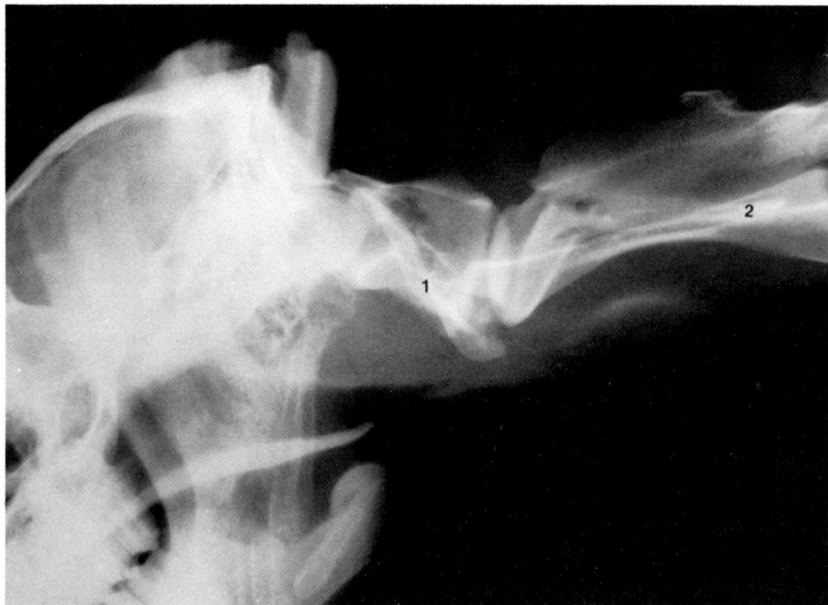

11.4 Lateral radiograph of caudal skull, C-1, and C-2.

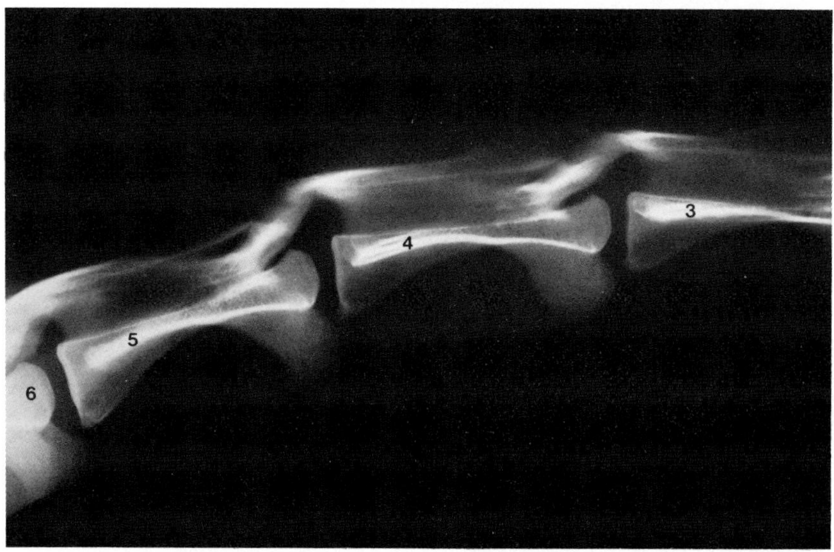

11.5 Lateral radiograph of cervical vertebrae, C-3 to C-6.

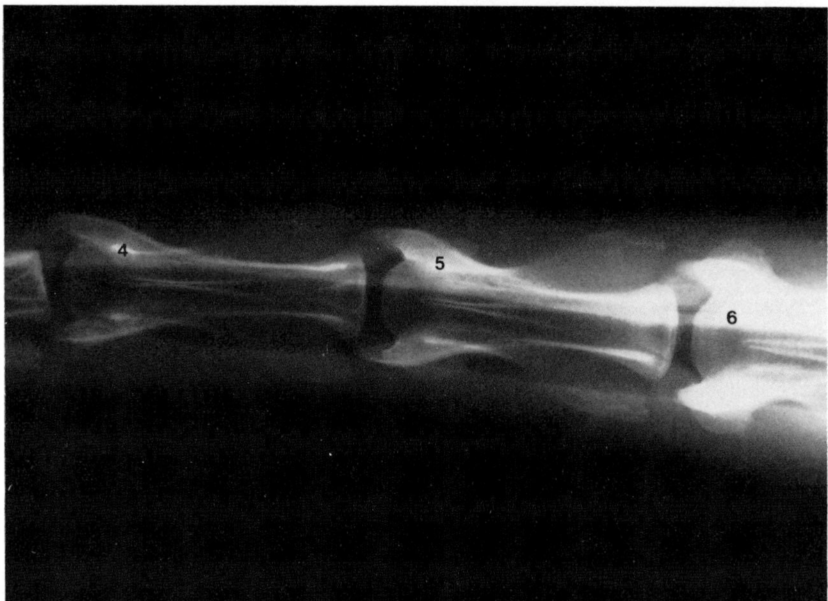

11.6 Dorsoventral radiograph of cervical vertebrae, C-4 to C-6.

radiograph (Fig. 11.7). Since C-7 lies deep within the neck, it is difficult to visualize radiographically. It has no ventral projections and is the shortest of the cervical vertebrae. The approximate length of each cervical vertebra is as follows: C-1, 5.5cm; C-2, 11cm; C-3, 10 cm; C-4, 9 cm; C-5, 9 cm; C-6, 8 cm; and C-7, 5 cm.

THORACIC. There are 12 thoracic vertebrae. The dorsal spinous processes are easily identified, but the bodies, articular facets, and spinal canal are more difficult to visualize because of the heavy vertebral muscle mass.

LUMBAR. There are seven lumbar vertebrae (Fig. 11.8). The transverse process of L-7 is shortened. The dorsal spinous processes are vertical.

SACRUM. There are five sacral vertebrae. The dorsal spinous process of S-1 is minimal. This clear demarcation of the lumbosacral space marks the preferred site for placement of the spinal needle (see Chap. 4).

Other Bones of the Trunk

There are 12 pairs of ribs. The lamoid pelvis is not unique. The sternebrae are flattened from side to side, as is characteristic of many artiodactylids. The skin over the sternum of an adult is highly calloused, giving an erroneous impression of soft-tissue pathology on a radiograph.

Limb Articulations

The radiographic appearance of the articulations of the forelimb are as follows: shoulder (Figs. 11.9–11.11), elbow (Figs. 11.12–11.15), carpus (Figs. 11.16–11.18), metacarpal phalangeal, and phalangeal joints (Figs. 11.19–11.22). Note that two sesamoid bones are associated with each first phalanx (P-1). For more details on the carpus, see Chapter 22.

The coxofemoral articulation of the adult is illustrated in Figures 11.23 and 11.24. The animal should be anesthetized for dorsoventral radiography. The femorotibial articulation is seen in Figures 11.25–11.30.

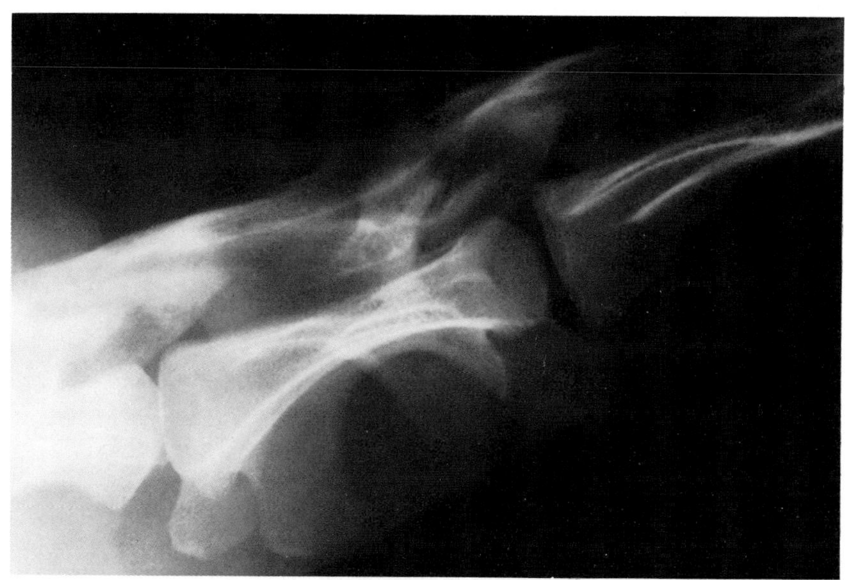

11.7 Lateral radiograph of C-6 illustrating pronounced ventral projections of the transverse processes.

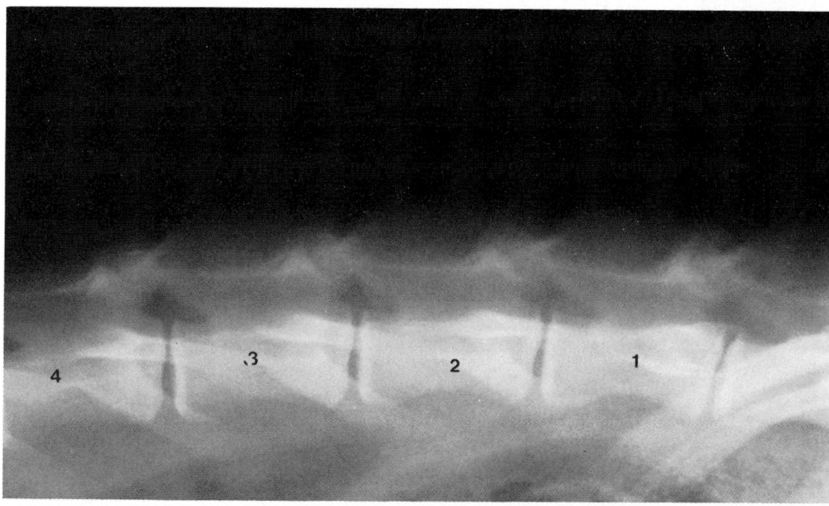

11.8 Lateral radiograph of lumbar vertebrae.

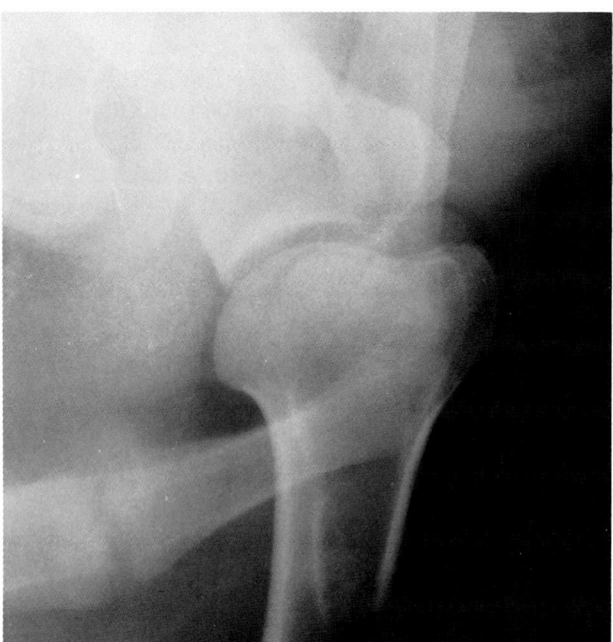

11.9 Lateral radiograph of llama shoulder.

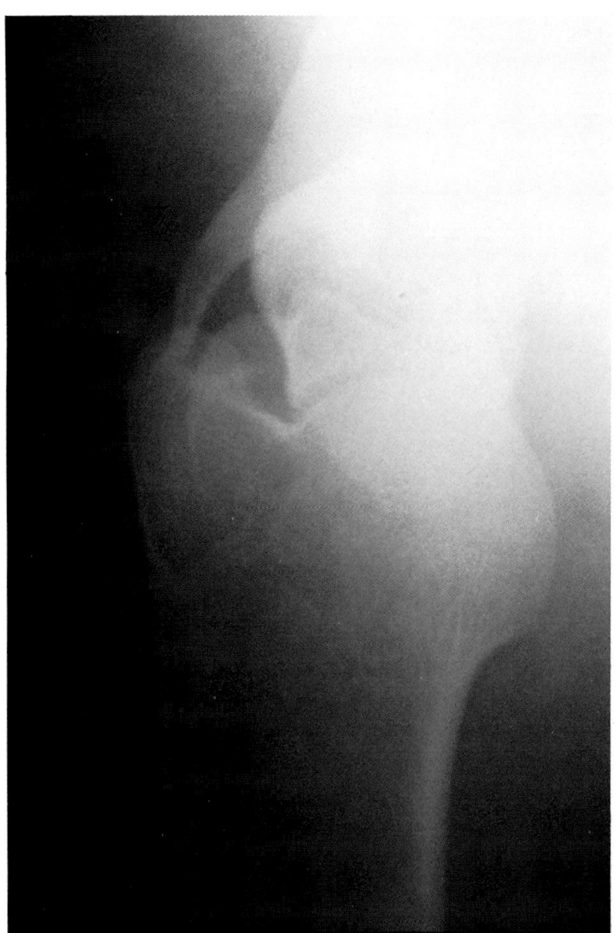

11.10 Craniocaudal radiograph of llama shoulder.

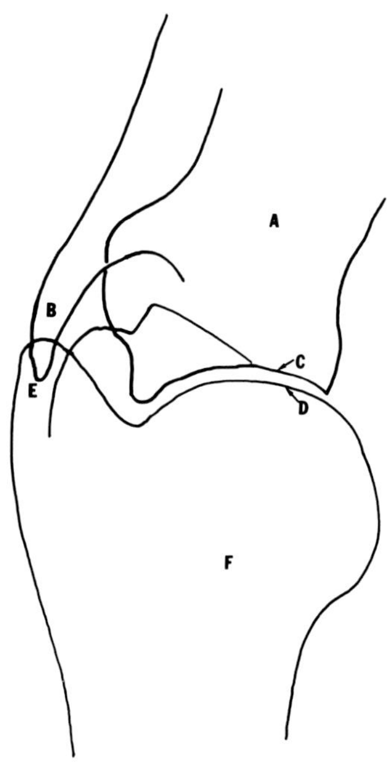

11.11 Diagram of craniocaudal radiograph of llama shoulder: **(A)** scapula, **(B)** acromion process, **(C)** glenoid cavity, **(D)** head of humerus, **(E)** major tubercle of humerus, **(F)** humerus.

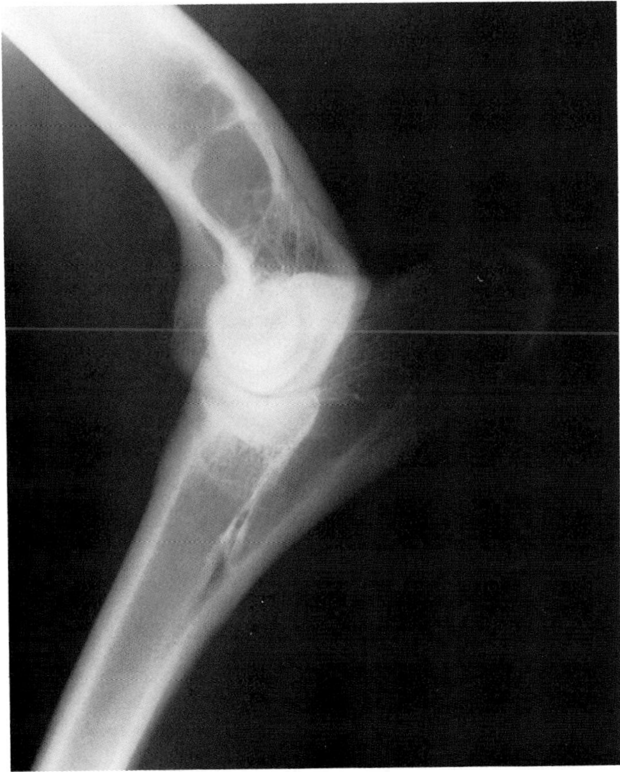

11.12 Lateral radiograph of llama elbow.

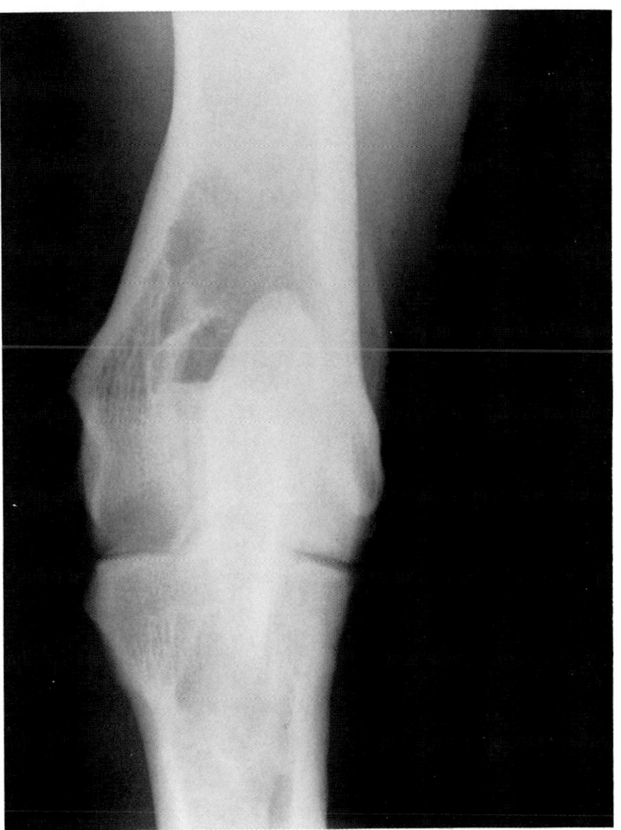

11.14 Craniocaudal radiograph of llama elbow.

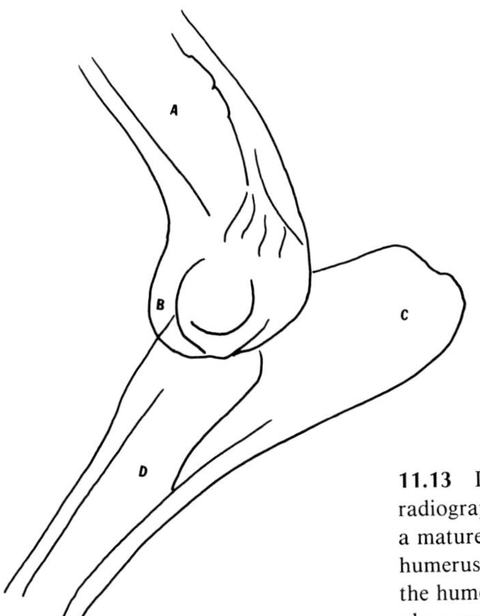

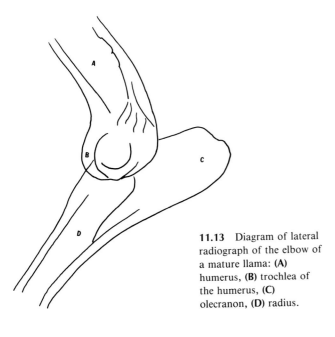

11.13 Diagram of lateral radiograph of the elbow of a mature llama: **(A)** humerus, **(B)** trochlea of the humerus, **(C)** olecranon, **(D)** radius.

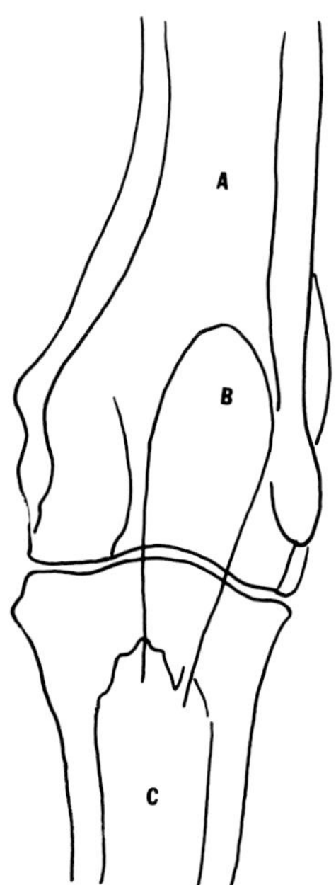

11.15 Diagram of craniocaudal radiograph of the elbow of a mature llama: **(A)** radius, **(B)** olecranon, **(C)** radius.

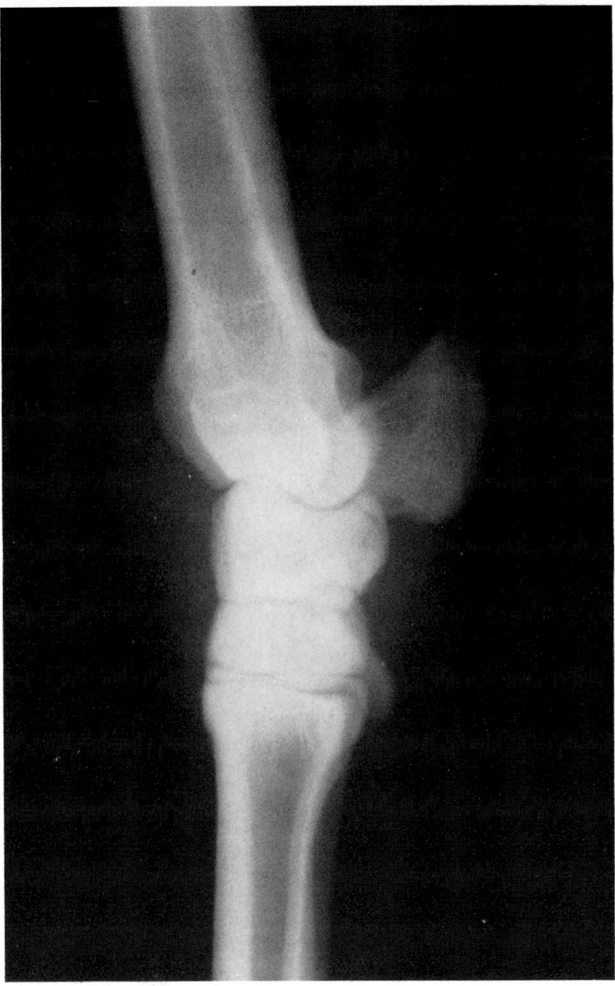

11.16 Lateral radiograph of llama carpus.

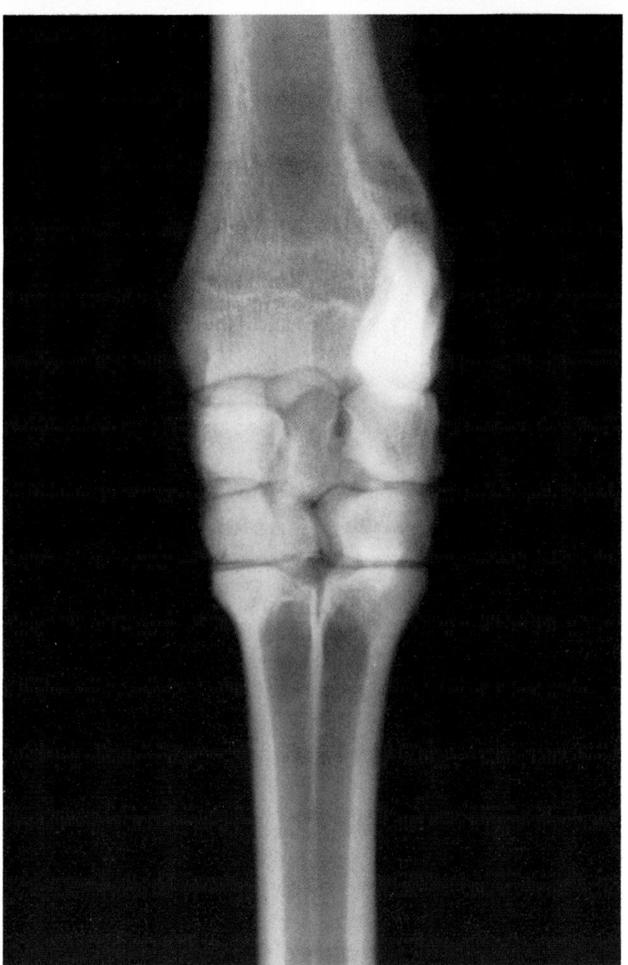

11.17 Dorsopalmar radiograph of llama carpus.

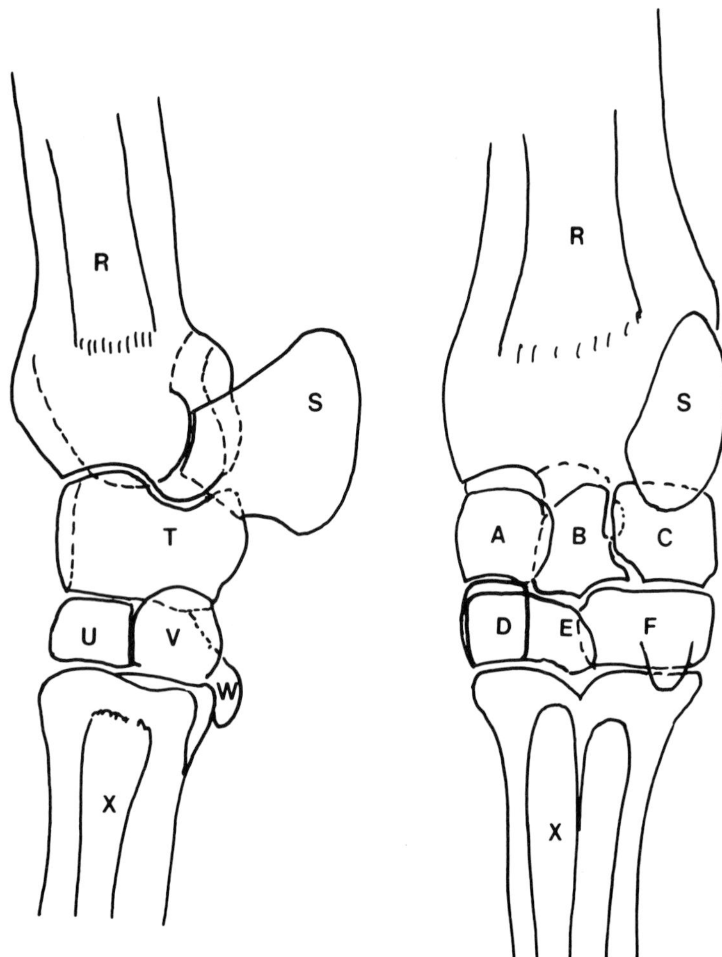

11.18 Diagram of mature llama carpus: **(R)** radius, **(S)** accessory carpal bone, **(T)** radial, intermediate, and ulnar carpal bones superimposed, **(U)** 3rd carpal bone, **(V)** 2nd carpal bone, **(W)** projection of the 4th carpal bone, **(X)** metacarpus, **(A)** radial carpal bone, **(B)** intermediate carpal bone, **(C)** ulnar carpal bone, **(D)** 2nd carpal bone, **(E)** 3rd carpal bone, **(F)** 4th carpal bone.

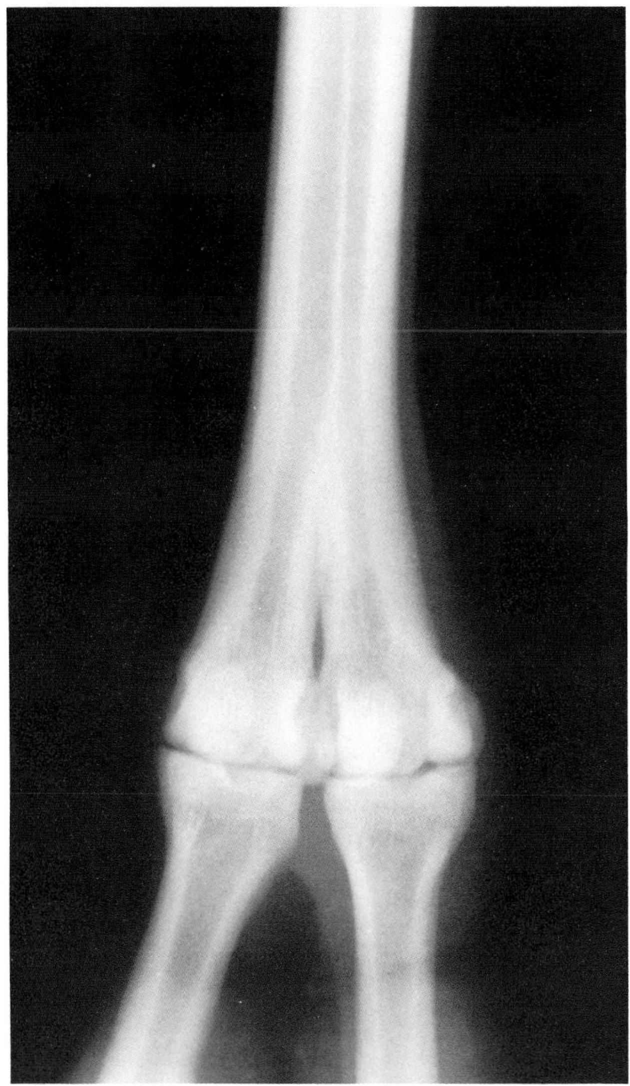

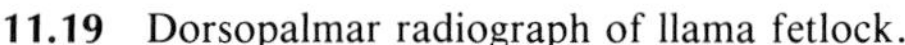

11.19 Dorsopalmar radiograph of llama fetlock.

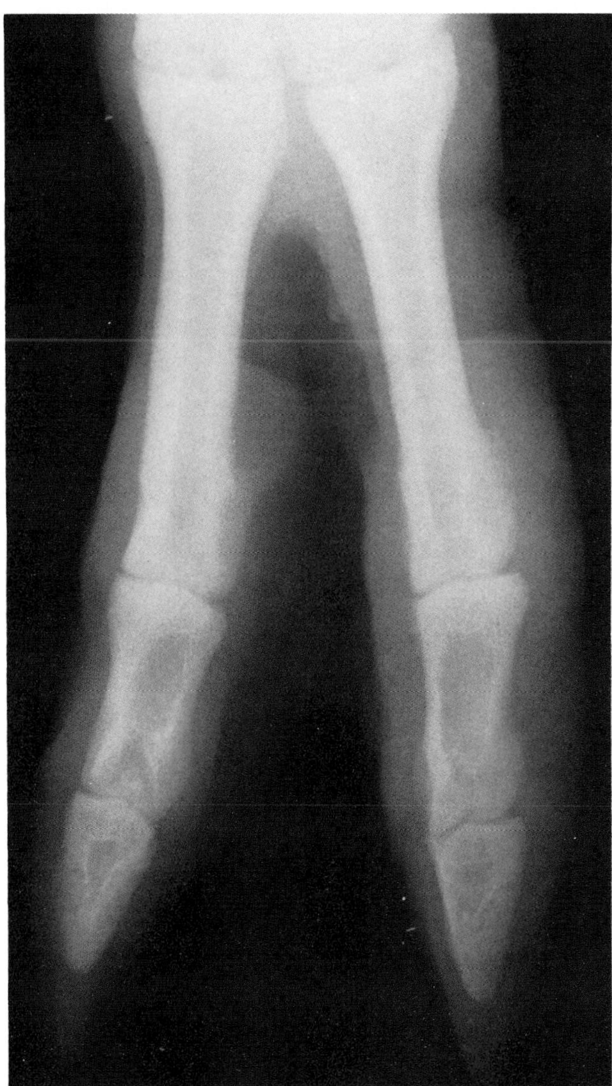

11.20 Dorsopalmar radiograph of llama pastern and foot.

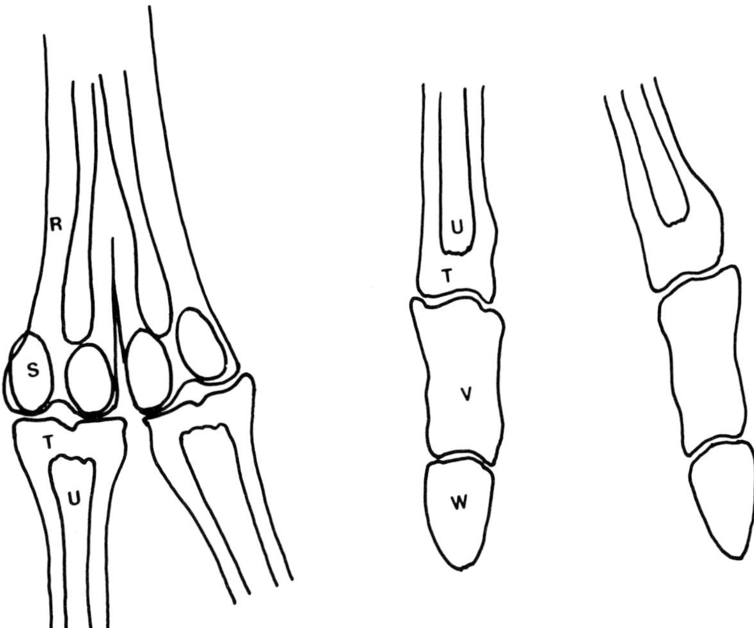

11.21 Diagram of the fetlock and phalanges: **(R)** metatarsus, **(S)** sesamoid bone, **(T)** P-1, **(U)** marrow cavity of P-1, **(V)** P-2, **(W)** P-3.

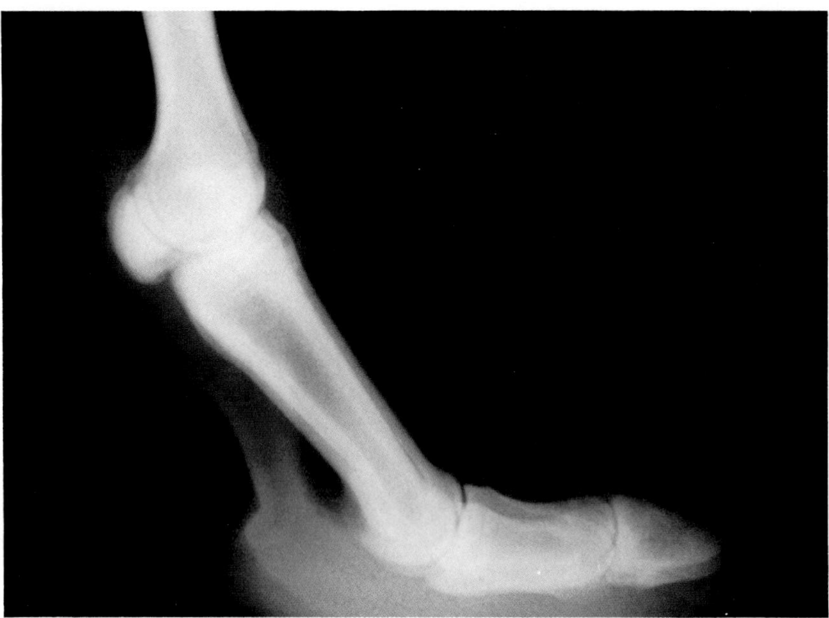

11.22 Lateral radiograph of llama fetlock and phalanges.

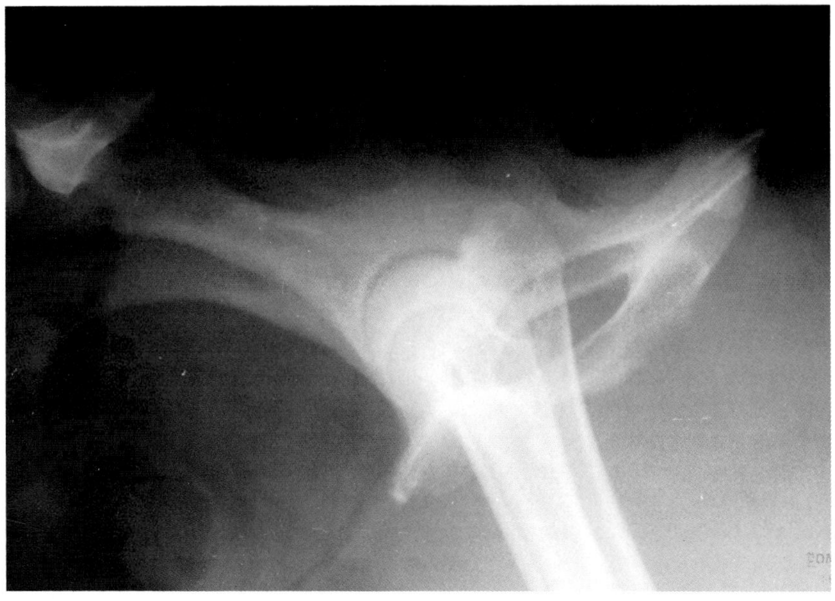

11.23 Lateral radiograph of llama pelvis and hip.

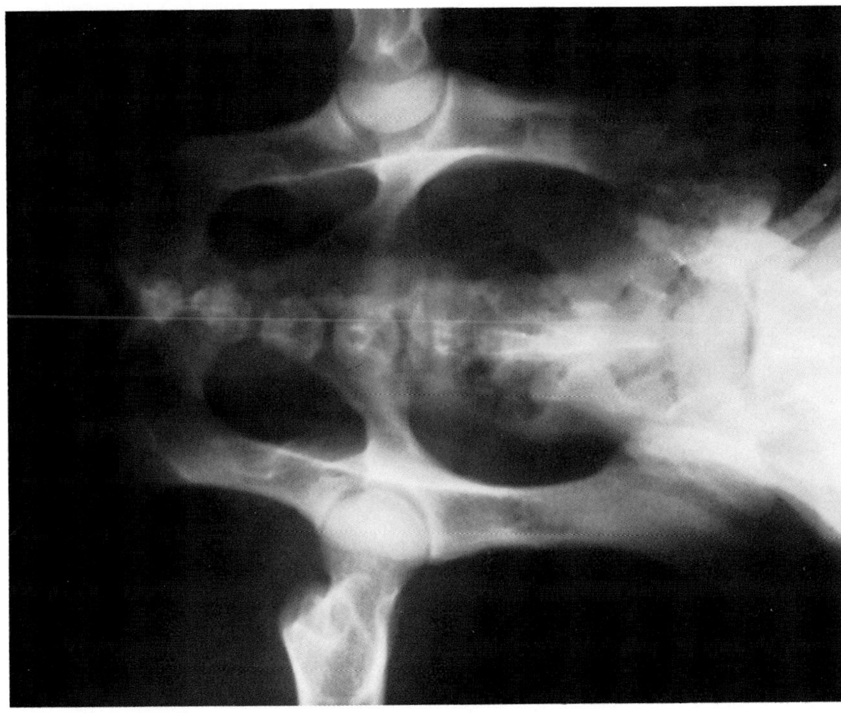

11.24 Dorsoventral radiograph of llama pelvis and hips.

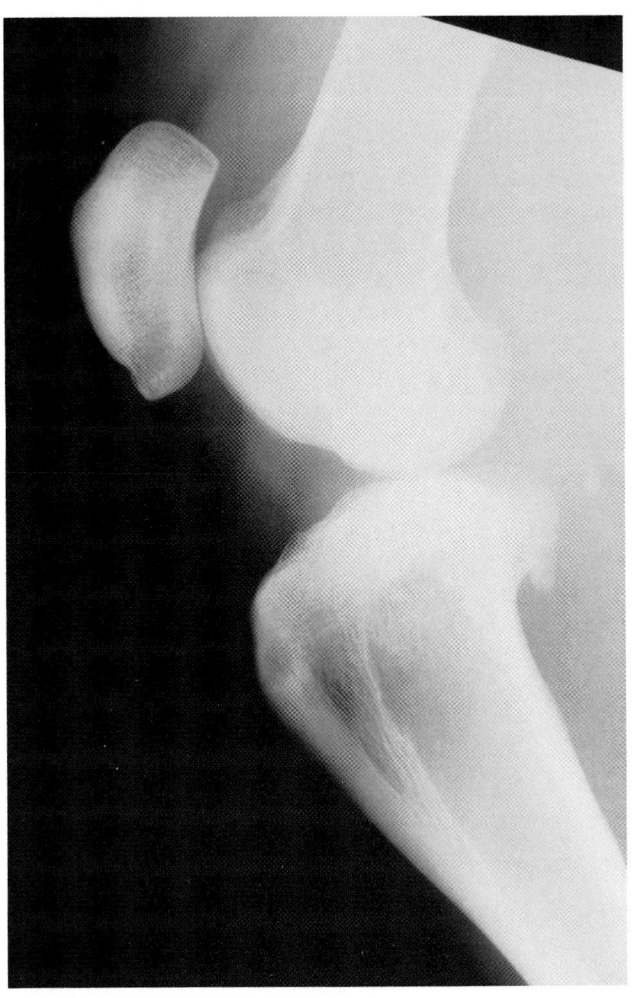

11.25 Lateral radiograph of llama stifle (patella in normal position).

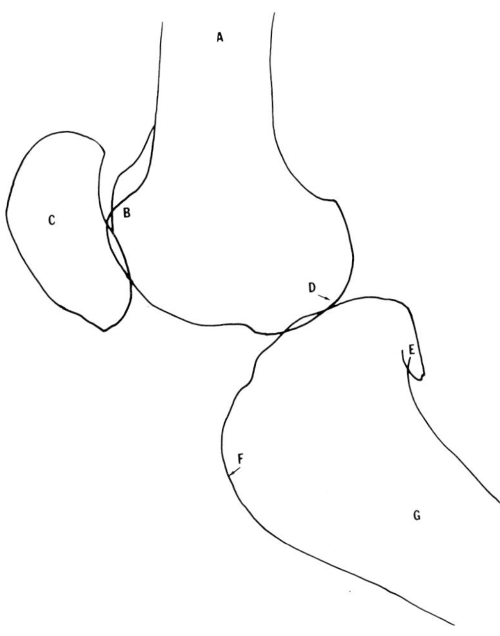

11.26 Diagram of Figure 11.25: **(A)** femur, **(B)** femoral trochlea, **(C)** patella, **(D)** femoral condyle, **(E)** fibula, **(F)** tibial crest, **(G)** tibia.

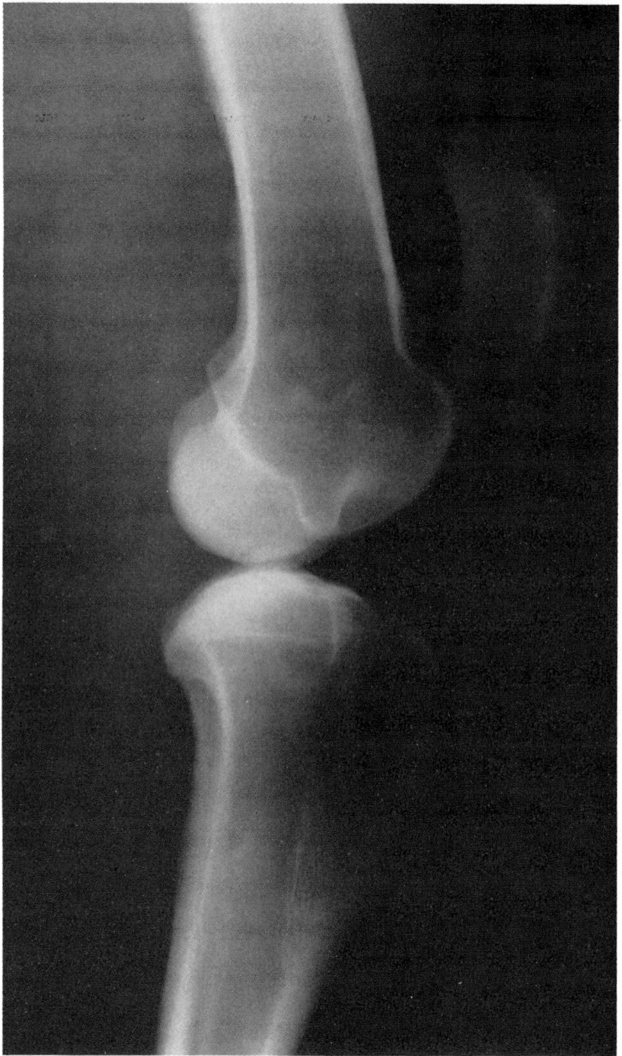

11.27 Lateral radiograph of llama stifle (patella riding too high on trochlea).

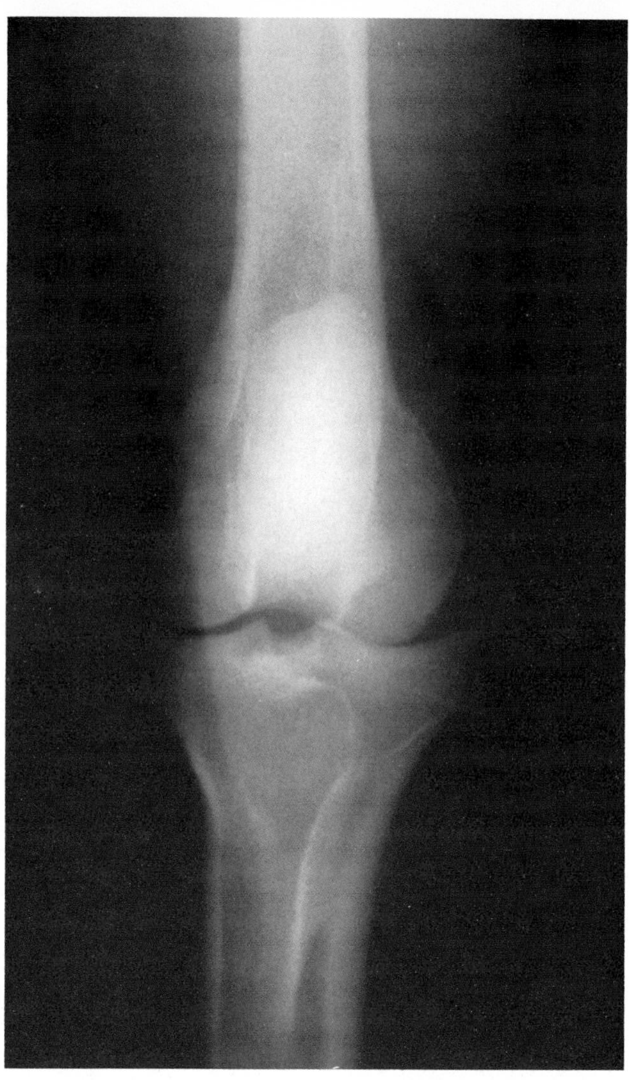

11.29 Craniocaudal radiograph of llama stifle.

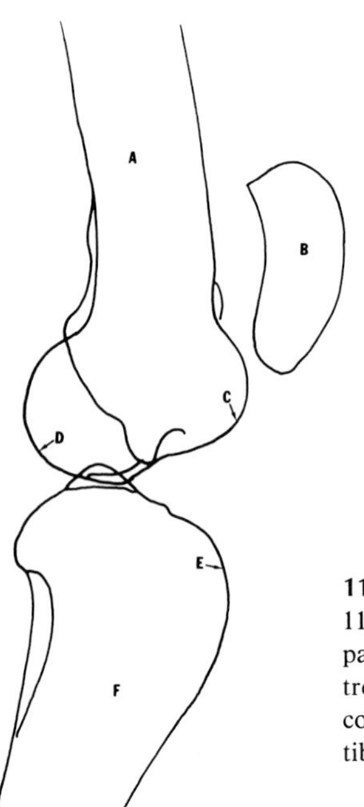

11.28 Diagram of Figure 11.27: **(A)** femur, **(B)** patella, **(C)** femoral trochlea, **(D)** femoral condyle, **(E)** tibial crest, **(F)** tibia.

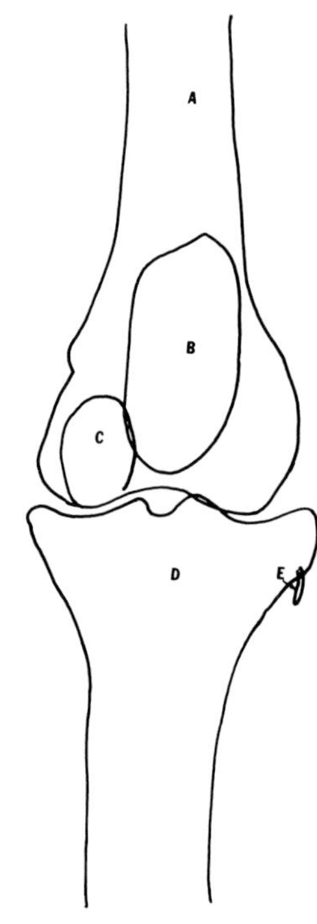

11.30 Diagram of Figure 11.29: **(A)** femur, **(B)** patella, **(C)** medial condyle of femur, **(D)** tibia, **(E)** fibula.

The relationship of the tarsal bones to the tibia and metatarsus is unique (Figs. 11.31–11.34). The lower limb articulations are similar to those of the forelimb. Figures 11.35–11.51 illustrate growth centers on neonate llamas.

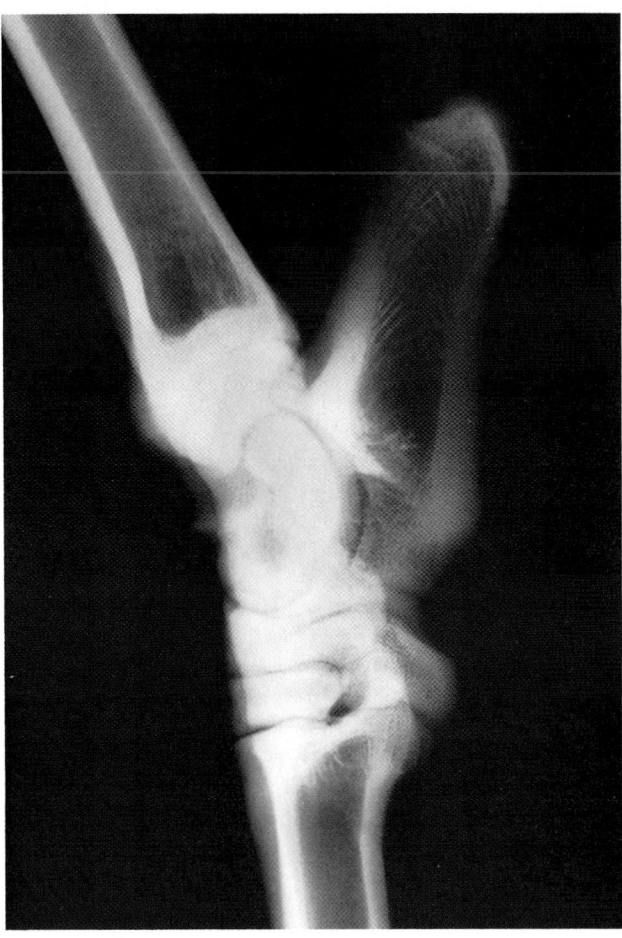

11.31 Lateral radiograph of a mature llama tarsus.

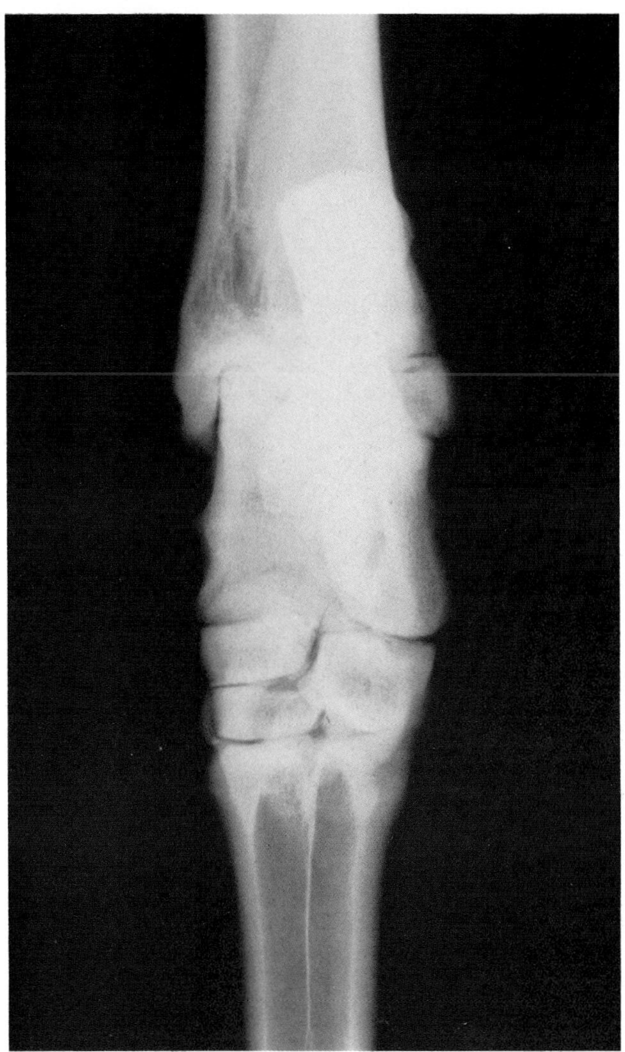

11.33 Dorsoplantar radiograph of a mature llama tarsus.

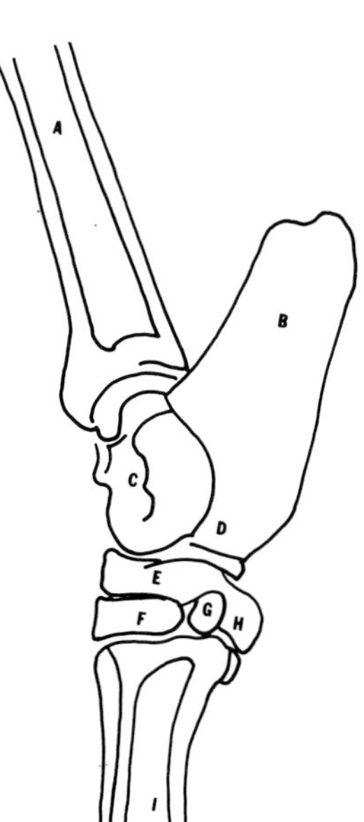

11.32 Diagram of Figure 11.31: **(A)** tibia, **(B)** tuber calcis, **(C)** tibial tarsal bone (talus), **(D)** fibular tarsal bone (calcaneus), **(E)** central tarsal bone, **(F)** 2nd and 3rd tarsal bones, **(G)** 1st tarsal bone, **(H)** 4th tarsal bone.

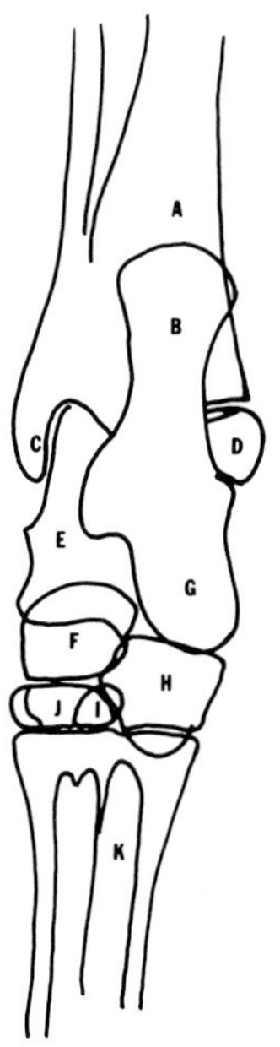

11.34 Diagram of Figure 11.33: **(A)** tibia, **(B)** tuber calcis, **(C)** lateral malleolus (distal tip of fibula) and medial malleolus, **(E)** tibial tarsal bone (talus), **(F)** central tarsal bone, **(G)** fibular tarsal bone (calcaneus), **(H)** 4th tarsal bone, **(I)** 1st tarsal bone, **(J)** 2nd and 3rd tarsal bones.

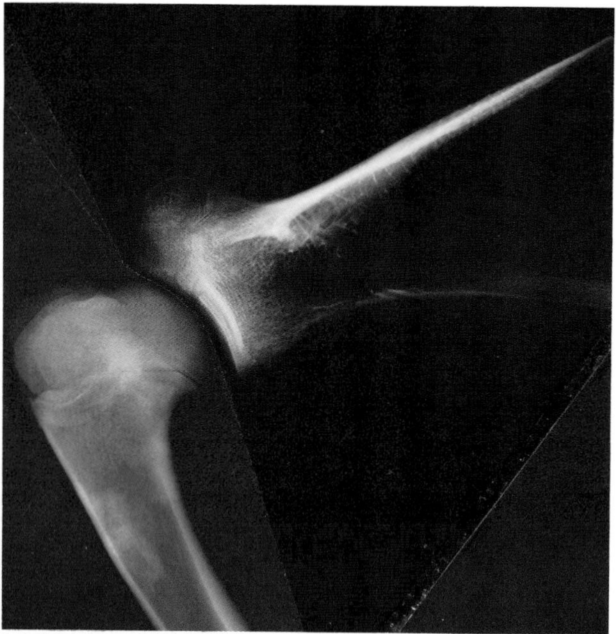

11.35 Lateral radiograph of neonate llama shoulder.

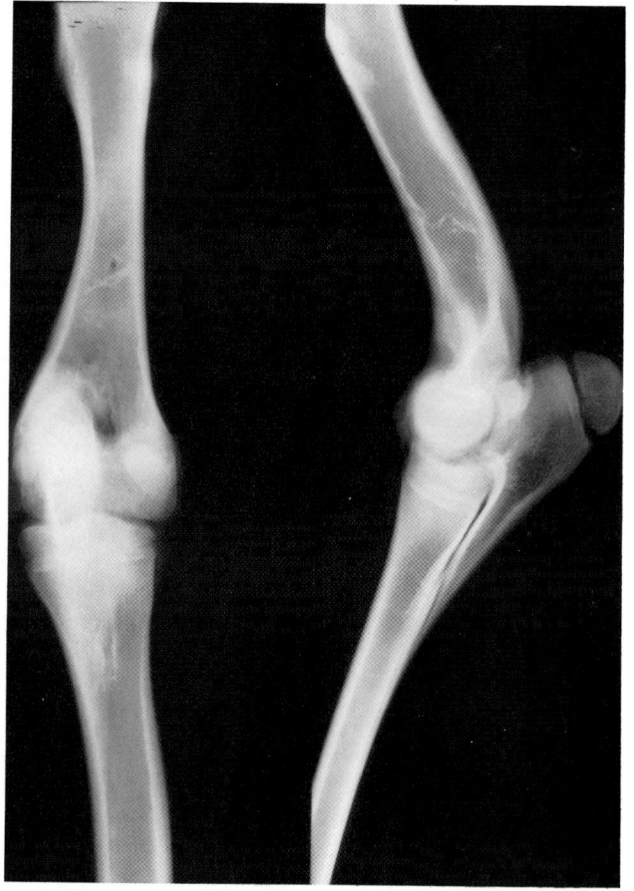

11.37 Lateral and craniocaudal radiographs of neonate llama elbow.

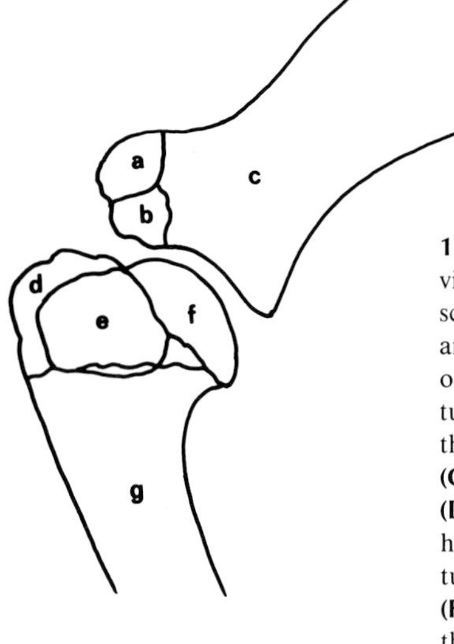

11.36 Diagram of lateral view of neonate llama scapulohumeral articulation: **(A)** epiphysis of the supraglenoid tubercle, **(B)** epiphysis of the cranial glenoid cavity, **(C)** neck of the scapula, **(D)** lateral tuberosity of the humerus, **(E)** medial tuberosity of the humerus, **(F)** proximal epiphysis of the humerus, **(G)** diaphysis of the humerus.

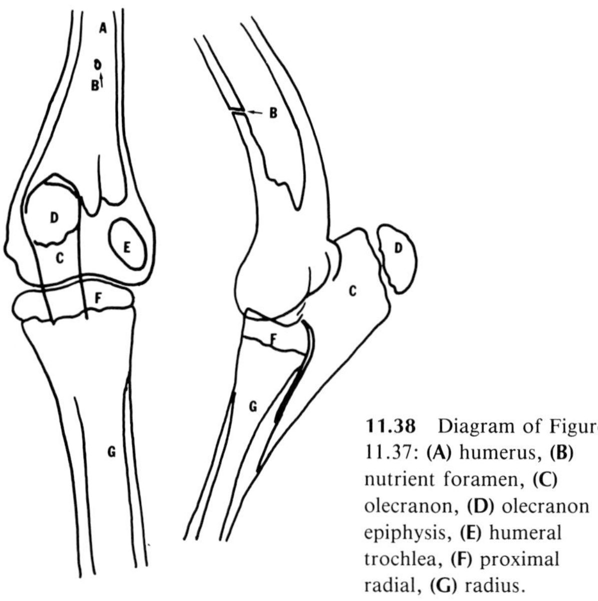

11.38 Diagram of Figure 11.37: **(A)** humerus, **(B)** nutrient foramen, **(C)** olecranon, **(D)** olecranon epiphysis, **(E)** humeral trochlea, **(F)** proximal radial, **(G)** radius.

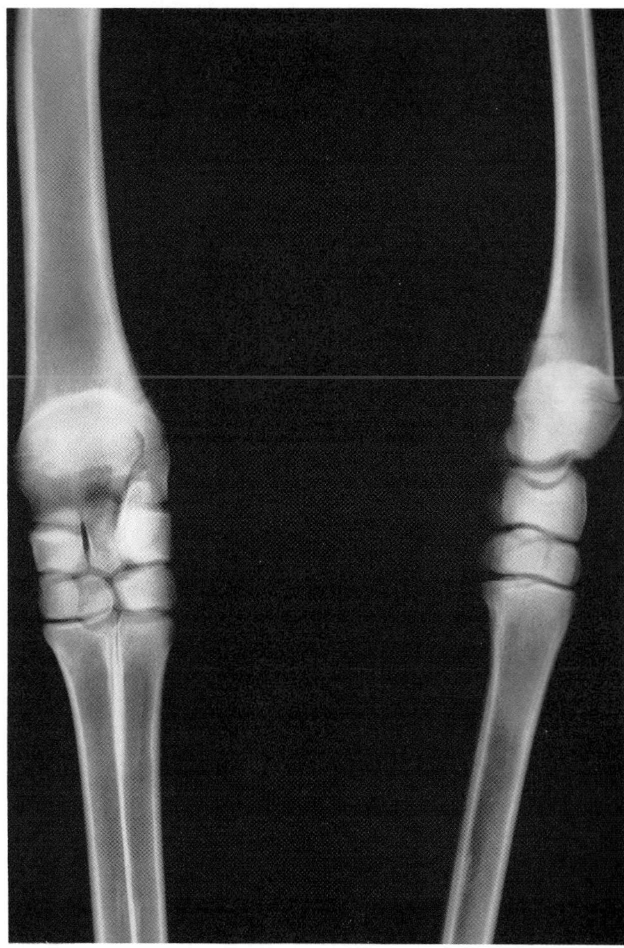

11.39 Lateral and dorsopalmar radiographs of neonate llama carpus.

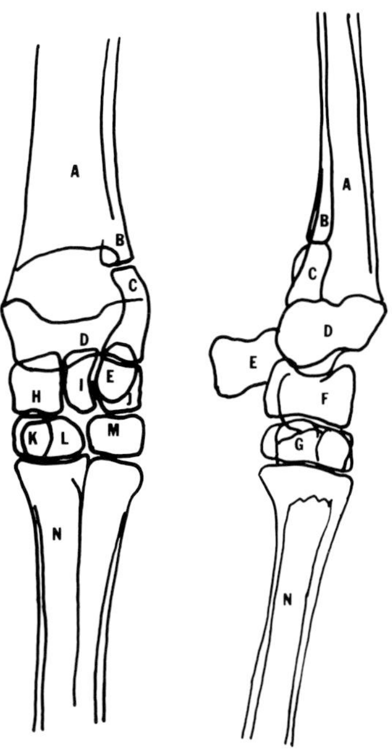

11.40 Diagram of Figure 11.39: **(A)** radius, **(B)** ulna, **(C)** ulnar epiphysis, **(D)** radial epiphysis, **(E)** accessory carpal bone, **(F)** combined ulnar, intermediate, and radial carpal bones, **(G)** combined 2nd, 3rd, and 4th carpal bones, **(H)** radial carpal bone, **(I)** intermediate carpal bone, **(J)** ulnar carpal bone, **(K)** 2nd carpal bone, **(L)** 3rd carpal bone, **(M)** 4th carpal bone, **(N)** metatarsus.

Radiographic Technique

Table 11.1 lists techniques used to obtain the foregoing radiographs. The film was 3-M, XDL general-purpose radiographic film in Kodak Lamex regular screen cassettes. The focal film distance was 100 cm (40 in.) and the exposure 1/10 sec.

Table 11.1. Radiographic technique used on adult llamas

Region	MAS	KVP	Approximate thickness in animals 115–127 kg(cm)
Head			
L-rostral	100	62	9
L-caudal	100	70	15
DV-rostral	100	70	13
DV-caudal	100	72	18
Vertebrae			
Cervical			
L	200	80	10
DV	100	66	15
Thoracic			
L	100	80	29
Lumbar			
L	200	84	23
DV	200	96	
Pelvis			
L	200	96	30
DV	200	96	30
Articulations			
Scapulohumeral	100	68	34
			23
Humeral-radioulnar			
L	100	66	9
DP	100	66	13
Carpus			
L	100	52	8
DPL	100	52	9
Metacarpal phalangeal	100	50	
Coxofemoral-DV	200	96	30
Femorotibial			
L	100	64	13
DPL	100	64	20
Tarsus			
L	100	50	7
DPL	100	68	9
Thorax–soft tissue	100	76	38

Note: L = lateral; DV = dorsoventral; DP = dorsopalmar; DPL = dorsoplantar.

MUSCULOSKELETAL DISORDERS

Congenital disorders of the musculoskeletal system are discussed in Chapter 22 and include angular limb deformities, choanal atresia, facial deformities, shortened long limb bones, arthrogryposis, polydactylae, syndactylae, medial luxation of the patella, dysgenesis of the maxilla and mandible, hemivertebrae, vertical talus, and contracted tendons. Nutritional myopathy and calcium-phosphorus-vitamin D imbalance are discussed in Chapter 2.

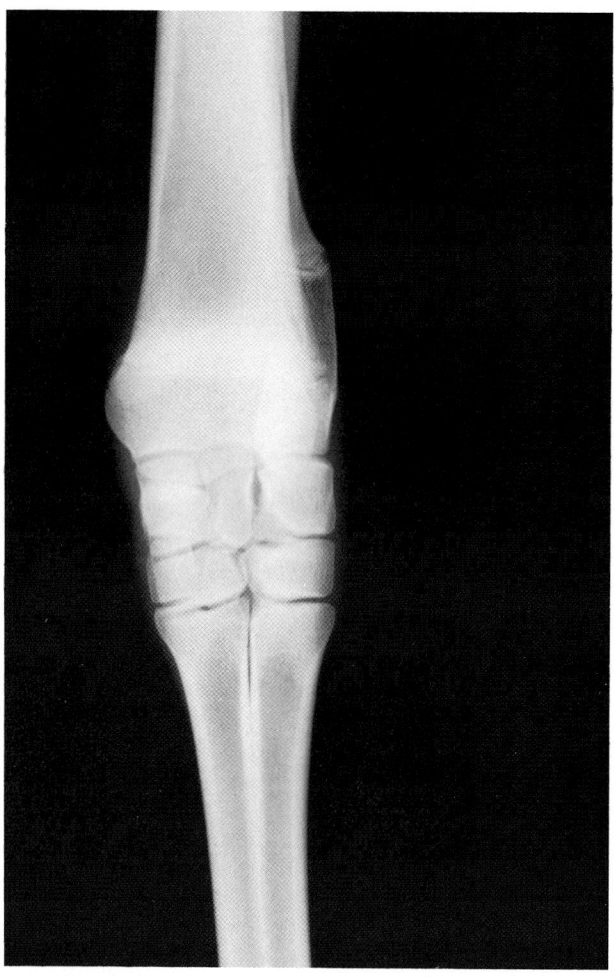

11.41 Dorsopalmar radiograph of a 6-week-old llama carpus.

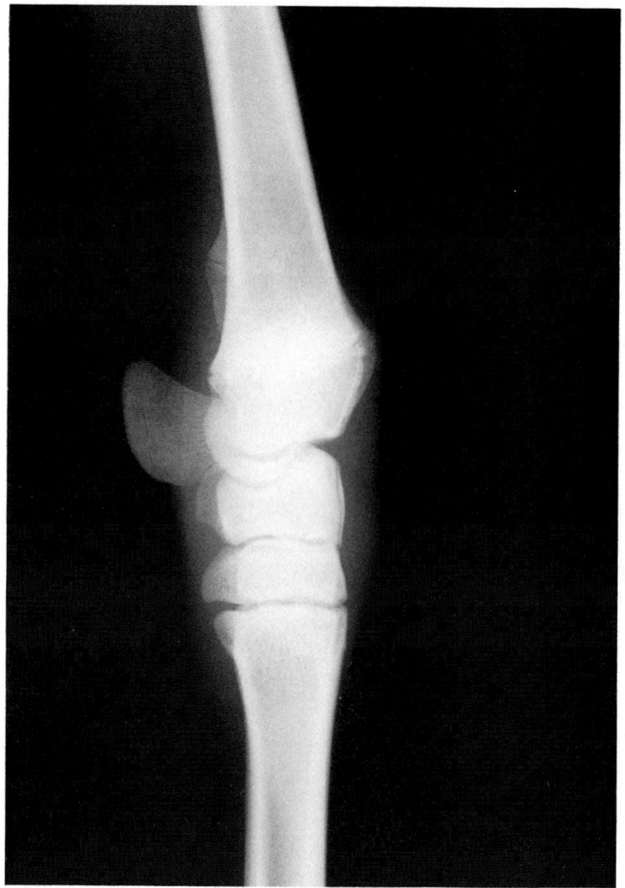

11.42 Lateral radiograph of a 6-week-old llama carpus.

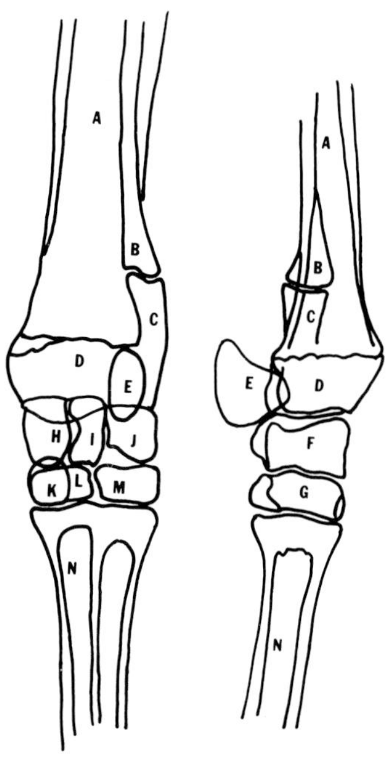

11.43 Diagram of Figures 11.41, 11.42: **(A)** radius, **(B)** ulna, **(C)** ulnar epiphysis, **(D)** radial epiphysis, **(E)** accessory carpal bone, **(F)** combined ulnar, intern, and radial carpal bones, **(G)** combined 2nd, 3rd, and 4th carpal bones, **(H)** radial carpal bone, **(I)** intermediate carpal bone, **(J)** ulnar carpal bone, **(K)** 2nd carpal bone, **(L)** 3rd carpal bone, **(M)** 4th carpal bone, **(N)** metatarsus.

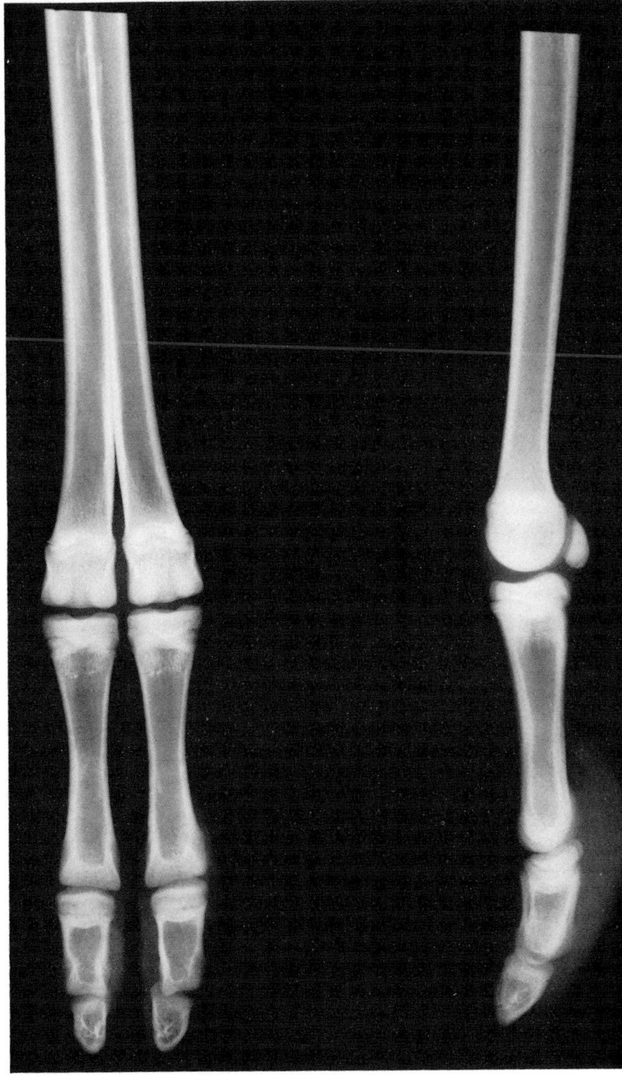

11.44 Lateral and dorsopalmar radiographs of neonate llama fetlock and foot.

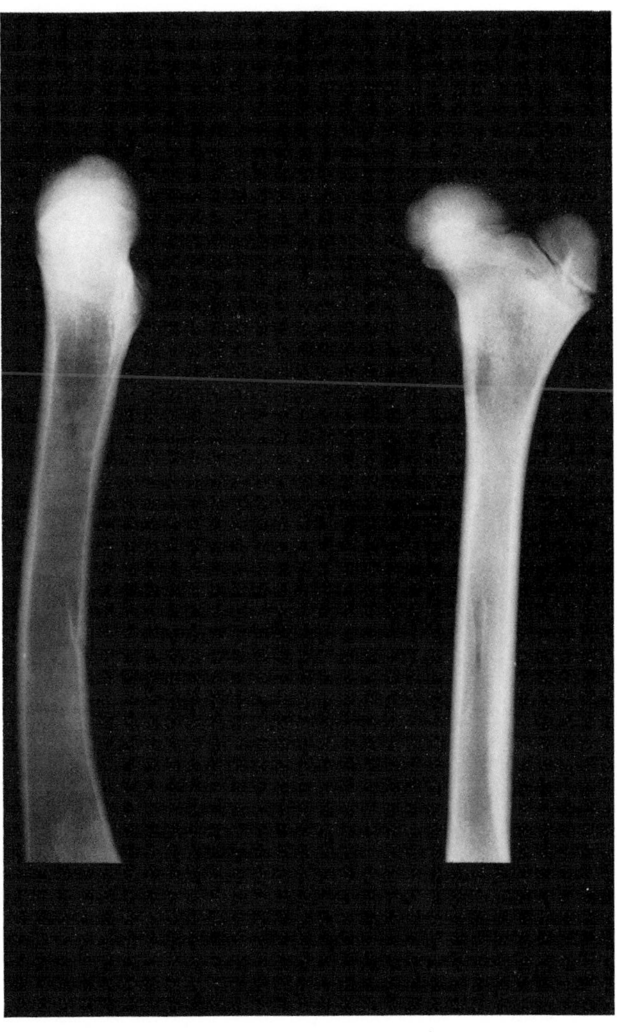

11.46 Craniocaudal and lateral radiographs of neonate llama proximal femur.

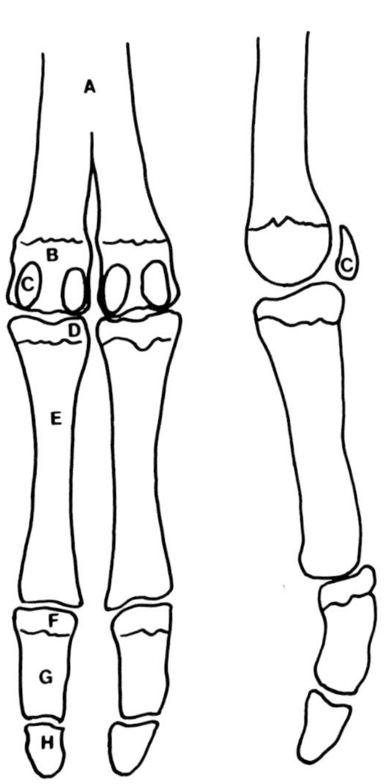

11.45 Diagram of Figure 11.44: (A) diaphysis of metacarpus, (B) distal epiphysis of metacarpus, (C) sesamoid bone, (D) proximal epiphysis of P-1, (E) diaphysis of P-1, (F) proximal epiphysis of P-2, (G) P-3, (H) P-3.

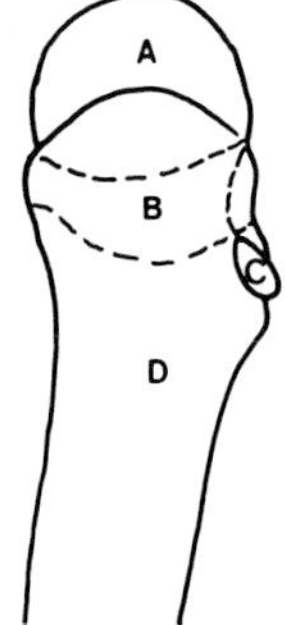

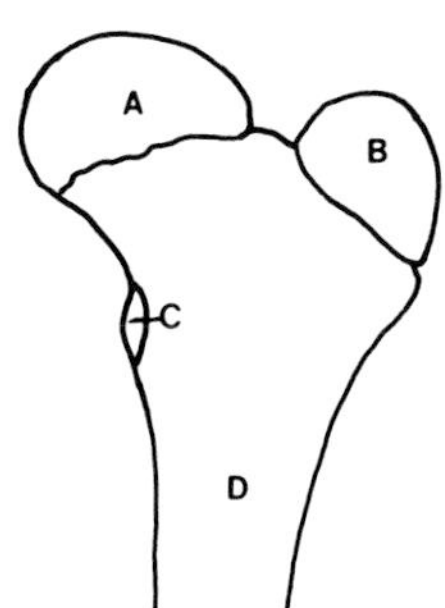

11.47 Diagram of Figure 11.46: (A) proximal epiphysis of femur, (B) trochanter major, (C) trochanter minor, (D) diaphysis of femur.

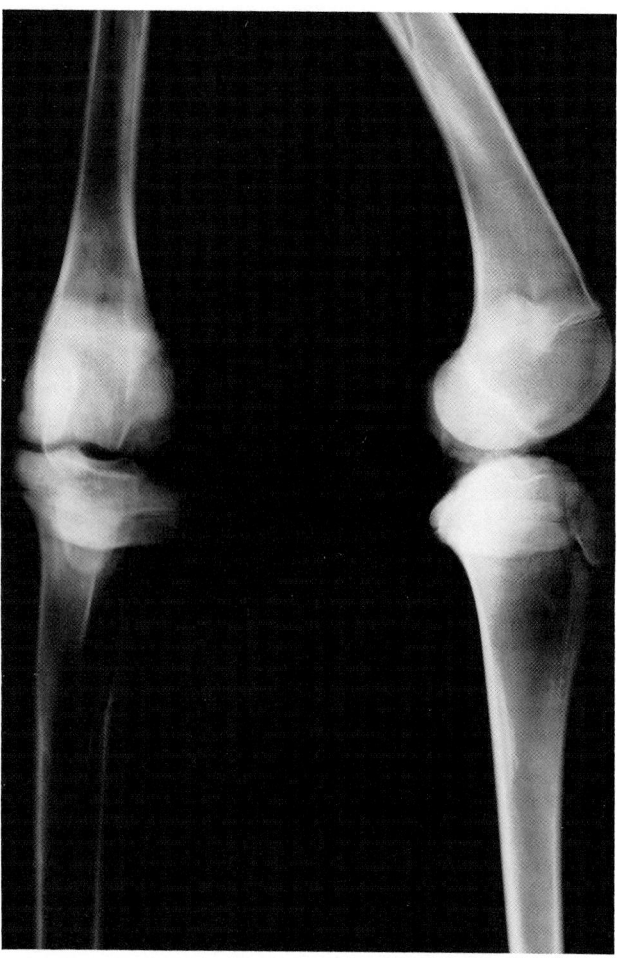

11.48 Craniocaudal and lateral radiographs of neonate llama stifle.

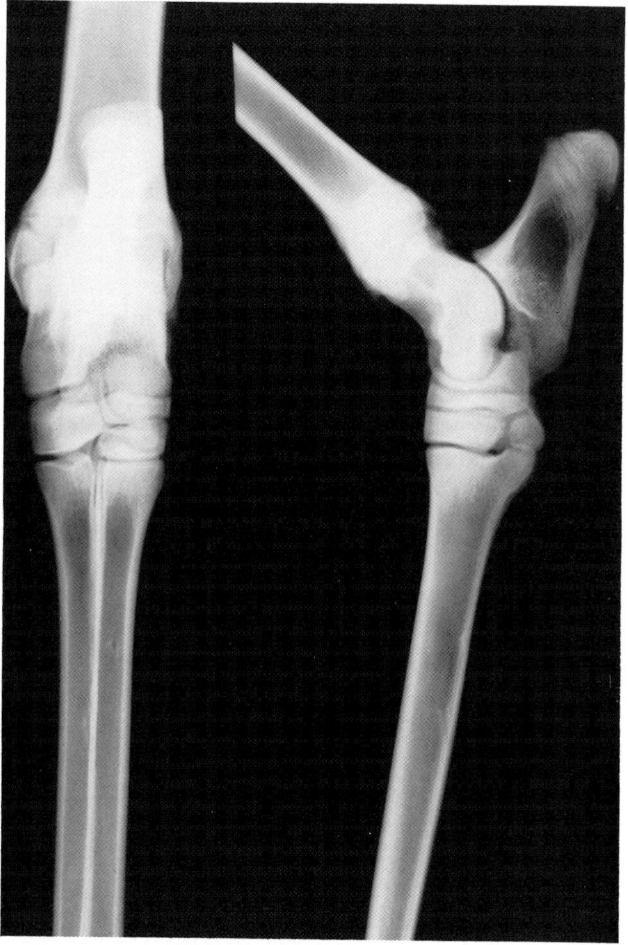

11.50 Dorsoplantar and lateral radiograph of neonate llama tarsus.

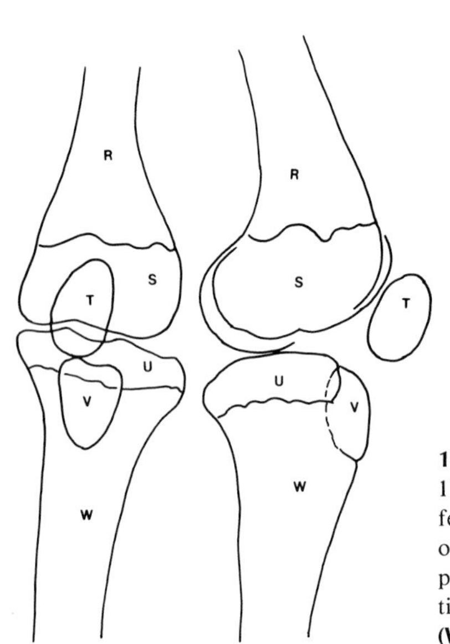

11.49 Diagram of Figure 11.48: **(R)** diaphysis of femur, **(S)** distal epiphysis of femur, **(T)** patella, **(U)** proximal epiphysis of tibia, **(V)** tibial tuberosity, **(W)** diaphysis of tibia.

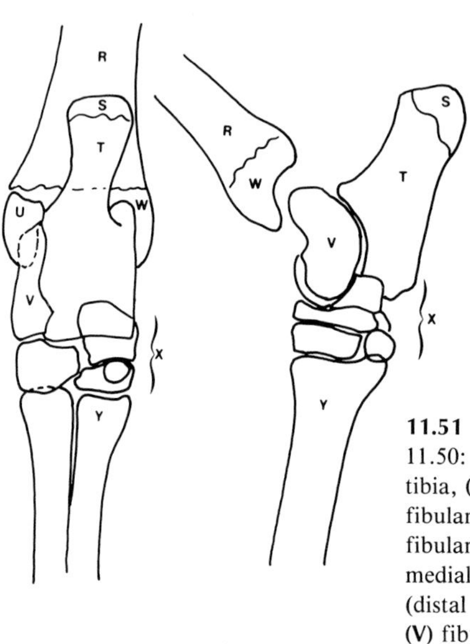

11.51 Diagram of Figure 11.50: **(R)** diaphysis of tibia, **(S)** epiphysis of fibular tarsal bone, **(T)** fibular tarsal bone, **(U)** medial malleolus of tibia (distal epiphysis of fibula), **(V)** fibular tarsal bone, **(W)** distal epiphysis of tibia, **(X)** tarsal bones, **(Y)** metatarsus.

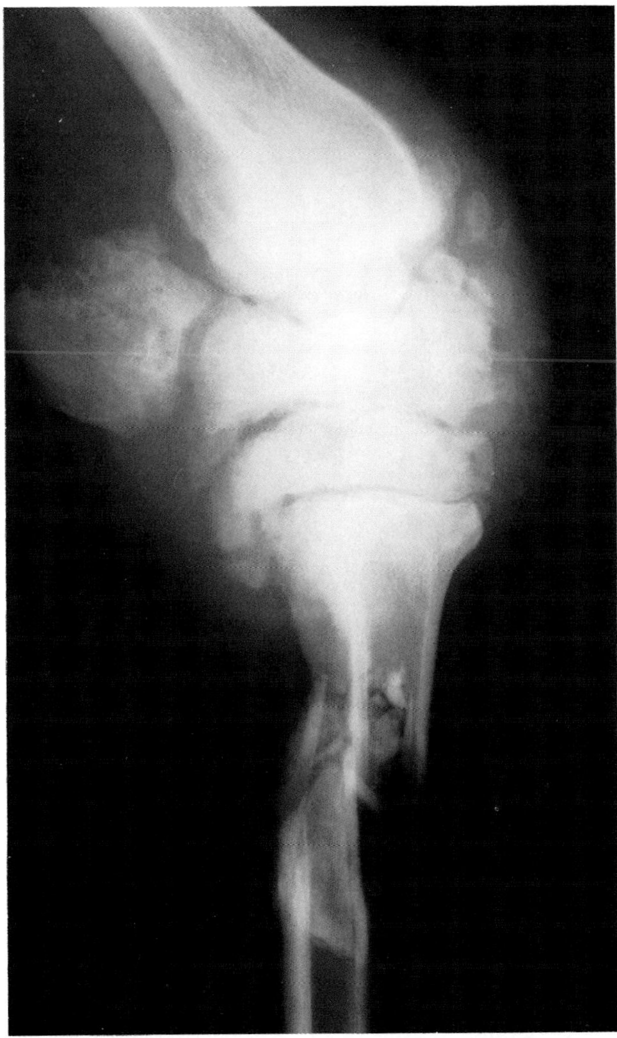

11.52 Radiograph of chronic osteoarthritis of carpus and recent metacarpal fracture.

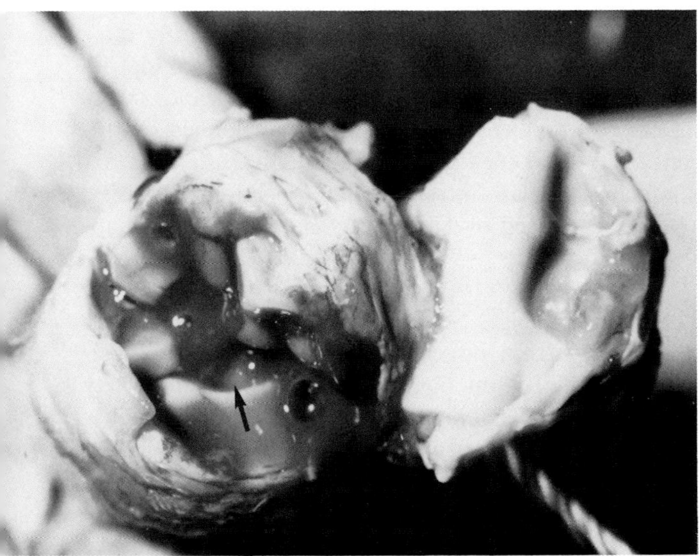

11.53 Suppurative carpitis.

Arthritis

No unique arthritic conditions have been reported in lamoids. Traumatic arthritis has been diagnosed in the author's practice. Degenerative osteoarthritis may be a sequel to angular limb deformity (Fig. 11.52) or result from other unknown etiologies. Infectious arthritis may follow omphalophlebitis or lacerations of the joint capsule or be caused by opportunistic bacteria (Fig. 11.53). No specific infectious arthritides have been reported.

Vertebral Fractures

Fractures occur in lamoids as they do in all species (13, 20) (see Chap. 6).

ETIOLOGY. Vertebral fractures are uncommon in lamoids. Probable cause of trauma to the cervical vertebrae and associated ligaments is a blow to the neck or a struggle against restraint when first being haltered and tied. Lumbar vertebral fractures may be caused by large animals rearing up and striking down on the back during intermale aggression or dominance behavior. A large breeding male may injure a small female as he attempts to force her to recumbency.

CLINICAL SIGNS. Variable degrees of ataxia, incoordination, paresis, and paralysis are observed in trauma that involves the vertebral canal and produces compression on the spinal cord or emerging nerves. Fractures of the articular facets of the cervical vertebrae (Figs. 11.54, 11.55) cause the head to be held in an abnormal position. There may be a palpable deformity at the fracture site and evidence of pain on digital pressure. Trauma to the intervertebral ligaments, intervertebral discs, and contiguous muscles produce signs indistinguishable from those caused by osseous lesions.

DIAGNOSIS. Radiography is required for definitive diagnosis. Figures 11.56 and 11.57 illustrate a luxation of the intervertebral disc. A complete fracture of the body of C-2 (Fig. 11.58) resulted in total paralysis, necessitating euthanasia.

MANAGEMENT. Vertebral fractures in large animals are difficult to manage. The cervical vertebrae of lamoids have no flat surface suitable for plating. A neck and body fiberglass cast was applied to a llama with an articular facet fracture of C-4, but euthanasia was elected by the client before evaluation of the cast could be made (Fig. 11.55).

Pressure on the spinal cord may be treated with steroids and analgesic antiinflammatory agents. Activ-

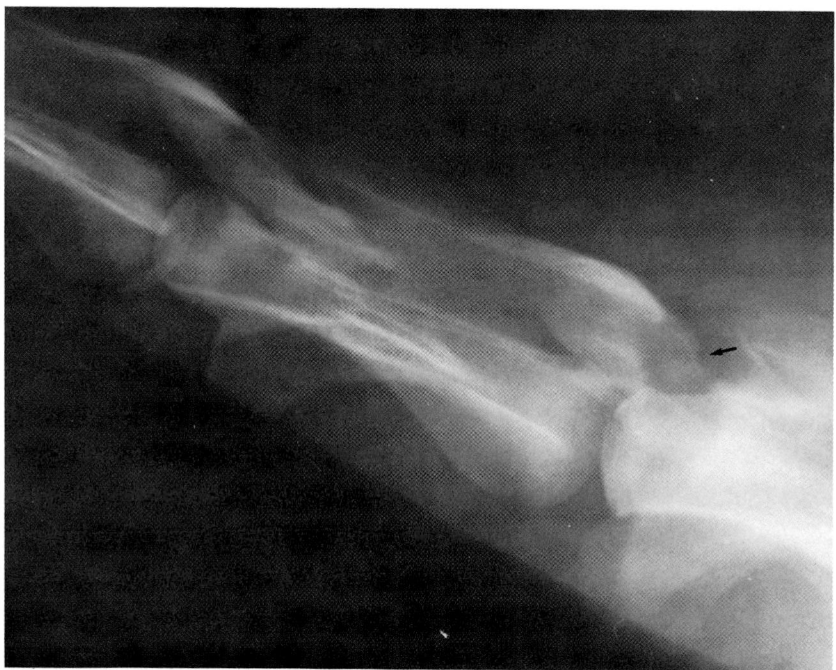

11.54 Radiograph of fracture of articular facet of C-6.

ity must be restricted, but lamoids do not tolerate slinging well.

Spondylosis

Spondylosis is periarticular hyperostosis with potential bridging between the vertebrae. Extensive spondylosis was seen at necropsy in a 21-year-old female llama (Fig. 11.59). Figures 11.60 and 11.61 are radiographs taken postmortem. This llama also had degenerative carpitis and thus was lame and spent most of the time in sternal recumbency. Whether the spondylosis contributed to reluctance to ambulate is unknown.

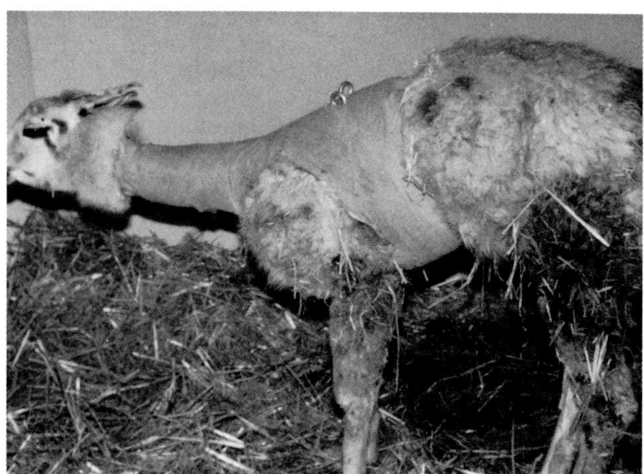

11.55 Body and neck fiberglass cast applied to fix fracture of an articular facet of C-6.

Spondylosis has been found as an incidental lesion in llamas as young as 9 years of age.

Myopathy

ETIOLOGY. Nutritional myopathy is discussed in Chapter 2. The cellular necrosis caused by nutritional myopathy cannot be differentiated from the lesions of exertional myopathy. Although llamas are usually not willing to exert themselves beyond endurance as pack animals or in a capture/restraint situation, an injured llama may overexert in a struggle to rise.

Muscle necrosis is frequently diagnosed on gross necropsy. Such a diagnosis should be made only after careful evaluation, because postmortem autolysis occurs quickly, giving muscles a whitish appearance. Muscle necrosis may ensue as a sequel to prolonged recumbency of a weakened llama (ischemic necrosis) or from a reaction to an intramuscular injection. Parasitic myositis is caused by *Sarcocystis aucheniae* (see Chap. 8).

CLINICAL SIGNS. Varying degrees of paresis or paralysis may be seen. Muscles may be hot, swollen, and painful on palpation. Chronic lesions may cause a loss of flexibility and resiliency of the muscle.

A common syndrome has been described as the "downer llama," in which the animal refuses to rise and is frequently hyperthermic. Prolonged recumbency in a lamoid prevents cooling via the thermal window (see Chap. 9). Muscle biopsies frequently indicate a mild to

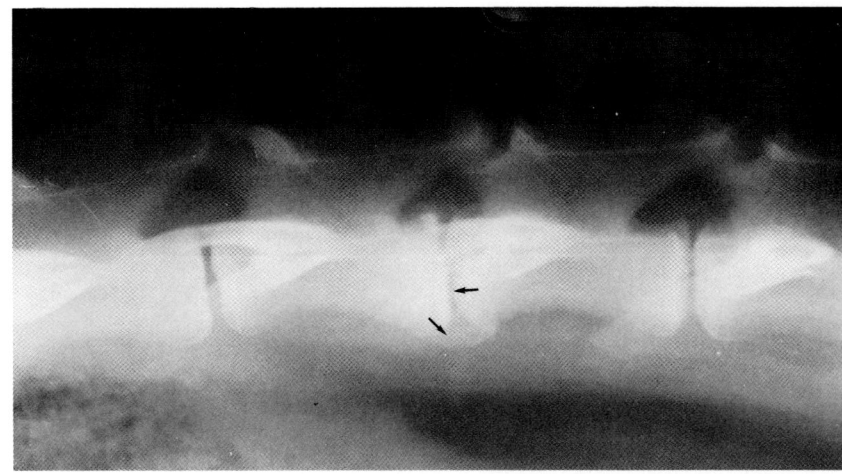

11.56 Lateral radiograph of lumbar area with chronic luxation of the intervertebral disc.

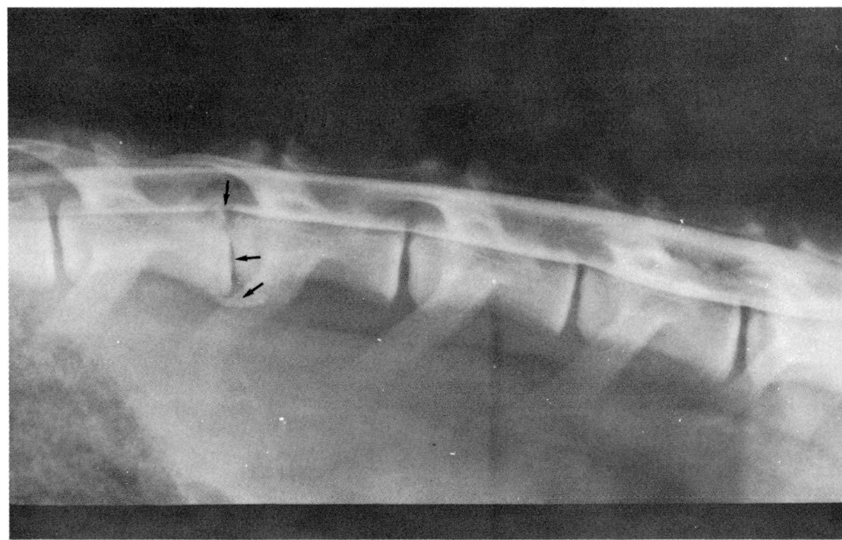

11.57 Lateral radiograph of lumbar area with contrast media in the subarachnoid space. Compare with Figure 11.56.

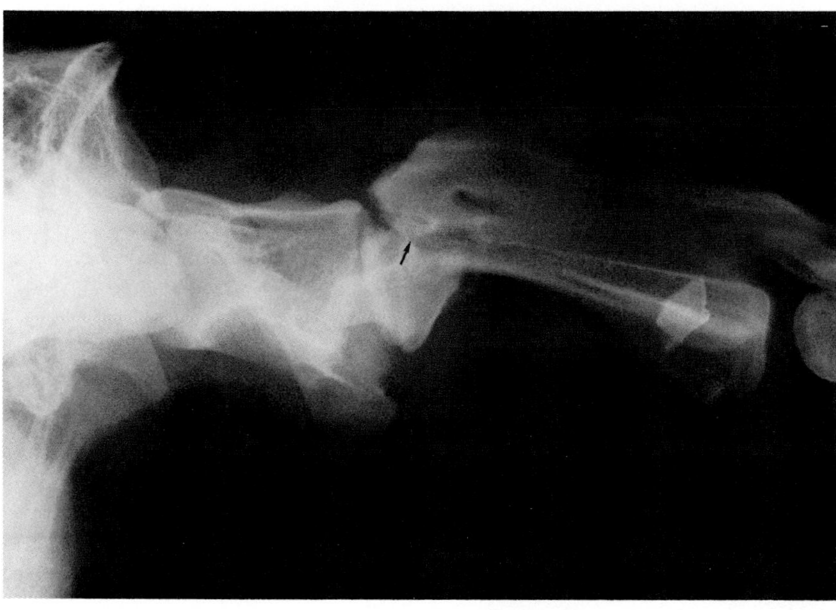

11.58 Radiograph of fracture of the dens of C-2.

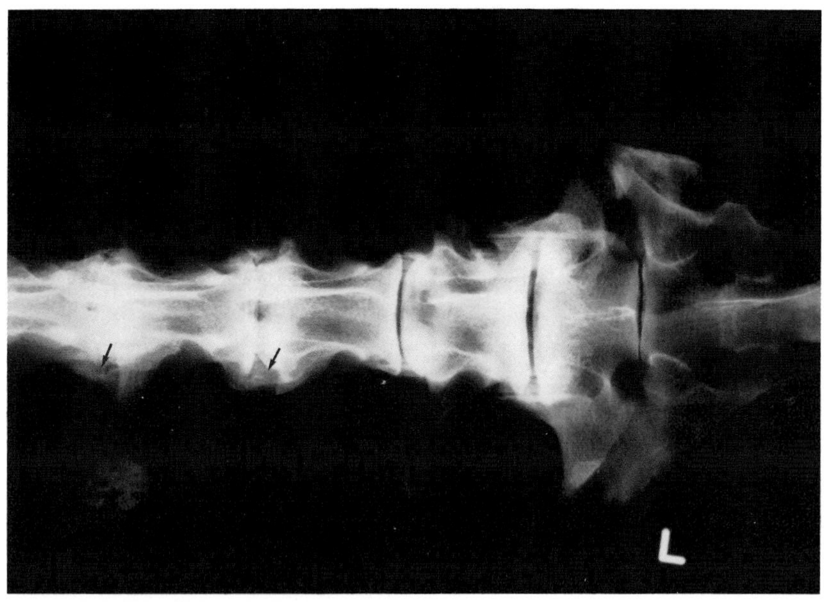

11.59 Dorsoventral radiograph of lumbosacral spine with spondylosis.

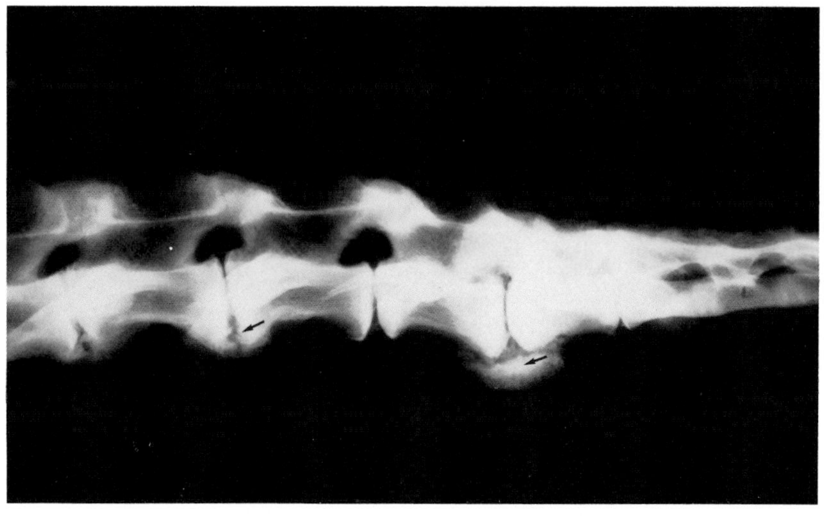

11.60 Lateral radiograph of lumbosacral spondylosis.

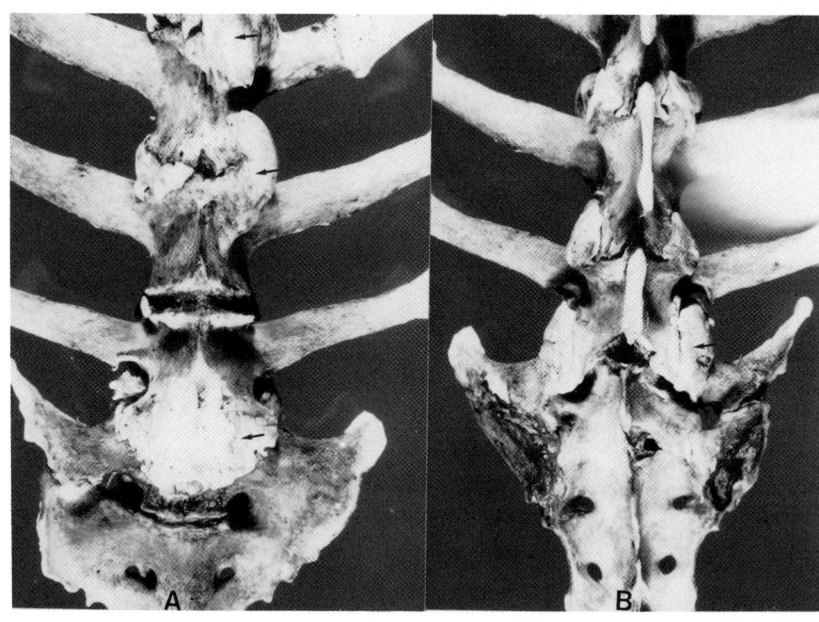

11.61 Spondylosis of llama lumbosacrum: **(A)** ventral view, **(B)** dorsal view.

moderate nonspecific myositis. Some of these animals die despite intensive therapy and support. Few other lesions have been seen at necropsy.

DIAGNOSIS. Muscle-specific serum enzymes may be elevated. However, prolonged recumbency and repeated intramuscular injections cause a mild to moderate elevation in serum enzymes. Diagnosis is made on the basis of clinical signs.

THERAPY. Nutritional myopathies may be prevented by appropriate use of selenium–vitamin E preparations, but these are not useful for therapy once the muscle has necrosed. Corticosteroid therapy is indicated for acute, noninfectious myositis. Hot packs applied over the affected muscles enhance circulation and healing. Physical therapy is appropriate, but exercises must be done gently.

Luxation of the Patella

ETIOLOGY. Both medial and lateral congenital patellar luxations have been diagnosed in llama crias. As in the horse, upward fixation of the patella also occurs, but with a different anatomic predisposition. Camelids have a single patellar ligament rather than the three ligaments of the horse. Fixation in the llama likely occurs when the patellar ligament is stretched or the bones of the rear limb are overly straight. This is accompanied by a stretching or rupture of the medial or lateral femoropatellar ligament, which allows the patella to move medially or laterally to catch the dorsal aspect of the ridges of the trochlea. Acquired medial and lateral patellar luxation usually follows a traumatic incident that ruptures the medial or lateral femoropatellar ligament.

Lamoids tend to have minimal angulation of the upper rear limb bones, but this may be exaggerated to produce a straight or post leg, which causes the patella to ride high on the trochlea. Trauma to the patellar ligament may cause weakening and stretching, which, in turn, allows the patella to ride higher. Such injuries have occurred when a llama attempted to jump a fence and the hind limbs failed to clear it. Stifle injuries may also occur as a result of twisting during chest butting episodes if one male catches the other slightly off balance. One llama jumped off a simulated bridge in an obstacle course of a show and traumatized the stifle.

CLINICAL SIGNS. Medial and lateral patellar luxation is evident on palpation. Lameness caused by pain or mechanical impairment is present. Congenital bilateral patellar luxation causes the cria to assume a crouched position, making ambulation difficult. Heat and swelling may be present. The various compartments of the stifle joint capsule may be distended, depending on the severity of the trauma.

If the patella is locked dorsally, the limb will be fixed in extension, and if forced to move, the llama must drag the limb (Fig. 11.62). With intermittent upward fixation, the signs may vary from an audible click as the patella momentarily locks during ambulation to a lock prolonged for a few seconds, followed by an exaggerated flexion of the limb as the lock is released. Lameness may be evident during periods of quiescence, depending on the cause of the upward riding of the patella.

DIAGNOSIS. Clinical signs and palpation are the primary means of diagnosis. Radiographs add little more than can be determined by palpation.

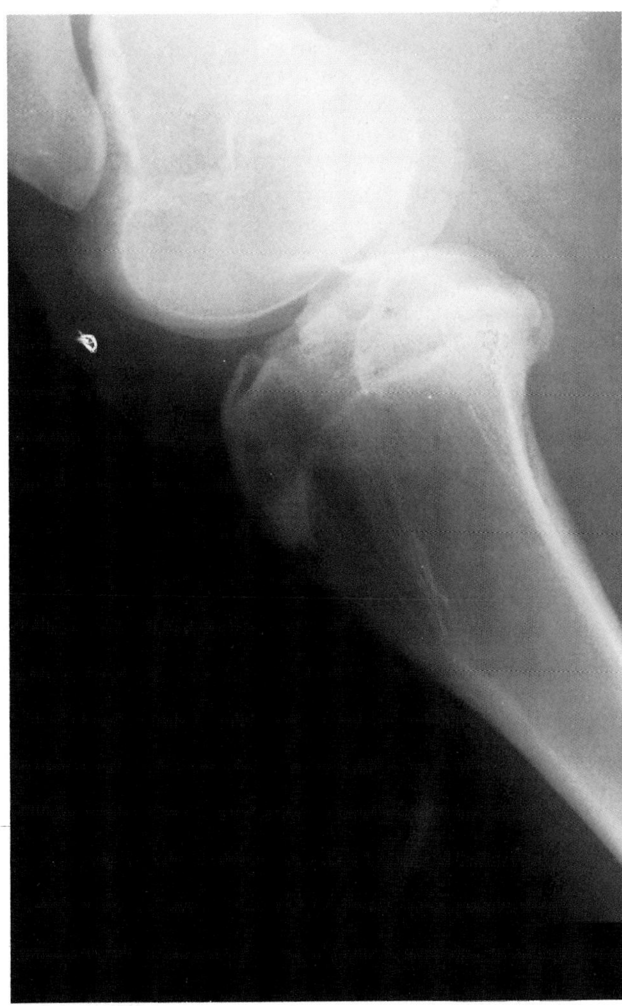

11.62 Lateral radiograph of upward subluxation of the patella.

TREATMENT. Upward fixation may be released by extending the limb fully while manipulating the patella. Mild upward fixation may be controlled by restricting activity to permit a stretched patellar ligament to heal. Surgical imbrication may be required in severe cases.

Acquired medial and lateral patellar luxations usually result from rupture of respective contralateral femoropatellar ligaments. Surgical correction may be necessary.

Tumors

Although only one osseous tumor has been reported (4), it is likely that, given time, all types may be diagnosed.

REFERENCES

1. Curaca Pena, A. A. 1970. (Determination of myohemoglobin in striated muscles of alpaca) Determinacion de miohemoglobina en musculo estriado de alpaca, *Lama pacos.* Arch. Inst. Biol. Andina 3:112–21.

2. Del Pozo, C. A. 1944. (Study of the bones of the head in the genus *Lama*) Estudio de la cabeza osea en el genero *Auchenia.* Rev. Univ. Cuzco 33(86):197–250.

3. ______. 1949. (The inferior posterior condilar tubercle in the genus *Auchenia*) La apofisis condilea postero inferior en el genero *Auchenia.* Asoc. Cient. Cuzco Bol. 1(1):64–66.

4. Fox, H. 1934. Fibroma of ulna in a llama. Rep. Penrose Res. Lab., pp. 17–26.

5. Fuentes, L. 1953a. (Contribution to the osteology of the alpaca) Contribucion a la osteologia de la alpaca, *Lama glama pacos.* Tesis, Fac. Med. Vet. (Lima), pp. 1–77.

6. ______. 1953b. (Contribution to the osteology of the alpaca) Contribucion a la osteologia de la alpaca, *Lama pacos.* Vet. Zootec. (Peru) 5(10):62–64.

7. Galotta, D. R., Freire, C. M., and Galotta, J. M. 1985. (Contribution to the anatomy of South American camelids. I. The digital cushions of the llama) Contributions a la anatomia de los camelidos sudamericanos I. Las almohadillas digitales la llama. Rev. Cienc. Agrar. 4(3, 4):5–13.

8. ______. 1986. (The digital cushions of the guanaco) Las almohadillas digitales del guanaco. Rev. Cienc. Agrar. 7(3, 4):28–36.

9. Galotta, D. R., Galotta, J. M., and Stover, E. 1985. (The quadrate plantar muscle of the llama) El musculo cuadrado plantar del llama. Rev. Cienc. Agrar. 6(3, 4):55–57.

10. Galotta, D. R., Stover, E., and Galotta, J. M. 1985. (Fusion of tarsal bones in a llama) Fusion de tarsianos en un llama. Rev. Cienc. Agrar. 6(3, 4):55–57.

11. Gulliver, G. 1842. Observations on the muscular fibers of the esophagus and heart of some vertebrate animals. Proc. Zool. Soc. Lond., vol. 63.

12. Manning, J. P. 1956. Fracture of the metacarpal bones in a llama. J. Am. Vet. Med. Assoc. 129:136.

13. Marelli, C. A. 1944. (Variations of the bones of the facial organs in the alpaca) Variaciones de los huesos del organo facial de la alpaca. Bol. Soc. Phys. (Buenos Aires).

14. Mohr, E. 1935. (The lamina of the bones of the New World camels) Die Hornplatten an den Beinen Neuweltlicher Kamele. Zool. Anz. 112:43–47.

15. Nunez, Q., and Sato Sato, A. 1960. (Superficial pectoral muscle of alpacas. Structure, origin, and insertion) Musculo pectoral superficial de alpacas. Estructura, origen y insercion. Rev. Fac. Med. Vet. (Lima) 15:41–47.

16. Poirson, J. 1970. (Osteology of the thoracic limb of the guanaco) Osteologie du membre thoracique due guanaco. Ph.D. these, Vet. Ec. Nat. Vet. d'Alfort.

17. Rodriguez Rodriguez, H. 1965. (Contributions to the study of the muscles of the forelimb of the alpaca, *Lama pacos*). Tesis, Fac. Med. Vet. Univ. Nac. Mayor San Marcos (Lima), pp. 1–52.

18. Roehrs, M. 1973. Quantitative changes of the skull from wild to domesticated animals. In J. Matolcsi, ed. (Domestication Research and History of Domestic Animals) Domestikationsforschung Geschichte der Haustiere. Int. Symp. Budapest, Hungary, Akademiai, pp. 127–33.

19. Scott, H. H. 1926. Report of the deaths occurring in the gardens in 1925 (fracture of leg bone in llama). Proc. Zool. Soc. Lond., p. 231.

20. Struch, J. 1943. (Comparative osteology of the Peruvian camelids) Osteologia comparada de los auchenidos peruanos. Univ. Arequipa Rev. 15(18):113–57.

21. Sueppel, R. 1926. (On the osteology of the llama) Zur Osteologie des Lama, *Auchenia lama.* Anat. Anz. 62(7):97–109.

22. Turner, H. N. 1849. On the evidence of affinity afforded by the skull in the ungulate mammalia. Proc. Zool. Soc. Lond., p. 147.

23. Vadet, A. 1970. (Contribution of the study of the skeleton of the head of a guanaco) Contribution a l'etude du squelette cephalique du guanaco. Ph.D. these, Ec. Nat. Vet. d'Alfort.

24. Willemse, J. J. 1958. The innervation of the muscles of the trapezius-complex in giraffe, okapi, camel and llama. Arch. Neerl. Zool. 12(4):532–36.

12 Respiratory System

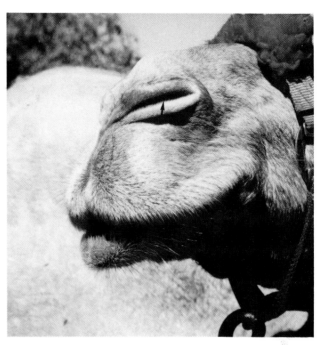

12.1 Nostril of a camel. Orifice can be closed tightly to exclude dust.

ANATOMY

The anatomy of the respiratory tract of lamoids has not been adequately described in the literature. No texts and only a few papers have been published (1–33). This presentation does not provide a complete anatomy; however, clinically important anatomic characteristics are described.

Nostril and Nasal Cavity

Nostrils of lamoids are not unique. Unlike their Old World cousins, the camels, lamoids are unable to completely close the nostrils to exclude dust (Fig. 12.1). The nasal cavity has a ventral, middle, and dorsal meatus (Figs. 12.1–12.3). Conchae (turbinates) are arranged in a pattern similar to those of cattle and sheep. The ventral aspect of the ventral meatus is 2–3 mm wide. A bulge in the septal mucosa partially occludes the lumen. The dorsal section of the ventral meatus is only 0.7–0.8 mm wide. The turbinates are delicate and easily traumatized, so passage of a nasogastric tube is not commonly practiced. Small fiber optic endoscopes may be inserted carefully to visualize the nasopharynx.

The nasal orifice of the nasolacrimal duct is located approximately 1 cm dorsal from the floor of the nostril at the junction of the mucocutaneous junction. The hard palate ends approximately 6 cm caudad to the leading edge of the first cheek tooth. The soft palate is elongated in lamoids and may lie either dorsal or ventral to the epiglottis, depending upon the stage of breathing or swallowing (Figs. 12.4, 12.5). See Chapter 5 for a more detailed discussion. Lamoids are obligate nasal breathers.

Sinuses

Maxillary and frontal sinuses are delineated in Figure 12.6.

Larynx

The larynx and hyoid bones (with their dimensions) of the llama are illustrated diagrammatically in Figure 12.7.

Trachea and Bronchi

The trachea and bronchi are not unique.

Lungs

Lamoid lungs are most similar to those of the horse. A cardiac notch separates the apical portion, but there are no lobes except for the small accessory lobe on the right lung that surrounds the caudal vena cava. Each main stem bronchus divides into an apical bronchus, a cardiac bronchus, and the larger diaphragmatic bron-

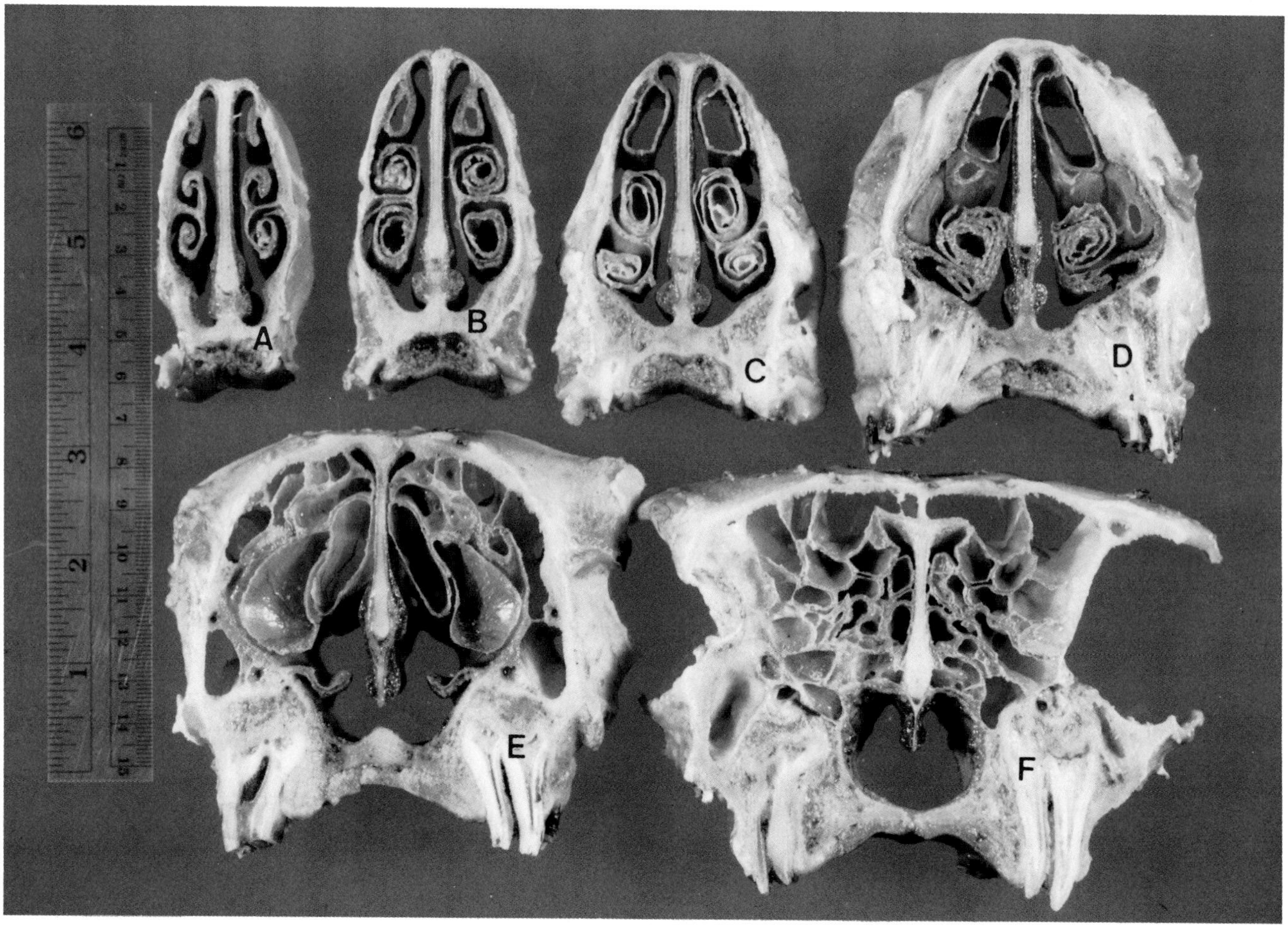

12.2 Serial cross sections of the nasal cavity of a llama: (A–F) locations are from Figure 12.3.

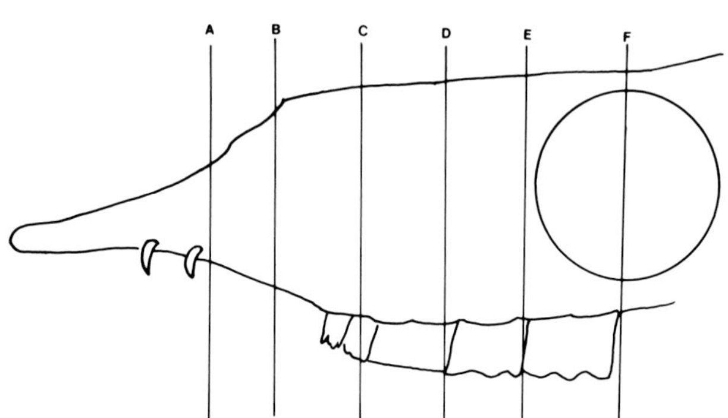

12.3 Locations of cross-sectional cuts are from Figure 12.2.

chus. The bronchus to the azygous lobe arises from the diaphragmatic bronchus (31).

The Clara cell is a nonciliated epithelial cell that occurs in the bronchioles of animals. It appears to be a secretory cell, but its function is unknown. The number of Clara cells per millimeter of bronchiolar epithelium is markedly different between llamas kept at high elevations (55–106/mm) and those kept at sea level (8/mm). Mountain air is dry and cold. The secretion of these cells may be of protective value in animals living at high altitude (19, 20).

The mediastinum is complete. The line of diaphragmatic pleural reflection follows a line approximately 2–3 cm cranial to the costochondral junction and crossing the midportion of the 12th (last) rib to finish dorsally approximately 4 cm caudal to the 12th rib.

PHYSIOLOGY

A study of anesthesia in five llamas provided baseline data on the following respiratory parameters (15). PaO_2 127 ± 8.9 mm Hg, $PaCO_2$ 34.1 ± 1.1 mm Hg, excess base −2.3 ± 1.1 mEq/L, and bicarbonate 21.3 ± 1.1 mEq/L.

The tidal volume of a 105 kg llama was 0.6 L and the calculated dead space 0.33 L. The ratio of dead space volume to the tidal volume of a llama is 0.55 compared

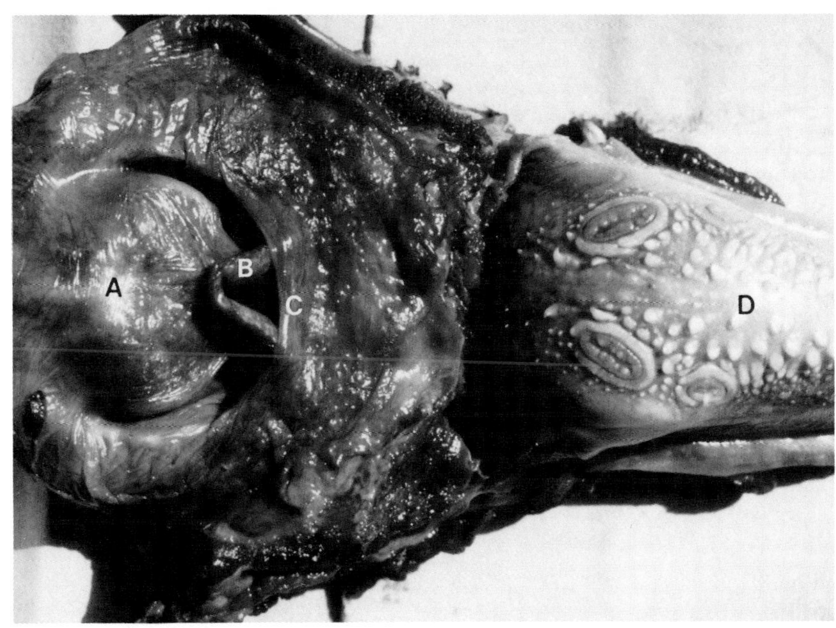

12.4 Anatomic dissection of the relationship of the soft palate to the larynx, dorsal view: **(A)** larynx, **(B)** arytenoid cartilage, **(C)** caudal margin of the soft palate, **(D)** tongue.

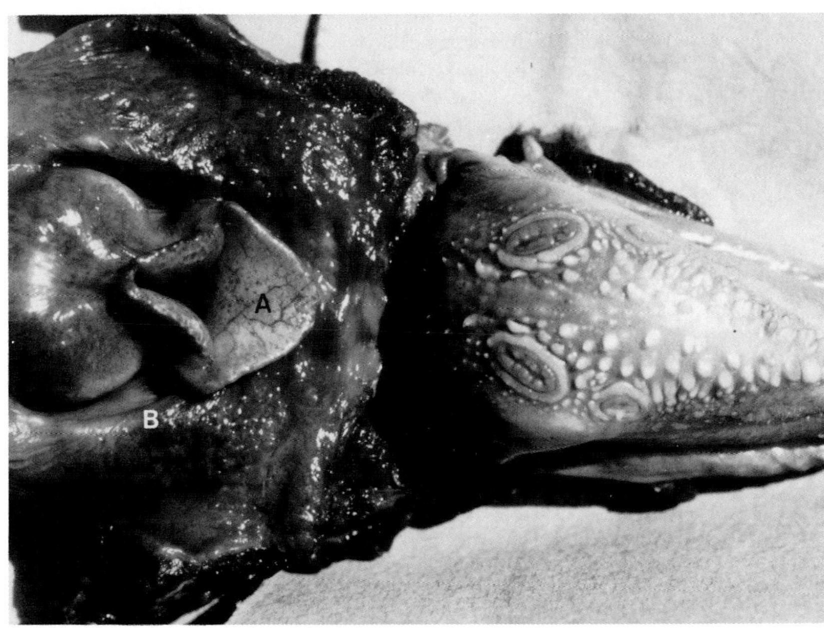

12.5 Soft palate situated ventral to the epiglottis: **(A)** epiglottis, **(B)** caudal margin of the soft palate.

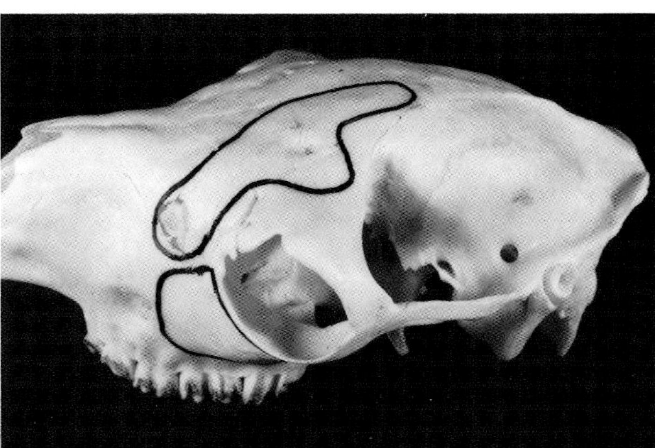

12.6 Skull, illustrating the outline of the maxillary and facial sinuses.

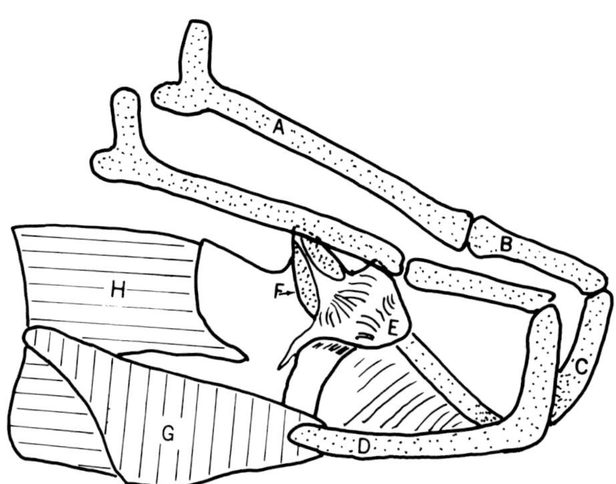

12.7 Diagram of larynx and hyoid apparatus of a llama (approximate size in an adult): **(A)** stylohyoid, 7 cm, **(B)** epihyoid, 4 cm, **(C)** ceratohyoid, 5.5 cm, **(D)** thyrohyoid, 5 cm, **(E)** epiglottis, 3.5 × 3.5 cm, **(F)** arytenoid cartilage, 2.5 × 1.5 cm, **(G)** thyroid cartilage, **(H)** cricoid cartilage.

with human 0.30, giraffe 0.36, and camel 0.25 (22). The minute volume of the 105 kg llama was 8.5 L/min.

Lamoids are known to be well adapted to the hypobaric environment of the high Andes. Numerous physiologists have studied this phenomenon in an attempt to establish the mechanism(s) for this adaptation. It is probable that a combination of mechanisms involving the respiratory, cardiovascular, muscular, and hemic systems are involved. Some of these mechanisms may have relevance to clinical syndromes and clinical evaluation of the respiratory system.

LAMOID ADAPTATIONS TO ALTITUDE

1. High hemoglobin concentration of blood.
2. Large numbers of erythrocytes.
3. Small ellipsoid, thin erythrocytes (greater surface area).
4. High mean corpuscular hemoglobin concentration, 45%.
5. Mild to moderate degree of pulmonary hypertension at altitude, which does not progress to right heart hypertrophy or thickening of the pulmonary arteries.
6. High affinity of lamoid hemoglobin for oxygen (2).
7. Efficient utilization of oxygen by the tissue (more efficient myoglobin).
8. Oxygen dissociation curves of the blood of lamoids are shifted to the left of species adapted to low altitudes (12, 13).

DIAGNOSTIC PROCEDURES

Auscultation is described in Chapter 4. The area available for auscultation is much more restricted than would be anticipated by the more caudal line of pleural reflection. Normal respiratory sounds are muted and may not be audible in the resting animal. Audible sounds are described as bronchovesicular, similar to cattle.

Thoracocentesis is described in Chapter 4.

Radiographic evaluation of the thorax is limited to the lateral view in the adult (Figs. 12.8, 12.9). Both lateral and dorsoventral projections are possible in neonates (Figs. 12.10, 12.11). The technique varies with the area of concern. When radiographing the dorsocaudal area, use an ffd 152 cm (60 in.), 1/50th sec., MAS 10, and KVP 100. In the cranial area use the same ffd, time 1/25th sec., 20 MAS, and 120 KVP. At Davis, a grid is placed on a Dupont Quanta 3 screen cassette, and Dupont Chronex 7 film is used.

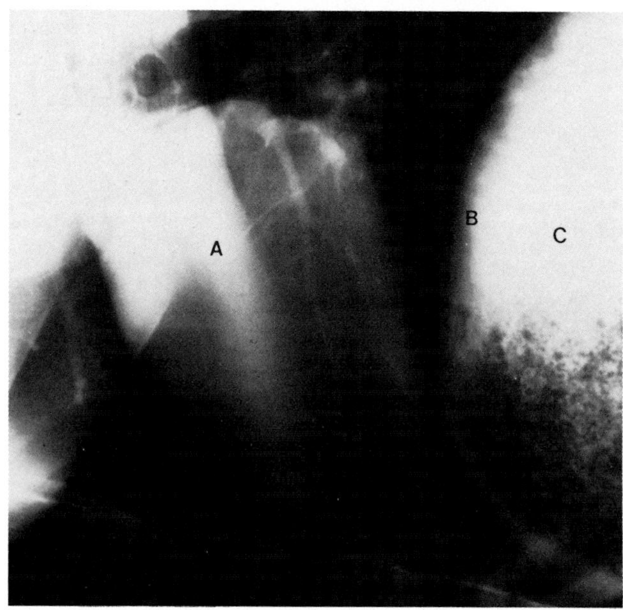

12.8 Lateral radiograph of the cranial thorax of a llama: **(A)** heart, **(B)** diaphragm, **(C)** C-1 of stomach.

INFECTIOUS DISEASES

Infectious diseases of the respiratory system include tuberculosis, coccidioidomycosis, actinobacillosis, and nonspecific ailments such as fusobacteriosis (Fig. 12.12) caused by opportunistic bacteria. Discussions of these diseases are found in Chapter 7. There are no known viral diseases of the lamoid respiratory system.

PARASITIC DISEASES

Lamoids are susceptible to lungworm, *Dictyocaulus viviparous,* and nasopharyngeal bots, *Cephenemyia* sp., both of which are described in Chapter 8. The lungs may also serve as a migratory route for larval parasites such as the meningeal worm, *Parelaphostrongylus tenuis.*

CONGENITAL DISORDERS

Congenital disorders include facial deformities, choanal atresia, and cleft palate, all discussed in Chapter 22.

MISCELLANEOUS DISEASES

Trauma

ETIOLOGY. Injuries to the muzzle (dog bite, contusion) or nasal cavity causing swelling of the tissue may occlude the passageways, resulting in dyspnea. Rat-

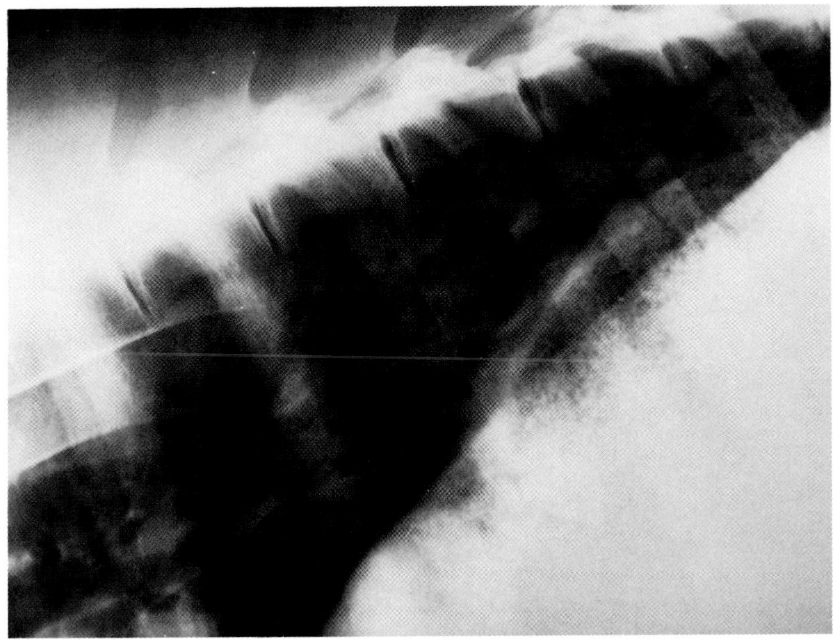

12.9 Lateral radiograph of the caudal thorax of an adult llama.

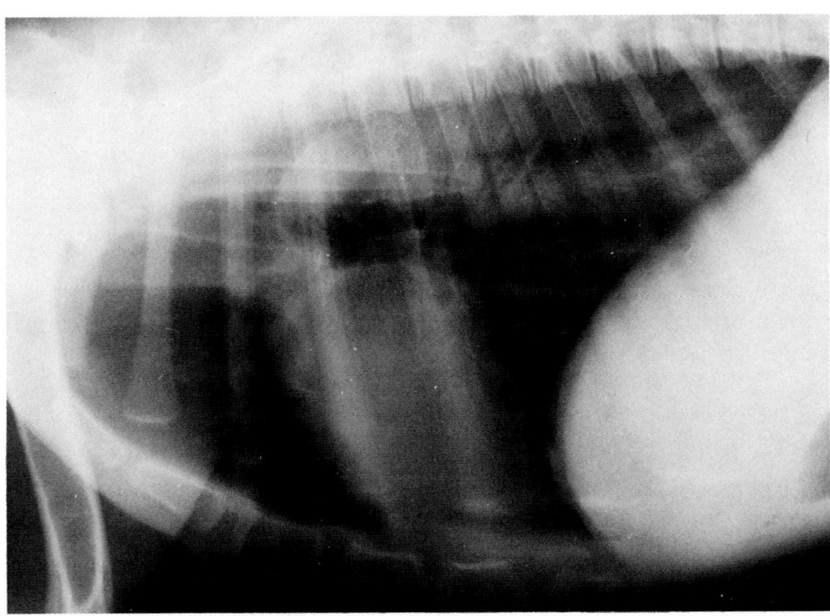

12.10 Lateral radiograph of a neonate llama thorax.

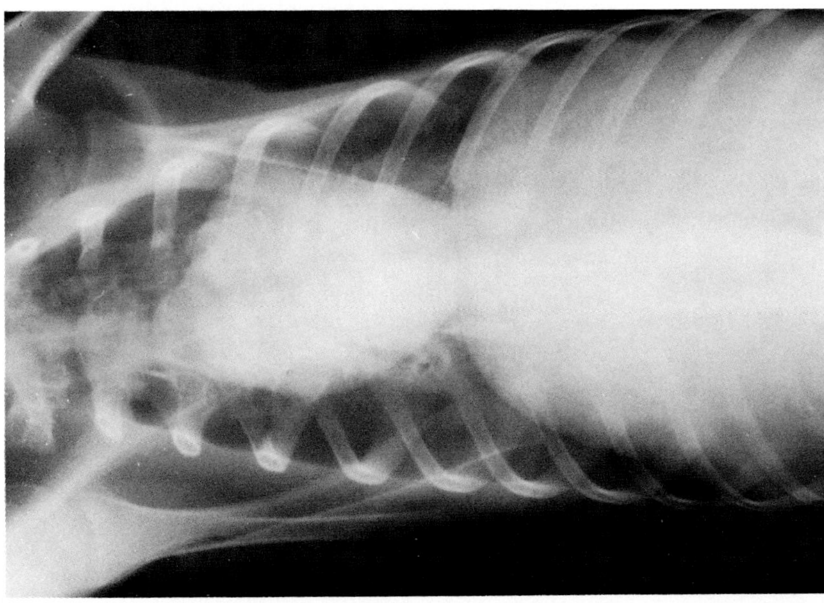

12.11 Dorsoventral radiograph of a neonate llama thorax.

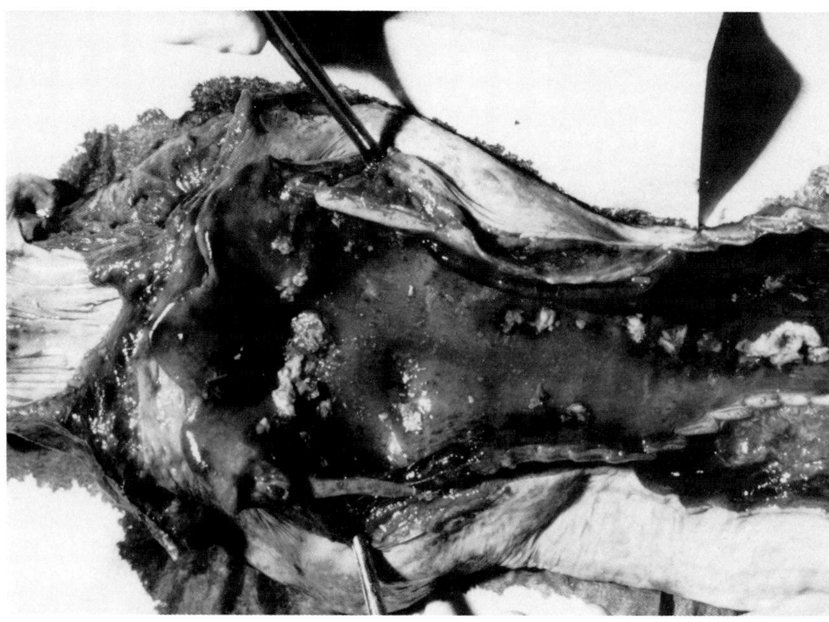

12.12 Necrotic laryngotracheitis.

tlesnake bites of the nose cause edema and occlusion of the nares. Llamas have strangled from occlusion of the nostril or trachea when they have become entangled in the halters and ropes used to secure them in trailers for transport. It is not desirable to tie llamas during transport.

One llama strangled as a result of a strange accident during trailering. The llama was tied over a bar at the front of a horse trailer. At some time during the trip the llama apparently was thrown forward, hitting the bar at the level of the larynx and upper trachea. The llama was found dead, hanging with the halter tightly occluding the nostrils and the mouth. A massive hematoma was found in the pharynx and larynx. The llama had apparently pulled backward, occluding the nostrils and mouth and restricting the flow of blood from the contused site.

Lacerations, contusions, and foreign body penetration of respiratory organs are similar to these accidents in other species. Llamas have been found upside down in ditches and other declivities, unable to extricate themselves. If left in this position for more than a few minutes, bloat or passive regurgitation and aspiration of stomach contents may occur, strangling the animal.

Bloat is rare in lamoids, but one case of esophageal obstruction caused by ingestion of a whole apple has been reported, with death resulting from bloat and internal pressure on the diaphragm and lungs.

CLINICAL SIGNS. Since lamoids are primarily nasal breathers, any impairment of air passage from the nostrils results in dyspnea and open-mouth breathing. Partial occlusion of the upper airways may result in stertorous breathing.

MANAGEMENT. Occlusive lesions may necessitate tracheostomy to preserve the life of the animal (see Chap. 6). The primary lesion must be dealt with as in any animal species.

Pneumonia

Pneumonia is often a presumptive diagnosis in llamas, especially neonates, based on increased respiratory sounds and some degree of dyspnea. Pneumonia is also a frequent diagnosis at a gross necropsy because the normal lung tends to be slightly edematous and hyperemic. That pneumonia occurs there is no doubt, but a thorough examination and evaluation are necessary to exclude diseases of other organ systems. Pulmonary edema is a common terminal lesion seen in animals dying from numerous diseases.

ETIOLOGY. The causal agents of lamoid pneumonia are similar to those causing pneumonia in livestock and horses, except that no viral agents are known to produce pneumonia in lamoids. Most infectious cases result from opportunistic bacteria. Septicemic animals usually develop pneumonia, and the most common agent isolated in the author's practice has been *Escherichia coli*. Other causes of pneumonia include inhalation of toxic vapors.

Aspiration of stomach contents occurs in the orphaned neonate being fed from a bottle or while being stomach tubed. Passive regurgitation during anesthesia is a significant risk. If surgery entails prolonged left lateral or dorsal recumbency, it is advisable to entubate the trachea with a cuffed tube and position the head and upper neck so that stomach contents can flow freely from the mouth.

CLINICAL SIGNS. Signs are exaggerated in the neonate and include dyspnea, coughing, elevated body temperature, variable nasal exudation, depression, and anorexia. Sounds heard at auscultation vary with the degree of exudation and consolidation.

DIAGNOSIS. A hemogram should be done. With bacterial or fungal infections, there will be an elevated leukocyte count and left shift. Radiographic evaluation is useful. A transtracheal wash can be used to collect material for culture and sensitivity. To do this, an area over the trachea in the midcervical region is prepared aseptically and a 15 gauge needle inserted between the tracheal rings. A sterile catheter is threaded through the needle. Position the neck to horizontal and flow 5–10 ml of nonbacteriostatic water or saline into the trachea with a pumping action of the syringe to aspirate exudate. Collected material should be examined for cytology and cultured.

THERAPY. Broad-spectrum antibiotic therapy is recommended until sensitivity results are available, since Gram-negative organisms are frequently involved. General nursing care and supportive treatment are indicated. Nebulization may be helpful in mobilizing exudates. Fifty percent dimethylsulfoxide (DMSO) in aqueous solution has been efficacious in the author's practice.

Pleural Effusion

ETIOLOGY. Pleural effusion is usually secondary to pleuritis, pericarditis, or right heart insufficiency. Generalized lymphosarcoma with mediastinal lesions resulted in incapacitating pleural effusion (14).

CLINICAL SIGNS. Inspiratory dyspnea is the most prominent sign. The absence of sounds in the lower thorax and a dull sound on percussion in the same area are diagnostic. A definitive diagnosis is based on radiography and thoracocentesis. It is imperative that the nature of the pleural fluid be determined, since it may be a modified transudate or exudate.

MANAGEMENT. Therapy will be determined by the etiology. Excess fluid may be removed via thoracocentesis, but the critical factor is to prevent recurrence. The prognosis for a neoplasm is grave. Infectious pleuritis should be treated with broad-spectrum antibiotics until results of culture and sensitivity tests are known.

Exercise Intolerance

ETIOLOGY. The llama was domesticated as a beast of burden in the high Andes. Many llama owners have purchased animals for the purpose of packing with them in the wilderness. A few llamas have either refused to carry a pack or have been unable to exert themselves sufficiently to make a worthwhile pack animal.

A number of defects within the respiratory system may contribute to exercise intolerance. Crias afflicted with congenital bilateral choanal atresia usually die, but unilateral or partial stenosis of the choanae could restrict air flow later in life. Congenital narrowing of the nasal cavity is recognized and causes stertorous breathing, particularly if the animal is excited or exercised. Lesions within the nasopharynx such as polyps, lymphoid hyperplasia, or granulomatous lesions caused by *Cephenemyia* sp. have caused restricted air flow. Hyperplasia of the soft palate (Fig. 12.13) of unknown etiology results in reduced air flow. Previous pneumonic episodes may have left areas of the lung fibrotic and nonfunctional.

Other nonrespiratory causes should be considered, such as ventricular septal defects, anemia, hepatic insufficiency, renal insufficiency, arthritis, and myopathy.

CLINICAL SIGNS. The primary sign is inability to work up to the potential for the animal's stage of training. Most llamas simply slow down or stop if the exertion is beyond their capability. Some animals may show open-mouth or audible breathing if the lesion is in the upper airway. Careful consideration should be given to the weights expected to be carried. Small animals (100 kg) should not be expected to start with more than 20–25 kg and should carry only 36 kg when trained and fit. Larger animals may carry 45 kg.

DIAGNOSIS. With the diversity of causes, a thorough physical examination is necessary, possibly including hematology, serum biochemistry, and radiography of the head and thorax. Lesions within the nasal cavity and the nasopharynx may be explored by endoscopy.

MANAGEMENT. Many of the lesions causing exercise intolerance are either congenital or chronic in nature. Little can be done to correct these, but an appropriate prognosis may be given. *Cephenemyia* sp. is treated with ivermectin (0.2 mg/kg). Surgery may be appropriate to correct hyperplastic lesions of the nasal cavity or nasopharynx.

Other Miscellaneous Conditions

The following conditions have been diagnosed, but no etiologic agent was identified: necrotic laryngotracheitis (Fig. 12.12), hyperplasia of the soft palate (Fig. 12.13), and subepiglottic mass (Fig. 12.14).

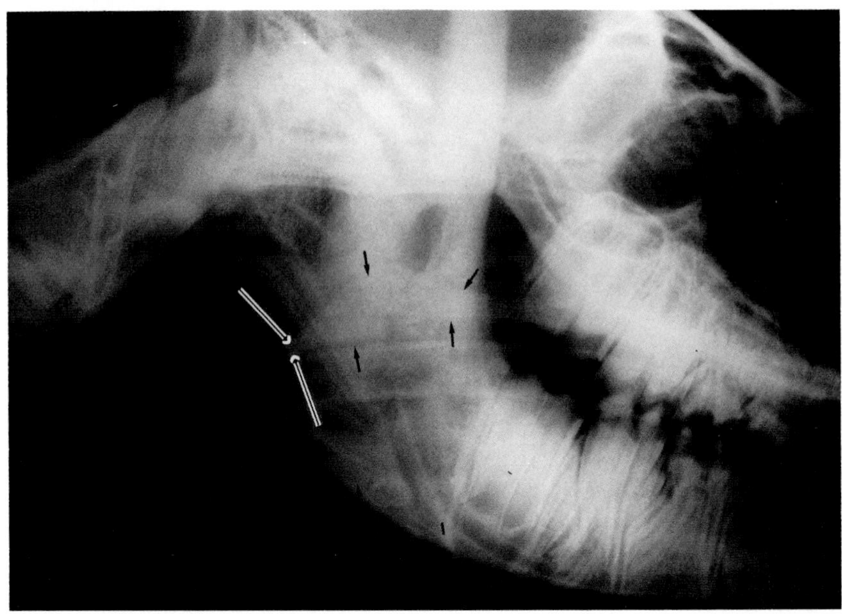

12.13 Hyperplasia of soft palate.

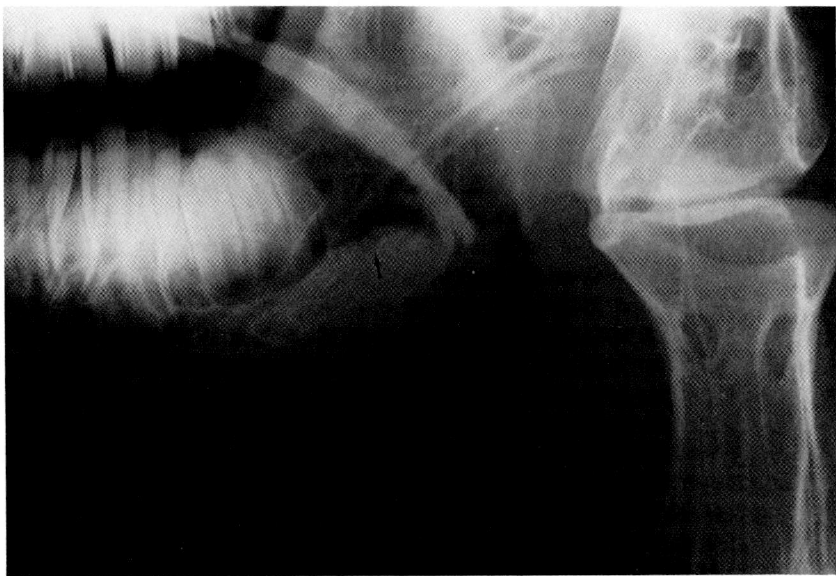

12.14 Subepiglottic mass.

REFERENCES

1. Banchero, N., and Grover, R. F. 1972a. Comparative aspects of oxygen transport in animals with hemoglobin of high (llama) and low (sheep) affinity for oxygen. Chest 61(2):155.

2. ______. 1972b. Effect of different levels of simulated altitude on oxygen transport in llama and sheep. Am. J. Physiol. 222:1239–45.

3. Banchero, N., Gee, M. H., and Maaske, C. A. 1969. Pulmonary circulation in the llama. Fed. Proc. 28(2):594.

4. Banchero, N., Will, J. A., and Grover, R. F. 1969. Oxygen transport in the llama. Physiologist 12(3):166.

5. Banchero, N., Grover, R. F., and Will, J. A. 1971. Oxygen transport in the llama (*Llama glama*). Respir. Physiol. 13(1):102–15.

6. Bartels, H., Hilpert, P., Barbey, K., Betke, K., Riegel, K., Lang, E. M., and Metcalfe, J. 1963. Respiratory functions of blood of the yak, llama, camel, Dybowski deer and African elephant. Am. J. Physiol. 205:331–36.

7. Braunitzer, G., Schrank, B., and Stangl, A. 1978. (Sequence of alpha chains of the hemoglobins of swine and llama, aspects of respiration at high altitude) Die Sequenz der Alpha-Ketten der Haemoglobine des Schweines und des Lames (Aspekte zur Atmung im Hochland). Hoppe-Seyler's Z. Physiol. Chem. 358(3):409–12.

8. Braunitzer, G., Schrank, B., Stangl, A., and Bauer, C. 1977. (Regulation of respiration at high altitudes and its molecular interpretation: The sequence of beta chains of hemoglobins from pigs and llama.) Hoppe-Seyler's Z. Physiol. Chem. 358(7):921–26. German

9. ______. 1978. (Hemoglobins Part 22: The interactions between phosphate and protein and the respiration of the llama, the human fetus and horse.) Hoppe-Seyler's Z. Physiol. Chem. 359(5):547–58. German

10. Brooks, J. R. III, and Tenney, S. M. 1968. Ventilatory response of llamas to hypoxia at sea level and high altitude. Respir. Physiol. 5(2):269–78.

11. Carlos Monge, C., and Whittembury, J. 1974. Increased hemoglobin oxygen affinity at extremely high altitudes. Science (Washington) 186:843.

12. Chiodi, H. 1970a. Comparative study of the blood gas transport in high altitude and sea level camelidae and goats. Fed. Proc. 29(2):591.

13. ______. 1970b. Comparative study of the blood gas transport in high altitude and sea level camelidae and goats. Respir. Physiol. 11(1):84–93.

14. Fowler, M. E., Gillespie, D., and Harkema, J. 1985. Lymphosarcoma in a llama. J. Am. Vet. Med. Assoc. 187:1245–46.

15. Gavier, D., Kittleson, M. D., Fowler, M. E., Johnson, L. E., Hall, G., and Nearenberg, D. 1989. Evaluation of the combination of xylazine, ketamine and halothane for anesthesia in llamas. Am. J. Vet. Res. 49:2047–55.

16. Hall, F. G. 1937. Adaptations of mammals to high altitudes. J. Mammal. 18:468–72.

17. Hall, F. G., Dill, D. B., and Guzman Barron, E. S. 1936. Comparative physiology at high altitudes. J. Cell. Comp. Physiol. 8(3):301–13.

18. Harris, P., Heath, D., Smith, P., Williams, D. R., Ramierez, A., Krueger, H., and Jones, D. M. 1982. Pulmonary circulation of the llama at high and low altitudes. Thorax 37:38–45.

19. Heath, D., Smith, P., and Harris, P. 1976. Clara cells in the llama. Exp. Cell Biol. 44(2):73–82.

20. Heath, D., Smith, P., and Biggar, R. 1980. Clara cells in llamas born and living at high and low altitudes. Br. J. Dis. Chest 74(1):75–80.

21. Herceg, M., Huber, I., and Gomercic, V. 1976. (Hyaline membranes in the lung of a newborn llama [*Lama glama*]) Hyaline Membranen in der Lunge eines neugeborenen Lama (*Lama glama*). Verhandlungsber. 18th Int. Symp. Erkr. Zootiere, Innsbruck 18:123–26.

22. Hugh-Jones, P., Barter, C. E., Hime, J. Am., and Rusbridge, M. M. 1978. Dead space and tidal volume of the giraffe compared with some other mammals. Respir. Physiol. 35(1):53–58.

23. Monkhouse, W. S., and Whimster, W. 1976. An account of the longitudinal mucosal corrugations of the human tracheobronchial tree with observations on those of some animals. J. Anat. 122(3):681–95.

24. Petschow, D., Wuerdinger, I., Baumann, R., Duhm, J., Braunitzer, G., and Bauer, C. 1977. Causes of high blood oxygen affinity of animals living at high altitude. J. Appl. Physiol. 42(2):139–43.

25. Reynafarje, C. 1971. Comparative study of the high altitude adaptation of human beings and of Auchenidae. Acta Cient. Venez. 22(2):28–31.

26. Reynafarje, C., Faura, J., Villavicencio, D., Curaca, A., Reynafarje, B., Oyola, L., Contreras, L., Vallenas, E., and Faura, A. 1975. Oxygen transport of hemoglobin in high-altitude animals (camelidae). J. Appl. Physiol. 38(5):806–10.

27. Sillau Gilone, H. 1965. (Hematologic variations of the blood oxygen capacity with different times of residency at sea level) Variaciones hematologicas de la capacidad de oxigeno de la sangre de alpacas con diferente tiempo de permanencia al nivel del mar. Tesis, Fac. Med. Vet. Univ. Nac. Mayor San Marcos (Lima), pp. 1–23.

28. Sillau G., H., Cueva, S., Chauca, D., Valenzuela, A., and Cardenas, W. 1972. (Some observations on oxygen transport in alpacas at altitude and sea level) Observaciones sobre el transporte de oxigeno en la alpaca en la altura y a nivel del mar. Rev. Invest. Pecu. 1(2):129–36.

29. Sillau G., H., Cueva, S., Valenzuela, A., and Candela, E. 1976. Oxygen transport in the alpaca, *Lama pacos,* at sea level and at 3300 meters. Respir. Physiol. 27(2):147–55.

30. Van Nice, P., Black, C. P., and Tenney, S. M. 1980. A comparative study of ventilatory responses to hypoxia with reference to hemoglobin oxygen affinity in llama, *Lama glama,* cat, rat, duck, *Anas platyrhynchos,* and goose, *Anser indicus.* Comp. Biochem. Physiol. 66(2):347–50.

31. Viera, R. F., Sato Sato, A., and Nunez, M. Q. 1968. (The lungs and bronchial tree in alpacas) Los pulmones y la arborizacion bronquial en las alpacas, *Lama pacos.* Tesis, Rev. Fac. Med. Vet. Univ. Nac. Mayor San Marcos (Lima) 22:54–60.

32. Williams, A., Heath, D., Harris, P., Williams, D., and Smith, P. 1981. Pulmonary mast cells in cattle and llamas at high altitude. J. Pathol. 134(1):1–6.

33. Zapata Quiroga, E. 1971. (Contributions to the macro and microscopic description of the nasal cavity and trachea and hyoid bones of the alpaca) Contribucion a la descripcion macroscopica y microscopica de la cavidad nasal, traquea y hioides de los camelidos Sudamericanos. Tesis, Fac. Med. Vet. Univ. Nac. Tec. Altiplano (Puno), p. 106.

13 Digestive System

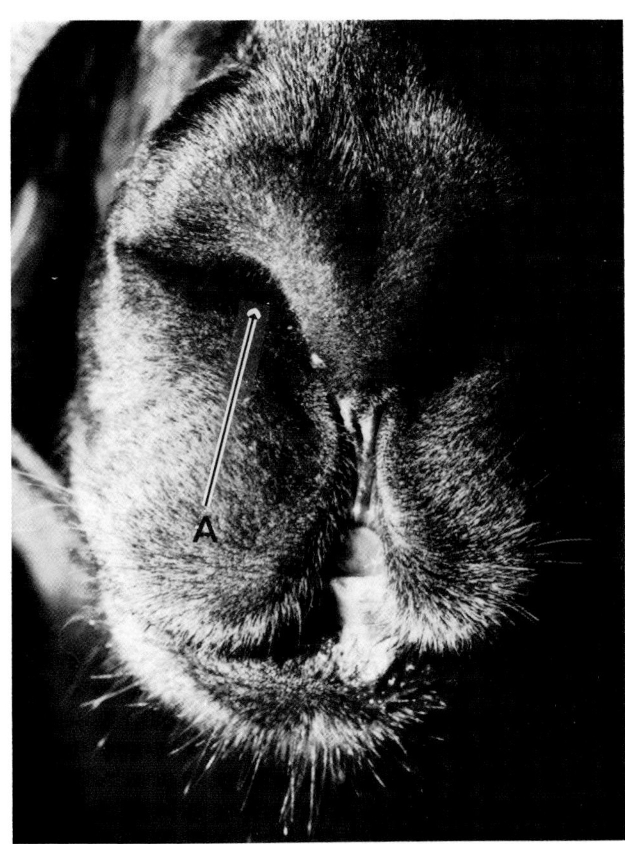

13.1 Philtrum in a llama: (A) approximate location of the nasolacrimal duct orifice.

THE DIGESTIVE AND REPRODUCTIVE SYSTEMS of camelids have been the most intensely studied of any of the organ systems. Both systems have unique characteristics, which constitute some of the major differences that separate camelids from true ruminants in the order Artiodactyla. Both Old and New World camelids evolved in harsh but differing environments. The two environments had in common a characteristic of sparse, poor-quality forage for at least part of the year.

In camelids, a foregut fermentation system and a rumination cycle evolved in parallel with the digestive systems of true ruminants, as it appears that the common ancestor of both lines was simple stomached. Numerous other morphologic differences of the digestive system affect diagnosis, treatment, and management of diseases in these animals.

ANATOMY AND PHYSIOLOGY

Lips

The upper lip of camelids is split by a philtrum (labial cleft) (Fig. 13.1). Each side of the lip can be manipulated independently by the elevator nasolabialis muscle under the control of the facial nerve. The upper lip is highly tactile, useful for fine discrimination, and the camelid uses it as a sense organ to investigate potential feed. As a result of this fastidious feeding behavior, gastric foreign bodies are rarely found in South American camelids (SACs). Old World camels are not so discriminating. The lower lip has no unique characteristic, but it is less mobile than the lower lip of the caprine or ovine.

Mouth

The oral cavity of the llama is small. The rami of the mandibles are set close together, and the tongue occupies the ventral space. The lips are tightly opposed to the teeth. It is rare for a cud to become trapped in the buccal cavity.

Tongue

The tongue of lamoids is relatively immobile. It is rarely extended beyond the lips and is not used for prehension of feed. The lamoid does not lick the neonate nor does it remove any attached fetal membrane. In a 150 kg llama male, the tongue was 20 cm long, 3 cm wide, and 2 cm deep in the anterior two-thirds. The caudal third had a pronounced dome (5 cm) (Fig. 13.2).

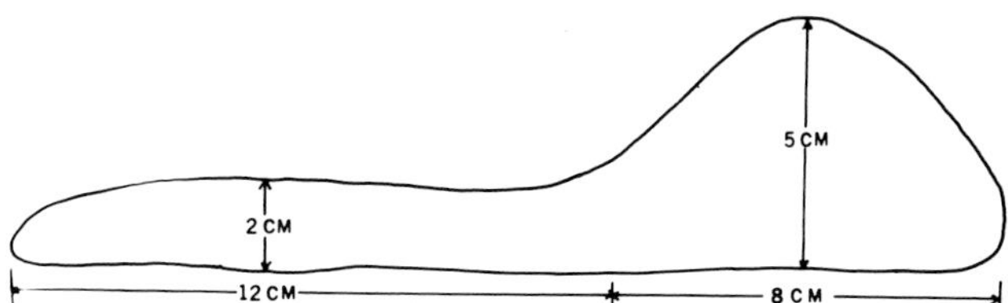

13.2 Diagram of the tongue of a llama.

Oropharynx

The major morphologic traits of this area that have clinical significance are the narrow oropharyngeal space, the elongated soft palate, and the domed base of the tongue. The llama is an obligate nasal breather, with inefficient mouth-breathing capabilities. With nasal obstruction, simultaneous eating and breathing are difficult. Breathing takes immediate precedence, and the animal will slowly starve if nasal obstruction persists.

Esophagus

The camelid esophagus is similar to that of ruminants. It is not known where the stimulus arises, but lamoids are more prone than the bovine to regurgitation during passage of a stomach tube.

Teeth

The dental anatomy of camelids sets them apart from ruminants. A comparison of the deciduous and permanent dental formulas for camelids and bovines is given in Table 13.1. The tabulation presents only part of the picture. The single upper incisor of both lamoids and camels has migrated caudally and evolved to a caniniform shape and function. With the mouth closed, this tooth rests just caudad to the corner lower incisor. All four canine teeth are present in adult males. Therefore, male lamoids appear to have two upper and one lower canine on each side.

Camels have more premolars than lamoids, but the first upper and lower premolars have also migrated forward in the jaw and become caniniform (47). Thus the camel appears to have three upper and two lower canines on each side. In contrast, cattle, sheep, and goats appear to have four lower incisors and no canines, but the corner incisor is actually a canine tooth that has migrated forward and become incisiform.

All lamoids have the same dental formula, but vicuña incisors differ in shape and structure from those of other artiodactylids, being more like the continuously erupting incisors of rodents. The permanent incisors of the vicuña are parallel sided, 10 times as long as they are wide, with a square cross section. The crown enamel is confined to the labial surface, extending down the root to within 2–3 mm of the wide, open base (Fig. 13.3) (55).

The deciduous teeth of vicuñas are more elongated than those of the llama, but they are spatulate. The base of the incisor remains open. There is no enamel on the lingual surface of the tooth, and the enamel of the labial surface extends halfway down the tooth (55).

Incisors of the llama and guanaco are spatulate, with the greatest width ranging from one-fifth to one-fourth the greatest length (Figs. 13.4–13.6). The root tapers rapidly to a closed base (Fig. 13.6) (55). Both labial and lingual surfaces of the crown are enameled, and on the lingual side the enamel extends one-third the length of the tooth. Deciduous and permanent incisors are similar in shape and structure but can be differentiated by size and amount of wear.

Incisors of alpacas seem to be intergrade between those of the vicuña and the llama (Fig. 13.3). This difference has caused some biologists to theorize that the alpaca developed from the vicuña and the llama from the guanaco. It has also been suggested that the vicuña should be placed in a separate genus on the basis of its dental structure.

The alpaca incisor is nonspatulate but has a rectangular cross section rather than the square cross section of the vicuña. The bases of the tooth remain open, and there is good clinical evidence that the incisor continues to grow throughout life. More dental anomalies have been reported in the alpaca than in other camelids. Overgrowth of the incisor teeth is common, caused either by genetic shortening of the premaxilla or failure to wear off the teeth, resulting from provision of too soft, succulent feed. See Chapter 22 on congenital anomalies.

The canines of the lamoids are adapted to intraspecies aggression, especially between breeding males. The deciduous canines are quite small and erupt rarely in females and in only about 5% of the males. The large canines of the mature male are formidable weapons (Fig. 13.7). Females and geldings vary as to whether or not the

Table 13.1. Dental formulas of some artiodactylids

	Lamoids	Camels	Cattle, sheep, goats
Deciduous	I 1/3, C 1/1 PM 2-3/1-2 × 2 = 20-22	I 1/3, C 1/1 PM 3/2 × 2 = 22	I 0/3, C 0/1 PM 3/3 × 2 = 20
Permanent	I 1/3, C 1/1 PM 1-2/1-2, M 3/3 × 2 = 30-32	I 1/3, C 1/1 PM 3/2, M 3/3 × 2 = 34	I 0/3, C 0/1 PM 3/3 M 3/3 × 2 = 32

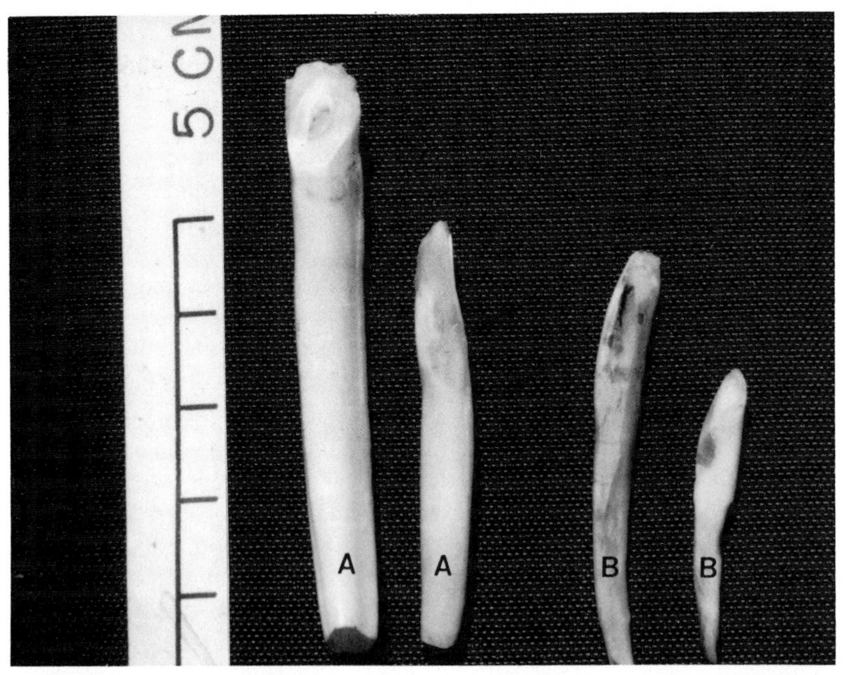

13.3 Incisor teeth of **(A)** vicuña, **(B)** alpaca.

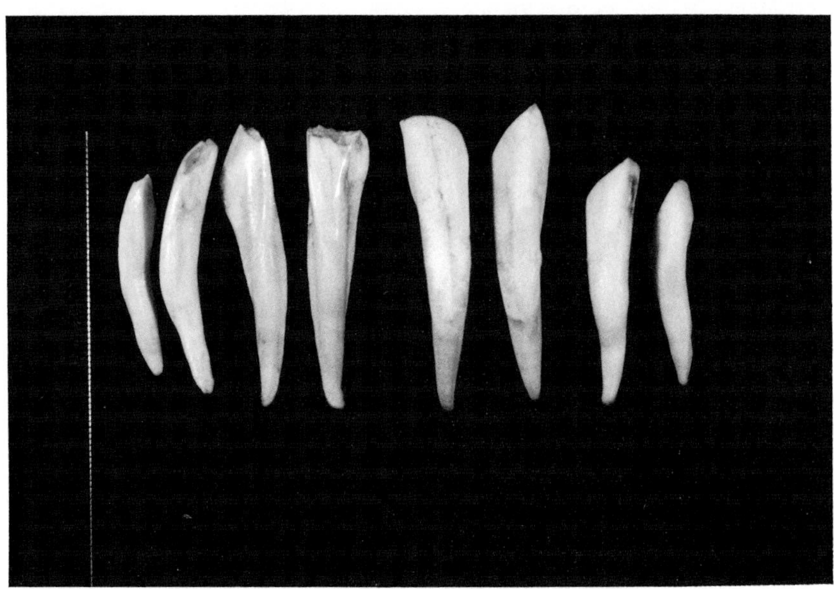

13.4 Incisor teeth of a mature llama.

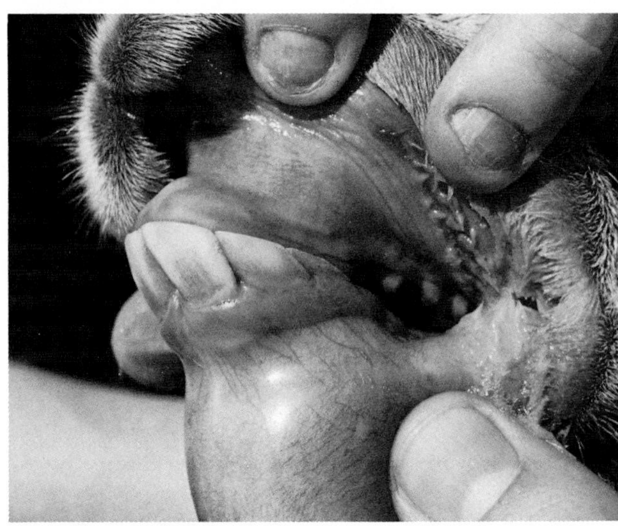

13.5 Incisors of a 5-month-old llama.

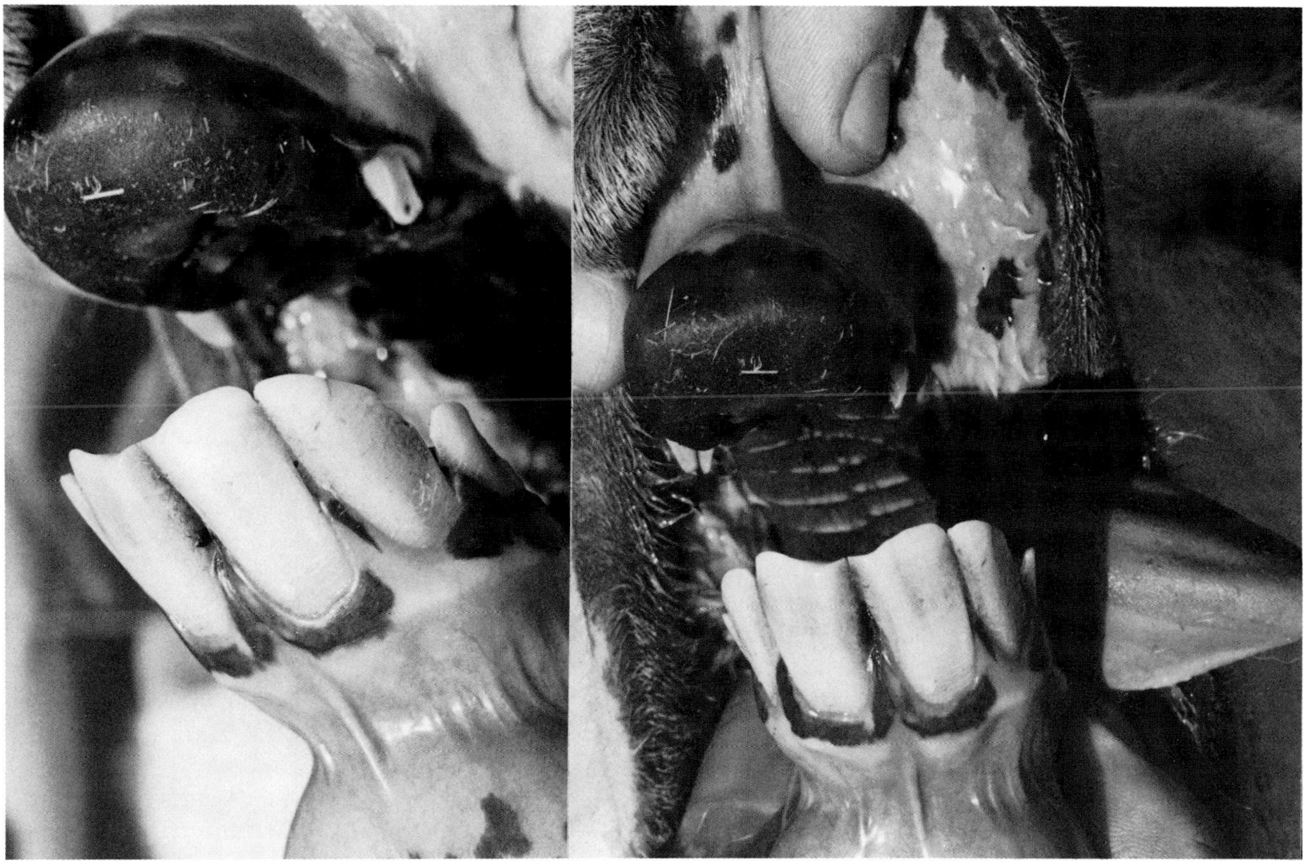

13.6 Incisors of a mature male llama.

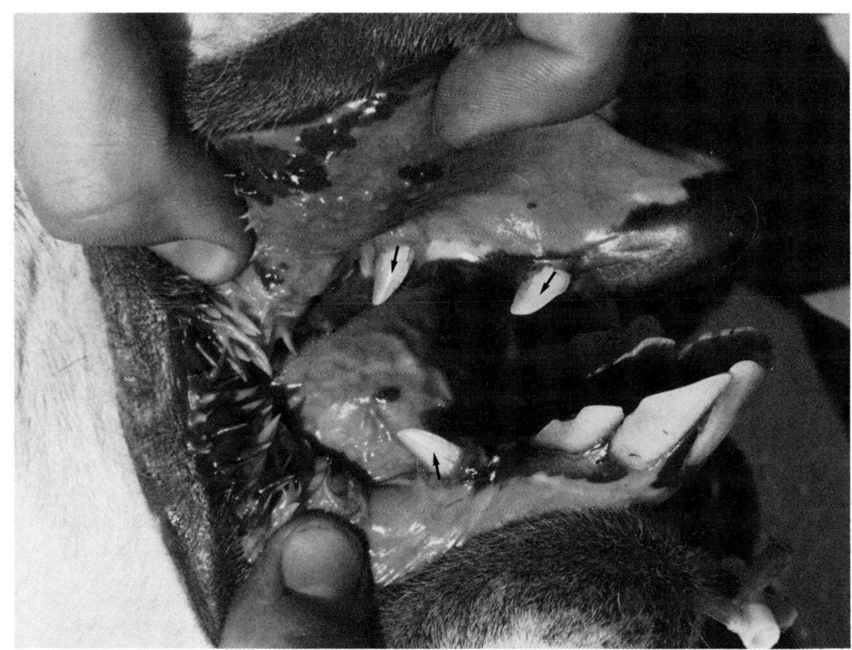

13.7 Male canine teeth.

permanent canines erupt. The teeth are sharp and are anchored into the jaw by a curved root.

The cheek teeth are selenodont (cusps have crescentic outline). It is sometimes difficult on clinical examination to identify where a tooth begins and ends. The table surface of the tooth exhibits the sharp ridges and points typical of a herbivore that is accustomed to eating harsh grasses, shrubs, and forbs. The cheek teeth of the lower jaw are slightly more narrow than those of the upper, but this does not seem to foster the excessive development of sharp enamel points on the lingual surfaces of the lowers and labial surfaces of the uppers as it does in the equine. The lamoid chews with a lateral motion that seems to keep wear even. The roots of the cheek teeth are closed, and there is no continuous growth.

Determining age by dental eruption times and wear of the teeth has been studied only in alpacas and llamas in South America. Eruption times may be controlled by a genetic trait, but wear is dependent upon the harshness of feedstuffs and the degree of grinding necessary to masticate them. An approximation of age in the living animal can be derived up to about 5 years (Table 13.2). After that, it is extremely difficult (25, 90).

Table 13.2. Eruption of lamoid teeth

Deciduous teeth

All three incisors are usually present in full-term neonates. In premature neonates I_2 and I_3 may be delayed up to 90 and 107 days, respectively.

Canines—only visible in 5% of males.

Premolars—present at birth.

Permanent teeth

I_1	2–2.5 yr
I_2	3–3.25 yr
I_3	3.1–6 yr
C	2–7 yr, but average is 2.5–3.5 yr
P_3	3.5–5 yr
P_4	3.5–5 yr
M_1	6–9 mo
M_2	1.5–2 yr
M_3	2.75–3.75 yr

Salivary Glands

There are three pairs of major salivary glands (parotid, mandibular, and sublingual). Four other glandular regions are less well defined but also contribute to salivary secretion (buccal, palatine, lingual, and labial) (59).

The salivary glands of camelids are similar in location, number, and histology to those of cattle, sheep, and goats. The parotid gland is much larger than the others and produces only a serous secretion, while the other salivary glands are both serous and mucous producers. For a detailed discussion of the histologic and histochemical anatomy of the salivary and intestinal glands, see Montalvo (50, 51) and Luciano (58). For a discussion of secretion, composition, and volume of salivary fluids, see Chapter 2.

The parotid duct arises on the ventral rostral border of the parotid salivary gland. The duct traverses the side of the face mesial to the platysmas muscle, approximately 1–1.5 cm dorsal to the facial vein (Fig. 13.8). The parotid duct empties into the oral cavity through an orifice on a flattened papilla that is located 1 cm dorsal to the gingiva at the junction of upper cheek teeth 2 and 3 (Fig. 13.9). The location of the orifice can be found by

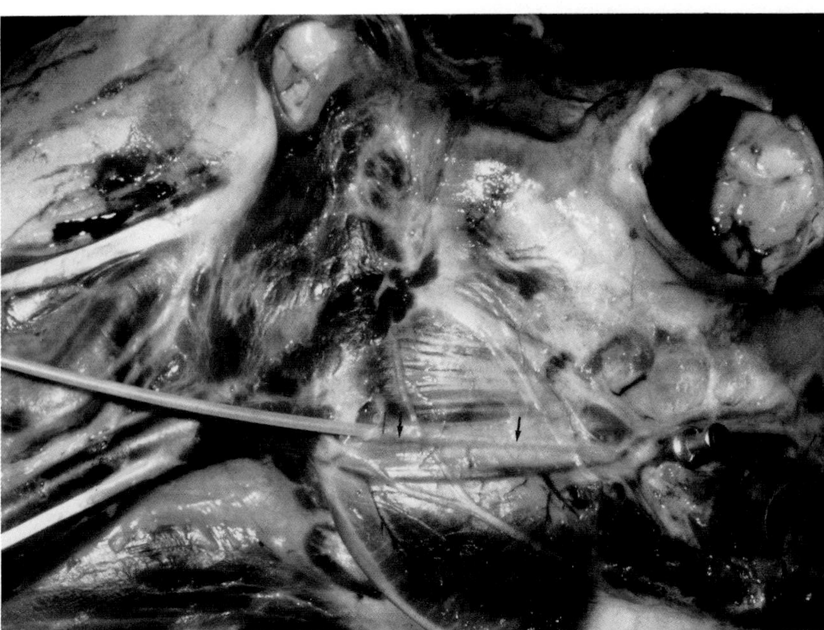

13.8 Course of the parotid salivary gland duct.

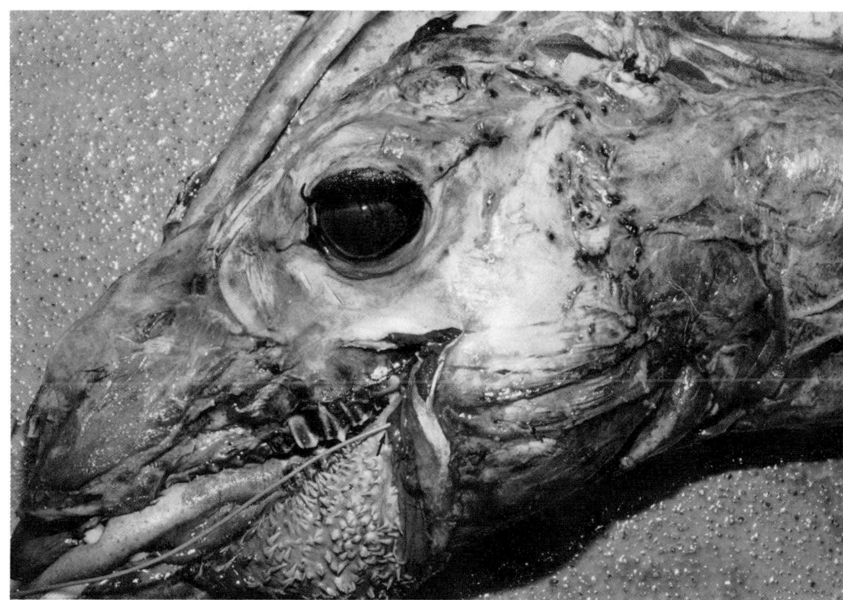

13.9 Parotid duct opening opposite upper cheek tooth 3.

dropping a perpendicular line from the rostral border of the orbit, which is also the rostral end of the facial crest. The duct may be cannulated with a 3.5 French catheter, but it is difficult to access it from the oral cavity because the mouth cannot be opened widely enough. The mandibular duct empties at the sublingual caruncle and the numerous ducts of the sublingual gland open alongside the tongue.

GASTROINTESTINAL TRACT

A diagrammatic representation of the digestive tract is illustrated in Figure 13.10.

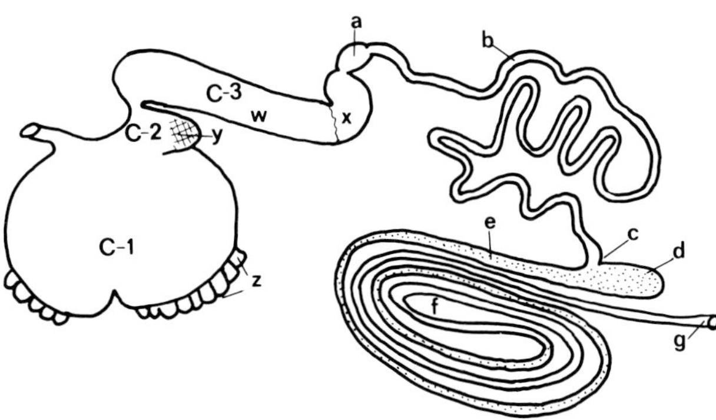

13.10 Diagram of the gastrointestinal tract of a camelid: (C-1 to C-3) compartments of the stomach, **(a)** ampula of the duodenum, **(b)** small intestine, **(c)** ileocecal orifice, **(d)** cecum, **(e)** proximal loop of the spiral colon, **(f)** spiral colon, **(g)** rectum, **(w)** general glandular area of C-3, **(x)** true stomach, **(y)** glandular divisions in C-2, **(z)** glandular saccules in C-1.

Stomach (23, 27, 52, 79, 84)

The anatomy of the forestomach of camelids differs significantly from that of true ruminants (Tables 13.3–13.5) (4, 5, 41). The three compartments of the camelid stomach (C-1, C-2, C-3) contrast with the four-compartmented stomach of the true ruminant. The compartments of the camelid stomach are not analogous, morphologically, to the rumen, reticulum, omasum, and abomasum (81, 83). There are no papillae in C-1 and C-2, but all three compartments have glandular areas. Motility patterns are markedly different in camelids, and the timing of rumination and eructation during the motility cycle also varies from that of the ruminant stomach (20, 78).

Table 13.3. Comparison of ruminant and camelid stomach

Ruminant	Camelid
4 compartments	3 compartments
Esophagus enters between rumen and reticulum	Esophagus enters C-1 only
Pillars pronounced, horizontal	Pillars minimal, horizontal
Glands in abomasum only	All compartments glandular
Esophageal groove double lipped	Esophageal groove single lipped
Rumen papillated	C-1 nonpapillated
Motility pattern 2–4/min	Motility pattern 3–5/min
Rumen—epithelium keratinized, stratified squamous	C-1—epithelium nonkeratinized, squamous
Abomasum—entirely covered with enzyme and acid-secreting epithelium	C-3—only distal one-fifth covered with enzyme and acid-secreting epithelium

Source: Bohlken 1960.

Table 13.4. Information about llama stomach compartments

Compartment	pH	Body weight of contents (%)	Retention time (hr) Liquid	Particles <0.2 cm	Particles >0.2 cm	Volume of stomach ingesta (%)	Function
C-1	6.4–7.0			20.3	>40	83	Fermentation, absorption of water, VFA and other solutes
C-2	6.4–7.0	10–15	9.6	20.3		6	Fermentation, absorption of water, VFA and other solutes
C-3	6.5 cranial <2–3 caudal	1–2	5.7	9		11	Absorption of water and solutes Proximal 4/5, digestive Distal 1/5, enzymes, acid

Table 13.5. Compartments of the ruminant stomach

Compartment	Epithelial covering	Volume of ingesta (%)	pH	Function
Rumen	Keratinized, stratified squamous-papillated	Cow–64 Sheep–69 Lamb–31	5.8–7.0	Fermentation chamber, major contractions 1–2/min
Reticulum	Stratified squamous		5.8–7.0	Fermentation chamber
Omasum	Stratified squamous	Cow–25 Sheep–8 Lamb–8	5.8–7.0	Reduce the particulate matter of the content of the omasum to a finer state
Abomasum	Glandular	Cow–11 Sheep–23 Lamb–61	3.0	Secretion of digestive juices that continue the digestive process

The evolution of the various regions of the stomach can be traced from the primordial simple stomach by the structure of the tunica muscularis (Fig. 13.11) (46). Basically, the anatomy of the stomach and intestines is the same in all camelids (Figs. 13.12–13.17). Similar to the ruminant, the camelid neonate has a poorly developed first compartment and a large true stomach (Fig. 13.13).

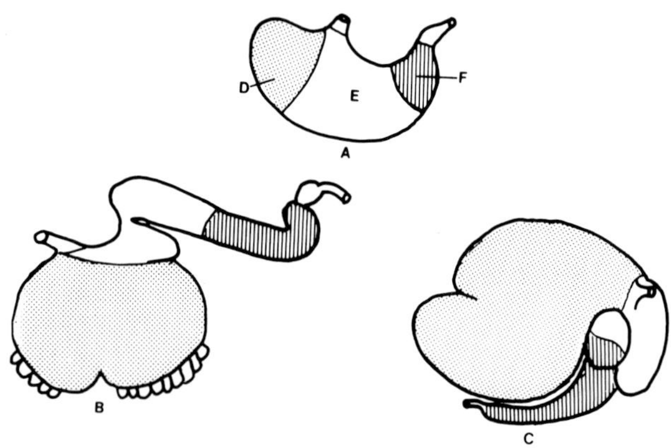

13.11 Comparative origins of different regions of the stomach: **(A)** simple stomach, **(B)** camelid stomach, **(C)** ruminant stomach, **(D)** fundal region, **(E)** body region, **(F)** pyloric region.

C-1 occupies the greater part of the left abdomen (Fig. 13.14). A cranial and caudal sac are weakly divided by a horizontal pillar. The esophagus enters C-1 on its craniodorsal midline. C-2 is situated on the right craniodorsal surface of C-1. The tubular C-3 arises on the cranial mesial aspect of C-2. It curves to the right, caudal and ventral to the liver, and lies on the right surface of C-1 in the right midventral abdomen.

The nonglandular mucosal surface of C-1 and C-2 is not papillated and is composed of unkeratinized, stratified squamous epithelium (13, 14, 50, 51). The ventral surfaces of both the cranial and caudal sacs of C-1 contain glandular saccules (Fig. 13.15). The epithelium varies slightly from the orifice to the depths of the saccule, but it is generally a mucinous glandular epithelium. In the camel, glandular epithelium is found only on the bottom and lower walls of the saccules.

In earlier studies, it was reported that this glandular epithelium was the source of sodium bicarbonate (19), but later studies, using a Pavlov pouch, did not confirm this (65, 66). Current studies indicate that the glandular epithelium also provides for rapid absorption of water and solutes (12, 50). For more information on the physiology of the stomach, see Chapter 2 and the references.

The mucosal surface of C-2 is glandular except for a small area on the lesser curvature that constitutes the

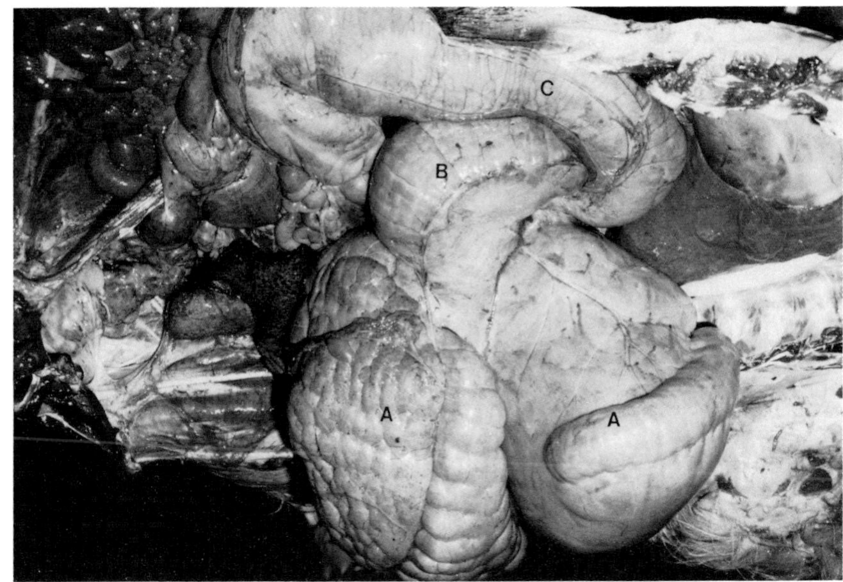

13.12 Stomach of a llama: **(A)** C-1, **(B)** C-2, **(C)** C-3.

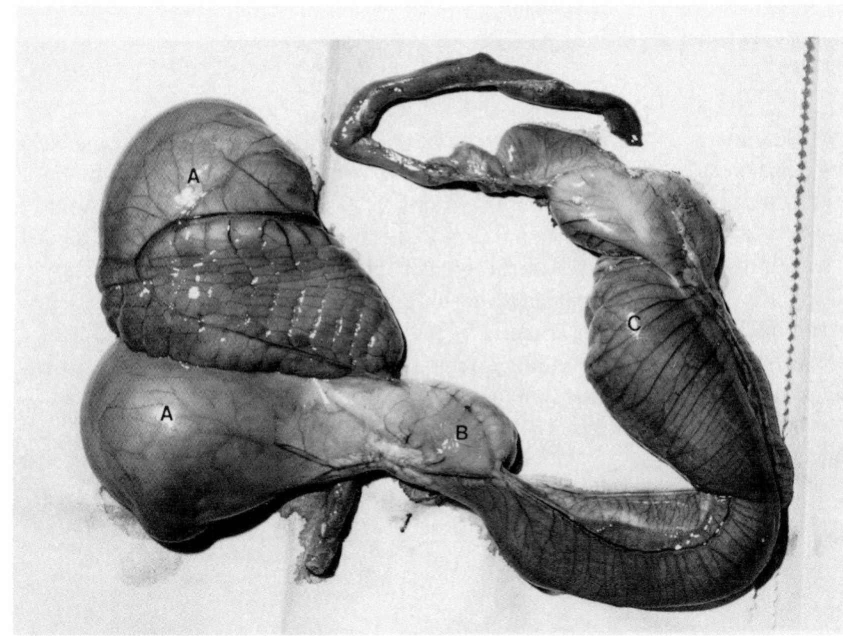

13.13 Stomach of a neonate llama: **(A)** C-1, **(B)** C-2, **(C)** C-3.

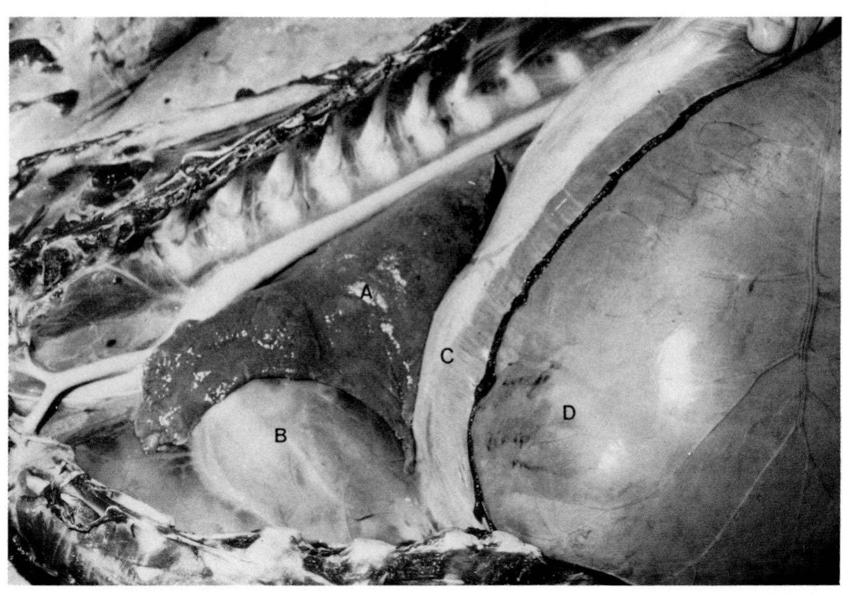

13.14 Relation of stomach to other organs: **(A)** lung, **(B)** heart, **(C)** diaphragm, **(D)** C-1.

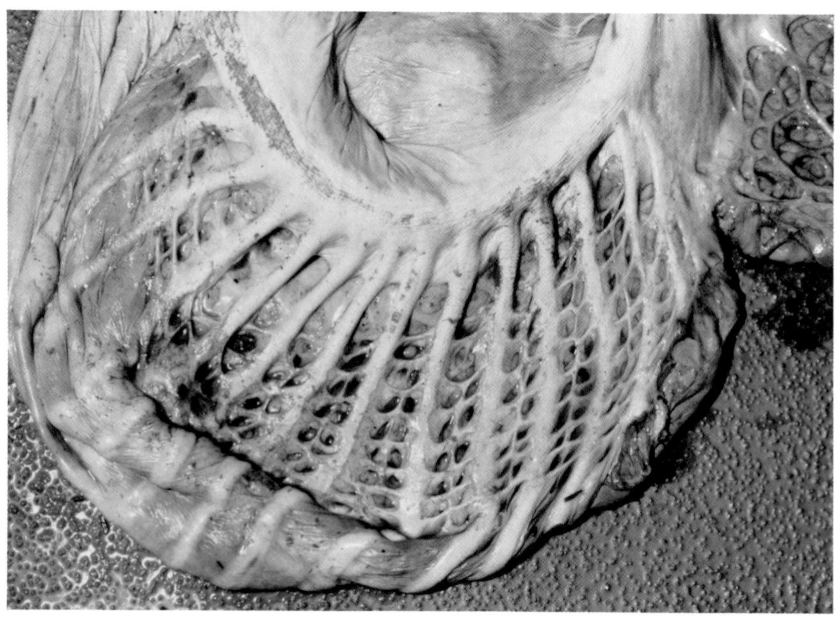

13.15 Glandular saccules of C-1.

esophageal or ventricular groove (Fig. 13.16). The glandular area is subdivided by a series of intersecting crests that produce a retiform pattern and is covered by a papillated glandular mucosa (68, 69). The retiform pattern is not analogous to the pattern seen in the reticulum of ruminants (81, 84). The primary crest margins are covered by stratified squamous epithelium extending from the ventricular groove, but the secondary crests are covered with glandular mucosa (81, 84). The depressions of C-2 are not deep and do not evert during the contraction phase of the motility cycle of the stomach.

The mucosa of C-3 is entirely glandular (Fig. 13.17). There are three pattern areas and two types of mucosa. On the lesser curvature of the first one-fifth is found a retiform pattern with short crests and shallow depressions. On the greater curvature of the first one-fifth are nonpermanent folds. The mucosa of the middle three-fifths consists of permanent longitudinal pleats (approximately 50). The epithelium of the proximal four-fifths is a mucinous glandular tissue, similar to the glandular tissue of C-1 and C-2.

The terminal one-fifth of C-3 contains the true gas-

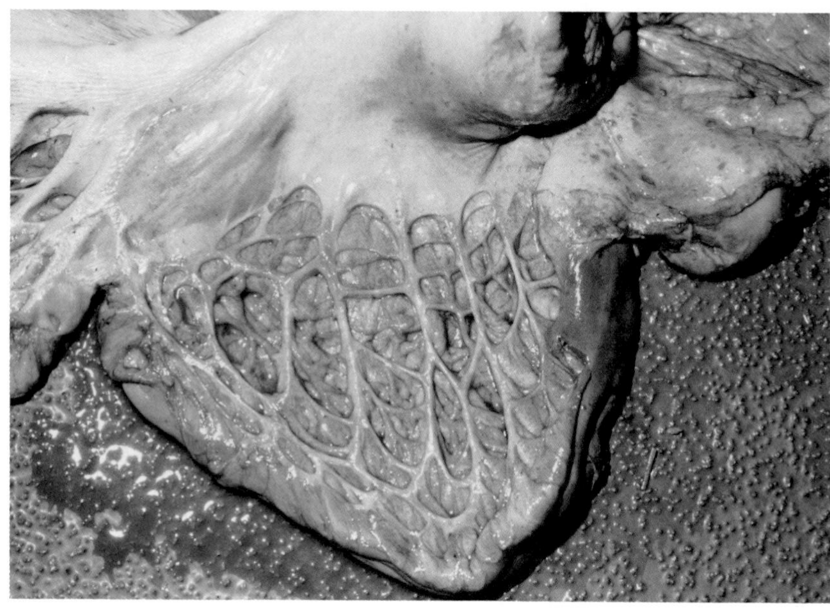

13.16 Glandular divisions of C-2.

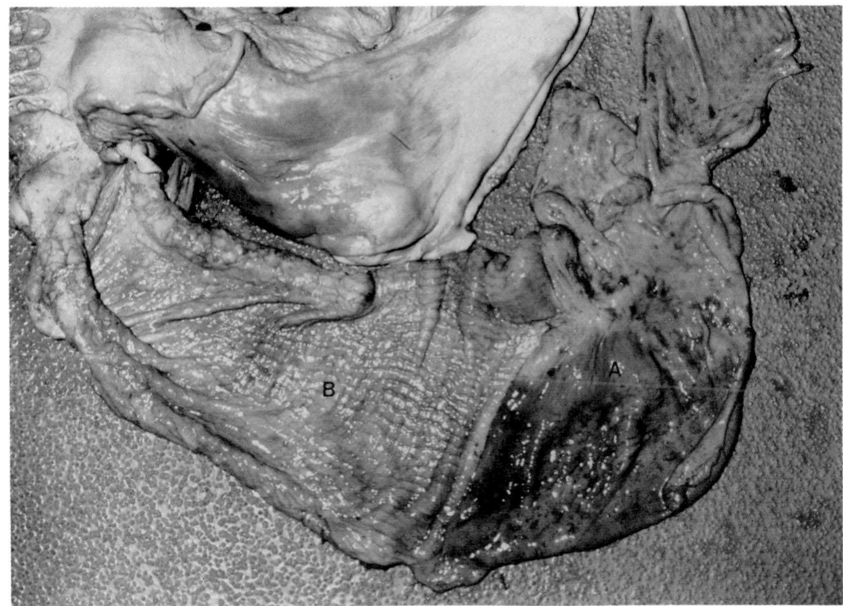

13.17 C-3 of stomach: **(A)** true stomach, **(B)** general glandular mucosa.

tric glands. The mucosa is reddish-brown in color, in contrast to the lighter pink color of the proximal four-fifths. The wall of this area is thickened and the mucosal surface smooth (81, 84). Digestive enzymes and acid are secreted by these glands. The pH in the cranial segment of C-3 is 6.5, which decreases to less than 2.0 in the terminal fifth (24). In Old World camels, the mucosa of the terminal fifth of C-3 may have coarse rugae (84).

The basic contraction cycle of the stomach of the llama and guanaco was established by Vallenas (20, 78, 82). A contraction cycle is initiated by a single rapid contraction in C-2, followed quickly by a contraction of the caudal sac of C-1. The direction of the contraction is from caudad to cranial. Next, the cranial sac of C-1 contracts in the reverse direction, cranial to caudad.

In the resting llama, the sequence of contractions of C-1 is repeated six to eight times before another contraction of C-2 occurs. The cycle is from one contraction of C-2 to the next (of C-2), and the average length of a cycle is 1.8 ± 2 minutes.

To the clinician, this equates to three or four audible contractions per minute in a resting animal and four to five contractions during feeding or the immediate post-feeding state. The amplitude of the contractions also increases during feeding.

The contents of the glandular saccules of the caudal sac are extruded just prior to the contraction of the caudal sac of C-1. The contents of the caudal sac and dorsal area of the cranial sac of C-1 are quite dry (Fig. 13.18). The more fluid and smaller particulate matter is

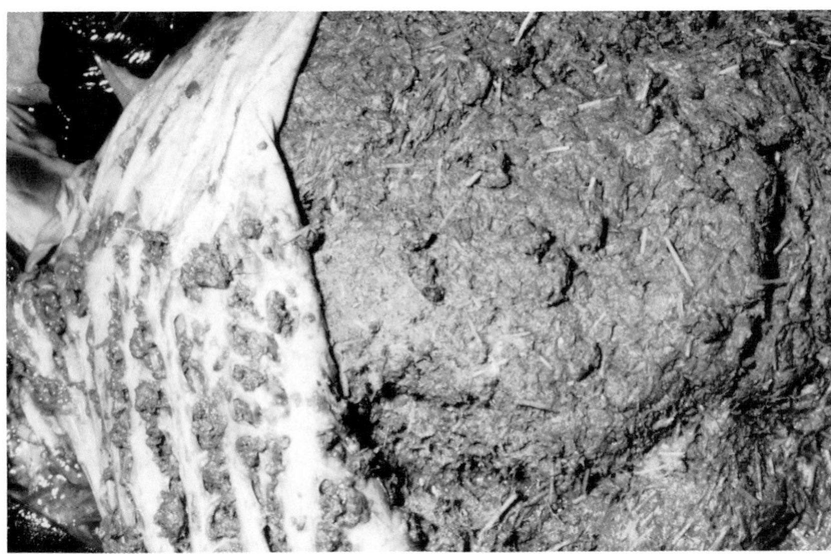

13.18 Homogeneous ingesta, characteristic of C-1.

found in the ventral cranial sac. The motility pattern tends to dump ingesta back and forth between the cranial and caudal sacs. This is a highly efficient mechanism for mixing the ingesta and enhancing the fermentation process. The ingesta in C-3 is rather dry, a result of the water absorption that takes place in the cranial four-fifths.

Volatile fatty acids (VFA) are rapidly absorbed from C-1, and in the case of VFA, perhaps at two to three times the rate of absorption from the rumen of sheep and goats (22–24, 80). Similar absorption of VFA occurs from the proximal four-fifths of C-3.

C-1 microflora and fauna are described by Harmeyer and Hill (35) and Sillau et al. (70) and in Chapter 2.

Camelids are capable of adapting to low-protein diets by recycling the urea produced as an end product of nitrogen metabolism (18, 36–38, 67). Urea is used by stomach bacteria to form their own protein. The bacteria will be subsequently digested and the protein absorbed further along the intestinal tract and utilized by the camelid. The presence of VFA enhances the efficiency of urea recycling; thus it is desirable for the camelid to consume a source of carbohydrate, if at all possible, when on a low-protein diet. When food is withheld from a llama for 48 hours, the plasma-urea (BUN) concentration will increase (36).

The esophageal groove of the camelid is not as well developed as in ruminants (76). There is only a single lip as contrasted with two in the ruminant. The functional groove extends from the cardia to and through the lesser curvature of C-2. See Vallenas (77) and Chapter 21 for a discussion of chemical stimulation and closure of the esophageal groove.

Transit times for ingesta have been studied (9), but no conclusions have been reached.

A study on eructated gas expulsion in alpacas was conducted in 1968 (17).

Omentum

The greater omentum is relatively smaller in the camelid than in cattle and sheep. In the adult ruminant, the greater omentum usually conceals all the intestines in a sling except for the descending duodenum. Again, in the ruminant, the omentum does not support the weight of the intestines, but merely rests on the abdominal floor.

In the camelid there is no omental sling. The greater omentum is attached along both the lesser and greater curvatures of C-2 and C-3 and along the right surface of C-1 (45). The epiploic foramen enters the sac formed by the greater omentum ventral to the liver, near the entrance of the post cava into the liver. Epiploic herniation of the jejunum has caused death in a llama.

Intestine

SMALL INTESTINE (39). There is a dilated ampulla at the entrance of the duodenum. The duodenum courses dorsally on the right side of C-1 to the dorsum of the abdominal cavity just caudad to the liver. The jejunum is folded around the root of the mesentery, in the right caudal abdomen. The ileum begins ventrally and courses mesially and dorsally to enter the large intestine at the cecocolic orifice.

LARGE INTESTINE. The cecum lies approximately on the midline and is directed caudally toward the pelvic inlet, or it may curve ventrally and laterally to the left. The camelid colon is similar to that of the bovine. The ascending colon begins as a proximal loop that courses cranially and ventrally to enter the spiral loop (Figs. 13.19a,b). The most proximal loop of the ascending colon is loosely attached by a mesentery to the more compact spiral colon. There are 5.5 centripetal coils (including the proximal loop) and 4.5 centrifugal coils (Figs. 13.19–13.20). There are only two coils in bovines and three in ovines. The centrifugal coils are buried within the spiral, deep to the centripetal coils. The spiral colon lies on the midventral abdominal wall and is likely to be the first organ encountered on a ventral midline laparotomy.

The colon narrows from a 5 cm diameter at its beginning to 2 cm within the first centripetal coil of the spiral loop. The spiral colon is the primary site of fecalith impaction in lamoids.

The distal loop of the ascending colon is juxtaposed to the proximal loop. The transverse colon passes from right to left cranial to the mesenteric artery and continues on as the descending colon to the rectum and anus.

LENGTH OF INTESTINAL SEGMENTS. The measurements of the intestines of a 140 kg llama were as follows: The small intestine was 11.5–12 m, of which the duodenum was less than 1 m, the jejunum 9.5–10 m, and the ileum 1 m in length. The large intestine was 7.5 m long, of which the cecum was 10 cm long and 5 cm in diameter, the large colon was 1.5 m long, diminishing in diameter from 5 to 2.5 cm in its course, and the small colon was 6 m long and approximately 2.5 cm in diameter.

PELLET FORMATION. Camelids void feces in pellet form (32). These begin to form in the proximal spiral colon. Desiccation of the pellet continues throughout the colon. Old World camels have the capacity to pass totally desiccated feces when water intake is restricted. In the Arabian desert during the summer, freshly passed feces can be used for fuel. The fecal pellets

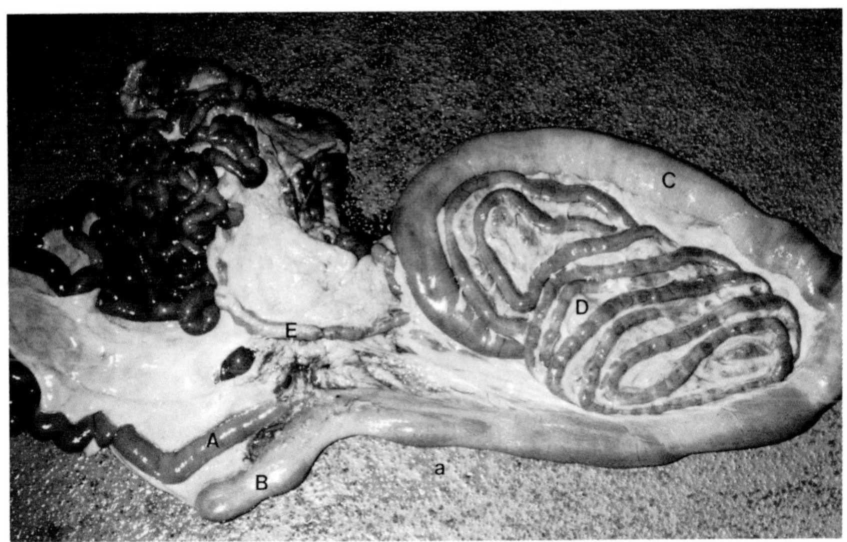

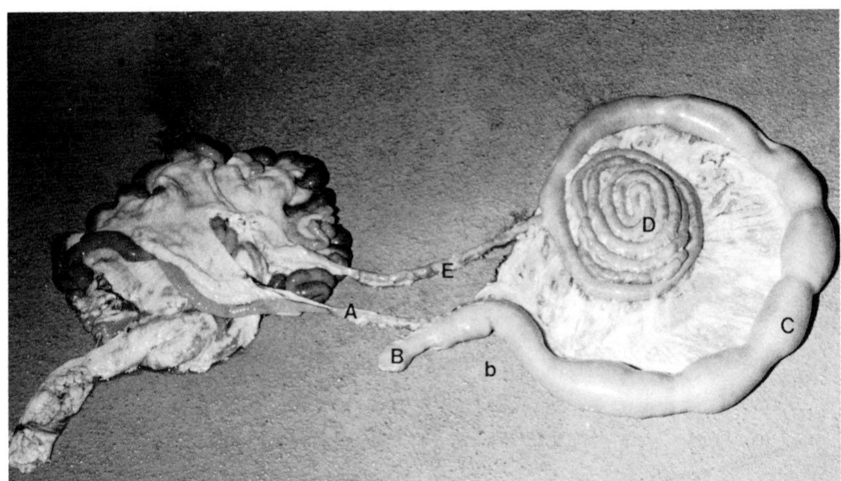

13.19a,b Intestines of a llama: **(A)** ileum, **(B)** cecum, **(C)** proximal loop of spiral colon, **(D)** spiral colon, **(E)** transverse colon.

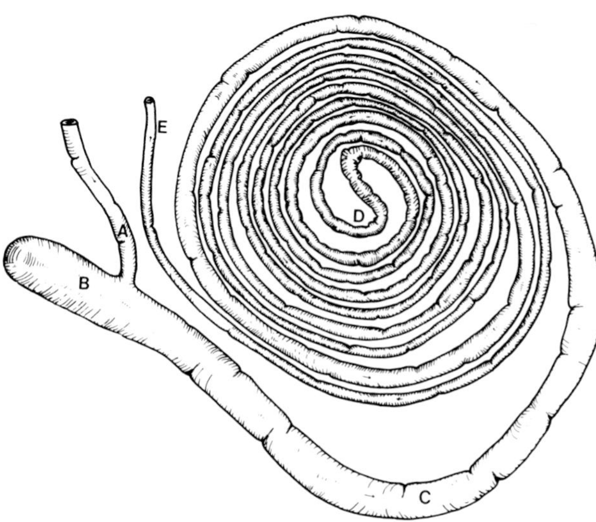

13.20 Diagram of the spiral colon of a llama: **(A)** ileum, **(B)** cecum, **(D)** proximal loop of spiral colon, **(D)** spiral colon, **(E)** transverse colon.

of SACs are also used for fuel, but they must be allowed to dry further.

The llama fecal pellet varies with the size of the animal, from 7 × 12 to 20 × 30 mm (Fig. 13.21). There is generally a sharp teat on one end of the pellet. Some individuals pass teardrop-shaped pellets (7 × 12 × 20 mm). The pellets of a healthy llama may be voided as separate pellets or in a compressed cylindric mass, which easily breaks apart into individual pellets. The color of the stool varies with the diet but is generally greenish-brown, blackening after voiding.

The stool of the dromedary camel is passed in irregularly shaped pellets. A medium-sized female may void pellets that range in size from 15 × 15 × 15 to 20 × 25 × 25 mm. A large male may pass pellets as large as 25 × 30 × 35 mm.

SACs generally use communal dung piles (Fig. 13.22). In inclement weather, a dung pile may be begun in a barn and the use of it continued into the summer.

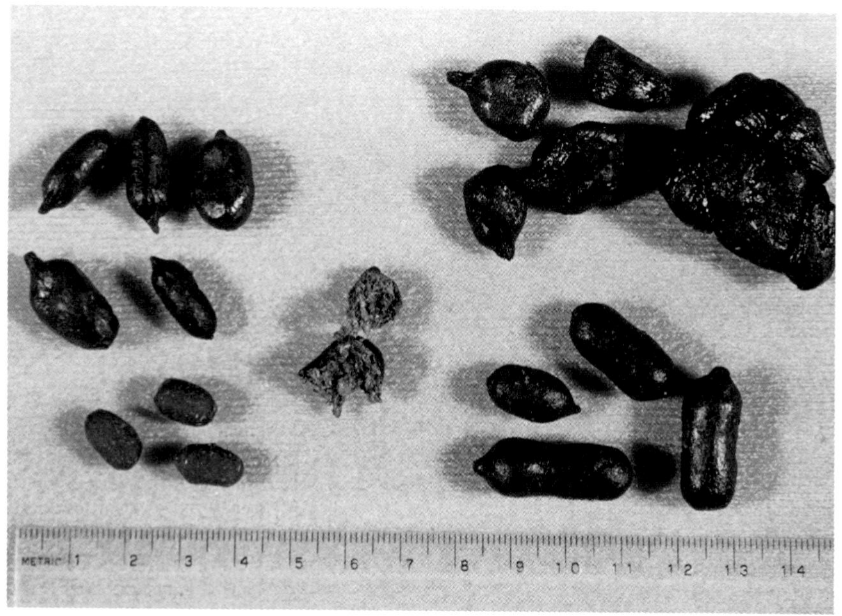

13.21 Fecal pellets from llamas.

Numerous methods have been tried by owners to change the location of a dung heap. Old World camels do not use a dung heap.

More details of the anatomy of the digestive system, including vascular supply, may be found in Langer (45), Vallenas (78), Montalvo (57–59), de la Vega (15), Cummings (12), and Galotta (27).

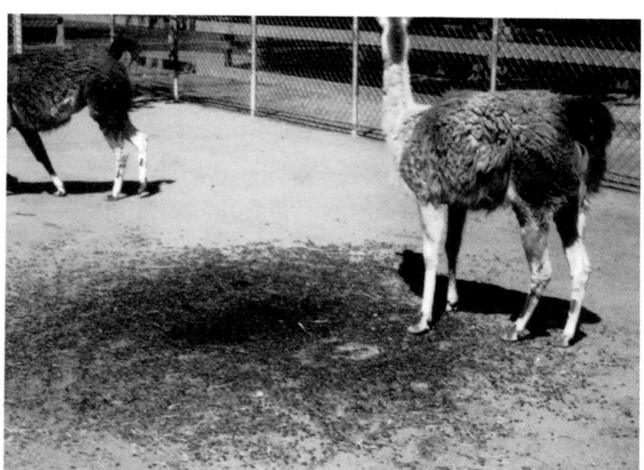

13.22 Dung pile utilized by llamas for urination and defecation.

Liver (2, 54, 85, 88)

The liver is located entirely on the right side (Fig. 13.23) (8). The dorsocaudal border extends caudad to the cartilage of the last rib. The liver covers C-2 and C-3 of the stomach, although there is a notch on the cranioventral border where a small portion of C-3 is visible. The caudal border of the liver is strikingly fimbriated (Fig. 13.24). Camelids have no gall bladder.

BILE DUCT. The collecting system ends in the major bile duct, 4 mm in diameter, at the caudal aspect of the liver. The duct is 3–4 cm long and penetrates the antimesenteric surface of a loop of duodenum that courses over toward the liver. The opening into the duodenum is 16–20 cm from the pylorus.

Pancreas

The pancreas lies caudal to the liver. It is a flattened gland, not well encapsulated in the duodenal mesentery. It is approximately 15–20 cm long and 3–6 cm wide. The pancreatic duct exits the cranial aspect of the gland and unites with the bile duct about 3 cm before it enters the intestine.

DIGESTIVE DISEASES

Signs Associated with Digestive Disorders

None of the signs suggesting disease of the digestive system are definitive. Nondigestive system diseases may produce similar signs. An overview of these signs and their multiple causes will help in establishing a tentative diagnosis and aid in formulating a diagnostic plan.

ANOREXIA. Anorexia is the lack or loss of appetite for food. Other words that are used, somewhat synonymously, to describe this condition include inanition (the physical condition resulting from the complete lack

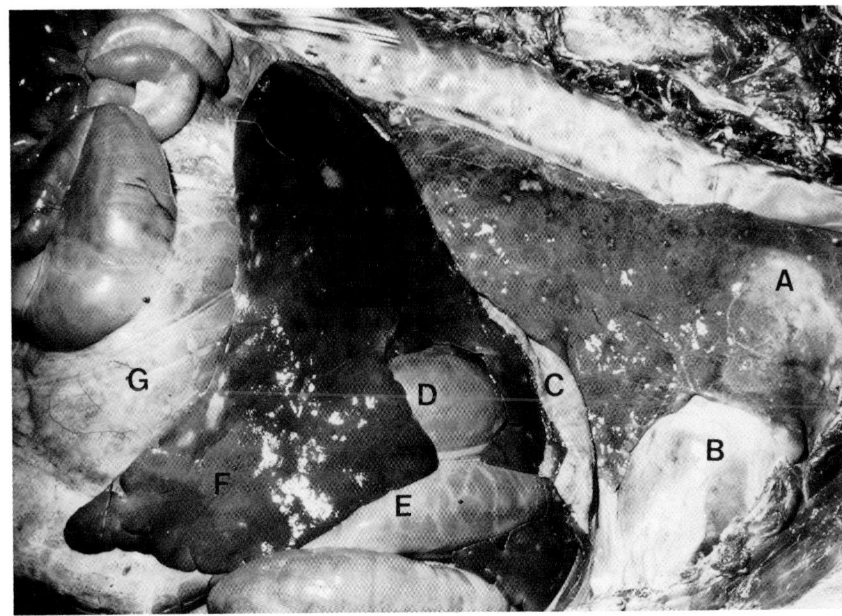

13.23 Liver of a llama in situ, right side: **(A)** lung, **(B)** heart, **(C)** diaphragm, **(D)** C-2, **(E)** C-3, **(F)** liver, **(G)** C-1.

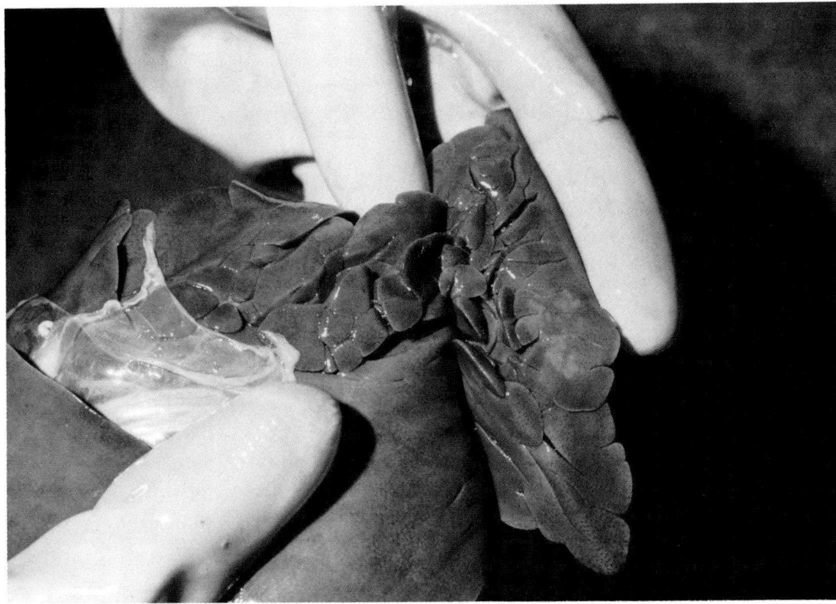

13.24 Fimbriated caudal border of a lamoid liver.

of food) and inappetence (lack of desire or appetite for food). It is difficult at times to determine whether there is a genuine lack of desire to eat or if there is an inability to eat because of weakness or an organic disorder that prevents eating. An attempt should be made to determine whether or not anorexia stems from an internal disorder or from external factors.

Internally caused factors include electrolyte imbalance, dental pain, stomatitis, temporomandibular arthritis, oral or pharyngeal abscesses, glossitis, colic, gastritis, central nervous system (CNS) injury, anemia, septicemia, and pyrexia. External factors that may contribute to anorexia include psychologic ostracism and unsuitable feed (not appropriate to the individual, moldy, too stemmy, or containing foreign material).

Herbivores normally consume feeds with low levels of sodium and an excess of potassium. The bovine kidney has a high concentration of renin to aid in the conservation of sodium. Potassium is poorly conserved since it is usually amply provided in the diet.

Anorexia will result in low potassium intake and, subsequently, development of hypokalemia, especially if the llama continues to drink or is given parenteral fluids lacking in potassium. Hypokalemia may also result from loss of ingesta via vomition or diarrhea or from prolonged diuretic or corticosteroid therapy. Hypokalemia may contribute to or result from an alkalosis.

Clinical signs of hypokalemia include muscular weakness, depression, and altered cardiac function. These are nonspecific signs often seen in an ailing llama, and a case must be carefully evaluated to determine the cause. Serum chemistry analysis may be necessary.

PREHENSION DIFFICULTIES. This sign may be closely related to anorexia, since anything that interferes with a llama's ability to take in food may result in anorexia. Some of the causes of prehension difficulty include facial nerve paralysis, glossal trauma, labioitis, dental pain, CNS disturbance, temporomandibular arthritis, trauma to the mandible/premaxilla/maxilla, infection or tumors of the same bone, congenital defects (brachygnathism of either the mandible or the maxilla), and foreign bodies in the oral cavity.

DYSPHAGIA. Reluctance or inability to swallow may be caused by hypoglossal or glossopharyngeal nerve paralysis, pharyngitis, esophagitis, pharyngeal abscesses, pharyngeal tumors, esophageal obstruction, stomach overload, bloat, infectious diseases (rabies, botulism), or congenital defects (agenesis of the soft palate, cleft soft palate). With choanal atresia, the infant cannot eat and breathe simultaneously. Fracture of the hyoid apparatus and a variety of CNS disorders may also cause dysphagia.

Signs of dysphagia include drooling of saliva (sialosis), retention of feed in the oral cavity, a fetid odor from the oral cavity, gagging, and retching.

REGURGITATION AND EMESIS. It is important to differentiate between regurgitation and emesis. Regurgitation may be voluntary in camelids. It is used as a threat or as a defense against aggression between males or by the female if she is pregnant or unwilling to submit to the male. This behavior can be anticipated if the ears lie back over the neck, followed by a gurgling noise in the pharyngeal region as the llama prepares to eject the bolus. On the left side, the bolus can be seen traversing the cervical region. Stomach contents can be spewed a distance of 3 m quite accurately.

Active regurgitation may occur as a result of esophageal stimulation as a gastric tube is passed or from laryngopharyngeal stimulation when an endotracheal tube is inserted. Passive regurgitation may occur from relaxation of the stomach cardia during anesthesia or from improper positioning during recumbency. If possible, the llama should lie on its right side. Abdominal pressure, either externally applied or as a result of bloat or other abdominal distention, may also cause regurgitation.

Emesis is the involuntary projection of stomach contents by a reflex action and consists of an initial deep inspiration followed by closing of the glottis to prevent aspiration of ingesta. At the same time, the soft palate should be automatically elevated to seal off the nasopharynx. Ingesta is ejected by a strong contraction of all the abdominal muscles and antiperistaltic contractions of the esophagus. In the llama, as in the horse, emesis is a grave sign because of the elongated soft palate. If the soft palate fails to seal off the nasopharynx, it is relatively easy for ingesta to be pushed into the nasal cavity, causing rhinitis, obstruction, or aspiration.

Some of the causes of emesis include overloading of C-1, gastritis, diaphragmatic hernia, arsenic poisoning, partial esophageal obstruction, and the ingestion of poisonous plants. A list of such plants includes oleander, *Nerium oleander;* corn lily, *Veratrum californicum* or *V. viridis;* lily of the valley, *Convallaria majalis;* foxglove, *Digitalis purpurea;* sneezeweed, *Helenium* sp.; and various members of the Ericaceae family, all containing the same andromedotoxin (a glycoside), including rhododendron and azalea, *Rhododendron* sp.; laurel, *Leucothoe* sp.; labrador tea, *Ledum* sp.; and kalmia, *Kalmia* sp.

The clinical evidence of regurgitation or emesis is obvious. The medical management of these conditions will depend on the primary cause. Any obstruction should be corrected and irritants removed from the stomach, which may require gastrotomy. In addition, C-1 electrolyte and microbial balance should be reestablished.

ABDOMINAL DISTENTION. Abdominal distention may be caused by excessive fat, presence of a fetus, excessive gas (flatus), accumulation of feces, or abdominal fluid (five "Fs" of abdominal distention). A thorough physical examination may lead to identification of the cause, but in lamoids, a thorough rectal examination is not possible.

Abdominal distention is frequently benign, caused by overeating. However, excessive or prolonged abdominal pressure pushes the diaphragm forward, causing dyspnea. Compression of the abdominal vessels interferes with circulation, and shock may ensue.

TENESMUS. Tenesmus is ineffectual straining to defecate. Nondigestive disorders may mimic this straining. Potential causes include diarrhea, parturition, rectal or vaginal prolapse, urethral calculus, cystitis, vaginitis, pyrrolizidine alkaloid poisoning, proctitis caused by irritation from a rough rectal examination, CNS derangements (spinal cord compression), and rabies.

The signs of tenesmus are obvious. Management requires correction of the primary cause. An epidural anesthesia may give temporary relief and possibly interrupt the painful cycle that perpetuates the tenesmus. Alcohol epidural blocks have proved to be efficacious when treating cattle with chronic tenesmus.

DIARRHEA. Diarrhea may be defined as the abnormally frequent passage of feces that are irregularly formed and more moist or fluid than usual. Diarrhea is such a frequently observed clinical sign that it cannot be considered to be definitive in differential diagnoses. However, some of the diseases in which it is important in making a tentative diagnosis should be discussed.

Enteritis is the most common cause of diarrhea and may be initiated by clostridial toxemia, parasitism, stomach overload (C-1 acidosis), or plant or other poisoning (arsenic, copper, lead, molybdenum). Additional causes are overhydration, consumption of too much lush feed, and sudden change in feed. Nondigestive tract causes of diarrhea include excitement, hepatopathy, and poisoning from organic phosphate insecticides. Infectious diseases causing enteritis, hence diarrhea, include salmonellosis, paratuberculosis, colibacillosis, rinderpest, and tuberculosis.

An overview of the pathogenesis of diarrhea may help in visualizing the many factors that may be contributors. There are five basic causes of diarrhea: (1) osmotic pressure imbalance, (2) inhibition of absorption of electrolytes, (3) derangement of the secretory function of the intestinal mucosa that may likewise adversely change the electrolyte balance, (4) changes in mucosal permeability caused by denudation of the epithelium or circulatory changes, and (5) derangement in the motility cycle of the intestine.

The signs of diarrhea are obvious. There are, however, numerous types of diarrhea, each of which has a bearing on the diagnosis. A detailed discussion, including the management of diarrhea, will be found under enteritis or specific diseases with diarrhea as the major clinical entity.

CONSTIPATION. Constipation is the abnormally infrequent or difficult evacuation of feces that have remained in the rectum and are usually more firm or dry than usual. The term obstipation is sometimes used instead, but the precise meaning of this term is intractable constipation. In the usual clinical sense, constipation refers to any slowness or absence of passage of feces. It is important to differentiate between true constipation, in which feces pass into the colon and rectum, but the rate of passage is slow and fluid is absorbed, making the feces hard and dry, and the more serious obstipation, in which an obstruction or other cause prevents passage of feces into the terminal colon.

Since camelids pass a relatively dry fecal pellet, the dryness of feces may be a difficult sign to interpret. The constipated llama is not likely to be straining. When feces are collected from the rectum, the pellets or the fecal mass may be covered with mucus, giving the feces a shiny appearance.

Some of the causes of constipation include malnutrition or starvation, dehydration, painful condition around the anus, pelvic abscess, pelvic fracture, pelvic tumors, acorn poisoning (*Quercus* sp. tannins), paralytic ileus, general debility, spinal injury, lack of exercise (downers), and toxicosis (lead, fluorine, chronic zinc poisoning).

ILEUS. Ileus refers to intestinal obstruction. True, or complete, ileus may be caused by external compression of the intestine from peritoneal adhesions, tumors, advanced pregnancy, torsions, or internal hernias. Such obstructions are referred to as mechanical ileus. Dynamic ileus may be spastic, caused by a constriction around an impaction or enterolith, or paralytic, a result of intrinsic disorders of bowel motility. Intestinal atony may be caused reflexively postoperatively as a result of peritonitis, ischemia, or overstretching of the intestine from ingesta or gas. Metabolic changes may also initiate an ileus (acidosis, hypokalemia).

STOMACH ATONY. Stomach atony does not occur as a primary disease but rather is a clinical sign caused by numerous disorders including grain overload (rare in llamas), simple indigestion, sudden changes of feed, prolonged antimicrobial therapy, spoiled feed, gastric ulceration, and obstruction of the cranial intestinal tract (89). Other causes might be hypomagnesemia, septicemia, and other types of colic.

Microflora and fauna activity is crucial to proper stomach activity, and any condition that destroys normal microorganisms predisposes to gastric atony. Atony is usually accompanied by anorexia.

Lack of motility is generally ascertained by auscultation with a stethoscope. The contractions of C-1 are not as pronounced as contractions of the rumen in the ruminant, so palpation in the left paralumbar fossa will not be helpful. The rate and rhythm of C-1 contraction vary with the proximity to feed ingestion. If the llama is eating or has recently consumed feed, the contractions will be frequent, two to four per minute, with no intervals between. If no rumination is taking place, the rate is slower. In the normal llama, the only abdominal sounds will be from C-1. With obstruction or delay of movement of ingesta along the intestinal tract, gas formation may mix with fluid and produce intestinal borborygmus.

Stomach atony is usually only a sign of other clinical problems, so medical management of atony should deal with the primary disorder. However, prolonged atony of C-1 (48–72 hours) may initiate a change in the pH of the ingesta, which in turn will destroy the microflora and fauna. Ultimate reestablishment of gastric motility may necessitate transfaunation.

COLIC. Much has been written about equine colic. The pathophysiology has been intensively studied, and great advances have been made in dealing with digestive disorders causing colicky or abdominal pain. Ruminants also have digestive disorders that cause obstruction and distention of the gastrointestinal (GI) tract, but ruminants react to pain differently. They are more passive and not so expressive of discomfort. Llamas seem to be more like the horse in expression of the pain of colic, but the digestive disorders of the llama resemble those of the ruminant because of the closer similarity of the digestive tract anatomy.

Normal GI mucosa is insensitive to touch, cutting, pinching, and tearing. GI pain arises from stretching of the muscular layer and serosa, as occurs with distention of the viscus or with powerful muscular contractions (42).

The sensory response is via the afferent visceral fibers accompanying the sympathetic pathway (42). An acute inflammation or vascular engorgement decreases the pain threshold. As a result, mild stimuli that would not initiate a pain response in the normal bowel cause pain. Tissue hypoxia also decreases the threshold, thus obstructive lesions compromising circulation cause significant pain. Excessive production of acid in C-1 may produce a direct inflammation of the gastric mucosa and initiate a pain response. Acid may also stimulate muscle spasms.

Most digestive tract disorders, at one time or another during the course of the disease, will produce colicky pain. What appears to be GI pain may arise from disorders of other organ systems, emphasizing the importance of careful evaluation in the initial examination. Uterine torsion, cystitis, urethral obstruction, liver diseases, back pain, and certain infectious diseases (salmonellosis, rabies, anthrax) should be considered. Even thirst or starvation may, in the early stages, cause stomach contractions that will be expressed as painful colic.

Signs of colic in the llama are similar to those seen in the equine and include groaning, grinding of the teeth, getting up and down, rolling, refusing to get up, kicking at the belly, peculiar stances, pressing into a corner, looking back at the belly, frenzy, depression, anorexia, arched back, tenesmus, tense abdomen, stomach atony, increased heart rate, frequent passage of small amounts of urine, tenseness of facial muscles, and a pained expression of the eyes. Signs of colic in the neonate may be caused by retained meconium, atresia ani or atresia coli, and incarceration of an intestinal loop in an inguinal or umbilical hernia.

Other conditions that may mimic signs of colic include normal rolling behavior, weakness, incoordination (insecticide poisoning, heavy metals, head injuries, spinal cord compression), septicemia, and arthritis. Other sources of abdominal pain may be pleuritis, peritonitis, ruptured liver, and ruptured bladder.

SPECIFIC DISEASES OF THE DIGESTIVE SYSTEM (40, 89)

Lip Disorders

Laceration of the lips may be caused by barbed wire or other sharp objects in the environment or by dog bites. The lips may also be lacerated by the incisor teeth as a result of a blow to the muzzle. Puncture wounds occur similarly. Labial swelling may result from dependent edema from hypoproteinemia or anemia, cellulitis, a tumor, constriction of venous drainage, contusion, or rattlesnake bite (see Chap. 23).

Erosions and ulcers of both the external and internal surface of the lips may be caused by vesicular diseases (foot-and-mouth disease, vesicular stomatitis), rinderpest, or grass awns (yellow bristle grass, *Setaria lutescens,* foxtails, *Hordeum* sp.). Caustic materials are known to cause labial ulcers in livestock and horses, but llamas are more cautious about ingestion of such materials.

Proliferative lesions of the lips may be caused by contagious ecthyma (see Chap. 7). Paralysis of the lips may follow damage to the facial nerve, as in listeriosis (see Chap. 7).

Stomatitis

The term "stomatitis" encompasses the inflammatory response to injury or disease of any oral tissue. Designation of a specific organ may be made, such as glossitis or gingivitis.

ETIOLOGY. Any of the factors causing lip problems may also affect the mouth. Additional damaging agents may include foreign bodies, candidiasis, actinobacillosis, trauma from gastric tube passage, cellulitis arising from focal infections within the mouth, and developmental defects (malocclusion).

SIGNS. Signs of oral ailments include inappetence, peculiar chewing motions, excessive salivation, odorous breath, hyperemia of the mucosa, erosions, ulcers, and vesicles.

DIAGNOSIS. Careful physical examination of the mouth will usually allow visualization of the lesions, although it may be difficult in lamoids because the mouth is narrow and will not open widely. The llama usually resents manipulation of the mouth, so sedation may be necessary to fully examine the mouth and carry out diagnostic procedures, including inspection, cultures, and biopsy. Since some oral diseases are foreign animal diseases, a definitive diagnosis is mandatory. Any case suspected of being a vesicular disease should be reported immediately to state or federal regulatory agencies. Procedures necessary to arrive at a definitive diagnosis will then be conducted by them.

TREATMENT. Correct the primary condition. Provide soft, palatable feed. The mouth may be flushed with water to cleanse it of feed particles or exudate, using a dose syringe with a long nozzle.

Tongue Disorders

No diseases specific to the tongue of the lamoid have been reported. Glossitis may be a part of a general stomatitis. Hypoglossal nerve paralysis may occur as a result of a blow to the intermandibular space or from fractures of the mandible and hyoid apparatus, abscesses at the base of the tongue, or lesions in the brain (encephalitis, rabies, tumor).

The tongue is rarely lacerated because it does not protrude from the mouth. Sharp dental enamel points could traumatize the tongue, but this is rare. The large canines in the male or the incisors of both sexes may puncture or lacerate the tongue if the llama should fall or strike the head in an attempt to flee from an aggressive enclosure mate or restraint attempts. The tongue may also be lacerated by overzealous pulling on the tongue when inserting an endotracheal tube.

DIAGNOSIS. Physical examination is necessary to establish the presence of a tongue disorder. In the instance of paralysis, more intensive investigation is necessary to ascertain the reason for the paralysis. This usually involves a neurologic evaluation.

Deglutition is usually inhibited with any lesion on the tongue. Bilateral hypoglossal nerve injury would allow the tongue to protrude from the mouth and possibly be secondarily traumatized.

TREATMENT. Lacerations should be sutured (probably requiring general anesthesia); otherwise, general nursing care is recommended.

Oral Abscess

ETIOLOGY. Oral abscesses may be caused by numerous opportunistic bacteria. The infection may enter through a break in the oral mucosa or be blood borne. *Corynebacterium pyogenes* is the organism most frequently cultured from oral abscesses in the author's practice, but streptococci, staphylococci, *Actinobacillus, Fusobacterium,* and *Actinomyces* have also been encountered.

In one case, an abscess on the lateral buccal surface ventral to the eye was repeatedly lanced. The organism isolated was an aberrant form of *Actinomyces* sp. Since the abscess complex was sited in the region of the passage of the facial nerve and the parotid duct, massive surgical extirpation was avoided until the failure of other measures to resolve the problem prompted drastic action. The abscessation had spread dorsally and caudally toward the ramus of the mandible. Radical surgery, followed by packing and irrigation with hydrogen peroxide and organic iodine finally eradicated the problem.

Necrobacillosis is a serious problem in lamoids in South America. The infection causes severe abscesses of the bones of the mandible and maxilla, but soft-tissue abscesses occur as well. See Chapter 7 for a full discussion of this disease.

Dental Problems

ETIOLOGY (53, 60, 68, 69). All of the dental problems seen in ruminants have been seen or are potential problems in camelids (10, 47). Conditions diagnosed by the author include dental plaque, pigmentation of the teeth, alveolar periostitis, pulpitis, fractures of the incisors and canines, fractures of the mandible, sharp enamel points caused by malocclusion, excessive wear, elongated teeth associated with superior brachygnathism, and other developmental defects causing malocclusion. The most common dental surgery is for canine tooth removal (43, 44, 73).

SIGNS. The signs of dental problems include inappetence, weight loss, abnormal chewing, dropping of a cud, swelling over the dental roots, mandibular fistulae, and sinusitis (molar roots are contiguous to the maxillary sinus).

DIAGNOSIS. Physical examination of the teeth is not easy and frequently necessitates anesthesia. Radiography is necessary, but high-quality, properly positioned films are required if radiography is to be of benefit. Oblique shots of the cheek teeth must be taken to prevent override from the opposite jaw. Radiographs of dental lesions of lamoids are evaluated in the same manner as those of other animals. Loss of the lamina dura dentes, radiolucent areas with abscessation, fractures and increased density with sclerotic bone, and osteomyelitis are conditions that may be seen.

TREATMENT. Plaque will rarely interfere with oral function and will not require removal unless it is causing gingivitis. Pulpitis and alveolar periostitis will necessitate extraction or repulsion of the tooth (see Chap. 6). If a dental fracture opens the pulp cavity, a pulpotomy may be done. If the pulp has become infected, the tooth should be removed.

Genetic defects can be eliminated only by a stringent breeding program, including culling. Elongated incisors may be cut off with a circular saw or an obstetric wire under anesthesia. The pulp cavities are rarely exposed. This should not be done to prepare a llama or alpaca for a show or sale. Elongated incisors is an unsoundness that should bar them from participation.

Salivary Gland Disorders

ETIOLOGY. The salivary glands of lamoids are affected by problems similar to those of ruminants. Abscesses within or next to the salivary glands are most common. *Corynebacterium pyogenes* is usually isolated from abscesses.

Generalized parotiditis has not been described. Salivary fistulae may occur from lacerations of the side of the face or abscessation and rupture of a duct. A laceration of the body of the gland is possible, but the skin thickness over the neck and face is such that a severe slashing blow would be required to penetrate the skin. A parotid salivary fistula may occur from a facial laceration.

SIGNS. The primary sign is swelling over the gland, either firm in the case of cellulitis or parotiditis or fluctuant with an abscess. The area is hot and the skin hyperemic. The llama would likely be reluctant to eat because of the pain in the angle of the jaw.

In the case of a salivary fistula, an excessive flow of saliva would be observed, especially while the llama is feeding or ruminating.

DIAGNOSIS. A physical examination will usually discover the problem. A needle may be inserted into a fluctuant swelling to establish the presence of an exudate, serum, or blood.

TREATMENT. Primary parotiditis requires broad-spectrum antimicrobial therapy. However, this is of little value in abscesses. It may be desirable to wait for an abscess to mature and localize before lancing, but otherwise a needle should be inserted at the ventral aspect of the abscess. When the exudate begins to flow, the needle should be left in place and an incision made along the needle in a vertical direction through the skin. If possible, blunt dissection should be continued with a hemostat to open the abscess. The cavity may be explored with a gloved finger and irrigated with a 1:4 dilution of povidone-iodine solution. The irrigation should be continued daily until the cavity has healed from the inside out.

Pharyngitis

Pharyngitis is any inflammation of the mucous membrane and surrounding tissue of the oro- or nasopharynx.

ETIOLOGY. Pharyngitis may be caused by acute or chronic bacterial infections, especially those of the respiratory system. Causes also include trauma from inept gastric intubation, abscesses, *Cephenemyia* sp. larvae infestation of the nasopharynx (see Chap. 8), and developmental defects such as agenesis of the soft palate or cleft soft palate (see Chap. 22).

SIGNS. Signs of pharyngitis include anorexia, weight loss, nasal discharge, coughing, fluctuant swelling behind the ramus of the mandible, extended head, pain response to palpation of the throat region, and hyperemia of the mucous membrane when examined with a laryngoscope or a Frick-type speculum.

DIAGNOSIS. The oropharynx may be visualized by insertion of a long-bladed laryngoscope, with the llama under anesthesia. Anesthesia is necessary because if examination is attempted without sedation or anesthesia, the llama may reflexively regurgitate. A Frick speculum is too large to insert into the mouth of any but the largest llama. The principle, however, may be applied by substituting an appropriately sized, smooth-ended piece of polyvinyl chloride pipe for the speculum. The nasopharynx may be explored with an endoscope via the nasal cavity, and the oropharynx, via the oral cavity.

TREATMENT. Soft, palatable feed and suitable quantities of water should be provided. Dehydration may be more of a problem than lack of food. If the problem is not resolved within a couple of days, with resumption of normal eating habits, it will be necessary to institute intravenous (IV) feeding. Parenteral antibiotics may be indicated.

It is usually necessary to lance abscesses. Sweating will help to bring an abscess to maturation. This may be done by frequent applications of moistened hot towels or by smearing the area with an irritant such as ichthammol. This would require that the wool in the upper neck be clipped, which most llama owners would resist.

Esophagitis

ETIOLOGY. Primary esophagitis is rare in camelids. They are apparently not susceptible to bovine virus diarrhea virus. There are no reports of rinderpest in SACs, but it has been reported in Old World camels, so lack of exposure is the probable reason the disease has not been reported in lamoids.

Esophagitis has been observed following repeated gastric intubation, especially with a rough-ended tube. Zinc deficiency or prolonged therapy with NaEDTA may result in esophageal parakeratosis.

SIGNS. Esophagitis is usually indicated by anorexia and a reluctance to swallow and/or regurgitate.

DIAGNOSIS. Diagnosis is difficult unless large-animal endoscopic equipment is available.

TREATMENT. The primary cause should be eliminated, then time allowed for healing.

Esophageal Obstruction (choke)

Obstruction of the esophagus is less common in camelids than in equines or bovines because of the ability of camelids to regurgitate freely. Camelids have more voluntary control of the esophagus than equines. However, choke related to apples and alfalfa pellets has been reported in the llama (29). Obstruction may be partial or complete. Any foreign body that becomes lodged in the esophagus will initiate muscular contractions with the purpose of moving the object one way or the other. If neither peristaltic nor antiperistaltic action is effective, the end result may be a spasm on either side of the obstruction that complicates the situation further and which may turn a partial into a complete obstruction.

ETIOLOGY. The only reported instance of choke in a llama involved the ingestion of apples falling from a tree in an orchard where the llama was corralled. In cattle, various feed items such as carrots, potatoes, or even boluses of grain have become lodged in the esophagus. The problem usually arises when a greedy animal bolts a mouthful of feed and attempts to swallow it without chewing.

SIGNS. Choke usually initiates alarming behavior that indicates the animal is in discomfort. The signs could be confused with colic, since they include retching, coughing, dysphagia, head shaking, salivation, nasal discharge, anxiety, and, if a blockage is prolonged, dehydration. If the animal continues to eat, food may pack in the pharyngeal area and subsequent retching may drive feed particles into the nasopharynx and out the nose. Aspiration of feed material into the trachea and lungs is a common sequel to choke.

The obstruction may be lodged anywhere from the origin of the esophagus to the cardia. If the object is in the cervical region, swelling may be observed over the esophagus. The esophagus of the lamoid lies deeper than that of other species and is somewhat obscured by the ventral tuberculum of the transverse process of the cervical vertebrae. Palpation may be necessary to locate the obstruction. The object causing the obstruction need not be larger than the bolus the animal would normally ingest or regurgitate for rechewing. The exact reason for initiation of a spasm causing an obstruction is not entirely known.

DIAGNOSIS. Clinical signs are characteristic in the early stages, but if the blockage persists, the animal will become depressed, and retching and coughing will diminish or cease. If blockage is suspected, a large gastric tube should be inserted into the esophagus and gently advanced to determine the patency of the esophagus (86). Vigorous force should not be used to push the object along. Radiography, both plain and contrast, is helpful, particularly in diagnosing obstructions within the thoracic esophagus. The diagnosis may also be aided by response to spasmolytic therapy.

TREATMENT. Objects in the upper esophagus cannot be retrieved by hand, as they may be in cattle. The narrowness of the throat of the llama does not allow this. Spasmolytics (atropine, regelen) should be given to relax the esophageal musculature and, hopefully, allow peristaltic activity to resume. Analgesics may be given, since this condition is certainly painful. Once the esophagus is relaxed, a large equine stomach tube may be used to gently push the object onward.

The foregoing stimulation of the pharynx and esophagus may initiate a reflex regurgitation attempt, and sedation or anesthesia may be necessary to continue. Aspiration of feed and saliva into the lungs is always a risk, and endotracheal intubation may be desirable when dealing with a difficult case.

Complete obstruction of the esophagus will prevent eructation, which may lead to the development of bloat. Bloat may be relieved by insertion of a large-bore needle into C-1 through the left paralumbar fossa, similar to the treatment of bloat in the ruminant.

Surgical intervention is rarely required to release an obstruction, but if it is necessary, reference to the equine literature will provide details of technique.

Esophageal Dilatation (megaesophagus, paralysis of the esophagus and esophageal achalasia, cardiospasm)

There are no literature citations on this condition, but the condition has been diagnosed in the author's clinic and elsewhere. The disease is characterized by dilatation of all or a part of the esophagus, especially the intrathoracic segment. In dogs, there may or may not be an associated failure or relaxation of the esophagogastric junction (34).

ETIOLOGY. The cause of esophageal dilatation (ED) is unknown in the llama. In dogs, it is considered to be a neuromuscular disorder that is seen most frequently in puppies but can be acquired later in life. The disorder may be congenital, but no hereditary transmission has been proven. In foals, it is felt to be caused by an uncoordinated opening of the cardia during the act of swallowing (16).

CLINICAL SIGNS. A llama with ED has recurring regurgitation. The material regurgitated may not have the normal odor of C-1 contents because it has never reached the stomach. Regurgitation is most likely to occur shortly after feeding and when the head is lowered to feed or drink. An affected animal fails to grow or will lose body condition. Aspiration pneumonia is a common sequel in the dog and foal and, presumably, in the llama. Dehydration may be a factor as well.

DIAGNOSIS. A greatly dilated esophagus is observed on plain radiographs of the thorax (Fig. 13.25). More definitive delineation is obtained by using contrast radiography. Fluoroscopy may also be used to evaluate the peristaltic activity of the esophagus. Figure 13.26 shows the dilated esophagus in situ at necropsy. Mild rhabdomyolysis of the skeletal muscle component of the distal esophagus was present on histologic examination.

TREATMENT. Insufficient cases have been managed to arrive at any conclusions as to treatment. Young dogs may improve as they mature. In dogs, more frequent ingestion of smaller quantities of food has been suggested to avoid overloading the esophagus.

Dietary management may be attempted in llamas, but the prognosis should be guarded to unfavorable. The presence of pneumonia may necessitate antimicrobial therapy. In foals, the cardiospasm is treated with promazine hydrochloride and spasmolytics such as dipyrone (Novin). If no response to drug therapy is obtained, surgical treatment is attempted (Ramsted operation) (16).

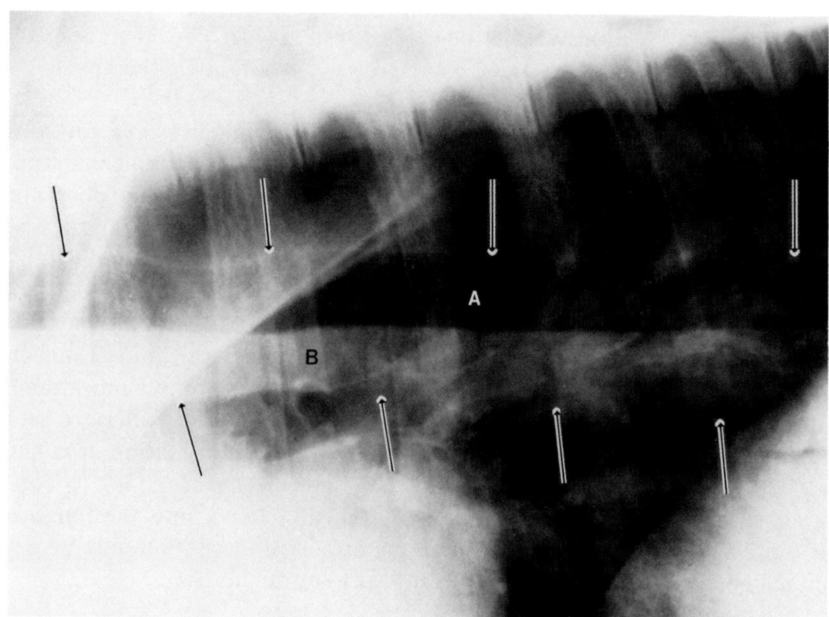

13.25 Lateral radiograph of dilated thoracic esophagus (arrows outline the wall of the esophagus): **(A)** gas, **(B)** food.

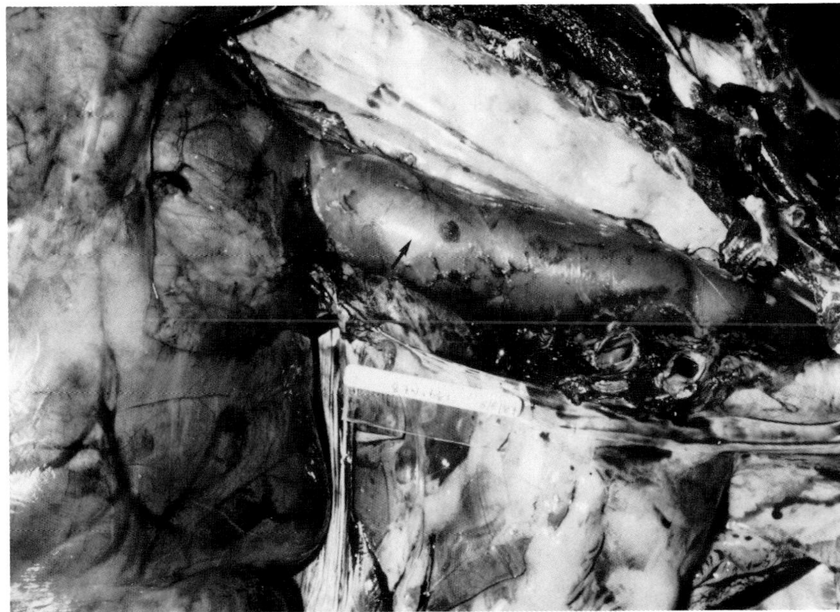

13.26 Thoracic esophageal dilatation in a llama.

Stomach Disorders

Disorders of the stomach may be primary or secondary to other diseases of the gastroenteric or other systems (75). The conditions seen by the author include simple indigestion (stomach atony) (74), gastritis, parasitism (see Chap. 8), and gastric ulceration with or without perforation. A llama will rarely engorge itself on grain or other concentrates, and bloat is not common. Lamoids are not troubled with displaced C-3 or traumatic gastritis, nor has vagal indigestion been described.

GASTRIC ULCERS. Primary gastritis is not usually diagnosed as a clinical condition but may be seen as a lesion at necropsy. Gastric ulceration, a common disorder, is not easily diagnosed but may contribute to serious problems in lamoids. Gastric ulcers may be seen in any of the stomach compartments. In C-1 and C-2, the ulcers are likely to involve the margins of the saccules in the glandular areas (Figs. 13.27, 13.28).

Ulceration of the mucous membrane of C-3 is common. The ulcers in the proximal four-fifths of C-3 tend to be linear along the ridges of the longitudinal pleats

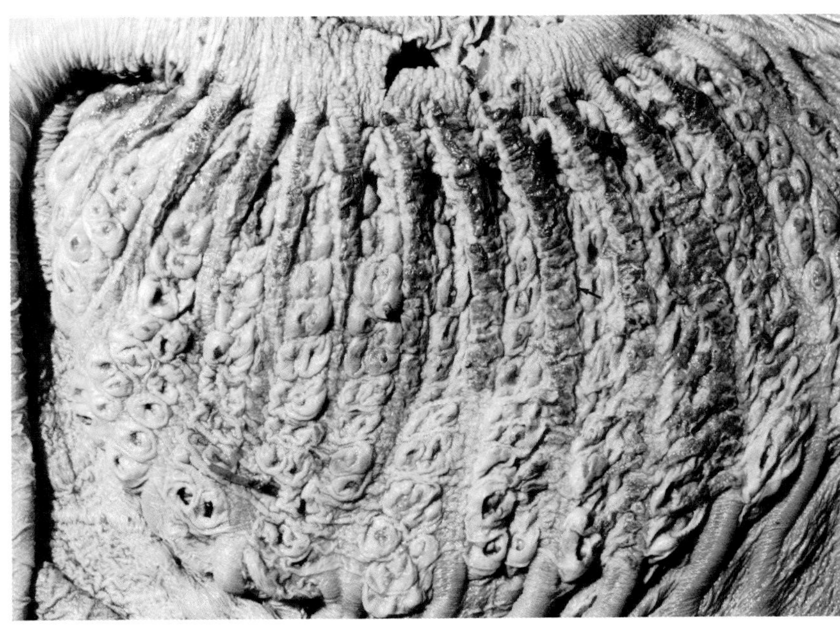

13.27 Mucosal ulceration of C-1 in a llama.

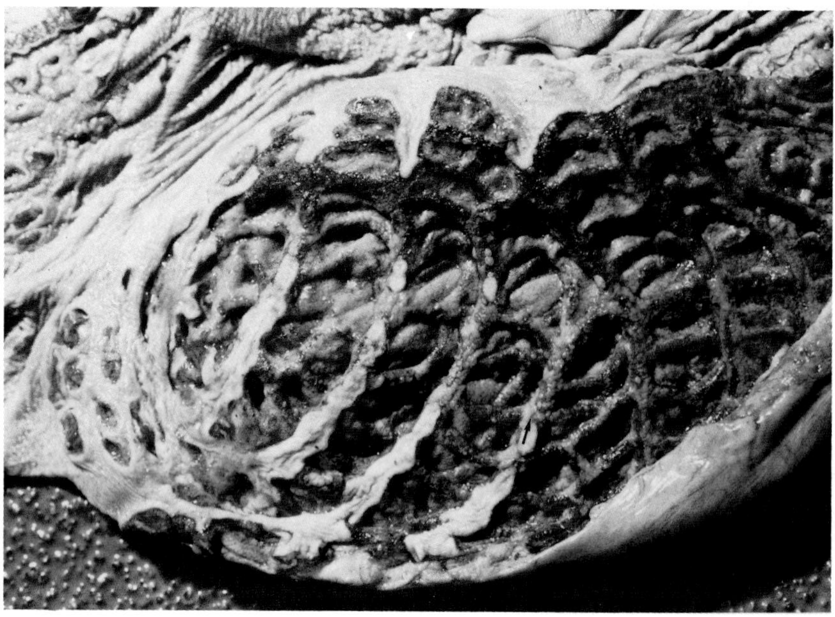

13.28 Mucosal ulceration of C-2 in a llama.

(Fig. 13.29). Ulcers of the distal one-fifth are more focal, deeper into the submucosa, and are more likely to perforate (Figs. 13.30, 13.31). Bleeding ulcers like those seen in ruminants, resulting in anemia and melena, have not been reported. Occult blood tests have been uniformly negative in the author's practice.

Etiology. The etiology of ulcers is unknown. The role of stress in the development of the syndrome is unknown as well (see Chap. 9). The condition has been diagnosed in animals on good rations as well as in those on poor rations. Some have been infested with parasites, while tests of others have been negative for parasitism.

Signs. Atony of C-1, with inappetence and scanty feces, may be the major syndrome. Nonperforating ulcers do not stimulate a hematopoietic tissue response or change the composition of the peritoneal fluid or blood serum. The temperature, heart rate, and respiratory rate are usually normal. The llama may be depressed and stand off from the herd, but colic is not a prominent sign. The owner will frequently comment about the llama off by itself, lying down and not coming up to feed in the usual manner. Unfortunately, these are the preliminary signs for most of the digestive and respiratory disorders. Animals exhibiting these mild signs should be given a thorough physical examination. If an ulcer has perforated, the signs of peritonitis will be seen.

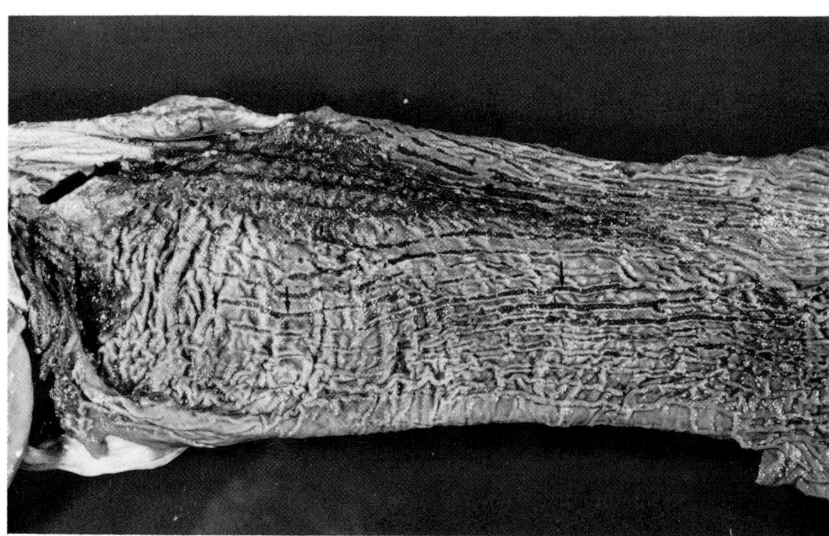

13.29 Linear mucosal ulceration of C-3 in a llama.

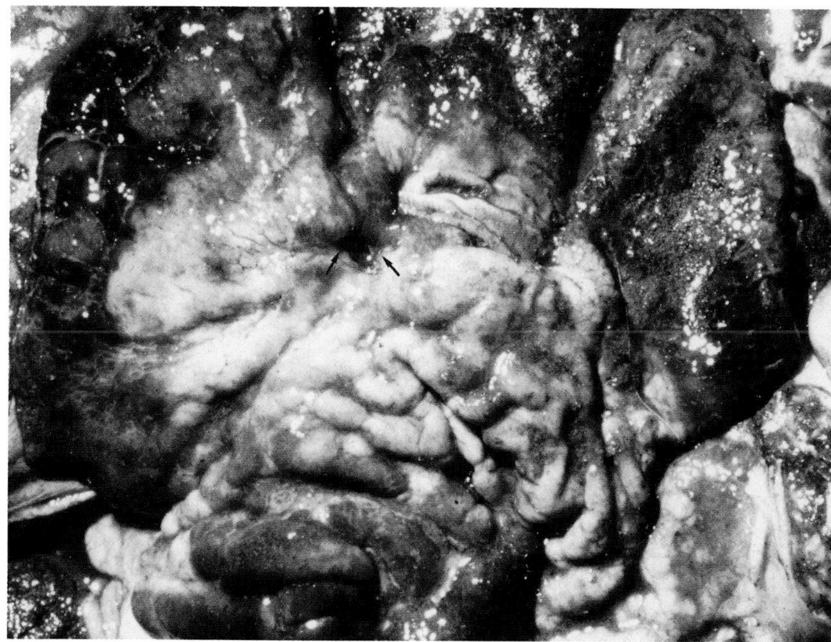

13.30 Perforating gastric ulcer in C-3.

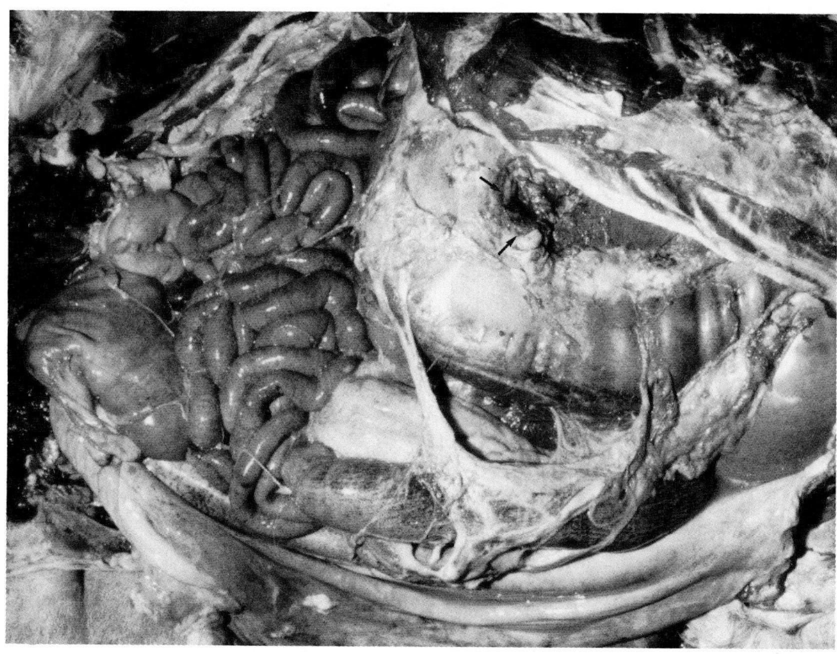

13.31 Acute, fibrinous peritonitis caused by perforating gastric ulcer.

Diagnosis. Simple gastric ulceration can be diagnosed only by elimination of other more serious digestive disorders. Tables 13.6–13.10 provide values for differential diagnosis.

Treatment. No studies have been conducted to establish the response of lamoids to most of the medications used in the treatment of ulcers. The effects of antacids on the lamoid stomach are unknown. Pharmacologic studies on true ruminants indicate that these species do not have the same type of acid receptors in the stomach as do simple-stomached animals. Therefore, ruminants would not be responsive to cimetidine. The type of acid receptor in the llama is not known, but empirical experience indicates that they do respond to cimetidine therapy. The recommended dosage regimen is 2.2 mg/kg, given twice daily subcutaneously. Oral cimetidine therapy in the adult ruminant is contraindicated because the drug is destroyed in the rumen. It is assumed that this is true in llamas also. If there is prolonged anorexia, no response to treatment, and no production of feces, it is the author's recommendation that an exploratory laparotomy be performed.

Different regimens may be indicated for treating a case of ulcers in C-1 as compared with treatment of ulcers in C-3. Oral medication given via stomach tube may take a long time to reach C-3.

Nourishment and fluid must be provided as appropriate. An IV catheter may be placed to hydrate the llama and give minimal nourishment. Electrolyte imbalance is not a major factor in gastric ulceration.

Table 13.6. Systematic examination of a colicky llama

Obtain a complete history—diet, stressors, pregnancy, recent acquisition
Clinical examination
- Temperature
- Heart rate—there are no good arteries to evaluate the pulse
- Respiratory rate and thoracic auscultation
- Palpation (if possible)—umbilicus, scrotum, abdomen (tenseness), rectal
- Auscultation of the abdomen
- Evaluation of colicky pain

Special diagnostic procedures
- Abdominocentesis—midline near the umbilicus
- Hematology
- Serum chemistry and electrolytes
- pH of C-1

Response to therapy

GASTRIC OVERLOAD. Although it is an uncommon disease of lamoids, when gastric overload is suspected, it must be dealt with immediately. Other names for this condition include acute gastric impaction, C-1 acidosis, grain overload, and engorgement toxemia.

Etiology. In one instance, a llama broke into a feed room and consumed a large quantity of grain.[1] The clinical signs were similar to those of a cow suffering from bloat.

The overingestion of highly fermentable carbohydrates, usually concentrates, may lead to lactic acidosis, dehydration, and depression. It is also possible to overingest highly fermentable proteinaceous feeds, such as soybean derivatives, resulting in excessive ammonium ion production, which causes alkalosis. Alkalosis produces signs of excitement and hyperesthesia. The latter syndrome has not yet been described in lamoids, but in the right circumstances, it could occur.

Pathogenesis. Diagnosis, therapy, and management of gastric overload require an understanding of the pathogenesis. The following discussion is based on ex-

1. S. Taylor, personal communication.

Table 13.7. Differential peritoneal aspirate parameters in acute abdominal disease in llamas

	Normal	C-3 perforation	Strangulated jejunum	Ruptured bladder
Gross appearance	Clear	Cloudy	Hemorrhagic	Cloudy
Protein g/dl	<2.0	4.2	3.8	<2.0
Specific gravity	1.0110	1.0185	1.0178	1.024
Leukocytes/μl	1–10	9700	1950	1–10
Potassium mmol/L	4.3 ± 0.78	4.3	4.3	185–400

Table 13.8. Differential hemograms

	Normal	C-3 perforation	Colonic perforation	Strangulated jejunum	Ruptured bladder
Erythrocytes × 10⁶/μl	12 ± 2	16	20	19	18
Hematocrit, %	33 ± 6	42	49	46	51
Fibrinogen, mg/dl	327 ± 96	100	800	300	700
Leukocytes/μl	14000 ± 3000	7,600	4,300	3,000	11,100
Metamyelocytes	0%	0	387	90	1,776
Bands	0–4%	3,192	645	930	3,330
Neutrophils	56–87%	2,356	989	690	1,554
Lymphocytes	3–22%	1,520	1,634	960	3,330

Table 13.9. Differential blood chemistry

	Normal	Stomach perforation	Strangulated jejunum	Ruptured bladder
Blood urea nitrogen mg/dl	22 ± 6	26	54	153
Sodium mmol/L	150 ± 3	152	155	
Potassium mmol/L	24 ± 0.78	3.3	2.7	
Chloride mmol/L	114	113	111	
Creatinine mg/dl				12.5

Table 13.10. Differential diagnosis of acute abdominal diseases of llamas

Definitive diagnostic parameters	Stomach atony	Intestinal obstruction	Stomach ulcers without perforation	Perforated ulcers	Retained meconium	Urinary obstruction without bladder rupture	Bladder rupture
Pain	−	+ + + +	+	+ + early + late	+ + +	+ + + +	±
Gastric atony	+ + + +	+ + + +	+ +	+ + + +	+	+	+
Shock	−	− early + late	−	+ + + +	−	−	+ + +
Abdominocentesis	Normal	Transudate, hemorrhagic, protein 3.8 g/dl, leukocytes +	Normal	Exudate cloudy, may have intestinal contents, protein 4.2 gm/dl, leukocytes +	Normal	Normal	Protein <2, few leukocytes, potassium 100 mmol/L
Hemogram	Normal	Leukocytes, left shift	Normal	Leukocytes, degenerative left shift	Normal	Normal or stress response	Leukocytes normal or elevated, left shift
Blood chemistry							
BUN mg/dl	Normal	54	Normal	Normal	Normal	Normal	100+
Potassium mmol/L	Normal	Decreased	Normal	Decreased	Normal		Decreased

trapolation from studies on cattle. The normal microflora of C-1 ferments carbohydrates, with short-chain VFA (acetic, propionic, butyric) as end products, which are absorbed and used for energy. If the llama consumes an overabundance of readily digestible carbohydrates, the fermentation pattern changes, a new microflora emerges as predominant, and lactic acid and other long-chain fatty acids are produced.

Lactic, formic, valeric, and succinic acids change the osmolarity of C-1, resulting in fluid being drawn in from the circulatory system and other tissues. Thirst also results in accumulation of excessive water in C-1. The pH of C-1 may drop to 4.0, and there is gastric stasis and destruction of the normal C-1 microflora. The excess fluid drawn into the GI tract produces a profuse, watery diarrhea. The acidic condition in C-1 also causes gastritis and permits bacterial invasion of the wall of C-1. A bacteremia may develop that may lead to development of abscesses on the liver.

Signs. Signs of toxic indigestion may not develop until 12–36 hours after engorgement. The timing depends on the nature of the food ingested and the amount consumed. This delay is important in the management of known engorgement, since it allows time to attempt to alleviate the problem. Signs of engorgement include weakness, incoordination, depression, anorexia, C-1 atony, colic (grunting, grinding teeth), abdominal distention, dehydration, a fetid diarrhea, and recumbency. The respiratory rate will increase because of the acidosis. Without treatment, death may occur in 24–48 hours. Some of the signs will persist during recovery. The mucosa of C-1 has received a severe insult, and time is required to relieve the gastritis. Since lamoids have no hoofs, they are not subject to laminitis, as may occur in ruminants and equines.

Diagnosis. The history of access to concentrates is vital to the diagnosis; however, it may be difficult to establish the amount consumed. Clinical signs are valuable in making a diagnosis. The ingesta from C-1 should not test below pH 5.

Treatment. In mild cases, the administration of antacids to correct the acidosis may suffice. Magnesium carbonate and magnesium hydroxide may be given in large volumes of warm water so as to disperse throughout C-1; 3 L may be used in an adult llama. The dose of the magnesium powder should be 1 g/kg in early acute cases and 0.5 g/kg if the stomach has been evacuated. Additional therapy should include thiamine HCl, IV fluids, antibiotics, and megulimide.

In consideration of the value of llamas and alpacas, a gastrotomy to remove the grain from the stomach may be prudent. The technique is the same as for rumenotomy. Parenteral therapy is also indicated to correct both acidosis and dehydration.

GASTRIC DILATION. All forms of overproduction of gas or eructation failure are rare in lamoids. The reasons for this are not understood. Obstructive lesions of the esophagus or neuromuscular disorders could theoretically cause gastric dilation, but such a case has not yet been reported. If the problem should arise, it may be handled as if in a ruminant.

Intestinal

Ailments of the intestinal tract of camelids will be similar in etiology to those of ruminants. However, the lamoid's response to colicky pain is more like that of the equine. Conditions that have been diagnosed in llamas include enteritis, obstruction, ulceration with and without perforation, colitis, proctitis, rectal prolapse, and GI parasitism.

ENTERITIS. The inflammatory response of the lamoid intestinal mucosa varies from hyperemic to catarrhal and hemorrhagic, progressing to necrosis of all the layers of the intestinal wall. Specific names may be given in reference to the specific area that is involved (duodenitis, jejunitis, ileitis, cecitis [typhlitis], colitis and proctitis).

Etiology. Enteritis may be primary or secondary to many other diseases (3). Infectious diseases that may involve enteritis include salmonellosis, colibacillosis, paratuberculosis, tuberculosis, rinderpest, and clostridial enterotoxemias.

Numerous parasitisms cause enteritis (see Chap. 8). All of the agents causing diarrhea may produce enteritis.

Secondary enteritis may occur with any of the obstructive lesions and also with septic metritis and mastitis. Proctitis may result from a too-vigorous rectal examination. The ultimate trauma associated with rectal abuse is a perforated rectal wall.

Signs. The primary manifestation of enteritis is diarrhea. The nature of the feces will aid in establishing the location and/or severity of the enteritis. The feces may have a fetid odor and contain excessive mucus, blood, undigested feed particles, and even shreds of sloughed mucosa.

Other signs of enteritis are dehydration, electrolyte imbalance, tenesmus, anorexia, colic, depression, stomach atony, plus or minus fever, and increased intestinal borborygmus. No intestinal sounds can be heard in the healthy llama. If sounds are present, fermentation has begun, resulting in a mixture of gas and fluid in the intestine.

Diagnosis. Clinical signs should determine diagnosis. An etiologic diagnosis will require cultures, fecal examination for cytology and parasitic ova, and hematology and blood chemistry evaluations. Colitis and proctitis may be evaluated by endoscopic examination. Colonic biopsies may be a diagnostic aid.

Treatment. In the management of enteritis, it is crucial to monitor and correct any fluid and/or electrolyte imbalance. It is particularly important to provide glucose and sodium. Acidosis is common, so giving sodium bicarbonate is usually necessary. Intestinal protectants are frequently given, but their use is of questionable value. These include kaolin, pectin, bismuth, and subsalicylate (Pepto-Bismol). *Lactobacillus acidophilus* therapy has not been found to be effective in ruminants. Broad-spectrum antibiotic therapy is indicated, not only to treat a primary infection, but to treat or prevent generalized secondary infections, since the permeability of the intestinal wall may be increased by enteritis, allowing invasion of the body by enteric bacteria.

OBSTRUCTION

Etiology. Either partial or complete obstruction of the intestine is a frequently seen clinical condition (30). While all the possible causes of obstruction have not been observed or diagnosed in llamas, it would be reasonable to assume that any of the types seen in ruminants may appear in lamoids.

Specific causes already described in lamoids include obstipation, impaction (sand, phytobezoars, enteroliths, fecaliths) (Fig. 13.22), torsion, intussusception, compression from the gravid uterus, strangulation from hernias, neoplasia, abscessation, infarction, and congenital defects (atresia coli and atresia ani).

Signs and Diagnosis. The signs of blockage vary with the location and completeness of the obstruction, the rapidity of development, the degree of enterotoxemia produced, the degree of vascular occlusion, and the production of gas. The major sign is colic, with little or no passage of feces.

When an obstruction involves interference with circulation, the ensuing sequence of events significantly alters the integrity of the bowel. In a partial vascular compression, the venous drainage will be adversely affected. Arterial blood will continue to flow into the area, causing edema. If compression is complete, there will be tissue anoxia and increased capillary permeability, followed by intramural and mucosal hemorrhage, with accompanying edema and loss of the integrity of the epithelium, which allows bacterial invasion of the intestinal wall and, ultimately, bacteremia and peritonitis (72). Ischemia will become complete and necrosis will occur. Tissue break-down products from the necrosis may be absorbed from the peritoneal cavity and contribute to cardiovascular collapse (shock).

Since this is an important clinical entity, characterized by a syndrome called the acute abdomen, a number of case reports will be presented to illustrate the signs, diagnostic procedures, and management of these cases.

Case 1. Strangulated jejunum

History: The patient was a 3-year-old pregnant female. Thirty-six hours before admission, she was noticed to be depressed and anorectic. She was generally recumbent, with her head pulled back over the side. *This clinical sign should not be given any specific clinical importance, since it is the usual position assumed by a weak or sick llama.* When encouraged to stand, she did so reluctantly and was somewhat ataxic. The owner reported that she frequently groaned. She refused water for 24 hours. Normal fecal pellets were excreted up to 4 hours before admission. Another female llama in this herd had died of a perforated gastric ulcer a few months previously.

Signs: When presented, the llama was recumbent and refused to rise. She was depressed, but respiration appeared to be normal. Rectal temperature was 36.1°C (97°F) and the heart rate 132 per minute. GI motility was absent. Mucous membranes of the mouth were pale.

The llama was in sternal recumbency most of this time. Intermittently, she would roll to lateral recumbency and throw her head back into opisthotonos. If stimulated, she would roll back up to the sternal position but was reluctant to hold her head up for more than a minute. Otherwise, the head and neck would curve around to the side. Periodically, the llama would struggle to her feet and wander around the stall in an ataxic manner. The head was carried low while standing. Then she would flop back into sternal recumbency.

Diagnosis: A standard battery of procedures was performed and the results tabulated (Tables 13.7–13.10).

Management: Therapy for shock was instituted, and on the basis of the results of abdominocentesis and the hemogram, an exploratory laparotomy was begun. The llama died during preparation for surgery.

Necropsy: Serosanguineous fluid was found in both peritoneal and pericardial sacs. The omental bursa had incarcerated approximately 2 L of fluid, which also contained floating specks of fibrin. Tags of fibrin were loosely adhered to the surface of C-1.

A 0.5 m segment of the proximal jejunum had herniated through the omental foramen and had become incarcerated and strangulated. The intestine was hemorrhagic and necrotic, but it had not ruptured. The colon was congested but contained normal fecal pellets.

Case 2. Perforated gastric ulcer

History: The llama was a 2-year-old male kept in a dry pasture with other llamas. On the morning of admission he had refused to get up, groaning as if in pain. The abdomen was distended.

Signs: Rectal temperature was 37.2°C (99°F); heart rate, 120 per minute; and respiratory rate, 50 per minute. Mucous membranes were cyanotic and capillary refill time was prolonged. There was no gastroenteric motility. The llama was unable or unwilling to stand.

Diagnosis: The high protein content (4.2 g/dl) and cloudy appearance of the abdominal aspirate were indicative of an acute abdominal disorder. Therapy for shock was instituted and an exploratory laparotomy was begun. Upon encountering GI contents in the peritoneal cavity, the llama was euthanized.

Necropsy: A perforating ulcer was found in C-3, accompanied by a generalized peritonitis. The ulcer was located 7 cm craniad from the pylorus. The serosal opening was approximately 4 mm, while on the mucosa there was a 10 mm craterous ulcer, with the surrounding mucosa thickened and hyperemic.

The thickened mucosa surrounding the ulcer was hyperplastic and was composed of a type of acid-secreting cells. Multifocal infiltrations of eosinophils and mononuclear cells were seen in the lamina propria. Excessive mucus and cellular debris covered the mucosal surface, and in this layer were embedded several adult trichostrongylid nematodes. Larval nematodes were noted in glands of the mucosa. The parasites were identified as *Ostertagia* sp. The remaining mucosa of C-3 was chronically inflamed and atrophic.

Case 3. Spiral colon impaction

History: An adult female llama was noticed by a caretaker to refuse feed one evening, and since she was alone in an enclosure he also noticed she was not passing feces. Treatment with milk of magnesia and banamine was not successful. Depression deepened, and the llama was admitted to the veterinary medical teaching hospital.

Signs: The llama was reluctant to rise, and when forced would move slowly. The rectal temperature was normal, as were heart and respiratory rates. Mucous membranes were normal. Abnormalities noted were a decrease in stomach motility, lack of feces, and depression. There were no overt signs of colic.

Hemogram and serum chemistry parameters were normal. Abdominocentesis was performed, but no fluid was obtained. Standard symptomatic treatment was begun with banamine and cimetidine for 3 days. No feces had been passed for 6 or 7 days. On day six, rumen contents (1 L) from a cow were given via stomach tube along with magnesium hydroxide. Another hemogram and chemistry panel was performed. All parameters remained normal.

The llama continued to be anorectic. She did drink

water, and it was noted that she had urinated. The temperature remained normal.

She spent most of the time in sternal recumbency. She would get up if harassed by treatment regimens but was reluctant to move around. Her abdomen was somewhat tense, and a general feeling of abdominal discomfort was noted.

Therapy: Seven days after the illness was noted, an exploratory laparotomy was performed (see Chap. 6). The small intestine and the proximal large intestine were distended with gas and ingesta. Gas was withdrawn from the distended intestine with a 16 gauge needle attached to an IV administration set. The terminal colon was empty of fecal pellets. The color of the viscera was normal. A small, hard mass (7 × 3 cm) was located within one of the loops of the spiral colon (Fig. 13.32). The loop of intestine could not be visualized without incising through a layer of mesentery. The mass was exteriorized, packed off, and an enterotomy performed.

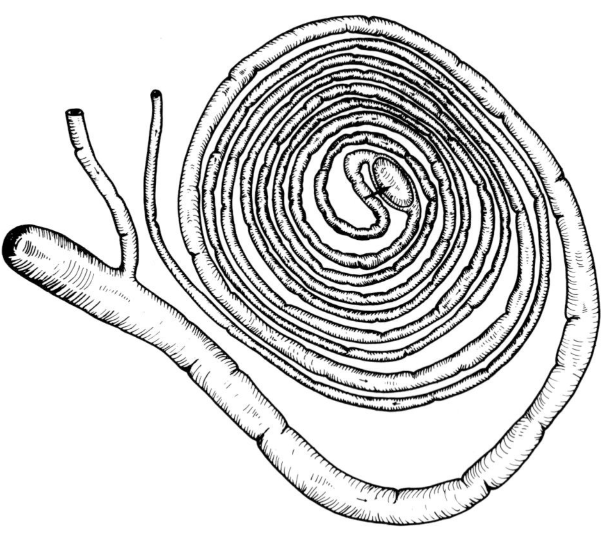

13.32 Diagram of spiral colon impaction in a llama.

The mass was not too large to have passed normally along the intestine. Why such a mass will impact is difficult to understand. It was composed primarily of dry, matted food particles, including a few large strands of straw, and was enveloped in a layer of mucus. Apparently, the consistency of the mass did not stimulate normal peristalsis but rather induced spasticity of the intestine on both sides of the mass. This phenomenon has also been seen in the horse and the hippopotamus. There was no evidence of ischemic necrosis of the intestinal wall as sometimes occurs in such cases.

The llama began to eat the day following surgery. Loose fecal material was passed within 12 hours, and within 48 hours pellets were being passed. Trimethoprim sulfa was administered daily for 4 days. The llama was discharged 1 week after admission.

Case 4. Perforating ulcer of the colon

History: The patient was a 1.5-year-old male kept with other llamas in a dry pasture. He had been ill for 5 days prior to admission. He was colicky, as evidenced by restlessness, continual recumbency, and vocalization.

Signs: Groaning was marked. Mucous membranes were cyanotic.

Diagnosis: Ingesta in the abdominal fluid indicated a grave prognosis, and the llama was euthanized. Laboratory parameters are listed in Tables 13.7–13.9.

Necropsy: Fibrinous adhesions were present over the serosal surfaces. Fecal material coated much of the intestine in the caudal abdomen, including the spiral colon. A thick-walled sacculation containing formed feces was found on the surface of the spiral colon. A 2 cm perforation was present just caudad to the sacculation. Another outpouching of the colonic wall was found in the inflamed area.

The sacculation was covered with a serosal membrane that was thickened by inflamed fibrovascular tissue. It is supposed that a previous perforation had penetrated through the mucosal and muscle layers of the colon and had then dilated but not ruptured the serosa. Fecal material had accumulated in the sacculation.

A summary of the laboratory data for these cases and a case of ruptured bladder are presented in Table 13.10. The table summarizes the diagnostic parameters used in analyzing acute abdominal diseases. It is important to remember that an etiologic diagnosis of any of the acute abdominal diseases cannot be made on the basis of clinical signs alone. The results of additional diagnostic procedures must be analyzed. These should include abdominocentesis and hemogram and blood chemistry evaluations.

Treatment. Successful therapy for many of the diseases causing the syndrome of acute abdomen requires surgery. The key is early diagnosis. Exploratory surgery and supportive therapy should not be delayed in order to establish the precise location of the lesion. The circulatory, electrolyte, and toxemic changes associated with obstructive lesions must be alleviated immediately. If the bowel perforates, death is inevitable unless the omentum successfully walls off the inflammatory response. The inability to conduct a thorough rectal examination precludes obtaining the diagnostic information that would be available in making a diagnosis in a cow or horse. In the llama, such information can be obtained only by exploratory surgery.

Supportive therapy may be supplied by cannulation of the jugular vein for administration of appropriate fluids. See Chapter 6 for details of the surgery.

Recommended procedures for conducting a complete physical examination of a llama with a suspected abdominal ailment are outlined in Table 13.6.

ULCERATION

Etiology. Ulceration of the intestinal mucosa may follow any severe enteritis and develop at any location from the duodenum to the rectum. The most common site is the small colon within the spiral colon. In many cases no indication of the cause can be determined, even at necropsy.

A unique ulcer is that seen resulting from ischemic necrosis caused by an intestinal spasm around an impaction of dried fecal matter. Multiple ulcers may develop in such a case, because the intestine may temporarily relax sufficiently for the impacted mass to move on, only to spasm again. This is sometimes seen in small colon impactions in horses, when chemotherapy results in temporary relaxation of the muscles. Such ulcers frequently necrose through the entire wall, perforating the intestine.

Diagnosis. It is extremely difficult to diagnose a primary ulcer. Elimination of other intestinal disorders should precede the tentative diagnosis, but an antemortem diagnosis of intestinal ulceration is always questionable.

GASTROINTESTINAL CONCRETIONS

Etiology. Concretions found in the GI tract of camelids are usually caused by precipitation of minerals around a nidus. Four types have been reported: (1) gastroenterolith (6, 31, 56), (2) phytobezoar (28, 49), (3) hair balls, and (4) sand.

Camelids form a unique gastrolith in the glandular saccules of C-1. Multiple saccules may contain the concretions, which vary in size from 1 mm in diameter to egg-shaped bodies 2 cm in diameter and 3.5 cm long (Figs. 13.33, 13.34).

No hypothesis has been formulated to explain the pathogenesis of the formation of these gastroliths because the saccules are supposed to evert their contents with each rumination cycle. A large, mineral-encrusted phytotrichobezoar caused obstruction of C-3 and ultimately killed a zoo llama (48).

The composition of GI enteroliths is unknown. Urinary tract stones can be analyzed by means of a variety of techniques, but the need for developing a similar technology for stones found in the bowel is not of sufficient clinical importance to warrant the time, money, and effort involved.

Signs. These concretions cause no impairment of C-1 function, as far as is known. The stones are seen as incidental findings on radiographs of the midventral abdomen or at necropsy. Other concretions may cause obstruction, ulceration, and perforation of the viscus wall (49).

Diagnosis. Concretions in C-1 may be seen on a radiograph of the abdomen (Fig. 13.35). Small concretions lying in a segment of the intestine overlaid by C-1 will be obscured. Signs of an intestinal obstruction may follow formation of an intestinal concretion.

Therapy. Concretions in C-1 require no therapy. If the concretion obstructs the intestine, it must be removed surgically. Recommended treatment for sand impaction is repeated doses of mineral oil or dioctyl sulfonate and neostigmine.

RECTAL PROLAPSE. Protrusion of the mucous membrane or the entire rectum through the anus is not common in lamoids, but it has been reported.

Etiology. The most common sign is tenesmus, associated with prolonged severe diarrhea. A mild protrusion, lasting only a few minutes, may be observed following defecation. A slight protrusion of both the rectal and vulvar mucosae has been noted in females near term, especially when lying down; pressure from the large fetus pushes organs into the pelvic canal.

Signs. A protrusion is obvious. The extent of the protrusion is important because of the potential disruption of the blood supply to the invaginated segment. The mucosa may be traumatized by laceration or abrasion from the tail or dirt when the animal is lying down. Edema is a likely result, and necrosis of the mucosa may occur.

Diagnosis. Obvious.

Treatment. This condition can be handled as the same condition in a ruminant. The inciting cause should be corrected. The mucous membrane should be cleaned and the edema reduced with glucose or sucrose. The protruding tissue should be gently replaced, avoiding point source pressure. It may be necessary to use epidural anesthesia to allow replacement. It is essential that the invagination be completely corrected. An equine glass or plastic vaginal speculum inserted into the rectum works well. A purse-string suture may be placed if necessary, but it should be remembered that a lamoid excretes pelletized feces and may need a proportionally larger orifice than a cow.

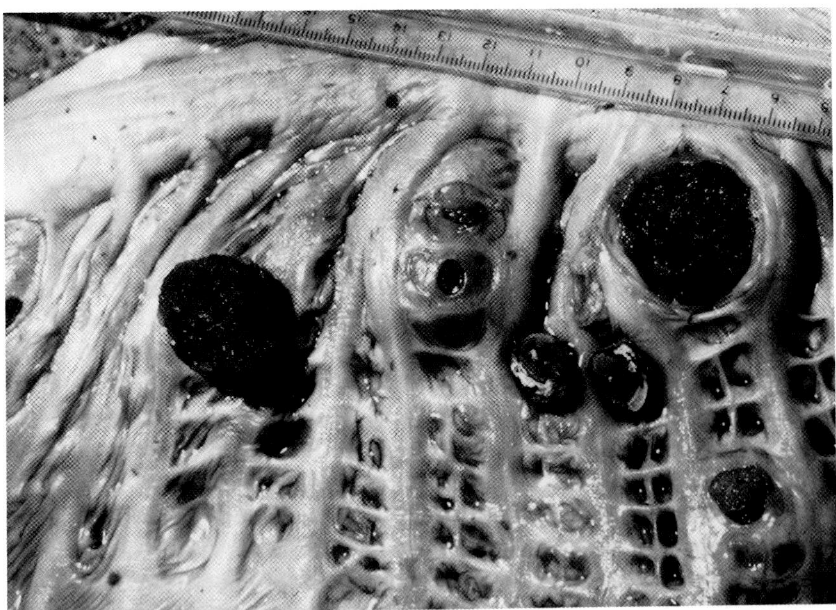

13.33 Gastroliths in the glandular saccules of C-1 in a llama.

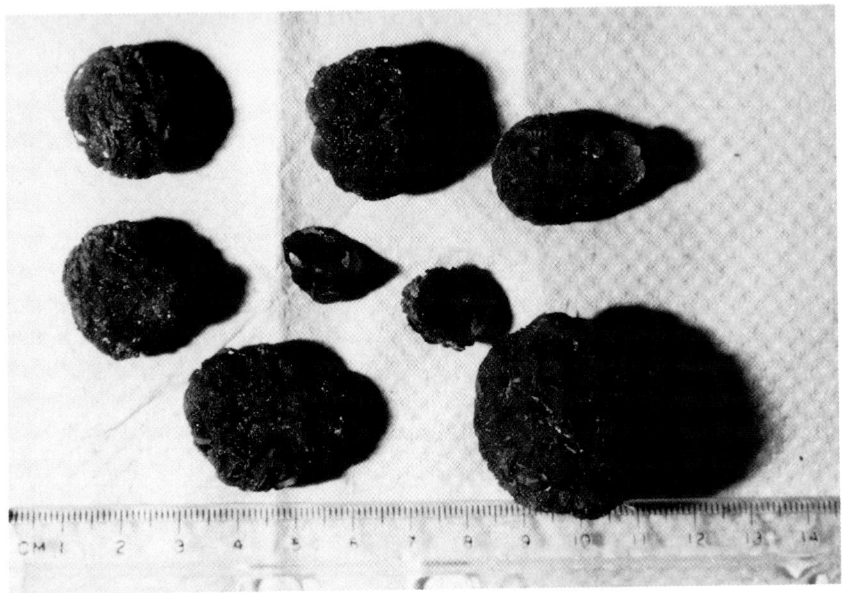

13.34 Gastroliths removed from the glandular saccules of C-1 in a llama.

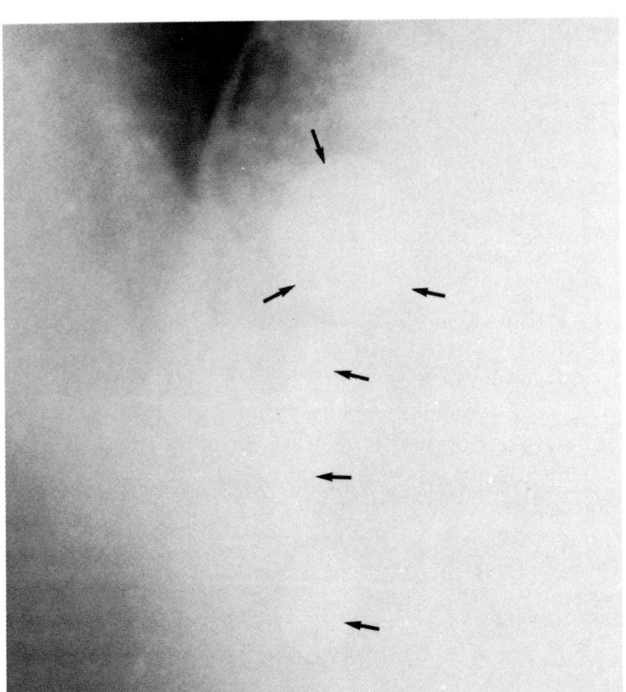

13.35 Lateral radiograph of gastroliths in situ.

The llama should be observed for recurrence of the problem or the buildup of feces behind a purse-string suture. Chronic rectal prolapse may require a submucous resection, similar to the procedure for cattle. If the protruding segment is necrotic, it may be amputated, using the same techniques as used in cattle (see Chap. 6).

RECTAL LACERATION

Etiology. A rectal tear may occur during breeding, but lamoid copulation is not accompanied by as vigorous pelvic thrusts as are seen in cattle or horses. Prolonged dystocia, especially with manual manipulation, may traumatize the rectal wall and allow either immediate or delayed rupture of the wall. The most likely cause of a rectal tear is an accident at the time of a rectal examination. The pelvis of even a large llama is small, and the size of the rectum is commensurate with the size of the animal. Persons with a glove size of over 7.5 will have difficulty performing a rectal examination in any but the largest animals.

Straining against an inserted hand and arm may be lessened by using an epidural anesthesia or by mixing xylocaine with the lubricant. Even under epidural anesthesia, a colonic spasm may trap an arm caudad to the wrist. It is necessary to wait until the spasm relaxes before removing the arm to avoid splitting the wall of the colon.

Diagnosis. The mucosal split may be felt at the time it is happening, but it is more likely that blood will be seen on the hand when it is withdrawn. Llamas are intermediate between mares and cows in terms of susceptibility to trauma of the rectal mucosa. It is not uncommon to see traces of blood on the back of the hand or wrist when finishing an examination as a result of tiny splits in the anus. Copious quantities of blood in the palm of the hand or on the fingers should alert the clinician to the possibility of a mucosal tear.

If a laceration is suspected, the rectum should be carefully explored with a speculum, under epidural anesthesia, to determine the extent of the laceration. The rectum should not be explored with a digit, since this may enlarge a tear.

Treatment. Lacerations that penetrate deeper than the mucosa should be sutured. This may be done through the anus, as described for diagnosis, if the laceration is caudal enough to be reached and there is sufficient space to manipulate the instruments. Tears occurring more craniad require suturing through a laparotomy. It is important to be aware that the pelvic reflection of the peritoneum extends approximately two-thirds the length of the pelvic canal, ventral to the uterus and bladder, but only half the length between the uterus and the rectum.

Peritonitis

Peritonitis is inflammation of the serosal surface of the abdominal viscera or the wall of the abdomen. The inflammation may be focal or diffuse. Adhesions are a natural sequence to an inflamed serosa.

ETIOLOGY. There are numerous causes of peritonitis, among which are uterine tears, ruptured bladder, abscessation, and GI perforation.

SIGNS. Signs include colic, tense abdomen, stomach atony, ileus, weakness, plus or minus fever, diarrhea, painful movement, recumbency, and death in 4–48 hours.

DIAGNOSIS. Of major diagnostic help is the collection of abdominal fluid by abdominocentesis. Since all forms of peritonitis produce fluid, if the lesion is focal or regional, the results of abdominocentesis may be negative. A diffuse peritonitis will cause a hemogram response.

At necropsy, peritonitis may be acute or chronic (Figs. 13.36, 13.37) and must be differentiated from serous atrophy of fat.

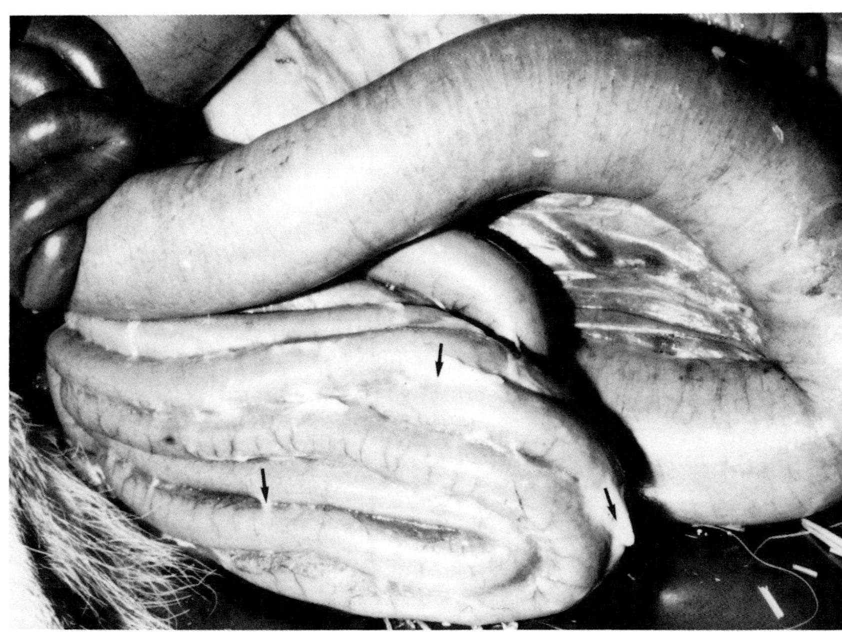

13.36 Acute peritonitis, with fibrin tags.

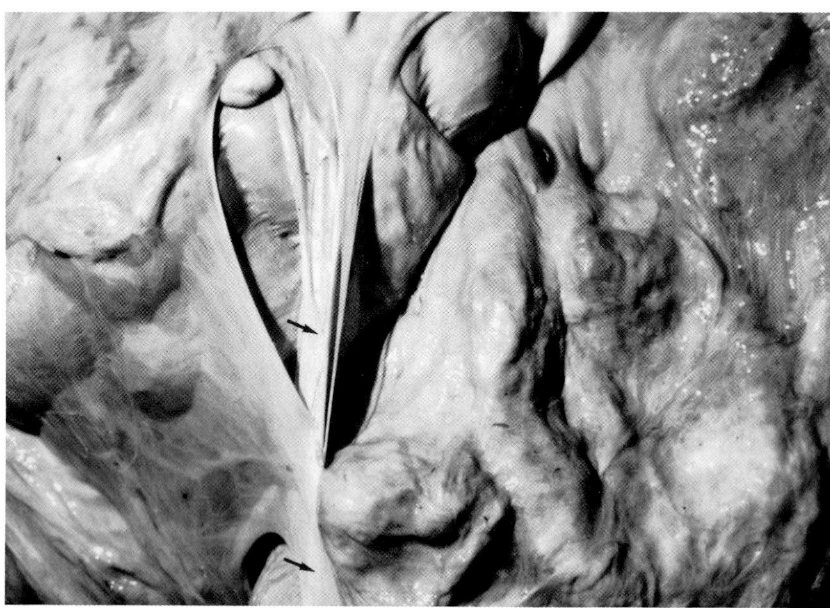

13.37 Chronic peritonitis, with fibrous bands that may incarcerate a loop of bowel.

TREATMENT. The prognosis for diffuse peritonitis is grave, especially if accompanied by perforation of the bowel. When that diagnosis is made, the llama should be euthanized. Otherwise, administration of broad-spectrum antibiotics and supportive therapy, including IV fluids, are recommended.

Intraabdominal Hemorrhage

ETIOLOGY. Hemorrhage may result from the rupture of any major vessel in the abdominal cavity or from extensive capillary oozing. Common sources of hemorrhage are a ruptured liver or spleen from abdominal trauma. The cranial uterine artery is in the freely moveable broad ligament and may be subject to trauma, particularly late in pregnancy. The umbilical arteries may rupture too close to the body wall in the neonate and retract into the abdomen without closing. If the spermatic cord is under excessive tension at the time of transection of the cord with an emasculator, the artery may retract into the abdomen and continue bleeding.

SIGNS. The severity and rapidity of development will vary with the rate of blood loss. The llama will first become weak. The heart rate will increase. There may be dyspnea and pallor of the mucous membranes and cool extremities. A hemogram will be of little help until 8–10 hours have passed.

TREATMENT. Even though results of a test for packed cell volume will not aid in initial diagnosis, it should be done to provide a base for monitoring to evaluate the response to therapy. Also, the blood should be checked for possible clotting defects. If blood loss is thought to be caused by rupture of an abdominal vessel, it may be necessary to investigate the site via laparotomy. In one case, the liver had been ruptured, and it was possible to correct this at surgery.

Blood transfusions are possible in lamoids. Numerous blood types have been identified in the llama and alpaca, but any llama's blood can be transfused to another, once. After that, there is risk of an incompatibility reaction.

Hepatic Insufficiency

Hepatic insufficiency is a syndrome common to all vertebrates. The liver has great reserves and will function even though severely insulted. However, once the critical threshold is reached, a process is set into motion that may cause the death of the animal in 36–48 hours. Lesions of the liver can be toxic, degenerative, proliferative, or inflammatory.

ETIOLOGY. The causes of hepatic injury are many and include parasites (71), infections, metabolic disorders, obstructive processes, and toxic agents. Additional causes include hematogenous abscesses, gastritis (C-1), septic metritis and mastitis, peritonitis, rupture of the liver, nutritional myopathy (selenium deficiency), adenoma (11, 26), carcinoma of the gall bladder (64), and mycotoxins. The syndrome produced by hepatic insufficiency is essentially the same, no matter what the initial cause. It is usually not possible to establish etiologic diagnosis based on gross necropsy findings. The liver may be large, small, soft, firm, yellowish, or blackened. Postmortem decomposition begins quickly in llamas, since they do not cool out well under the heavy woolly coat. The liver is one of the first organs affected. It is not uncommon for a snap diagnosis of hepatopathy to be changed after microscopic examination.

SIGNS. The author has not dealt with a case of primary hepatopathy in a llama. Cases described by colleagues indicate that the hepatic insufficiency syndrome in a llama more resembles that of the ruminant than of the horse. In the horse the central nervous signs are more exaggerated, with violent pushing, ataxia, aimless walking, leaning on objects, and falling. Chewing at objects or attempting to grasp feed or a fence with the mouth opened in a yawn is also characteristic of hepatic insufficiency in the horse. All these CNS manifestations would cause alarm in rabies-endemic areas.

The ruminant and camelid appear to be depressed. Coma, rather than violent, active signs, may be associated with hepatoencephalopathy. When a camelid becomes weakened and toxic, it will lie down and refuse to rise rather than stumble about and push against objects in its environment.

Photosensitization is a sign seen in some hepatopathies. Normally, the liver degrades chlorophyl through a step producing phylloerythrin, which is further degraded to inactive substances. In hepatic insufficiency, the liver fails to decompose phylloerythrin, which then accumulates in the peripheral circulation. Phylloerythrin is a photodynamic agent. For a llama to be photosensitized, nonpigmented skin must be exposed to the ultraviolet rays of sunshine. Heavily wooled areas of the body would be free of risk, normally protected from photosensitization.

The clinical signs of photosensitization are similar to those of sunburn. Photosensitization is only one sign of hepatic insufficiency and is relatively insignificant in the overall management of the case. Placing llamas inside a barn will prevent progressive skin damage from the effects of sunlight.

Hemoglobin, bile pigments, or both may be seen in the urine of llamas suffering from hepatic insufficiency. Hemolysis is not of a magnitude to produce anemia.

Although icterus is the most consistent sign associated with hepatic insufficiency, it may be absent in a small percentage of cases. Diseases other than primary hepatic disease, such as hemolytic conditions and obstructive intestinal disorders, also produce icterus.

DIAGNOSIS. Distinctive clinical signs, plus evaluation of clinical pathology parameters, will be the primary diagnostic tools. Urinalysis and liver biopsy may be definitive in establishing the etiology.

It should be mentioned that studies to establish which of the enzymes are specific for hepatic injury have not been done. Extrapolation from ruminant data is being currently used. Enzyme changes are likely to be seen only when there is active necrosis. In pyrrolizidine alkaloid poisoning, where there is fibrosis and atrophy, a bromosulfothalein clearance test may be necessary to evaluate hepatic function.

TREATMENT. The prognosis for acute hepatic necrosis is unfavorable. In mild cases, the therapeutic rationale is to supply glucose and lipotropic substances such as choline and methionine to spare the need for hepatic action. Since secondary bacterial infection is frequently seen in any hepatopathy, broad-spectrum antibiotics are indicated.

Pancreatitis

There have been no reports of pancreatitis in camelids. This may reflect failure in diagnosis, or in documenting diagnoses, but pancreatic disease is also rare in cattle. Only a few cases of diabetes mellitus have been reported in camelids, but those animals showed the classic signs, i.e., hyperglycemia, glucosuria, polydypsia, polyuria, and weight loss.

Lamoids normally show a higher serum glucose (100–200 mg/dl) than cattle (45–75 mg/dl). During many digestive diseases, glucose levels may elevate to 200–300 mg/dl. This may cause some erroneous diagnoses of diabetes to be made. The precise reason for the elevated serum glucose is not known.

REFERENCES

1. Altman, N. H., Small, J. D., and Squire, R. A. 1974. Squamous cell carcinoma of the rumen and thymic amyloidosis in a guanaco, J. Am. Vet. Med. Assoc. 165(9):820–22.

2. Arnao, I., Ore, R., and Villavicencio, M. 1981. Some properties of alpaca liver microsomal glucose and phosphatase. Fed. Proc. 40(6):1776.

3. Blair, W. R. 1908. Report of the veterinary pathologist—Toxic enteritis in a guanaco. 13th Annu. Rep. N.Y. Zool. Soc.

4. Boas, J. E. V. 1890. (The anatomy of the stomach of camelids and tragulids) Zur Morphologie des Magens der Cameliden und der Traguliden. Morphol. Jahresber. Leipz. 18:494–524.

5. Bohlken, H. 1960. Remarks on the stomach and the systematic position of the Tylopoda. Proc. Zool. Soc. (Lond.) 134:207–15.

6. Bullock, D. S. 1929. Stones from the stomach of a guanaco. J. Mammal. 10(2):170–71.

7. Cavero Robbiano, J. O. 1970. (Chemical composition of the parotid saliva of the alpaca and titrated alkalinity) Composicion quimica de la saliva parotida de la alpaca *Lama pacos* ($PO_4H=$, CO_3H-) y alcalinidad tituable. Tesis, Fac.

Med. Vet. Univ. Nac. Mayor San Marcos (Lima), pp. 1–24.

8. Ciprian Rodriguez, C. 1972. (Micro and macroscopic description of the liver of the alpaca). Descripcion macro y microscopica del higado de la alpaca *Lama pacos.* Tesis, Fac. Med. Vet. Univ. Nac. Tec. Altiplano (Puno).

9. Clemens, E. T., and Stevens, C. E. 1980. A comparison of gastrointestinal transit time in ten species of mammal. J. Agric. Sci. (UK) 94(3):735–37.

10. Colyer, F. 1931. Abnormal condition of the teeth of animals and their relation to similar conditions in man. Dent. Board U.K. (London), pp. 1–167.

11. Cuba C., A., and Mestanza, W. A. 1950. (A case of hepatic adenoma in an alpaca) Sobre un caso de adenoma de higado en una alpaca. Rev. Fac. Med. Vet. (Lima) 4:115–18.

12. Cummings, J. F., Munnell, J. F., and Vallenas, A. 1972. The mucigenous glandular mucosa in the complex stomach of two New World camelids, the llama and guanaco. J. Morphol. 137(1):71–110.

13. De la Vega, D. E. 1950a. (Digestive system of alpacas) Aspectos histologicos del aparato digestivo de la alpaca. Rev. Fac. Med. Vet. (Lima) 5:163–87.

14. ______. 1950b. (Histologic aspects of the digestive apparatus and the urogenital system of the alpaca) Aspectos histologicos del aparato digestivo y systema urogenital de la alpaca. Tesis, Fac. Med. Vet. Univ. Nac. Mayor San Marcos (Lima), pp. 1–58.

15. ______. 1951. (Histologic aspects of the digestive apparatus and the urogenital system of the alpaca) Aspectos histologicos del aparato digestivo y sistema urogenital de la alpaca. Rev. Fac. Med. Vet. Univ. Nac. Mayor San Marcos (Lima) 6:145–70.

16. Dietz, O., and Wiesner, E., eds. 1984. Diseases of the Horse, 3 vols., transl. A. S. Turner. Basel: Karger.

17. Dougherty, R. W., and Vallenas, P. A. 1968. A quantitative study of eructated gas expulsion in alpacas. Cornell Vet. 58(1):3–7.

18. Duran Zuniga, A. H. 1970. (Comparative digestibility between sheep and alpacas. Consideration of the equivalents of sheep units) Digestibilidad comparada entre ovions y alpacas. Consideraciones en las equivalencias a unidades ovinos. Tesis, Ing. Agr. Univ. Nac. Tec. Altiplano (Puno), pp. 1–76.

19. Eckerlin, R. H., and Stevens, C. E. 1973. Bicarbonate secretion by the glandular saccules of the llama stomach. Cornell Vet. 63(3):436–45.

20. Ehrlein, H. J., and Engelhardt, W. von. 1971. (Investigations on stomach motility in the llama) Untersuchungen uber die Magenmotorik beim Lama. Zentralbl. Veterinaermed. [A] 18:181–91.

21. Engelhardt, W. von. 1972. Use of isotopes in studies on fluxes across the forestomach wall of ruminants. In A. Guillon, ed. 1972. Isotope Studies on the Physiology of Domestic Animals. Proc. Symp. Int. At. Energy Agency, Athens, pp. 273–84.

22. Engelhardt, W. von, and Sallmann, H. P. 1972. (Absorption and secretion in the rumen of the guanaco, *Lama guanacoe*) Resorption und Sekretion im Pansen des Guanakos (*Lama guanacoe*). Zentralbl. Veterinaermed. [A] (2):117–32.

23. Englehardt, W. von, Harmeyer, J., Hoernicke, H., and Hill, H. 1965. (Investigation on rumen physiology in tylopods) Untersuchungen zur Pansenphysiologie der Tylopoden. Naturwissenschaften 52:91–92.

24. Engelhardt, W. von, Ali, D. E., and Wipper, E. 1979. Absorption and secretion in the tubiform forestomach compartment three of the llama. J. Comp. Physiol. [B] 132 (4):337–42.

25. Fernandez Baca, S. 1961–62. (Some aspects of the dental development of the alpaca) Algunos aspectos del desarrolio dentario de la alpaca, *Lama pacos.* Rev. Fac. Med. Vet. Univ. Nac. Mayor San Marcos (Lima) 16–17:88–103.

26. Fox, H. 1912. Neoplasms in wild animals (adenocarcinoma of liver in alpaca). J. Comp. Pathol. 17:217–31.

27. Galotta, D. R., and Galotta, J. M. 1987. (Arterial and venous circulation of the stomach of the llama) Irrigacion arterio-venosa del estomago del llama. Rev. Cienc. Agrar. 8(1, 2):27–33.

28. Galotta, D. R., Nuevo Freire, C. M., and Galotta, J. M. 1987. (Bezoars of guanaco) Bezoares de guanaco. Rev. Cienc. Agrar. 8(1, 2):20–24.

29. Goldsmith, B. 1984. Some notes on environmental hazards (choke). 3 L Llama (21):7.

30. Greth, F. 1981. Bowel-colon impaction in baby llamas. 3 L Llama 9:5–6.

31. Grunberg, W., and Preisinger, A. 1974. (Magnesium phosphate concretion of the forestomach of llamas) Bobierrit-newberyit-Konkremente in den Drusensachen des Vormagens von *Lama lama.* Experientia 30(9):1047–48.

32. Guerrero, R. J., and Franco, E. 1966. (Observations of the behavior of alpacas during defecation) Observaciones sobre la conducta de las alpacas durante la defecacion. Gac. Vet. 1(3):12–15.

33. Guerrero, R. J., and Villavicencio, M. 1971. Glucose oxidation in the submaxillary gland of the alpaca. Peru Soc. Quim. Bol. 3(2):49–50.

34. Guffy, M. M. 1975. Esophageal disorders. In S. Ettinger, ed. Textbook of Veterinary Internal Medicine, vol. 2. Philadelphia: W. B. Saunders, pp. 1101–4.

35. Harmeyer, J., and Hill, H. 1964. The volume of protozoa in the rumen of goat and the guanaco. Zentralbl. Veterinaermed. [A] 11(6):493–501.

36. Hinderer, S. 1978. (Kinetics of urea-metabolism in llama on protein-poor diet) Kinetik des Harnstoff-Stoffwechsels beim Lama bei proteinarmen Diaeten. Diss., Hoenheim Univ.

37. Hinderer, S., and Engelhardt, W. von. 1975. Urea metabolism in the llama. Comp. Biochem. Physiol. [A] 52:619–22.

38. Hinderer, S., and Engelhardt, W. von. 1976. Entry of blood urea into the rumen of the llama. In Tracer Studies on Non-protein Nitrogen for Ruminants. Vienna: Int. Atomic Energy Agency, pp. 59–60.

39. Holgado Montufar, R. 1972. (Macro and microscopic description of small intestine of the alpaca) Descripcion macro-microscopica del intestino delgado de la alpaca, *Lama pacos.* Tesis, Fac. Med. Vet. Univ. Nac. Tec. Altiplano (Puno), p. 25.

40. Howard, J. L., ed. 1986. Current Veterinary Therapy: Food Animal Practice, 2nd ed. Philadelphia: W. B. Saunders.

41. Johnson, L. W. 1983. The llama stomach: Structure and function. Llama World 1(4):33–34.

42. Kirsner, J. B., and Winans, C. S. 1979. The stomach. In W. A. Sodeman, Jr., and T. M. Sodeman, eds. Sodeman's Pathologic Physiology, 6th ed. Philadelphia: W. B. Saunders, p. 907.

43. Kock, M. 1984. Canine tooth extraction and pulpotomy in the adult male llama. J. Am. Vet. Med. Assoc. 185:1304–6.

44. Kress, P. J. 1979. Dental surgery in the llama. Llama Newsl. 4:1–2.

45. Langer, P. 1973. (Comparative anatomical investigations on the stomach of artiodactylids. II. Investigations on the stomach of tylopoda and ruminantia) Vergleichend anatomische Untersuchungen am Magen der Artiodactyla. II. Untersuchungen am Magen der Tylopods und Ruminantia. Gegenbaurs Morphol. Jahrb. 119:663–95.

46. ______. 1974. Stomach evolution in the artiodactyla. Mammalia 38(2):295.

47. Leon, J. A. 1937. (The age of the South American camelids) La edad de los auquenidos. Vida Agric. (Peru) 14:725–32.

48. Loring, S. H., and Wood, A. E. 1969. Deciduous premolars of some North American tertiary camels, family Camelidae. J. Paleontol. 43(5):1199–1209.

49. Loupal, G. 1982. (Gastrolithiasis in a llama) Gastrolithiasis bei einen Llama. Berl. Muench. Tieraerztl. Wochenschr. 95(1):1416.

50. Luciano, L., Voss-Wermbter, G., Behnke, M., Engelhardt, W. von, and Real, E. 1979. (The structure of the stomach mucosa in the llama) Die Struktur der Magenschleimhaut beim Lama, *Lama guanacoe* und *Lama lamae*. I. Vormagen. Gegenbaurs Morphol. Jahrb. 125:519–49.

51. Luciano, L., Reale, E., and Engelhardt, W. von. 1980. The fine structure of the stomach mucosa of the llama (*Llama guanacoe*). II. The fundic region of the hind stomach. Cell Tissue Res. 208(2):207–28.

52. McCandless, E. L., and Dye, J. A. 1950. Physiological changes in intermediary metabolism of various species of ruminants incident to functional development of the rumen. Am. J. Physiol. 162:2.

53. McIntosh, W. C. 1929. On abnormal teeth in certain mammals, especially in the rabbit. Trans. R. Soc. (Edinburgh) 56:333–407.

54. Marcelo, A., and Villavicencio, M. 1980. Purification and properties of pyruvate carboxylase from alpaca liver. Fed. Proc. 39(6):2526.

55. Miller, G. S. 1924. A second instance of development of rodent-like incisors in the artiodactyla. Proc. Smithson. Inst. 66:1–3.

56. Milton, C., and Axelrod, J. M. 1957. Calculi and other stones found in mammals. J. Mammal. 38:279–80.

57. Montalvo Arenas, C. 1966. (Contributions to the study of the morphology of the alpaca: Histologic and histochemic study of the bowel) Contribucion al estudio de la morfologia de la alpaca, *Lama pacos,* estudio histologico e histoquimico del intestino. Tesis, Fac. Med. Vet. Univ. Nac. Mayor San Marcos (Lima), pp. 1–55.

58. ______. 1970. (Some advances in the histology of the alpaca) Advances sobre histologia de la alpaca. Primera Conv. Camelidos Sudam. (Auquenidos), Puno, Peru, pp. 49–57.

59. Montalvo Arenas, C., Ploog Werner, H., and Copaira, B. M. 1967. (Contributions of the study of morphology of the alpaca, histologic and histochemic study of the salivary glands and bowel) Contribucion al estudio de la morfologia de la alpaca, *Lama pacos.* Bol. Extraordinario 2:47–61.

60. Neuville, M. H. 1931. (Some dental peculiarities of camelids) De certaines particularities dentaires des Camelides. Bull. Mus. Nat. Hist. (Paris) Ser. 2, 3(1):77–81.

61. Ortiz Velarde, C. F. 1971. (Contributions to the study of the parotid saliva of the alpaca) Contribucion al estudio de la saliva parotidea de alpaca (fluid, pH, Na, K. y Ca). Tesis, Fac. Med. Vet. Univ. Nac. Mayor San Marcos (Lima), pp.1–27.

62. Ortiz, C., Cavero, J., Sillau, H., and Cueva, S. 1974. The parotid saliva of the alpaca, *Lama pacos.* Res. Vet. Sci. 16(1):54–56.

63. Ploog Werner, H. 1966. (Contribution to the study of the morphology of the alpaca; anatomic study, histology, histochemistry of the salivary glands) Contribucion al estudio de la morfologia de la alpaca, *Lama pacos,* estudio anatomico, histologico, histoquimico de las glandula. Tesis, Fac. Med. Vet. Univ. Nac. Mayor San Marcos (Lima), pp. 1–59.

64. Ratcliffe, H. L. 1933. Incidence and nature of tumors in captive wild animals and birds (haemangioma of liver in camel, carcinoma of gall bladder in llama.) J. Cancer Res. 17:116–35.

65. Rubsamen, K., and Engelhardt, W. von. 1978. Bicarbonate secretion and solute absorption in forestomach of the llama. Am. J. Physiol. 235(1):E1–E6.

66. ______. 1979. Morphological and functional peculiarities of the llama forestomach. Communications Digestive Physiology Metabolism. Ann. Rech. Vet. 10(2):473–75.

67. Ruckebuseh, Y., ed. 1974. Digestive Physiology and Metabolism in Ruminants—Short Communications. 5th Int. Symp. Ruminant Physiol. 10(2):157–502.

68. Rusconi, C. 1930. (Numeric dental anomalies in some living guanacos, *Lama guanacoe*) Sobre anomalias dentarias numericas en algunos guanacos vivientes (*Lama guanaco*). Physis (Buenos Aires) 10(35):199–203.

69. Shklair, I. L. 1980. Dental decay, llamas, livestock, *Streptococcus mutans* natural occurrence of caries in animals—animals as vectors and reservoirs of carcinogenic flora. Proc. Anim. Models Cardiol., pp. 41–51.

70. Sillau, H., Chauca, D., and Valenzuela, A. 1973. (Evaluation of microbial activity in the ruminal fluid of sheep and alpacas) Evaluacion de la actividad microbiana del fluido ruminal del ovino y la alpaca. Rev. Invest. Pecu. 2(1):15–21.

71. Sillau, H., Llerena, L., Esquerre, J., Rojas, M., and Alva, J. 1973. (Liver function tests in young alpaca infected or uninfected with *Lamanema chavezi*) Pruebas functionales hepaticas en crias de alpaca normales y infectadas experimen-

talmenta con *Lamanema chavezi*. Rev. Invest. Pecu. 2(1):103–5.

72. Sodeman, W. A., Jr., and Sodeman, T. M. 1979. Sodeman's Pathologic Physiology, 6th ed. Philadelphia: W. B. Saunders, p. 833.

73. Taylor, S. 1981. Male llamas—removal of "fighting teeth." 3 L llama 9:6–7.

74. Temple, R. M. S., and Temple, C. M. 1983. Rumenal atony. Llama World 1(4):23.

75. Vallenas P., A. 1956. (Fistula closure of the rumen of the alpaca) Fistula cerrada en el rumen de alpaca. Rev. Fac. Med. Vet. Univ. Nac. San Marcos (Lima) 7(11):172–77.

76. ______. 1958. (Preliminary study on the reflex closure of the esophageal groove in alpacas as viewed through a rumen fistula) Estudio preliminar sobre el clerre reflejo del surco esofagico de las alpacas a traves de una fistula abierta en el rumen. Vet. Zootec. (Lima) 10(26)7–12.

77. ______. 1958–59. (Study of some chemical substances which produce closure of the groove of the esophagus in alpacas) Estudio de algunas substancias quimicas que peuden provocar el clerre del surco esofagico en alpacas. Rev. Fac. Med. Vet. Univ. Mayor San Marcos (Lima) 13–14:49–65.

78. ______. 1960. (Some aspects of the motility of the stomach of alpaca) Algunos aspectos de la motilidad del rumen de alpaca. Rev. Fac. Med. Vet. Univ. Nac. Mayor San Marcos (Lima) 15:69–79.

79. ______. 1965. Some physiological aspects of digestion in the alpaca, *Lama pacos*. In R. W. Daugherty, ed. Physiology of Digestion in the Ruminant. Washington, D.C.: Butterworth, pp. 147–58.

80. ______. 1970a. (Physiology of digestion of South American camelids) Fisiologia de la digestion de los auquenidos. Primera Conv. Camelidos Sudam. (Auqenidos), Puno, Peru, pp. 69–78.

81. ______. 1970b. Structural and functional studies of the llama and guanaco stomach. Cornell Univ. Diss. Abstr. 31(6):3682.

82. Vallenas P., A., and Stevens, C. E. 1971. Motility of the llama and guanaco stomach. Am. J. Physiol. 220(1):275–82.

83. Vallenas P., A., Cummings, J. F., and Munnell, J. F. 1971. A gross study of the compartmentalized stomach of two New World camelids—the llama and guanaco. J. Morphol. 134:399–424.

84. Vallenas P., A., Sillau, H., Cueva, S., and Esquerre, J. 1974. (Outlines of anatomic and physiologic science) Linea de ciencias fisiologicas y morfologicas. Bol. Divulg. 151:118–22.

85. Vasquez, R., Guerra, R., Ore, R., and Villavicencio, M. 1978. Purification and properties of fructose 1,6,biophosphatase from alpaca liver. Fed. Proc. 37(6):1525.

86. Vetter, R. L. 1982. The use of stomach-tubes in llamas. Llama World 1(2):25.

87. Villavicencio, M., Guerra, R., and Vasquez, R. 1971a. Glucose oxidation in the alpaca liver. Peru Soc. Quim. Bol. 37(2)52.

88. ______. 1971b. Glucose oxidation and glucose neogenesis in alpaca liver. Acta Cient. Ven. [Suppl. 2] 22:65.

89. Wass, W. M., Thompson, J. R., Moss, E. W., Kunesh, J. P., and Eness, P. G. 1981. Diseases of the ruminant stomach. In J. L. Howard, ed. Current Veterinary Therapy: Food Animal Practice. Philadelphia: W. B. Saunders, pp. 877–910.

90. Wheeler, J. C. 1982. Aging llamas and alpacas by their teeth. Llama World 1(2):12–17.

14 Endocrine System

ANATOMY AND PHYSIOLOGY

Other than a few anatomic and physiologic studies describing the glands and hormones involved with reproduction, few discussions of the endocrine system of lamoids have been published (1–17).

Pituitary Gland

The pituitary gland of lamoids is not unique. It is located at the base of the brain in the pituitary fossa of the basic sphenoid bone, similar to the location in the bovine. The gross anatomy, histology, and histochemistry of the gland have been studied (10). The growth hormone of the alpaca has been isolated and characterized and found to be chemically similar to other mammalian growth hormones (1). Unfortunately, this hormone has not been studied in a clinical setting to determine if it is involved in a dwarf syndrome that has been reported by clinicians at conferences.

Thyroid Gland

The paired thyroid glands are situated on the dorsolateral surface of the trachea. They are approximately 4 cm long and 2 cm wide and occupy the space from the cricoid cartilage of the larynx to the third or fourth tracheal ring. Blood is supplied by a cranial and caudal thyroid artery directly from the carotid artery (12).

Reference ranges for triiodothyronine (T-3) and thyroxine (T-4) in llamas have been established using radioimmunoassay techniques.[1] The range of T-3 for 8 llamas less than 1 month of age at the 95 percentile limit is 274–686 ng/dl, while for 81 llamas of all ages, the range was 48–468 ng/dl. Similar ranges for T-4 were 18–39 μg/dl in 7 llamas less than 1 month of age and 9.8–30 μg/dl for 75 llamas of all ages. These levels are higher by 10 times than those reported for any other species in which values have been determined. The significance of this is unknown.

Parathyroid Glands

The parathyroid glands are imbedded in the caudal pole of each thyroid gland, as they are in other ungulates. No parahormone levels or disorders of parathyroid function have been reported.

Adrenal Glands

The right adrenal gland is elongated (1 × 4.5 cm) and lies medial and 3–4 cm craniad to the cranial pole of the right kidney. The left adrenal gland lies in approximately the same position relative to the left kidney but has a squarish shape (2.5 × 3 cm and 1 cm thick). Lamoid adrenal function has not yet been studied.

Gonads

Gonadal anatomy and physiology are discussed in Chapter 17.

DISEASES

Diseases of the gonads are discussed in Chapter 17. No other diseases of the endocrine system have been definitively diagnosed. Stress, as it relates to lamoids, is discussed in Chapter 9.

Failure to Grow

Although there are no references to lamoid dwarfism in the literature, clinicians who see numerous animals have described individuals that do not grow normally. These crias, with normal birth weights, fall behind same-age farm mates. No correlation with lack of milk from the female or any identifiable nutrient has been established. Four- and 5-month-old affected crias may be the size of a 1-month-old normal cria. Body condition is usually adequate, and the cria seems to eat sufficiently,

1. M. Fowler, personal research data.

but it simply does not grow. Physical and laboratory examinations of a number of these individuals have failed to identify a common denominator. Thyroid function seems adequate. Other biochemical and hematologic parameters are within normal limits.

The condition has been identified in guanacos and llamas in North America. Dwarfism has not been recognized in lamoids in Peru. Body size is an inherited trait in all species of animals. There is no evidence that this is a hereditary defect, but, contrarily, there is no evidence that it is not, except that the condition has not been repeated on the same farm. Occurrence seems to be random. More investigations must be carried out on animals with a tendency to dwarfism.

Llamas from lines with past alpaca infusion may produce offspring with the body size of an alpaca, even though the parents are large. This is not dwarfism.

REFERENCES

1. Biscoglio, M. J., Cascone, O., Arnao D. N., A. I., Santome, J. A., Sanchez, D., Ore, R., and Villavicencio, M. 1981. Isolation and character of alpaca growth hormone. Int. J. Peptide Protein Res. 17:374–79.

2. Bonino, M. J. B. D., Cascone, O., De Nue, A. I. A., Ore, R., Villavicencio, M., Santome, J. A., and Sanchez, D. 1981. Isolation and characterization of alpaca, *Lama pacos,* growth hormone. Int. J. Peptide Protein Res. 17 (3):374–79.

3. Cascone, O., Biscoglio, M. J., Pena, C., Santome, J. A., Arnao D. N., A. I., Sanchez, D., Ore, R., and Villavicencio, M. 1984. Amino acid sequences around cystine residues in alpaca growth hormone. Acta Physiol. Pharmacol. Latinoam. 34:21–28.

4. Chavez M., A. 1956. (Histologic aspects of the alpaca, glands of internal secretion) Aspectos histologicos de la alpaca, glandulas de secrecion interna. Tesis, Fac. Med. Vet. Univ. Nac. Mayor San Marcos (Lima).

5. El-Nouty, F. D., Yousef, M. K., Magdub, A. B., and Johnson, H. D. 1976. Thyroid secretion hormones in Camelidae and Equidae. Fed. Proc. 35(3):216.

6. ______. 1978. Thyroid hormones and metabolic rate in burros, *Equus asinus,* and llamas, *Lama glama:* Effects of environmental temperature. Comp. Biochem. Physiol. [A] 60(2):235–38.

7. Huaman, J., Villavicencio, M., Guerra, R., and Ore, R. 1975. Effect of insulin and hydrocortisone on the activity of glycolytic and gluconeogenic enzymes of alpaca liver. Fed. Proc. 34(3):659.

8. Malaga M., A. 1970. (Attraction of radioactive iodine to the thyroid gland of the alpaca) Captacion del yodo radioactive (I-131) por la glandula tiroides de *Lama pacos* (alpaca). Tesis, Fac. Med. Vet. Univ. Nac. Tec. Altiplano (Puno), pp. 1–29.

9. Matusita, A., and Manrique, J. 1970. (Preliminary observations of the pars intermedia of the pituitary in alpacas) Observaciones preliminares de la pars intermedia de hipofisis en alpacas. 1st Conv. Camelidos Sudam. (Auquenidos), Puno, Peru, pp. 61–62.

10. Montalvo A., C., and Copaira, B. M. 1968. (Contributions to the study of the morphology of the alpaca. Histologic and histochemical study of the endocrine glands. I. Pituitary) Contribucion al estudio de la morfologia de la alpaca, *Lama pacos.* Estudio histologica y histoquimico de las glandulas endocrinas. I. Hipofisis. Rev. Fac. Med. Vet. (Lima) 22:70–85.

11. Samuel, C. A., Sumar, J., and Nathanielsz, P. W. 1979. Histological observations of the adrenal glands of new born alpacas, *Lama pacos.* Comp. Biochem. Physiol. [A] 62(2):387–96.

12. Sato S., A., Tawata N., H., and Kian, T. O. 1979. (Anatomical study of the thyroid glands of the alpaca) Estudio anatomico de la glandula tiroides de la alpaca. Rev. Invest. Pecu. 4(1):3–11.

13. Silva Grey, L. J. 1965. (Anatomichistologic variations of the future of alpacas by action of pitocin) Variaciones anatomicohistologicas del futuro de alpacas por accion del pitocin. Tesis, Fac. Med. Vet. Univ. Nac. Mayor San Marcos (Lima), pp. 1–25.

14. Smollich, A. 1965. (Bone production in the adrenal cortex of llamas) Knochenbildungen in der Nebenniereurende eines Lamas. Zentralbl. Allg. Pathol. 107:214–17.

15. Stohl, G. 1973. (The thyroid of naturally living and domesticated South American tylopods). In J. Matolcsi, ed. Domestikationsforschung und Geschichte der Haustiere. Int. Symp. Budapest: Akademiai Kiado, pp. 141–49.

16. Sumar, J., Smith, G. W., Mayhua, E., and Nathanielsz, P. W. 1978. Adrenocortical function in the fetal and newborn alpaca. Comp. Biochem. Physiol. [A] 59(1):79–84.

17. Wiesner, H. 1973. (Use of the anabolic steroid [zeranol] in zoo animals) Beitrag zur Anwendung des anabolicums Ralgro bei Zootieren. Tieraerztl. Umschau 28(4):186–89.

15

Hemic and Lymphatic Systems

ANATOMY AND PHYSIOLOGY

Numerous investigations have been carried out on camelid blood (1, 2). The unique oval erythrocyte of camelids was first described over 100 years ago (23), and ever since, researchers have been attempting to establish the role played by blood constituents in the adaptation of camels to life in a desert environment and of South American camelids (SACs) to life at high altitudes. Though a complete physiology of hemic systems will not be reviewed here, facts having relevance to evaluation of a diseased state or to therapy will be discussed.

HEMATOLOGY

Only one study of hematologic values for llamas in North America has been reported (20). Reference ranges are listed in Table 15.1. Studies carried out in South America have reported results for llamas, alpacas, and vicuñas that are so similar that hematologic values for one species may be assumed to be applicable to the others (Tables 15.2, 15.3) (3–11, 15, 16, 21, 29). Hematologic parameters for camelids are compared with those of dromedaries, cattle, and horses in Table 15.4. Certain values are significantly different and should be considered in evaluating a hemogram of a diseased lamoid.

Hemoglobin values for lamoids are higher than for cattle, the same as for horses. Camelid erythrocytes are small (Table 15.2), ellipsoid in shape, and circulate in larger numbers than in other mammalian species (14, 24). The small size and shape result in a lower packed cell volume (PCV). Camelid erythrocytes are oriented with the long axis in the direction of the blood flow and are able to traverse small capillaries, resulting in fewer problems of sludging when the viscosity of the blood increases during dehydration (31, 32). One study determined that alpaca blood had a large oxygen-carrying capacity and a low viscosity, which ideally suited this animal to living in an environment with low oxygen tension (35).

The normal mean corpuscular volume (MCV) of llamas is lower than that found in livestock species because of the lower PCV. The mean corpuscular hemoglobin concentration (MCHC) is higher with llamas (44.5) than in livestock (30–35). The MCHC measures the ratio of the weight of hemoglobin (Hb) to the total volume of the erythrocytes. Since normal Hb levels in llamas are higher than those of livestock species and the PCV is slightly lower, a higher MCHC index results. A low MCHC in llamas is indicative of a hypochromic anemia.

The mean corpuscular hemoglobin (MCH) expresses the weight of Hb in an average erythrocyte. Normal MCH levels of llamas are slightly lower than those of other livestock species because the erythrocytes are smaller. An excessively low value indicates anemia.

The leukocyte count is significantly higher in llamas than in other domestic mammals. The neutrophil-lymphocyte ratio is similar to that of the horse, with the majority of cells being neutrophils. High eosinophil numbers have been reported in the European, North American, and South American literature (19). Attempts have been made to correlate this with parasite burdens, but no controlled studies have been conducted.

SERUM BIOCHEMISTRY

Reports of reference ranges for biochemical parameters are few in number, usually limited to a few parameters or small numbers of animals. Most biochemical parameters are similar to those of cattle, with the exception of serum glucose, which is twice that of cattle (Table 15.5). There are no established reference ranges for a number of parameters (liver function other than enzymes and the liver-specific enzymes, kidney function, glucose tolerance, amylase, xylose absorption).

Serum protein levels in alpacas have been studied in South America (12, 34) (Table 15.6). Reference ranges for llamas in North America are listed in Table 15.7. Insufficient numbers of protein electrophoresis patterns

Table 15.1. Hematologic values in llamas

	<1 mo. n = 20	2–6 mo. n = 30	6–18 mo. n = 35	All young n = 85	Adult female n = 54	Adult male n = 35	All adults n = 89	All llamas n = 174
Erythrocytes ($\times 10^6/\mu l$)	9.8–14.2[a] (12)[b]	10.6–17.2 (13.9)	10.8–15.9 (13)	9.9–16.8 (13.3)	10.2–17.7 (13.9)	9.6–17.6 (13.6)	9.9–17.7 (13.8)	
Hemoglobin (g/dl)	10.1–15.4 (12.7)	11.6–18.2 (14.9)	11.0–17.9 (14.4)	10.6–17.8 (14.2)	9.9–17.9 (13.9)	11.3–19.4 (15.3)	11.5–19.5 (15.5)	10.8–18.0 (14.4)
Hematocrit (%)	24–36 (30)	27–43 (35)	26–41 (33)	25–41 (32)	26–47 (36)	25–45 (35)	25–46 (35)	22–46 (34)
Mean corpuscular (vol. fl)	21.7–26.3 (24)	20.8–29.3 (25)	22.0–28.2 (25.1)	21.3–28.4 (24.8)	22.5–30.0 (26.3)	21.4–30.0 (25.7)	22.0–30.1 (26)	21.4–29.0 (25.2)
Mean corpuscular hemoglobin concentration (g/dl)	39.0–44.8 (41.9)	39.8–46.0 (42.9)	39.4–46.4 (42.4)	34.3–46.0 (39.9)	39.2–46.6 (42.9)	36.6–51.5 (43.9)	37.7–49.0 (43.3)	38.3–47.0 (42.6)
Mean corpuscular hemoglobin (pg)	8.9–11.2 (10)	9.4–12.3 (10.8)	9.3–12.3 (10.3)	9.1–12.1 (10.1)	9.8–12.8 (10.8)	10.0–12.5 (11.2)	9.8–12.7 (11.2)	9.4–12.0 (10.7)
Leukocytes ($10^3/\mu l$)	5.4–20.1 (12.7)	8.0–23.5 (15.7)	8.9–24.8 (16.8)	7.1–23.8 (15.4)	7.8–19.9 (13.8)	7.3–22.2 (14.7)	7.5–20.9 (14.2)	7.2–22.2 (14.2)
Bands (per μl)	0–487[c] (243)	0–99 (49)	0–90 (45)	0–215 (107)	0–145 (72)	0–21 (10)	0–169 (84)	0–128 (64)
Neutrophils (per μl)	1031–15743 (8387)	2799–14575 (8692)	4021–14009 (9015)	2819–14697 (8758)	3659–13826 (8743)	2785–16985 (9885)	3130–15254 (9192)	2966–15005 (8986)
Lymphocytes (per μl)	1156–4972 (3064)	1470–9860 (5665)	1456–7901 (4679)	764–8493 (4629)	645–4739 (2692)	982–4922 (2952)	689–4848 (2769)	963–7642 (4302)
Monocytes (per μl)	0–1268 (624)	0–1235 (617)	0–1151 (575)	0–1016 (508)	0–977 (488)	0–895 (492)	0–955 (477)	0–1091 (545)
Eosinophils (per μl)	0–983 (491)	0–2234 (1117)	0–6220 (3110)	0–4863 (2431)	0–4696 (2348)	369–4085 (2227)	16–4471 (2244)	0–4722 (2861)
Basophils (per μl)	0–132 (66)	0–234 (117)	0–321 (165)	0–250 (125)	0–246 (123)	0–352 (186)	0–293 (146)	0–275 (137)

[a]Range = (± #2 standard deviations).
[b]Mean.
[c]Range (95th percentile).

Table 15.2. Erythrocyte factors for South American camelids in Peru

	At 4200 m[a]			At 3900 m[b]	
Parameters	Llama (12)	Alpaca (12)	Vicuña (12)	Alpaca (116)	Vicuña (12)
Erythrocytes (mil)	13.7 ± 0.59	14.4 ± 0.37	13.1 ± 0.34	13.96 7.98–21.39	14.50 11.78–19.06
Erythrocyte size (μ)					
Length	6.48 ± 0.47	6.56 ± 0.41	6.30 ± 0.51		
Width	3.30 ± 0.21	3.30 ± 0.18	3.26 ± 0.25		
Hemoglobin (g/dl)	15.1 ± 0.45	13.8 ± 0.27	13.5 ± 0.51	14.25 9.50–20.50	14.29 11–18.50
Hematocrit (%)	38.1 ± 1.21	35.5 ± 0.86	36.0 ± 0.85	35.55 24–45	37.20 31–43
MCV	28.0 ± 0.37	24.8 ± 0.30	27.4 ± 0.57	25.45 17.37–32.31	25.83 21.64–29.36
MCHC	39.7 ± 0.52	38.8 ± 0.40	37.5 ± 0.52	39.69 33.33–48.43	38.38 35.36–44.04
MCH	10.8 ± 0.40	9.5 ± 0.30	10.2 ± 0.30	10.06 7.69–13.43	9.81 8.26–11.15

[a]Data from Reynafarje 1968.
[b]Data from Copaira 1949, 1953.

Table 15.3. Leukocyte factors for South American camelids in Peru

	At 4200 m[a]			At 3900 m[b]	
Parameters	Llama (12)	Alpaca (12)	Vicuña (12)	Alpaca (113)	Vicuña (12)
Leukocytes × $10^3/\mu l$	11.7 ± 1.20	11.6 ± 0.85	12.2 ± 0.81	15.79 5.68–28.48	12.76 8.08–22.76
Neutrophils (%)	59.0 ± 3.90	58.5 ± 3.90	46.8 ± 3.10	52.24 25.5–86.00	55.16 41–67
Lymphocytes (%)	27.7 ± 4.30	33.5 ± 4.20	33.8 ± 3.00	36.21 11.8–69.00	28.81 17.50–42.50
Monocytes (%)	3.3 ± 0.50	3.0 ± 0.60	2.4 ± 0.30	1.50 0–9.80	6.85 1–26.80
Eosinophils (%)	10.0 ± 2.90	5.0 ± 1.10	14.6 ± 2.20	8.24 0–28.00	8.49 0.5–22.50

[a]Data from Reynafarje 1968.
[b]Data from Copaira 1949, 1953.

Table 15.4. Comparative hemogram of the llama, camel, cow, and horse

	Llama	Camel	Cow	Horse
Erythrocytes ($10^6/\mu l$)	9.9–17.7	7.22–11.76	5–10	6.8–12.9
Hemoglobin (g/dl)	10.8–18.0	7.8–15.9	8–15	11–19
PCV (%)	25–44.5	25–34	24–46	32–53
MCV (fl)	21.4–29.0	35–60	40–60	37–58
MHCH (g/dl)	38.3–47.0	36.5–50.9	30–36	31–38.6
MCH (pg)	9.4–12.0	17–22	11–17	12.3–19.7
Leukocytes ($10^3/\mu l$)	7.2–22.0	11.5–16.5	4–12	5.4–14.3
Neutrophils ($10^3/\mu l$)	2.9–15.0	51%	0.6–4	2.3–8.6
Lymphocytes ($10^3/\mu l$)	0–7.4	40%	2.5–7.5	1.5–7.7
Monocytes ($10^3/\mu l$)	0–1.1	4%	0.025–0.84	0–1.0
Eosinophils ($10^3/\mu l$)	0–4.7	4%	0–2.4	0–1.0
Basophils ($10^3/\mu l$)	0–0.3	4%	0–0.2	0.029

Source: Schalm et al. 1985.

have been performed on North American llamas to allow statistical computation, but Table 15.7 provides means and ranges for various age groups on a limited number of llamas. Precolostrum neonates have low total protein and relatively low globulin. With the absorption of colostral immunoglobulin, the A-G ratio is lowered and the total protein and globulin levels elevated. Globulin levels decrease at about 3 weeks of age, as passively acquired globulin wanes, remaining low until production of globulins by the maturing immune system of the cria makes up the loss. This may be a critical time in the life of the lamoid neonate, since it may be more susceptible to infectious diseases at this stage of life (33).

There is a wide range of values for both calcium and phosphorus in llamas, with some apparently normal ratios showing more phosphorus than calcium (Table 15.5). The significance of either high or low calcium and/or phosphorus levels is unknown. In a study of 188 alpacas in Peru, calcium levels ranged from 7.6 to 11.6 mg/dl and phosphorus, 4.2–9.7 mg/dl (27, 28). This same investigator noted that alpacas did not become hypocalcemic shortly before or following parturition, as do other domestic ungulates. No cases of clinical postpartu-rient hypocalcemia (milk fever) in lamoids have been reported. In one study, neonate alpacas, up to 3 weeks of age, had higher calcium levels than adults (27).

Miscellaneous biochemical parameters for SACs kept at 4200 m are listed in Table 15.8. Prenursing neonate biochemical and hematologic values differ from those of adults. See Chapter 21 for a full discussion of important parameters. Comparative serum biochemistry values are listed in Table 15.9.

Coagulation factor reference ranges have been reported in only one llama and one guanaco (26). Clotting time was 10 seconds for the guanaco and 14.5 seconds for the llama, prothrombin time was 120 seconds for the llama, partial thromboplastin time was 36.4 seconds for the guanaco and 26.4 seconds for the llama, and the platelet count in the llama was 370,000, with a platelet diameter of 2 μm.

There is disagreement between two studies of the life span of erythrocytes in lamoids. In one study, utilizing erythrocytes labeled with 51 Cr in vitro, the life span was approximately 60 days in 12 llamas, 12 alpacas, and 12 vicuñas (29). In another study of two guanacos, using glycine-2-^{14}C, the life span was 225 days (17). The life

Table 15.5. Serum biochemistry parameters in llamas

	<1 mo. n = 20	2–6 mo. n = 30	6–18 mo. n = 35	All young n = 85	Adult female n = 54	Adult male n = 35	All adults n = 89	All llamas n = 174
Total protein	3.8–6.9[a]	4.2–6.9	4.9–7.3	4.4–7.2	5.2–7.4	5–7.4	5–7.4	4.7–7.3
(g/dl)	(5.4)[b]	(5.6)	(6.1)	(5.8)	(6.3)	(6.2)	(6.2)	(6)
Albumin	2.6–4.2	3.3–4.6	3–5.1	2.8–4.9	2.9–5.2	2.9–5	2.9–5.1	2.9–5
(g/dl)	(3.4)	(4)	(4.1)	(3.9)	(4.1)	(4)	(4)	(4)
Globulin	0.8–3.1	0.7–2.8	1.2–2.9	0.9–2.9	1.2–3.2	1.4–2.9	1.3–3.1	1.1–3
(g/dl)	(2)	(1.8)	(2.1)	(1.9)	(2.2)	(2.2)	(2.2)	(2.1)
Fibrinogen	100–400[c]	100–400	100–400	100–400	100–500	100–500	100–500	100–400
(g/dl)	(150)	(150)	(150)	(150)	(200)	(200)	(200)	(150)
Icteric	2–5[c]	2–5	2	2–5	2	2	2	2–5
index	(3.5)	(3.5)	(2)	(3.5)	(2)	(2)	(2)	(2)
Serum urea	6–22	13–29	14–34	8–33	13–38	10–34	10–37	9–35
nitrogen (mg/dl)	(14)	(21)	(24)	(21)	(26)	(22)	(24)	(22)
Creatinine	0.3–2.7	1–2.4	0.9–2.7	0.7–2.7	0.9–2.7	1.4–2.8	1.1–2.9	0.9–2.8
(mg/dl)	(1.5)	(1.7)	(1.8)	(1.7)	(1.8)	(1.6)	(2)	(1.9)
Glucose	90–190	97–159	95–160	93–168	82–157	83–155	82–156	86–163
(mg/dl)	(140)	(128)	(128)	(131)	(120)	(119)	(119)	(125)
Cholesterol	17–127	0–208	0–115	0–157	13–89	11–68	10–82	0–128
(mg/dl)	(72)	(104)	(57)	(78)	(51)	(40)	(46)	(64)
T-3	178–706	0–445	42–330	0–528	58–221	87–282	57–244	0–423
nanogram (ng/dl)	(442)	(222)	(186)	(264)	(140)	(185)	(153)	(211)
T-4	14.4–41.8	4.4–28.6	9.7–20.9	4.7–31.7	7.8–20	11.8–21.4	8.3–20.8	5.2–27.3
microgram (μg/dl)	(28.1)	(16.5)	(15.3)	(18.2)	(13.9)	(16.6)	(14.6)	(16.3)
Bilirubin	0–0.6[c]	0–0.2	0–0.1	0–0.2	0–0.2	0–0.2	0–0.2	0–0.2
(mg/dl)	(0.2)	(0.1)	(0.1)	(0.1)	(0.1)	(0.1)	(0.1)	(0.1)
CK	0–115	0–108	0–46	0–83	0–58	0–110	0–56	0–70
(IU/L)	(57)	(54)	(23)	(41)	(29)	(55)	(28)	(35)
SGOT (AST)	123–485	137–547	175–417	141–482	137–413	114–429	127–420	128–450
(IU/L)	(304)	(342)	(296)	(312)	(275)	(272)	(274)	(289)
SGPT (ALT)	0–12	1–10	0–14	0–12	0–16	0–14	0–15	0–14
(IU/L)	(6)	(6)	(7)	(6)	(8)	(7)	(7)	(7)
SGGT	1–29	0–30	7–22	1–27	8–30	8–21	7–27	3–28
(IU/L)	(15)	(15)	(15)	(14)	(19)	(15)	(17)	(16)
SDH	0–17	0–19	0–17	0–16	0–4	0–4	0–4	0–10
(IU/L)	(80)	(9)	(80)	(8)	(2)	(2)	(2)	(5)
LDH	111–855	135–813	115–651	103–768	0–602	41–531	0–572	10–695
(IU/L)	(483)	(474)	(383)	(436)	(301)	(286)	(286)	(356)
ALP	170–1000	0–638	0–362	0–680	0–222	6–93	0–179	0–500
(IU/L)	(585)	(369)	(181)	(340)	(111)	(50)	(89)	(200)
Calcium	9.2–10.9	8.6–10.8	8.5–11	8.7–10.9	7.6–10.1	7.1–10.6	7.4–10.2	7.8–10.8
(mg/dl)	(10.1)	(9.7)	(9.8)	(9.8)	(8.9)	(8.9)	(8.9)	(9.3)
Phosphorus	7–12.2	4.5–11.2	2.8–9.9	3.4–11.9	2.1–7.9	2.3–7.3	2.3–7.6	2–10.7
(mg/dl)	(9.6)	(7.9)	(6.4)	(7.7)	(5.5)	(4.8)	(5)	(6.4)
Sodium	146–156	149–155	149–157	148–156	149–158	146–159	148–158	148–158
(meq/L)	(151)	(152)	(153)	(152)	(154)	(153)	(153)	(153)
Potassium	4.4–6	3.8–6.6	3.9–5.7	3.9–6.2	3.8–6.3	3.3–5.6	3.6–6	3.6–6.2
(meq/L)	(5.2)	(5.2)	(4.8)	(5.1)	(5.1)	(4.5)	(4.8)	(4.9)
Chloride	97–115	98–114	98–119	98–117	97–117	105–123	99–121	98–120
(meq/L)	(107)	(106)	(109)	(108)	(108)	(114)	(110)	(109)
Total CO_2	21–34	21–29	21–35	19–34	22–32	10–31	11–35	14–34
(m M/L)	(28)	(25)	(28)	(27)	(27)	(21)	(23)	(24)

[a]Range = (± 2 standard deviations).
[b]Mean.
[c](95th percentile).

Table 15.6. Serum protein and fractionation in alpacas

		Crias				
	Adults (100)	1 day	8 days	15 days	22 days	120 days
Total protein	5.22–8.92 (6.79)	6.36	5.70	5.82	5.95	5.92
Albumin	2.05–4.78 (3.19)	2.32	2.69	3.21	3.13	1.19
Globulin	1.76–5.47 (3.55)	4.03	3.00	2.60	1.27	4.72
Alpha	0.18–2.70 (1.24)	1.56	1.42	1.08	2.82	3.34
Beta	0.03–2.79 (1.04)	1.21	0.59	0.75	0.62	0.55
Gamma	0.66–2.32 (1.42)	1.37	0.98	0.76	0.79	1.02
A/G ratio	0.44–1.80 (0.90)	0.52	0.90	1.28	1.14	0.26

Source: Vallenas 1957.

Table 15.7. Serum protein electrophoresis patterns in llamas

Age group	Parameter	Total protein (g/dl)	Albumin (g/dl)	Globulin (g/dl)	Alpha (g/dl)	Beta (g/dl)	Gamma (g/dl)	A:G ratio
<1 month	Mean	5.6	3.3	2.3	0.7	1.0	0.7	1.4:1
n = 6	Range	5.1–5.9	3.1–3.5	1.9–2.7	0.5–0.9	0.8–1.1	0.4–1.1	1.1–1.7:1
1–5 months	Mean	5.9	3.7	2.2	0.7	0.9	0.6	1.7:1
n = 6	Range	5.4–6.4	3.3–4.0	1.4–2.7	0.4–1.0	0.7–1.1	0.3–1.0	1.4–2.8:1
6–18 months	Mean	6.1	3.8	2.3	0.7	0.9	0.8	1.6:1
n = 11	Range	5.5–6.9	3.1–4.4	1.8–3.0	0.5–0.8	0.6–1.1	0.4–1.1	1.3–2.4:1
Mature male and female	Mean	6.3	3.5	2.9	0.7	1.0	1.1	1.2:1
n = 7	Range	5.9–6.8	3.1–3.7	2.3–3.3	0.5–0.9	0.9–1.1	0.8–1.5	1.1–1.6:1
All llamas >1 month	Mean	5.9	3.5					
n = 24	Range	5.4–6.9	3.1–4.4					

Note: n = number of animals tested.
Source: Author's unpublished data.

Table 15.8. Miscellaneous biochemical and hematologic parameters of llamas, alpacas, and vicuñas maintained at altitude (4200 m)

Parameter	Llama	Alpaca	Vicuña	Horse	Cow	Human	Camel
Plasma iron (μg/dl)	192 ± 11[a]	156 ± 11	113 ± 6.6	73–140	57–162 (62–133)	94 ± 3.8	98.5
Iron uptake (%)	84.8 ± 3.6	82.4 ± 4.4	90.6 ± 3.3	74–77	55	92 ± 2.4	
Plasma iron turnover rate (mg Fe/day/kg)	0.59 ± 0.12	0.52 ± 0.04	1.11 ± 0.32	0.45–0.65	0.27	0.39 ± 0.01	
Red cell iron turnover rate (mg/Fe/day/kg)	0.52 ± 0.10	0.43 ± 0.04	1.03 ± 0.34				
Total blood volume (ml/kg body weight)	65.2 ± 4.1	72.0 ± 5.3	86.6 ± 2.1	68.8–109.6	62.5–81.1	88.1 ± 1.5	
Plasma (ml/kg body weight)	40.2 ± 2.1	45.3 ± 3.4	56.0 ± 1.4				
Erythrocytes (ml/kg body weight)	25.0 ± 1.4	24.3 ± 4.2	31.3 ± 0.9				
Hemoglobin (ml/kg body weight)	9.9 ± 0.8	9.7 ± 0.8	11.9 ± 0.3				
Arterial (%) oxygen saturation	80.2 ± 2.31	91.5 ± 0.1					
Bilirubin							
Direct mg/dl	0.07 ± 0.004	0.10 ± 0.015	0.06 ± 0.004				
Indirect mg/dl	0.06 ± 0.01	0.04 ± 0.01	0.02 ± 0.01				
Total mg/dl	0.13 ± 0.03	0.14 ± 0.01	0.08 ± 0.01				

[a]Standard error.

Table 15.9. Comparative serum biochemistry of the llama, camel, cow, and horse

Parameter	Llama	Camel	Cow	Horse
Total protein (g/dl)	4.7–7.3	6.3–8.7	6.7–7.5	5.2–7.9
Albumin (g/dl)	2.9–5	3–4.4	3–3.6	2.6–3.7
Globulin (g/dl)	1.1–3	2.8–4.4	3–3.5	2.6–4
A:G ratio	1.1–1.6:1		0.84–0.94:1	0.62–1.46:1
Calcium (mg/dl)	7.6–10.9	6.3–11	9.7–12.4	11.2–13.6
Phosphorus (mg/dl)	1.6–11	3.9–6.8	5.6–6.5	3.1–5.6
Sodium (meq/L)	148–158	129.3–160.7	132–152	132–146
Potassium (meq/L)	3.6–6.2	3.6–6.1	3.9–5.8	2.4–4.7
Chloride (meq/L)	98–120		99–109	97–111
Total CO_2 (mm/L)	14–34		24–32	21.2–32.2
T-3 (ng/dl)	0–423			
T-4 (μg/dl)	9.8–30		4.2–8.6	0.9–2.8
SGOT (IU/L)	128–450		78–132	226–366
SGPT (IU/L)	0–14		14–38	3–23
SGGT (IU/L)	3–28			3–13.4
SDH (IU/L)	0–15		4.3–15.3	1.9–5.8
LDH (IU/L)	10–695		692–1445	162–412
ALP (IU/L)	0–610		0–488	143–395
CPK (IU/L)	0–137		4.8–12.1	2.4–23.4
Creatinine (mg/dl)	0.9–2.8	1.2–2.8	1–2	1.2–1.9
Urea N (mg/dl)	9–36	15.7–48.5	20–30	10–24
Cholesterol (mg/dl)	0–128	20.8–79.2	80–120	75–150
Glucose (mg/dl)	76–176	37–67	45–75	75–115

span of erythrocytes in humans is 120 days, horses 140–150 days, and cattle 135–162 days (25). The shorter life span in Reynafarje's study may be the result of adaptation to chronic hypoxic conditions, reflected also in the higher rates of red cell iron turnover in lamoids as compared with other domestic animals (29).

Bone marrow biopsies were performed on 6 alpacas, 8 llamas, and 12 vicuñas kept at 4200 m (29). The myeloid-erythroid (M-E) ratio was approximately 0.5:1. In humans living at sea level, the M-E ratio is 3:1 and for those living at high altitudes, 1:1. In cattle, the M-E ratio is 0.71:1 and in horses 2.43:1 (30). In the author's clinic, healthy llamas usually have an M-E ratio of 1:1 or 1.2:1.

Blood volumes for lamoids have been calculated to be between 6.5 and 8.6% of body weight (Table 15.8).

LYMPHATICS

Lymph vascular patterns and sites of the lymph nodes in lamoids are the subjects of two dissertations in Peru, but, otherwise, little is known about this lymphatic system (13, 22). These authors report that the distribution of lymph nodes is similar to that of cattle and sheep. However, on the basis of anatomic and pathologic dissection by the author, the nodes of lamoids are small and may be difficult to locate. Multiple small nodes may be found, rather than a single large node at certain sites such as the superficial inguinal or prefemoral locations. It is possible to palpate these nodes on emaciated animals. The mediastinal and mesenteric nodes are present but are small and may be easily overlooked. Aggregations of lymphoid tissue (Peyer's patches) are located along the antimesenteric border of the large intestine.

DIAGNOSTIC PROCEDURES

Constituents of the blood are easily measured in the laboratory, facilitating diagnoses. Standard procedures are employed for lamoids. There are no reference ranges for some parameters, but these will be developed as more attention is paid to individual animal medicine. The technique for bone marrow aspiration is described in Chapter 4.

DISEASES

Infectious Diseases

Infectious diseases of vascular systems, discussed in Chapter 7, include leptospirosis, bacillary hemoglobinuria, and septicemia caused by miscellaneous bacteria.

Parasitic Diseases

The only parasitic disease of the blood of lamoids is trypanosomiasis, which is discussed in Chapter 8. Immature stages of other parasites may be found in the blood, as a stage of the life cycle or while being transported to preferred locations within the body. *Parelaphostrongylus tenuis* matures in the venous sinuses of the meninges of the white-tailed deer, and ova are transported to the lungs via the jugular vein. This strongyle is an aberrant parasite of llamas and may not reach maturity in this host (see Chap. 8).

Noninfectious Diseases

Lymphosarcoma is the only neoplasia as yet reported from the hematopoietic or lymphatic system (see Chap. 9). With more critical necropsies and more complete reporting, it is probable that tumors similar to those affecting other domestic animals will be found.

ANEMIA. Generally, anemia is a secondary disease caused by numerous primary agents. Anemia is reduced ability of the blood to supply oxygen to the tissues and may be the result of a reduction of erythrocyte numbers, hemoglobin concentration or hematocrit (see Table 15.1 for normal values).

Etiology. Basically, anemia is caused by either an excessive loss of erythrocytes and/or hemoglobin or by decreased production of vital blood constituents. Excessive loss of blood constituents may be caused by hemorrhage (lacerations, hematoma, extensive contusion, gastrointestinal ulceration, coagulopathy), parasitism, ingestion of spoiled yellow sweet clover hay or anticoagulant rodenticides, or hemolytic crisis (copper toxicity, leptospirosis, bacillary hemoglobinemia).

Iron deficiency is the most common cause of decreased hemoglobin production, but other nutrient deficiencies (copper, vitamin B_{12}) may contribute. Bone marrow suppression may be caused by renal disease, irradiation, myelotoxins (bracken fern toxicity), mild chronic inflammatory diseases (infections), or hypothyroidism.

Hepatopathy may interfere with serum protein production, causing hypoproteinemia and changes in the osmolarity of the blood. Two toxicities inhibit oxygen transport and utilization, but they are not considered to cause anemia. Methemoglobinemia prevents oxygen binding to hemoglobin, hence oxygen transport. The most frequent cause of methemoglobinemia is the ingestion of excessive nitrate, which is reduced to nitrite in the forestomach and absorbed, producing the toxic effect. The lamoid stomach provides the chemical environment for reduction of nitrate to nitrite, and toxicity is possible. There is one report of vicuñas dying from nitrite poisoning following consumption of silage.

The cyanide ion interferes with the cytochrome oxidase enzyme system and inhibits utilization of oxygen at the tissue level. The body becomes starved for oxygen, and death ensues quickly if immediate therapy is not forthcoming.

Clinical Signs. Anemic animals exhibit variable signs, depending on the etiology (18). Basically, dyspnea, depression, and pallor of mucous membranes are seen. If anemia is caused by a hemolytic crisis, additional signs will include icterus, hemoglobinuria, and elevated body temperature (a result of hemolysis). Anemia associated with hypoproteinemia results in ventral edema, with no inflammatory component.

Chronic blood loss may produce the basic signs of anemia, but acute blood loss has a more serious prognosis. Loss of one-third of the blood volume is serious in all animals, and further loss may result in death. Acute blood loss may produce hypovolemic shock, with tachycardia and dyspnea. Hemorrhage inside the calvarium may cause paresis, ataxia, and sudden death. Pericardial hemorrhage may produce cardiac tamponade. Hemorrhage into any organ may interfere with the function of that organ and result in signs of organ malfunction.

Chronic to mild blood loss may be reflected in a regenerative anemia response, demonstrated in hematologic parameters and bone marrow evaluation. Acute blood loss is not easily evaluated in the laboratory (hours elapse before the hematocrit changes, since the body attempts to reestablish blood volume by shifting tissue fluid to the blood). Clinical signs provide the vital clues to establish a diagnosis of peracute hemorrhage.

Methemoglobinemia causes cyanosis, with a chocolate discoloration of the blood and mucous membranes. Cyanide poisoning causes ataxia, muscle tremors, convulsions, and rapid death. Venous blood is bright red because the tissues are unable to accept oxygen bound to hemoglobin. This diagnosis should be made with caution, because lamoid venous blood is normally a brighter red than that of other domestic animals.

This has been a somewhat superficial discussion of anemia as it may appear in a lamoid. Most anemias of lamoids encountered by the author have been mild, secondary to infectious diseases. The anemia disappeared once the primary disease was managed. The reader should obtain more detailed information when faced with a difficult diagnosis (30).

Therapy. The underlying cause of the anemia should be corrected. Proper nutrients should be supplied in the diet or given parenterally in acute cases. Blood transfusion is indicated in life-threatening situations (i.e., a hematocrit level less than 15%). Blood compatibility testing is possible, but in an emergency, any lamoid blood may be given once with little risk. Thereafter, the risk of a transfusion reaction increases.

REFERENCES

1. Abdelgadir, S. F., Wahbi, A. G. A., and Idris, O. F. 1874a. Some blood and plasma constituents of the camel. In W. R. Cockrill, ed. The Camelid—An All Purpose Animal. Uppsala, Sweden: Scandinavian Institute of African Studies p. 438.

2. ______. 1984b. A note on the haematology of adult Sudanese dromedaries. In W. R. Cockrill, ed. The Camelid—An All Purpose Animal. Uppsala, Sweden: Scandinavian Institute of African Studies p. 444.

3. Anonymous. 1966a. (Hematologic values in the domestic animals— erythrocytes) Constantes hematologicas en los animales domesticos, serie roja. Bol. Extraordinario 1:72–73.

4. ______. 1966b. (Hematologic values in the domestic animals—leukocytes) Constantes hematologicas en los animales domesticos, serie blanca. Bol. Extraordinario 1:74–75.

5. ______. 1974. (Hematologic values in the domestic animals in high altitudes) Constantes hematologicas de algunas especies animales domesticas en la altura. Bol. Divulg. 15:71–75.

6. Aste Salazar, H. 1964. (Differentiation of hemoglobin in sheep, llamas and alpacas at high altitude and in vicuña at sea level) Diferenciacion de hemoglobinas en carneros, llamas y alpacas en las grandes alturas y en vicuñas al nivel del mar. Proc. 2nd Congr. Nac. Vet. Zootec., Lima, pp. 332–39.

7. Barreto D., R. 1949. (Hematologic studies in normal domestic animals) Estudios hemotalogicos en animales domesticos normales. Rev. Fac. Med. Vet. (Lima) 4:66–72.

8. Bendezu, H. 1957. (Histologic aspects of the alpaca. Hematopoietic organs) Aspectos histologicos de la alpaca. Organos hemtopoyeticos. Tesis, Fac. Med. Vet. Univ. Nac. Mayor San Marcos (Lima).

9. Bernengo, M. G. 1970. (Observations on the morphology of blood cells in Tylopoda and their relative serum values). Inst. Lombardo Accad. Sci. Lett. Rend. Sci. Biol. Med. [B] 104(1):33–45. Italian

10. Bustinza Menendez, J. A. 1970. (Some physiologic values of the blood of the South American camelids) Algunos valores fisiologicos de la sangre de los camelidos Sudamericanos. Proc. 1st Conv. Camelidos Sudam. (Auquenidos). Puno, Peru, pp. 79–81.

11. Butcher, P. D., and Hawkey, C. M. 1977. Comparative study of haemoglobins from the artiodactyla by isoelectric focusing. Comp. Biochem. Physiol. 568(3):335–39.

12. Capurro, L. F., and Silva, F. 1960. (Chromatographic studies and electrophoretic studies in South American camelids) Estudios cromatographicos y electroforeticos en camelidos Sudamericanos. Invest. Zool. Chil. 6:49–63.

13. Carrasco V., A. A. 1968. (Vessels and superficial lymph nodes of the pelvic limb of the alpaca) Vasos y centros

linfaticos superficiales del miembro pelvico de la alpaca *Lama pacos*. Tesis, Fac. Med. Vet. Univ. Nac. Mayor San Marcos (Lima), pp. 1–16.

14. Carter, R. H., Parkin, J. D., and Spring, A. 1972. Scanning electron microscope studies of vertebrate red cells. Pathology 4(4):307–10.

15. Copaira B., M. A. 1949. (Hematologic studies in South American camelids) Estudios hematologicos en auquenidos. Rev. Fac. Med. Vet. (Lima) 4(C-73; A-85):49–52.

16. ______. 1953. (Hematologic studies in South American camelids) Estudios hematologicos en auquenidos. Fac. Med. Vet. Zootec. (Lima) 5(7):78.

17. Cornelius, C. E., and Kaneko, J. J. 1962. Erythrocyte life span in the guanaco. Science 137:673.

18. Dabrowski, J. 1976. (Anemia in alpacas in the zoological garden of Lodz) Anaemie bei Alpakas (*Lama pacos* L.) im Zoologischen Garten Lodz. Verhandlungsber. 18th Int. Symp. Erkr. Zootiere 18:121–22.

19. Duran-Jordan, F. 1951. The eosinophil cell as seen in the llama. Nature (London) 168:1129.

20. Ellis, J. 1982. The hematology of South American camelidae and their role in adaptation to altitude. Vet. Med. Small Anim. Clin. 77:1796–1802.

21. Ezquerra A., W. G. 1968. (Construction of the normal hemogram in order to determine some hematologic constants in alpacas and llamas) Construccion de un nomograma para determinar algunas constantes hematologicas en alpacas y llamas. Tesis, Fac. Med. Vet. Univ. Nac. Tec. Altiplano (Puno), pp. 1–32.

22. Gambirazio, C. 1967. (Superficial lymphatic vessels and lymph nodes of the forelimb of the alpaca) Vasos linfaticos superficiales y centros linfaticos del miembro anterior de la alpaca, *Lama pacos*. Tesis, Fac. Med. Vet. Univ. Nac. Mayor San Marcos (Lima), pp. 1–14.

23. Gulliver, G. 1875. Observations on the sizes and shapes of the red corpuscles of vertebrates. Proc. Zool. Soc. Lond., pp. 474–95.

24. Jain, N. C., and Keeton, K. S. 1974. Morphology of camel and llama erythrocytes as viewed with the scanning electron microscope. Br. Vet. J. 130(3):288–91.

25. Kaneko, J. J. 1980. Clinical Biochemistry of Domestic Animals, 3rd ed. New York: Academic Press, p. 134.

26. Lewis, J. H. 1976. Comparative hematology—studies on camelidae. Comp. Biochem. Physiol. [A] 55:367–71.

27. Lombardi, L. M. 1957. (Calcium and inorganic phosphorus of the blood serum of alpacas, some physiologic variations) El calcio y el fosforo inorganico del suero sanguineo de las alpacas. Algunas variaciones fisiologicas. Rev. Fac. Med. Vet. Univ. Nac. Mayor San Marcos (Lima) 12:70–95.

28. ______. 1958. (Calcium and inorganic phosphorus of the blood serum of alpacas, some physiologic variations) El calcio y el fosforo inorganico del suero sanguines de las alpacas; algunas variaciones fisiologicas. Vet. Zootec. 10(25):17–18.

29. Reynafarje, H. C., Faura, J., Paredes, A., and Villavicencio, D. 1968. Erythrokinetics in high-altitude-adapted animals (llama, alpaca, and vicuña). J. Appl. Physiol. 24(1)93–97.

30. Schalm, O. W., Jain, N. C., and Carroll, E. J. 1985. Veterinary Hematology, 3rd ed. Philadelphia: Lea & Febiger, pp. 271–75.

31. Smith, J. E., Mohandas, N., Clark, M. R., and Shohet, S. B. 1979. Variability in erythrocyte deformability among various mammals. Am. J. Physiol. 236(5):H725–30.

32. Smith, J. E., Mohandas, N., Clark, M. R., Greenquist, A. C., and Shohet, S. B. 1980. Deformability and spectrin properties in three types of elongated red cells. Am. J. Hematol. 8(1):1–14.

33. Vallenas P., A. 1956. (Some physiologic constant values in alpacas) Algunas constantes fisiologicas en alpacas. Rev. Fac. Med. Vet. (Lima) 7(11):172–77.

34. ______. 1957. (Total protein and fractionation of the blood serum of alpacas. Some physiologic variations) Las proteinas totales y fraccionadas del suero sanguineo de las alpacas. Algunas variaciones fisiologicas. Rev. Fac. Med. Vet. (Lima) 12:40–59.

35. Whittembury, J., Lozano, R., Torres, C., and Monge, C. 1968. Blood viscosity in high altitude polycythemia. Acta Physiol. Latinoam. 18(4):355–59.

ADDITIONAL READING

Gelbhaar, H. 1966. (Hematologic findings in Tylopoda) Haematologische Befunde bei Tylopoden. Giessen, Univ. Vet. Med. Fak. Diss.

Gilone, A. 1965. (Hematologic variations and the capacity of oxygen in the blood of alpacas with different lengths of time at sea level) Variaciones hematologicas y de la capacidad de oxigeno de le sangre de alpacas con diferent tiempo de permanencia al nivel del mar. Tesis, Fac. Med. Vet. Univ. Nac. Mayor San Marcos (Lima).

Gloeckner, G. 1958. (The blood of llamas) Das Blutbild des Lamas. Leipzig, Vet. Med. Diss.

Goniakowska-Witalinska, L., and Witalinski, W. 1977. Occurrence of microtubules during erythropoiesis in llama, *Lama glama*. J. Zool. 181(3):309–13.

Gonzalez M., E. J. 1971. (Determination of clotting and bleeding time in alpacas) Determinacion del tiempo de coagulacion y sangria en la especie *Lama pacos*. Tesis, Fac. Med. Vet. Univ. Nac. Tec. Altiplano (Puno), pp. 1–49.

Gudat, E. 1963. (Blood investigations in camelids) Blutuntersuchungen bei Kameliden. Vet. Med. Diss. Humboldt Univ., Berlin.

______. 1964. (Investigations on the blood of camelids) Untersuchungen zum Blutbild der Kameliden. Monatsh. Med. Vet. 19 822 (8):26.

Gurmendi R., J. 1966. (Osmotic fragility and mechanics in red cells) Fragilidad osmotica y mecanica en hematies. Lima Inst. Biol. Andina Arch. 1(5):299–310.

Hawkey, C. M. 1975. Comparative Mammalian Haematology. London: Heinemann Medical Books (Camelids), pp. 170–77.

Hebbel, R. P., Eaton, J. W., Berger, E. M., Zanjani, E. D., Kronenberg, R. S., and Moore, L. G. 1978. Human, llamas adaptation to altitude in subjects with high hemoglobin oxygen affinity. Clin. Res. 26(3):554A.

Hebbel, R. P., Eaton, J. W., Kronenberg, R. S., Zanjani, E. D., Moore, L. G., and Berger, E. M. 1978. Human, llamas adaptation to altitude in subjects with high hemoglobin oxygen affinity. J. Clin. Invest. 62(3):593–600.

Hoepfner, D. 1957. (The blood picture of the guanaco) Das Blutbild des Guanaco. Inaug. Diss., Leipzig.

Iniguez R., L., Gutierrez, N., and Gourdin, D. 1974. (Electrophoretic analysis of hemoglobin in llamas) Analisis electroforetico de hemoglobinas en llamas. Reun. Nac. Invest. Ganad. Segunda, Estac. Exp. Chipiriri Mem., La Paz, Bolivia, pp. 31–34.

Ipinza, J. 1968. Haematological studies in the llama, *Lama glama*. Rev. Soc. Med. Vet. Chil. 18:29–33.

Kapff, E. 1925. (A llama serum) Ein Lamaserum gagen lues. Munch. Med. Wochenschr. 72(85).

Khodadad, J. K., and Weinstein, R. S. 1980. Band 3 protein-rich membranes of *Llama glama* red blood cells. J. Cell Biol. 87(2):202A.

______. 1981. Comparison of association number of band 3 oligomers in llama and human red cell membranes. Fed. Proc. 40 (3):484.

______. 1983. The band-3-rich membrane of llama erythrocytes: Studies on cell shape and organization of membrane proteins. J. Membr. Biol. 72:161–71.

Konuk, T. 1970. The microscopic appearance of camel and llama erythrocytes. Vet. Fak. Derg. Ankara Univ. 17:518–22.

Krotlinger, F., and Thiele, O. W. 1977. Transfer of blood group determinants from bovine serum nonlipids to erythrocyte lipids of various mammals. Naturwissenschaften 64(11):596.

Ladera, T. L. A. 1973. (Neutrophil index of alpacas) Indice neutrofilo de alpacas. An. Cien. (Peru) 2:405–9.

Lewis, J. H. 1973. Variation in abilities of animal fibrinogens to clump staphylococci. Thromb. Res. 3(4):419–24.

______. 1976. Comparative hematology: Ultrastructure of mammalian platelets. Fed. Proc. 34(3):806.

Malan, A. 1930. Studies on the mineral metabolism 13. The phosphorous partition of the blood of some animals. 16th Rep. Vet. Res. S. Afr., pp. 327–28.

Manrique L., L. 1968. (Some physiologic variations of the osmotic fragility of erythrocytes in alpacas) Algunas variaciones fisiologicas de la fragilidad osmotica de los eritrocitos en la especie *Lama pacos*. Tesis, Fac. Med. Vet. Univ. Nac. Tec. Altiplano (Puno), pp. 1–16.

Medvedev, Z. A. 1973. Biochemical mechanisms of aging of nucleated and anucleated erythrocytes. Tsitologiya 15(8):963–75.

Miller, J., Gudat, E., and Lindner, H. 1965. (Comparative electrophoretic investigations on the serum of camelids and cattle) Vergleichende papierelektrophoretische Untersuchungen an Seren von Kameliden und Rindern. Arch. Exp. Veterinaermed. 19(4):1027–36.

Montero R., R. 1970. (Determination of platelet numbers, reticulocytes and eosinophils in alpacas and some variable factors) Determinacion de numerode plaquetas, reticulocitos y eosinofilos en especie *Lama pacos* y algunos factores variables. Tesis, Fac. Med. Vet. Univ. Nac. Tec. Altiplano (Puno), pp. 1–40.

Montes, G., Stutzin, M., Correa, J., and Glade, A. 1983. (Hematologic studies of total protein, and fibrinogen in alpacas of the province of Parainacota, Chile) Estudio hematologico, de proteinas totales y fibrinogeno en alpacas de la Provincia de Parainacota, Chile. Arch. Med. Vet. 15:37–41.

Oulevey, J., Bodden, E., and Thiele, O. W. 1977. Quantitative determination of glyco-sphingo-lipids illustrated by using erythrocyte membranes of various mammalian species. Eur. J. Biochem. 79(1):165–268.

Palomino, H., Castellanos O., A., and Copaira B., M. 1964. (Hematologic modifications in alpacas moved to sea level) Modificaciones hematologicas en alpacas trasladadas a nivel del mar. Proc. 2nd Cong. Nac. Vet. Zootec., Lima, p. 331.

Pasquier, M. 1947. (Level of calcium in the serum and whole blood of some mammals) Teneur en calcium du serum et du sang total de quelques mammiferes. Bull. Mus. Nat. Hist. (Paris) 19:249–51.

Ponder, E., Franklyn, Y., and Charipper, H. A. 1928. Hematology of the Camelidae. N.Y. Zool. Sci. Contrib. 11(1):1–7; Q. J. Exp. Physiol. 19(2):115–28.

Portocarrero P., M. A. 1971. (Determination of the prothrombin time in alpacas) Determinacion del tiempo de protrombina en la especia *Lama pacos*. Tesis, Fac. Med. Vet. Univ. Nac. Tec. Altiplano (Puno), pp. 1–26.

Rewell, R. E. 1948. Microcytic anemia in a vicuña. Report of the pathologist for the year 1947. Proc. Zool. Soc. Lond. 118:501–14.

Rodman, G. P., and Ebauch, F. G., Jr. 1957. Electrophoresis of animal hemoglobins. Proc. Soc. Exp. Biol. Med. 95:397.

Rojas T., B. L. 1971. (Determination of the serum iron in alpacas) Determinacion del hierro serico en la especie *Lama pacos*. Tesis, Fac. Med. Vet. Univ. Nac. Tec. Altiplano (Puno), pp. 1–24.

Rosado M., C. E. 1969. (Study of plasma turnover with radioactive iron in alpacas) Estudio de depuracion plasmatica con fierro radiactivo (Fe 59) in alpacas. Tesis, Fac. Med. Vet. Univ. Nac. Tec. Altiplano (Puno), pp. 1–60.

Sillau G., H., and Llerena, B. L. 1968. (Plasma and cellular sodium and potassium in alpacas) Sodio y potasio plasmatico y globular en alpacas (*Lama pacos*). Bol. Extraordinario 3:46–49.

Sosnowski, A. 1972. (Morphological studies of the blood of Old and New World camelidae) Badania morfologiczne krwi wielbladow starego I nowego swiata. Med. Weter. 28(5):292–95.

Stone, H., and Thompson, H. K. 1966. The effect on blood viscosity of red cell size and shape. Fed. Proc. 25:236.

Tillman, A. 1978. Blood chemistry and hematology in llamas. Llama Newsl. 1:1–2.

Umminger, B. L. 1975. Body size and blood sugar concentrations in mammals. Comp. Biochem. Physiol. [A] 52(3):455–58.

Urbain, A. 1936. (Level of breakdown products of nitrogen in serum of several ungulates) Teneur en derives de degradation de l'azote de serum de quelques ongules. C. R. Acad. Sci. (Paris) 203:343–45.

______. 1938a. (Freezing point of serum of mammals)

Point cryoscopic du serum mammiferes. C. R. Acad. Sci. (Paris) 206:1596.

______. 1938b. (Level of cholesterol in several mammals) Teneur en cholesterol en quelques mammiferes. C. R. Acad. Sci. (Paris) 127:475.

______. 1983c. (Level of serum chloride in several wild or domestic mammals) Teneur en chlore du serum de quelques mammiferes sauvages ou domestiques. C. R. Acad. Sci. (Paris) 128:144.

______. 1941a. (The freezing point of total serum and plasma for several wild mammals) Point cryoscopic due serum total et du plasma de quelques mammiferes sauvages. Bull. Mus. Nat. Hist. (Paris) 13:218.

______. 1941b. (Level of total blood potassium from red blood cells and from the serum of several wild mammals) Teneur en potassium du sang total des globules et du serum de quelques mammiferes sauvages. C. R. Acad. Sci. (Paris) 213:83.

______. 1941c. (Whole blood level of reducing sugars of several wild mammals) Teneur en sucres reducteurs du sang total de quelques mammiferes sauvages. C. R. Acad. Sci. (Paris) 212:510.

Vallenas P., A. 1952–56. (Glucose in the alpaca) La glucemia en la alpaca. Rev. Fac. Med. Vet. (Lima) 7–9:142–56.

______. 1959. (Some aspects of the physiology of the alpaca) Algunos aspectos sobre la fisiologia de la alpaca. 1st Ciclo. Conf. Med. Vet., Lima.

Villavicencio, M., and Izquierdo, D. 1971. Electrophoretic characteristics of alpaca hemoglobin. Peru Soc. Quim. Bol. 37(2):48.

Wedding, W. 1979. (Blood picture, in first 3 months of life of Bactrian camels and a lama in Berlin Zoo) Das Blutbild in den ersten drei Lebensmonaten von drei Kamelen *Camelus bactrianus,* und einem Lama, *Lama glama,* des Zoologischen Berlin. Inaug. diss., Freie Univ., Berlin.

Zavaleta G., J. M. 1973. (Effects of experimental acute hemorrhage in alpaca) Efectos de la hemorrhagia aguda experimental en la especie, *Lama pacos* (alpaca). Tesis, Fac. Med. Vet. Zootec. Univ. Nac. Tec. Altiplano (Puno), p. 40.

16 Cardiovascular System

ANATOMY

The heart and arterial system are not unique in lamoids. The distribution of arteries in the limbs vary slightly, but they do not present any clinical problems. To obtain more detail, a limited number of references are available (1–30).

The jugular vein is unique. See Chapter 4 for a discussion of superficial veins for collection of blood samples and intravenous medication.

The arterial supply and venous drainage of the lower limb are different than in horses and cattle. The major vessels are on the medial aspect of the metacarpus and metatarsus and are then directed to the palmar and plantar surfaces of the tendons and are distributed to the digits from the interdigital space.

PHYSIOLOGY

A study of anesthesia in five llamas provided baseline data on the following cardiovascular parameters (9):

Cardiac output 8.2 ± 0.8 L/min; stroke volume 146 ± 20 ml/beat; mean systemic arterial pressure 137 ± 8 mm Hg; mean pulmonary arterial pressure 14 ± 0.8 mm Hg; mean right atrial pressure 2.6 ± 0.7 mm Hg; total peripheral resistance 1470 ± 183 dyne.sec/cm^3; left ventricular work 15.7 ± 0.9 kg m/min; cardiac output per kilogram 73 ± 9 ml/min/kg; PaO_2 127 ± 8.9 mm Hg; $PaCO_2$ 34 ± 1.1 mm Hg; base excess 2.3 ± 1.1 mEq/L; and bicarbonate 21.3 ± 1.1 mEq/L.

Cardiovascular adaptations contribute to hypobaric tolerance in lamoids. Lowland-adapted species, including humans, respond to high-altitude hypoxia with pulmonary artery constriction, resulting in pulmonary hypertension and subsequent right heart hypertrophy. Although llamas and alpacas may have a light to moderate pulmonary hypertension at high altitude, they do not respond with pulmonary arterial hypertrophy and right heart hypertrophy. Lamoids also do not respond to chronic hypoxia by enlargement of the carotid bodies and changes in their cellular components as do lowland-adapted animals (10, 11).

The blood volume in llamas and alpacas averages 63.5 ml/kg body weight, or 6.35% of the body weight (25). This is lower than the 7–10% body weight of most other mammals.

SPECIAL DIAGNOSTIC PROCEDURES

The diagnosis of cardiovascular disorders requires special procedures, including auscultation, electrocardiography, angiography, cardiac catheterization, cinefluoroscopy, and ultrasonography. The principles are the same in lamoids as in other species. Employment of these procedures requires special technical help, special equipment, and interpretation by a specialist.

DISEASES

Congenital Defects

Congenital defects of the heart include ventricular septal defects, atrial septal defects, patent ductus arteriosus, transposition of the aorta and pulmonary artery, persistent aortic trunk, and persistent right aortic arch. These are described in Chapter 22. Septal defects are not unusual, and a familial tendency may be suspected, but proof of such is lacking. The author has seen two transpositions of the aorta and pulmonary artery, a rare defect in any other species.

Infectious Diseases

No unique infectious diseases of the cardiovascular system have been reported. Valvular endocarditis has been diagnosed, but the causal organism was not isolated. Fibrinous pericarditis and epicarditis occur in septicemic conditions (Fig. 16.1).

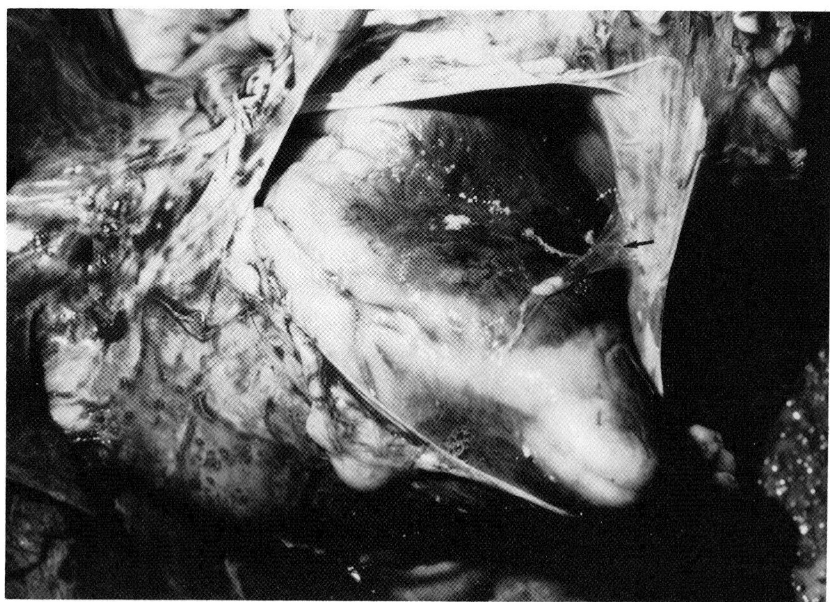

16.1 Fibrinous pericarditis and epicarditis in a llama.

Parasitic Diseases

Cysts of *Sarcocystis* sp. have been found in the myocardium (see Chap. 8). Larval forms may be found in the vascular system transiently. Llamas may be infested with larvae of *Parelaphostrongylus tenuis*. The adult parasites are found in the subdural venous sinuses of the brain of the white-tailed deer. It is not known whether the parasite completes its life cycle in the llama, an aberrant host.

Miscellaneous Diseases

Selenium–vitamin E deficiency may cause necrotic myocarditis with cardiac failure or fibrosis, which may decrease the efficiency of the heart.

Ischemic gangrene of the extremities, including the tail, ears, and limbs, may occur with frostbite or ingestion of ergot.

REFERENCES

1. Bego, U. 1960. (Comparative anatomy of blood supply and nerves of the foreleg in the camel, llama, giraffe, and cattle) Divergleichende Anatomie der Blutgefas se und Nerven der vorderen Extremitaten bei Kamel, Lama, Giraffe, und Rind. Acta Anat. 42(3):261.

2. Bustinza, G. 1961a. (Descriptive study of the carotid arteries of the alpaca) Estudio descriptivo de las arterias carotidas de la alpaca *Lama paco*. Tesis, Fac. Med. Vet. Univ. Nac. Mayor San Marcos (Lima).

3. ______. 1961b. (Descriptive study of the carotid arteries of the alpaca). Estudio descriptivo de las arterias carotidas de la alpaca *Lama pacos*. Vet. Zootec. (Peru) 13(37):33–36.

4. ______. 1964. (In a specimen of alpaca the minor circulatory incursion in the major circulation) En un especimen de alpaca la circulacion meno incursiona en la circulacion mayor. Proc. 2nd Congr. Nac. Vet. Zootec., Lima.

5. Calsin Colquehuanca, A. 1968. (Determination of the blood volume by the T-1824 method in alpacas) Determinacion de la volemia por el metodo T-1824 en alpacas. Tesis, Fac. Med. Vet. Univ. Nac. Tec. Altiplano (Puno), pp. 1–28.

6. Cueva, S., and Sillau, H. 1972. (Relative weights of the right ventricle of the heart in alpacas and llamas at high altitude and at sea level) Peso relativo del ventriculo derecho en alpacas y llamas en la altura y a nivel del mar. Rev. Invest. Pecu. 1(2):145–49.

7. Fowler, M. E. 1983. The jugular vein of the llama—a clinical note. J. Zoo Anim. Med. 14:77–78.

8. ______. 1984. Clinical anatomy of the head and neck of the llama. In O. A. Ryder and M. L. Byrd, eds. One Medicine—A Festschrift for K. Benirschke. Heidelberg: Springer.

9. Gavier, M. D. 1987. Evaluation of the combination of xylazine, ketamine and halothane for anesthesia in llamas. M. S. thesis, Univ. California, Davis.

10. Heath, D., Castillo, Y., Arias-Stella, J., and Harris, P. 1969. The small pulmonary arteries of the llama and other domestic animals native to high altitudes, cat, dog, cow. Cardiovasc. Res. 3(1):75–78.

11. Heath, D., Smith, P., Williams, D., Harris, P., Arias-Stella, J., and Kruger, H. 1974. The heart and pulmonary vasculature of the llama (*Lama glama*). Thorax 29(4):463–71.

12. Kerstetter, H. 1983. Blood collection from the ear. 3 L Llama 19:24.

13. Laos V., A. 1973. (Arterial circulation of the small and large intestine of the alpaca) Irrigacion arterial de los compartimentos del estomago de la alpaca (*Lama pacos*). Te-

sis, Fac. Med. Vet. Univ. Nac. Mayor San Marcos (Lima).

14. Leva, S., and Sillau, H. 1972. (Relative weight of the right ventricle in alpacas and llamas at heights and sea level) Peso relativo del ventriculo derecho en alpacas y llamas en la altura y a nivel del mar. Rev. Invest. Pecu. 1(2):145–49.

15. Lopez Jimenez, E. A. 1972. (The ascending aortic arch, the thoracic aorta and their collaterals in the alpaca) Arteria aorta ascendente, arco aortico y toraxico y sus colaterales de la alpaca, *Lama pacos*. Tesis, Fac. Med. Vet. Univ. Nac. Mayor San Marcos (Lima), pp. 1–19.

16. Manrique Meza, J. 1969. (Macro and microscopic description of the heart of the alpaca) Descripcion macro y microscopica del corazon de alpaca, *Lama pacos*. Tesis, Fac. Med. Vet. Univ. Nac. Tec. Altiplano (Puno), pp. 1–53.

17. Manrique Meza, J., and Matusita, A. 1970. (Observations on the myocardium of alpacas) Observaciones sobre el miocardio del alpaca. Primera Conv. Camelidos Sudam. (Auquenidos), Puno, Peru, pp. 58–59.

18. Miller, P. D., and Banchero, N. 1971. Hematology of the resting llama. Acta Physiol. Latinoam. 21(1):81–86.

19. Miller, P. D., Alexander, A. F., Lebel, J. L., and Banchero, N. 1972. Iatrogenic myocardial infarction and mitral valve insufficiency in a llama, *Lama glama*. Am. J. Vet. Res. 33(3):639–47.

20. Mongrut Munoz, O. G. 1973. (Lateral circulation of the head of the alpaca) Irrigacion lateral de la cabeza de la alpaca, *Lama pacos*. Tesis, Fac. Med. Vet. Univ. Nac. Mayor San Marcos (Lima), pp. 1–28.

21. Myczkowski, K. 1968. Topography of the arteries of the pelvic limbs of the camel and llama. Acta Anat. 69(1):41–42.

22. Olivos E., R. E. 1974. (Arterial circulation of the small and large intestine of the alpaca) Irrigacion arterial del intestino delgado y grueso de la alpaca (*Lama pacos*). Tesis, Fac. Med. Vet. Univ. Nac. Mayor San Marcos (Lima).

23. Rejas Mendoza, H. S. 1972. (Study of the abdominal aorta and its branches in the alpaca) Estudio de la arteria aorta abdominal y sus colaterales de la alpaca (*Lama pacos*). Tesis, Fac. Med. Vet. Univ. Nac. Mayor San Marcos (Lima), pp. 1–29.

24. Traverso S., C. R. 1968. (Arteriosclerotic complex in the aorta and coronary arteries of the llama) Complejo arteriosclerotico en arterias aorta y coronarias de llama (*Lama glama*). Tesis, Fac. Med. Vet. Univ. Nac. Mayor San Marcos (Lima).

25. Vallenas, A., and Sillau, G. H. 1968. (Cardiac output in South American camelids by the color dilution method) Gastro cardiaco en camelidos Sudamericanos por elmetodo de dilucio del colorante. Rev. Fac. Med. Vet. (Lima) 22:100–110.

26. Vera Colona, O. F. 1975. (Descriptive anatomical study of the external jugular vein of the alpaca) Estudio anatomo-descriptivo de la vena yugular externa de la alpaca. B.S. tesis, Univ. Nac. Mayor San Marcos, Programa Acad. Med. Vet.

27. Vergara Harniz, V. M. 1965. (Arteries of the forelimb of the alpaca) Arterias del miembro anterior de la alpaca, *Lama pacos*. Tesis, Fac. Med. Vet. Univ. Nac. Mayor San Marcos (Lima), pp. 1–32.

28. Will, J. A., and Bisgard, G. E. 1972. Cardiac catheterization of unanesthetized large domestic animals. J. Appl. Physiol. 33(3):400–401.

29. Zakheim, R., Mattioli, L., Hertzog, R., Molteni, A., and Svoboda, D. 1976. Angiotensin 2 and angiotensin converting enzyme in animals native to high altitude and native to sea level. Fed. Proc. 35(3):480.

30. Zakheim, R. M., Bodola, F., Park, M. K., Molteni, A., and Mattioli, L. 1978. Renin angiotensin system in the llama. Comp. Biochem. Physiol. [A] 59(4):375–78.

17 Reproduction

SOUTH AMERICAN CAMELIDS (SACs) occupy some of the most inhospitable habitats in the world. The progenitors of the four species now found in the Andean countries developed unique reproductive strategies that enabled them to survive and flourish. Reproductive anatomy and behavior are similar in all the lamoids, but little is known of the fundamental physiology of the reproductive cycle. Nonetheless, the available information is useful for the clinician attempting to solve some of the problems that arise with lamoid reproduction.

Consideration of the reproductive strategies of vicuñas and guanacos may aid in understanding problems of llamas and alpacas. The anatomy and physiology of the reproductive system will be addressed, followed by a discussion of infertility.

REPRODUCTIVE STRATEGIES

Vicuñas

Vicuñas are limited to ranges at high elevations in the Andes of Peru, Bolivia, and the border between Argentina and Chile. They are nonmigratory. Family groups are highly territorial. The dominant male defends a family feeding territory against intrusion by strangers, either male or female. The borders of the territory are strictly delineated. The family group also maintains a sleeping territory, to which the family retreats in the evening. Corridors between sleeping and feeding territories may be neutral territory for several family groups.

Vicuñas are seasonal breeders in Peru, with 90% of all births occurring between mid-February and early April (71). Though females will be bred within 2 weeks of parturition, only approximately half of the females will give birth the following year.

Vicuña social structure consists of family groups of 2–5 females and their crias, which are dominated by a single breeding male, and male groups (bachelor herds), varying from 2–100 animals. Both male and female offspring are driven from the family group by the dominant male (males at 4–9 months of age, females at 10–12 months). Females rarely conceive before they are 2 years old, but a few become pregnant at 12–14 months (71).

Males driven from the family group form temporary associations with other males and do not attempt to establish their own territories until 4 years of age. Juvenile females that are driven from the family group may attempt to enter another family group, but they may be repulsed by the male so as to maintain the optimum size of the group. Unattached females will ultimately become part of a new male's family group.

In the Andes, over 90% of vicuña births occur in the morning hours. This is probably an evolutionary adaptation to the weather patterns of that area (71). The frequent afternoon storms could interfere with adequate drying of the cria before the nightly drop to near-freezing temperatures occurs.

Guanacos (71, 117)

Reproductive strategies and the social organization of guanacos are similar to those of the vicuña. However, guanacos have a broader distribution in more diverse habitats, from sea level to 3000 m (71). Guanacos are more flexible than vicuñas, some populations being sedentary, while others are migratory. Migratory behavior necessitates some modifications of family group and male group patterns. In addition to these, aggregates of females may form during the winter, while each breeding male remains alone in the family group territory. There may even be mixed groups of males and females that come together during the winter.

Reproduction takes place only within the family group. Juvenile males and females are evicted from the family group, as in the vicuña strategy, but the age differs at which dispersal occurs. In guanacos, juvenile males and females are weaned at approximately 7 months but will begin nursing again when the next cria is born, continuing until both are evicted at 13–15 months of age. Thus both juveniles and the crias of the

year are present in a family gr
is thought that enhanced socia.
this biologic strategy (71).

penile s
ma

NORMAL REPRODUCTION
Male Llama and Alpaca (32–3…

ANATOMY (31, 35, 102, 103). The penis o…
lamoid has a prescrotal sigmoid flexure (Fig. 1…
The nonerect penis of a small llama, 135 kg (300 lb), may vary in length from 36 to 45 cm (14–18 in.), measured from the tip to the ischial arch. The diameter is relatively small, 0.8–1 cm (0.3–0.4 in.), at the region of the preputial reflection, increasing to 1.2–2 cm (0.5–0.8 in.) at maximum diameter near the ischial arch. The penis does not expand appreciably in diameter during erection but becomes firm and elongated. The erect alpaca penis varies from 35 to 40 cm (14–16 in.) in length (137).

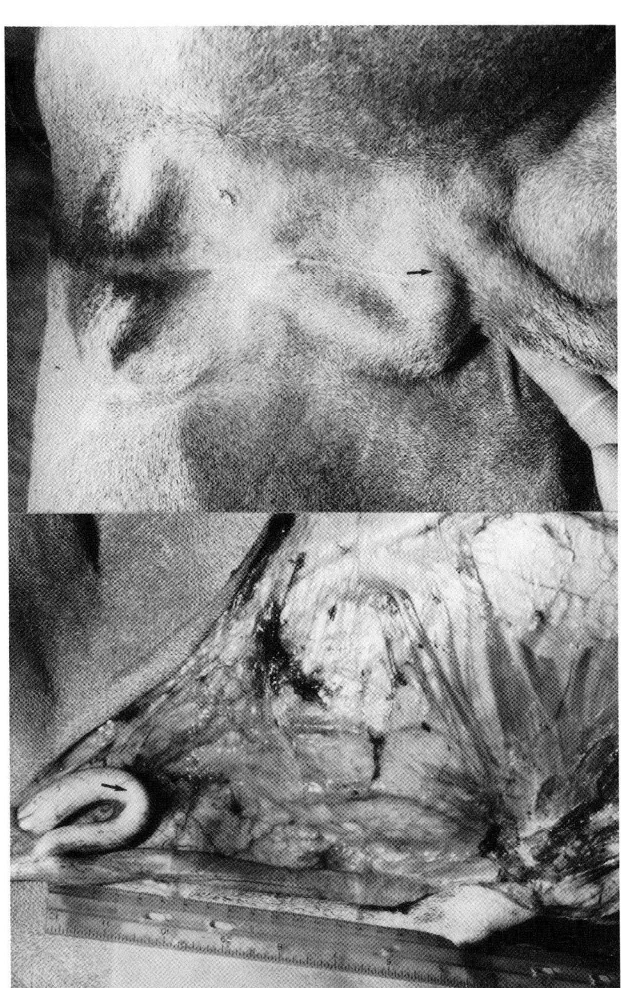

17.1 Sigmoid flexure of llama penis.

…male, the glans is long (9–12 cm) and
…merging into a firm cartilaginous pro-
…ht clockwise curvature (Fig. 17.2).
…tip to the preputial reflection is
…in.). It is assumed that the
…nd deposits semen into the
…laginous tip may be an
…the penis through the

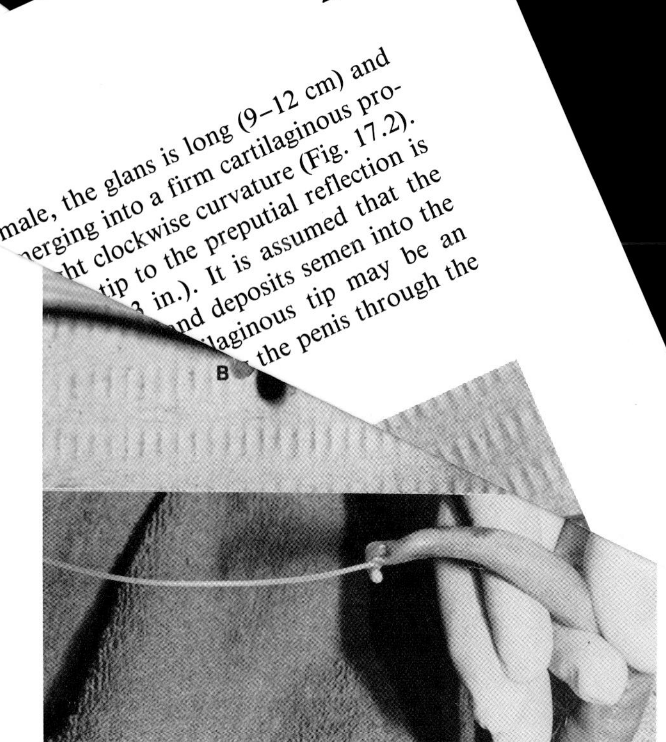

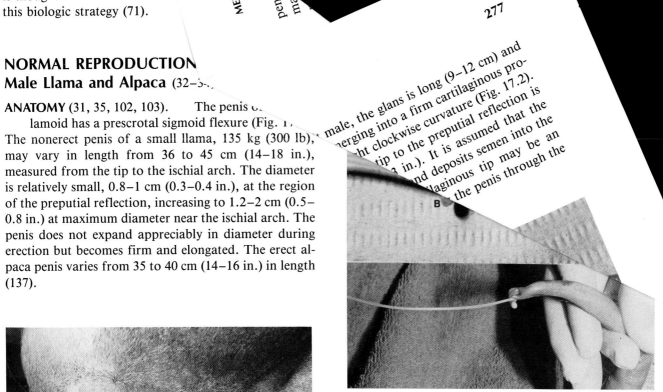

17.2 Tip of penis: **(A)** urethral orifice, **(B)** fibrocartilaginous projection.

The prepuce of the lamoid is triangular and nonpendant. In an unaroused male, the prepuce is directed caudally, and urine is projected backward between the hind limbs from a semisquatting position. When the male is sexually aroused, the cranial preputial muscles pull the prepuce cranially and the penis is extruded in the same manner as in the bull. Movement is controlled by a double set of preputial muscles, cranial and caudal. Both arise from the cutaneous trunci muscle and lie on either side of the linea alba. These muscles are relatively larger in lamoids than in domestic livestock.

The prepuce of the neonate and juvenile male adheres to the glans penis, making it impossible to extrude the penis from the prepuce until as late as 2–3 years of age (Fig. 17.3). In a study of male alpacas, only 8% were free of adhesions at 1 year of age, 70% were free at 2 years, and by the age of 3, all were free of adhesions (137). When selecting future alpaca sires in Peru, early maturation is desirable, and yearlings that are free of adhesions are preferred (137). If a male is castrated prior to the onset of testosterone production, these adhesions may not be released or may be only partially released.

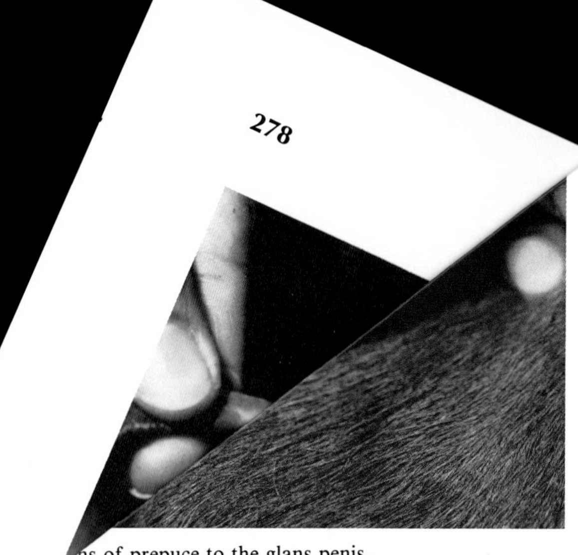

ns of prepuce to the glans penis.

Urethral catheterization is difficult in the lamoid male neonate because the glans cannot be isolated. Under sedation, the urethral opening may be protruded through the folds of the prepuce. At this stage of development, the cartilaginous process of the adult male glans penis is not present, and the tip of the penis is blunt. Attempts to peel the prepuce from the glans will usually cause hemorrhage. Successful catheterization may be accomplished by gently probing for the urethral orifice with a number 3 French urinary catheter.

In the adult, the urethral opening on the glans is located adjacent to the cartilaginous projection (Fig. 17.2) and will accommodate passage of a number 5 or larger French catheter. The pelvic urethra is approximately 5 mm in diameter, narrowing as it enters the egment. The urethra narrows further at approxi- ely the level of the preputial reflection. Uroliths may lodge at this site.

It is impossible to pass a catheter through the tip of the penis into the bladder because of a dorsal urethral diverticulum just cranial to the ischial arch. A catheter would automatically be directed into the diverticulum. Even with a finger inserted into the rectum to deflect the catheter ventrally, it would be strictly fortuitous to bypass this recess.

Accessory sex glands are limited to a pair of bulbourethral glands and a small prostate (Fig. 17.4). There are no seminal vesicles. The bulbourethral glands lie dorsally and laterally to the pelvic urethra at the ischial arch and are approximately 2 cm (0.8 in.) in diameter. The prostate gland is small (3 × 3 × 2 cm), situated on the dorsum of the urethra near the trigone of the bladder.

The retractor penis muscles arise from the anal sphincter muscle and pass around the ischial arch in close association with the body of the penis. When conducting a pelvic urethrostomy, the paired muscles must be parted or pulled to one side to enhance exposure of the urethra. The distal insertion of the muscle on the tunic of the penis is at the level of the preputial reflection.

The testicles of llamas and alpacas are roughly ovoid (Fig. 17.5), but a few tend to be globose. There is great variation in the size of the testicles, which may be an important factor in the fertility of the male. Measurements of a few adult male llama testicles are as follows: length 5–7 cm (2–3 in.), width 2.5–3.5 cm (1–1.5 in.), and depth 3–4 cm (1.2–1.6 in.).

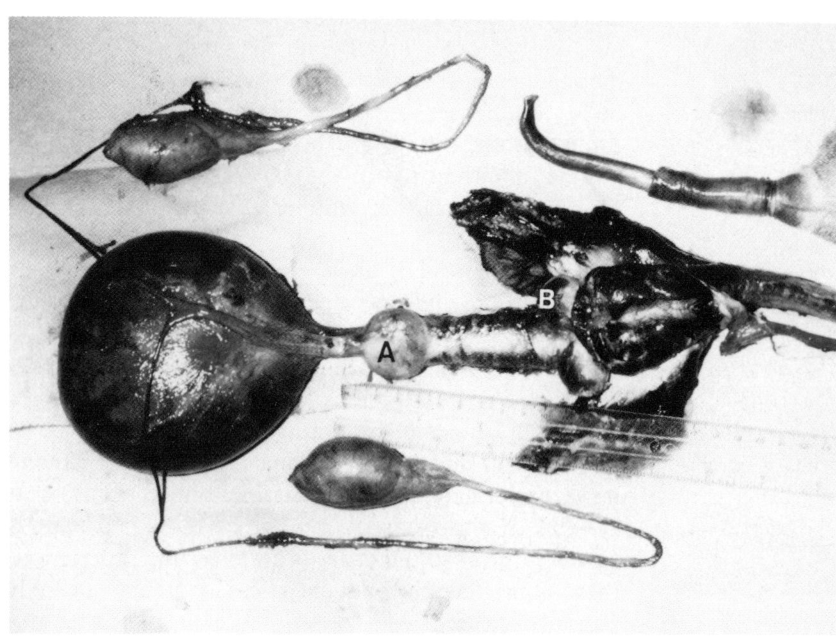

17.4 Male lamoid genitalia: **(A)** prostate gland, **(B)** bulbourethral gland.

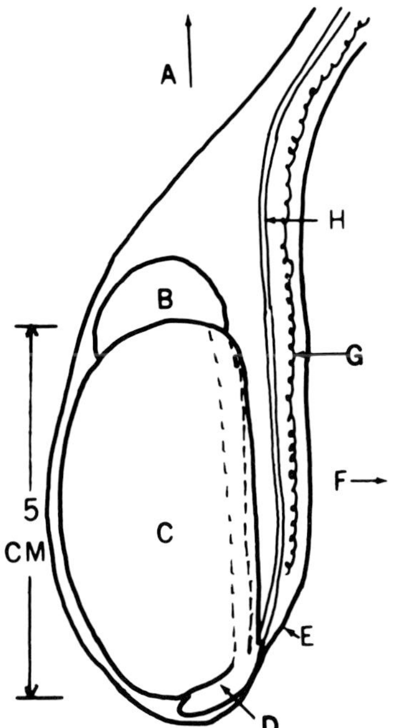

17.5 Diagram of a llama testicle: (A) cranial, (B) head of epididymis, (C) testicle, (D) tail of epididymis, (E) common tunic, (F) toward body, (G) blood vessels, (H) ductus deferens.

In a study of 25 adult Peruvian alpacas, the testicles were 3.98 ± 0.4 cm long (range 3.2–4.8), 2.59 ± 0.31 cm wide (range 1.9–3.2), and weighed 17.72 ± 3.65 g (range 13.15–28) (137). In Peru, future alpaca sires are selected at 1 year of age. The length of the testicles at this time ranges from 1.1 to 1.4 cm. The males with larger testicles are chosen (141). Testicular size is also important in bulls (124).

The nonpendant scrotum is situated at the level of the ischial arch. The testicles and the scrotum protrude only slightly from the surrounding surface. Having the testicles closely apposed to the body may be an important adaptation to prevent accidental castration during male-male fighting. Also, the skin over the scrotum is thick, providing additional protection for the testicles. Scars are often seen on the scrotum, a result of lacerations from the bites of other males. The testicles are usually in the scrotum at birth but are tiny, flabby, and difficult to palpate. The adult testicles should be turgid, not mushy, and freely moveable within the scrotum. The epididymis is closely attached to the testicle, and the head, body, and tail can be palpated after some practice. The epididymis should be resilient, with no nodules.

The microscopic characteristics of the testicles and epididymis are essentially the same as for other livestock species (25–27, 35, 64, 110, 125). The shape of lamoid spermatozoa is similar to that of livestock (93, 96, 112, 149). Size ranges of lamoid spermatozoa from some limited studies are noted in Table 17.1.

Table 17.1. Size of llama spermatozoa

Total length	49.47 ± 2.18 μ
Head length	5.33 ± 0.52 μ
Head width	3.81 ± 0.08 μ
Midpiece length	5.33 ± 1.6 μ
Tail length	36.64 ± 1.8 μ

PHYSIOLOGY (118, 145). To understand lamoid breeding behavior and physiology, the general biology of the wild species should be reviewed (see also Chap. 1). Wild lamoid males are basically territorial polygamists (71). A successful breeding male will defend a territory and a set number of females against all intruders, male or female. Fights between males may be vicious (Figs. 17.6–17.8). Although domestication of the llama and alpaca has diminished territorial behav-

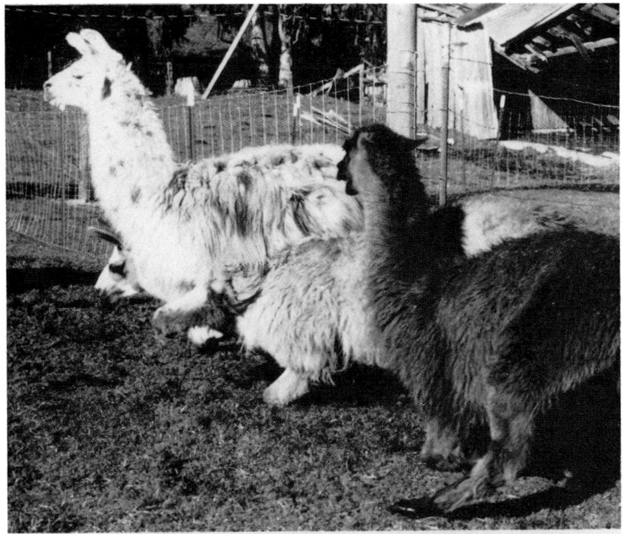

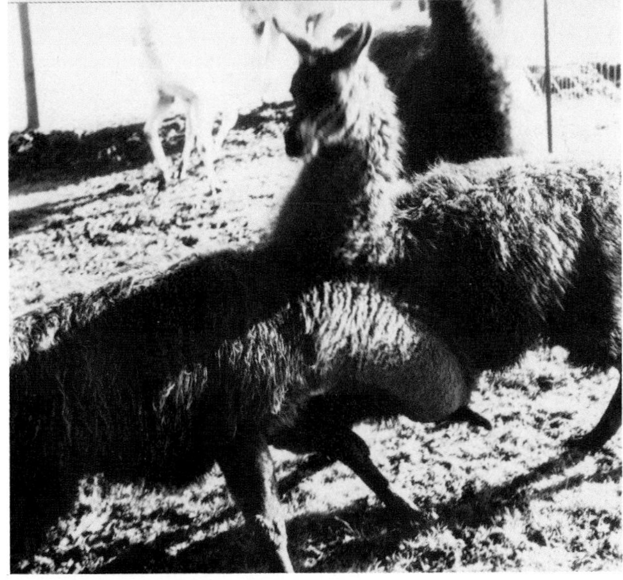

17.6 Male llamas fighting.

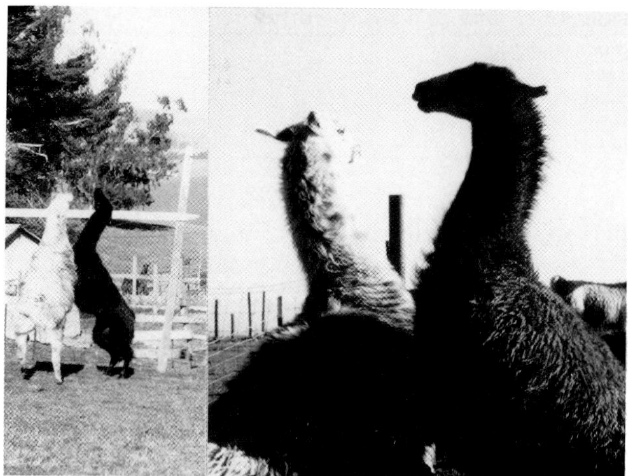

17.7 Male llamas chest butting.

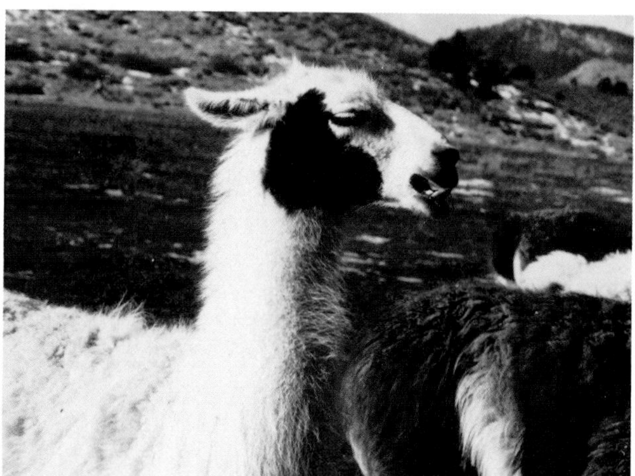

17.8 Open-mouth stance assumed by male llama after aggressive encounter with another male.

ior, if males are kept near vicuñas they revert to wild behavior and become difficult to manage with a herd of alpacas or llamas.

Male llama neonates begin play fighting at a few weeks of age (Fig. 17.9). Some precocious weanlings will rear up on females, and, if they can catch a non-pregnant female lying down, may attempt to mount her. Weanling males and females should be kept separate from each other because, in a few instances, males less than a year of age have impregnated females. Llama breeders in North America may tend to push young males into breeding too soon. Some individuals are anatomically capable of breeding when they are 1.5–2 years old, but most individuals lack sufficient libido and the body weight necessary to force the female down and breed vigorously until they are 3 years old. In some very young males, the testicles do not produce viable sperm, and there may still be preputial adhesions that prevent full extension of the penis.

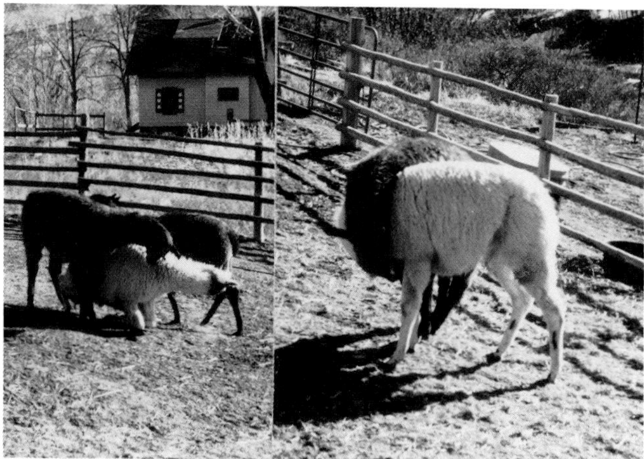

17.9 Young male llamas play fighting.

Guanaco males do not become territorial until they are 4–6 years of age (71). This does not mean that male guanacos are physically incapable of breeding earlier than this, but social and behavioral restrictions prevent earlier breeding.

In Peru, male alpacas are put into breeding service at 3 years of age (137). It would be unwise to pronounce a male llama or alpaca as infertile (precluding any anatomic defects) before the age of 3.5–4 years.

Both male and female (to a lesser extent) lamoids exhibit flehmen, but in a slightly different manner than other mammals (Fig. 17.10). A male approaches a dung heap recently used by a female. He sniffs the area and

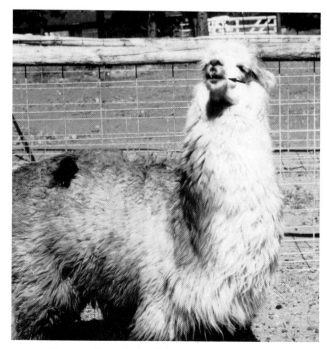

17.10 Alpaca male exhibiting flehmen.

then lifts his head and elevates the upper lip and opens the mouth slightly. The upper lip does not curl back as it does in other artiodactylids. Neither does the male sniff the perineal area of the female.

The usual breeding behavior of a male llama placed in the same enclosure with a receptive female begins with pursuit of the female. Some females become recumbent immediately, but most move away from the male until he rears up and puts pressure on the hindquarters in an attempt to force the female to lie down (Fig. 17.11). He may do this repeatedly if she continues to move away. The rearing is not an attempt to copulate but merely to force the female to lie down. The size and body weight (not fat) of the male is important in successful copulation, as is the libido of the male. A male with good libido will chase a female for at least 10 minutes before giving up.

Once the female is recumbent, the male positions himself at her rear, in a half-sitting position, and begins intromission (Fig. 17.11). The pelvic thrust of lamoids is not as vigorous as it is in other domestic livestock. It may be difficult to ascertain whether or not intromission has actually occurred unless the penis is palpated or the fiber coat (wool) is pulled to the side to allow observation.

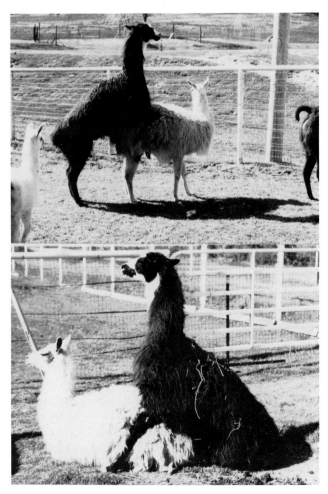

17.11 (Top) Male llama attempting to force a female to sternal recumbency prior to copulation. (Bottom) Copulation position of llamas.

With some experience, it is possible to perceive whether or not the male is in proper position. The male may be too far behind the female's pelvis. This is often observed when the male first mounts a recumbent female. At this stage, erection begins and the tip of the penis may be visible. As the male begins to adjust his position by shifting from side to side or forward, working closer to the female, erection is completed. The perineal area of the female will be probed with the penis, almost as if the male is exploring to find the vulva. Upon close observation of the penis at this stage, it should be noted that the glans may alternately assume a corkscrew and a straight shape. This alternate configuration of the glans also occurs during electroejaculation and should not be construed as penile malformation. Perhaps this shape changing aids in penetration of the vulva and in threading the penis through the cervix.

When intromission has occurred and effective copulation is under way, the male will be positioned with his pelvis close to the pelvis of the female. The male constantly vocalizes during copulation with a guttural sound that is called "orgling."[1] The exact source of the sound is unknown, but it may be the result of vibrations of the relaxed, elongated soft palate as air rushes past during rapid breathing.

Copulation may continue from 5 to 50 minutes, with an average time of 20–30 minutes. The elapsed time of copulation and conception rates have not been correlated. It is impossible to ascertain exactly when ejaculation occurs. There is no tail flagging, as in the stallion, or hyperpelvic thrust, as in the bull. It is not known whether there is a single ejaculation or an extended release of semen, sometime described as "dribble ejaculation." It is common to see the male reposition himself from side to side during copulation. He may be ejaculating into the other horn; it has been demonstrated that the penis reaches the uterine horns (69).

Occasionally, a male will cease copulation for no apparent reason, stand up, and begin the positioning sequence once again. When copulation is completed, the male rises and wanders off. The penis will have been retracted into the prepuce. The female may remain recumbent for a few minutes or may arise and move away also.

If the male and female are left together, copulation may be repeated the same day, but usually not until the

1. The term used in Peru is cutuneo.

next day, and, perhaps, a third day. If ovulation has occurred, the female will refuse to lie down and will spit at the male to discourage him. This is called "spitting off."

If other receptive females are in the enclosure, a vigorous male may breed as many as five or six females in 1 day. Reports from Peru indicate that a vigorous alpaca male may breed as many as 18 times in 1 day, but this activity quickly drops off on subsequent days, and if the male is left with the females for 10–14 days, he will ignore newly receptive females (137).

It has been observed that a male llama may take a dislike to a particular female and refuse to breed her. He may even become somewhat aggressive with her. Varying degrees of aggressiveness have been observed in breeding males. Some will even "rape" pregnant females. Others are so shy that they almost have to find a female lying down before they will attempt to copulate. Shy males may be intimidated by dominant females. Libido may be an inherited trait, so it may be undesirable to use a shy breeder.

Intermale aggression can be violent and damaging to both combatants, especially if each has a full complement of canine teeth. The objective of the fight is to establish dominance. The males may run at each other, rear up, and ram chests, each trying to knock the other off balance. If an advantage has been gained, the stronger will try to position himself to the side, with his neck over the neck of his opponent, in an attempt to force him to the ground. If the weaker animal cannot dislodge the stronger, he may reach around and bite the leg of his opponent. This "necking" may continue for some time, with each alternating at being the stronger.

Males may position themselves side by side in a head to tail position. Each male may try to bite the other on the hind legs and the scrotum. As one male is being bitten, he may lean into the aggressor and almost sit down on the aggressor's head. Severe wounds may be inflicted by intact canine teeth.

Particularly aggressive males may charge from the side in an attempt to knock an opponent down or rear up and come down on the body to force recumbency. They may also bite at the neck, ears, or jaws of an opponent. During the fight, the animals may constantly spew stomach contents at one another.

The interaction is over when one of the males remains recumbent in a subordinant posture. Both males will stand with their mouths partly open for several minutes after breathing has returned to normal (Fig. 17.8). This is not a form of open-mouth breathing, necessary to increase air flow into the lungs, but rather a behavioral trait exhibited after any aggressive or disagreeable interaction. The author has also observed this behavior after a strenuous restraint episode.

Female (13, 22, 43, 44, 46–48, 52, 56, 57, 61, 67, 73, 75, 84, 87–89, 91, 92, 103–109, 126, 131, 148)

ANATOMY (1–4, 6, 8, 10, 16–18, 40, 66, 92, 130). The female reproductive tract is illustrated in Figures 17.12–17.15. See Table 17.2 for a comparison of measurements of llama and alpaca reproductive organs.

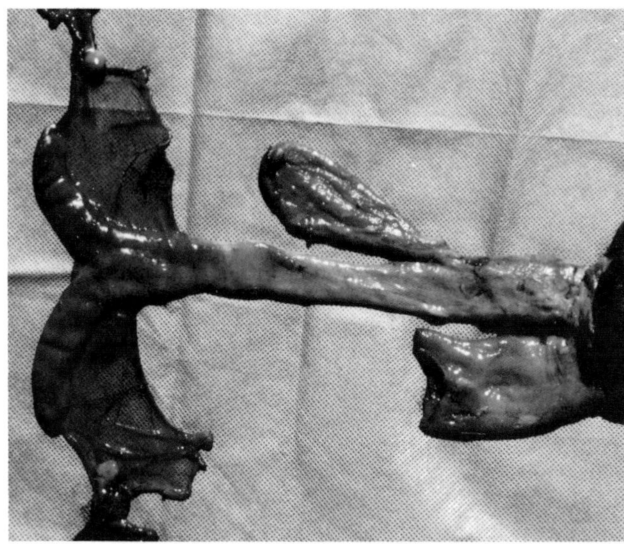

17.12 Female reproductive tract of a nulliparous alpaca.

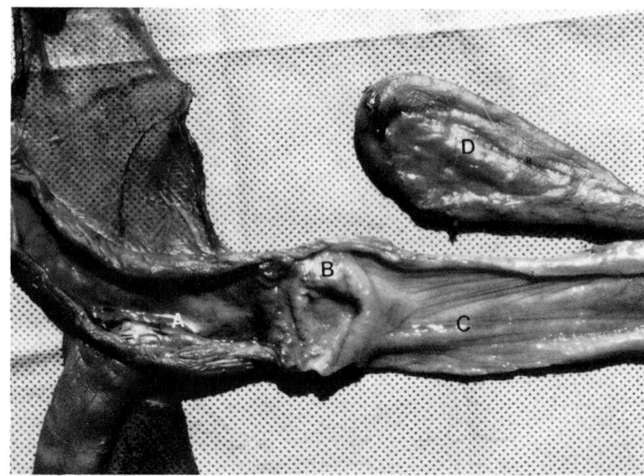

17.13 Female reproductive tract of a nulliparous alpaca: **(A)** intercornual septum, **(B)** cervix, **(C)** vagina, **(D)** bladder.

Vulva. The labia of the vulva lie in a slightly slanted to vertical position approximately 4–6 cm ventral to the anal orifice (Fig. 17.16). In aged or emaciated llamas or those with congenital malformations of the reproductive tract, the labia may lie in a more horizontal plane (vulvar shelving) (Fig. 17.17). The vulvar orifice (a slit) is approximately 3–5 cm long. The labia do not swell during the reproductive cycle. The depth of the vulva, to the hymen, varies from 6 to 8.5 cm.

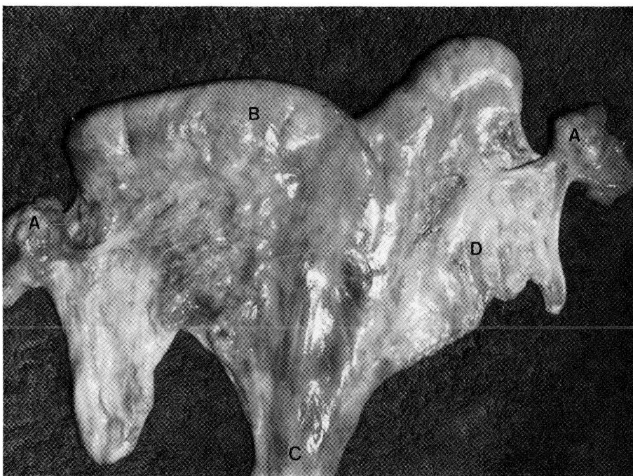

17.14 Uterus and adnexa of a multiparous llama: **(A)** ovary encased with the ovarian bursa, **(B)** left uterine horn, larger than the right, **(C)** cervix, **(D)** mesosalpinx.

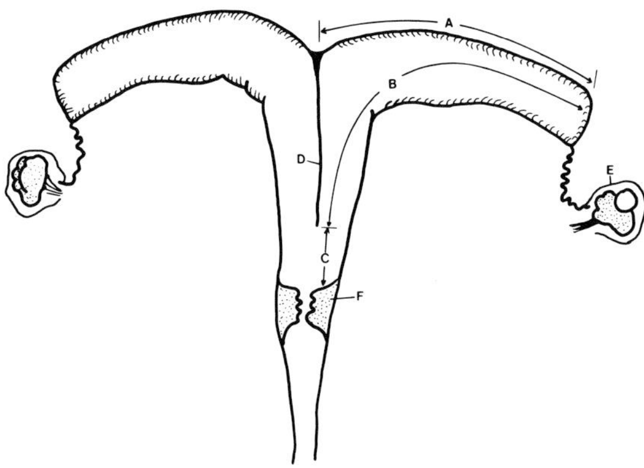

17.15 Diagram of lamoid female reproductive tract: **(A)** palpatable length of uterine horn, **(B)** actual length of uterine horn, **(C)** body of uterus, **(D)** intercornual septum, **(E)** ovarian bursa, **(F)** cervix.

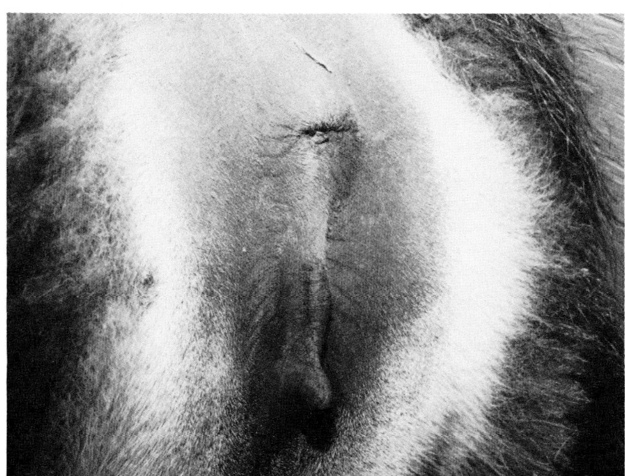

17.16 Llama perineum.

Table 17.2. Measurements of female lamoid reproductive organs

	Llama[a] (*cm*)	Alpaca[b] (*cm*)
Vulva		
Length of labia	5	
Depth of hymen	6–8.5	
Vagina		
Hymen to cervix		
Length	15–21	13.4 ± 2
Diameter	5	3.4 ± 0.7
Cervix		
Length	2–5	
Diameter	2–4	
Rings	2–3	2–3
Body of uterus		
Length to septum	3–5.5	3.05 ± 0.71
Diameter	3–5	
Horns of uterus		
Tips of septum to tip of horn	21–22.5	
Bifurcation to tip of horn	8.5–15	7.9 ± 1.3
Diameter	2.5–4	
Oviduct	10.5–18.3	20.4 ± 4.2
Ovary		
Right		
Length	1.3–2.5	1.6 ± 0.3
Depth	1.4–2	1.1 ± 0.2
Width	0.6–1	1.1 ± 0.2
Weight		1.87 ± 0.94 g
Left		
Length	1.5–2.5	1.6 ± 0.3
Depth	1.5–2.5	1.1 ± 0.2
Width	0.5–1	1.1 ± 0.2
Weight		2.4 ± 1.34 g

[a]Measurements collected at University of California, Davis.
[b]Data from Bravo and Sumar 1984.

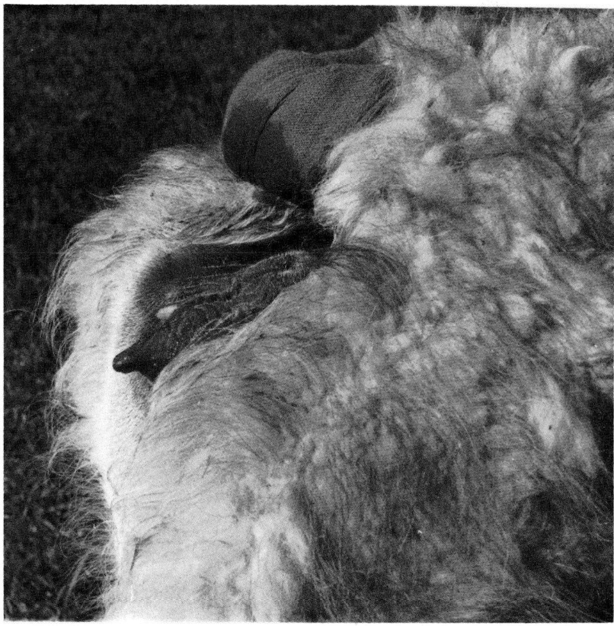

17.17 Perineum of llama with abnormal, near horizontal relationship of vulva to anus (shelving).

Vagina (23, 29, 30, 132). The vagina, from the hymen to the cervix, varies in length from 15 to 25 cm (6–10 in.) and is approximately 5 cm in diameter.

Cervix. The llama cervix is 2–5 cm long and 2–4 cm in diameter. The cervix has two to three spiral rings (Fig. 17.18). The cervix relaxes with estrogen stimulation but will never open as it does in the mare.

Uterus. The lamoid uterus is bicornate. The body of the uterus is short (3–5.5 cm) and approximately the same diameter (3–5.5 cm) throughout. Externally, the length is not apparent because the horns are fused together for a short distance, being separated by a septum (Fig. 17.15).

The left uterine horn may be slightly larger than the right, especially after the first pregnancy. The uterine horns of a llama, from the end of the septum to the tip of the horn on the convex surface, vary from 20 to 22.5 cm in length. The proximal segments of the horns diverge at approximately 180 degrees. The distance from the notch at the divergence to the tip of each horn varies from 8.5 to 15 cm (3.3–6 in.). The diameter of the horns varies with age and the number of previous pregnancies, from 2.5 to 4 cm. The tip of the uterine horn is rather blunt.

Uterine mucosa is similar to that of other species, consisting of a columnar epithelial layer (148). The fibrous tissue of the submucosa is more dense than in the mare, and there are fewer and smaller uterine glands (115). There are no glands in the cervical submucosa, and the epithelial layer is more cuboidal. This information is necessary to enable differentiation of the site from which a biopsy specimen has been taken.

Oviducts (133, 135). The oviducts are rather long and tortuous and are embedded within the mesosalpinx. The duct measured 10.5 cm in one llama, with a diameter of 3 mm. Bravo and Sumar measured the ducts of alpacas at 20.4 ± 4.2 cm. The oviduct empties into the tip of the uterine horn on a papilla that contains a sphincter (Fig. 17.19) (137). It is impossible to flush fluid retrograde into the oviduct from the uterus, but the reverse is possible.

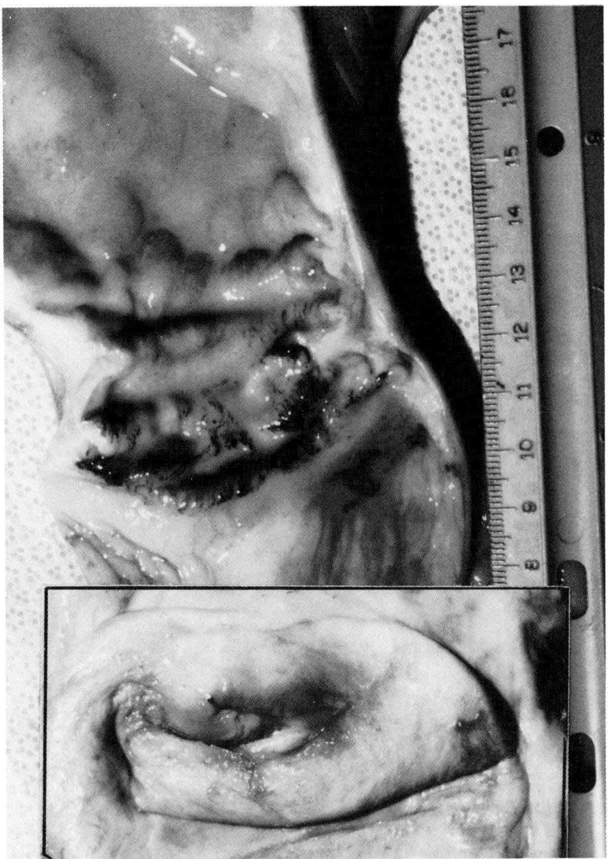

17.18 Llama cervix: (top) incised cervix illustrating spiral rings, (bottom) external cervical os.

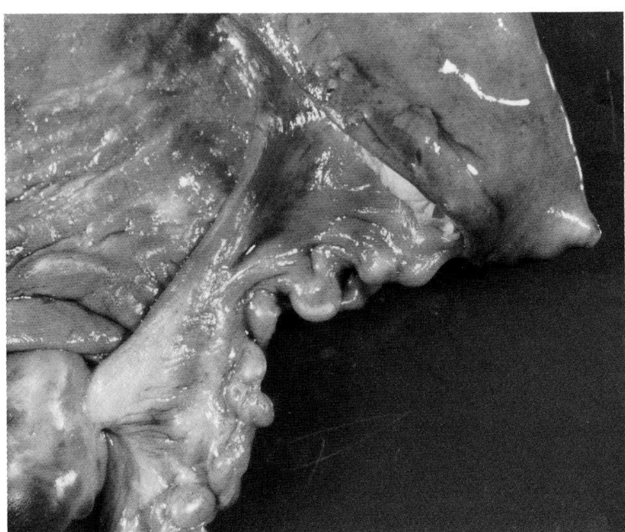

17.19 Tip of uterine horn everted to expose oviduct papilla.

The ovarian bursa is large (2.5 × 2.5 × 5 cm) and completely surrounds the ovary (Fig. 17.18). Ovarian structures must be palpated through the bursa, or the bursa may be gently moved to expose the surface of an ovary. At laparoscopy, the bursa is lifted off the ovary with forceps.

Ovary (113, 128). The ovaries of the llama are ellipsoid to globular, while those of the alpaca are more globular (Table 17.2). Numerous follicles, varying in size from 2 to 5 mm, can be seen on the surface of the mature, normal ovary (Fig. 17.20). A follicle ready for ovulation may reach 12 mm. Any follicle larger than 12 mm is considered to be pathologic (137). Measurements of the ovaries from six llamas are as follows: length 1.3–2.5 cm, depth 1–2 cm, and width 0.5–1 cm. These measurements may be compared with those of alpacas (Table 17.2). Llama ovaries have not been weighed, but alpaca ovaries weigh approximately 2 g.

PHYSIOLOGY (24, 37, 39, 58, 111, 127, 129, 138, 139, 143). Camelids have a unique ovarian cycle; they are induced ovulators but differ from other induced ovulators such as the rabbit or cat (95). The typical cycle is charted in Figure 17.21.

There may be seasonal or periodic anestrus. At this

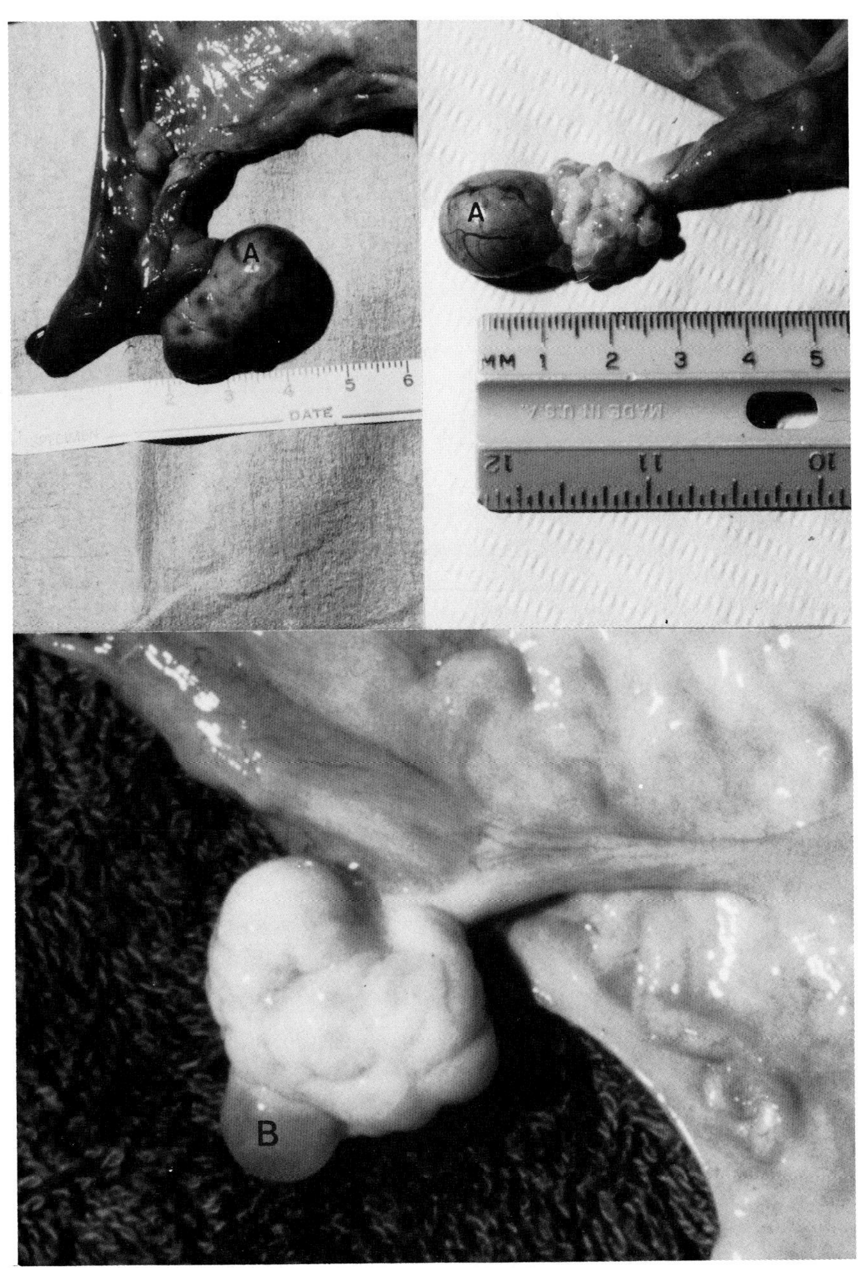

17.20 Llama ovaries: **(A)** corpus luteum, **(B)** follicle.

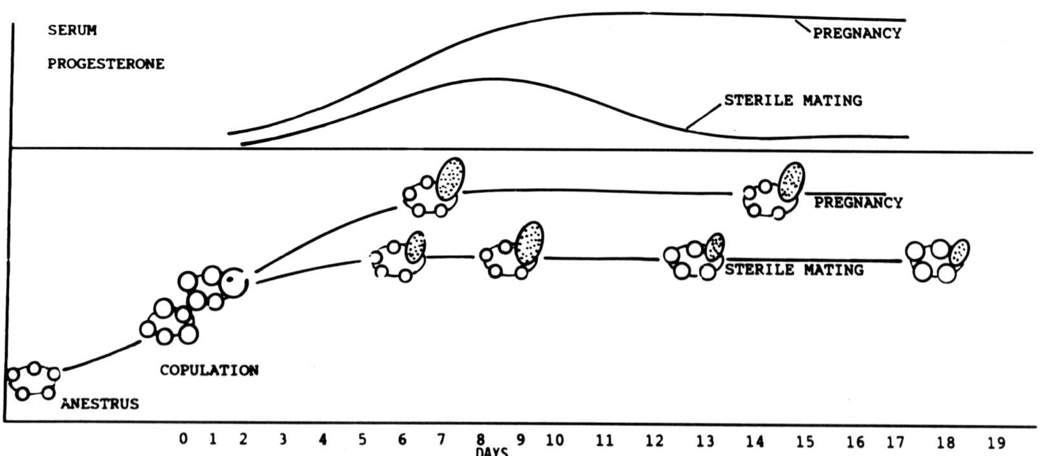

17.21 Reproductive cycle of lamoids.

stage, the ovary contains numerous small follicles (less than 3 mm in diameter), and the female is not receptive to a male. At an appropriate time, the follicles will enlarge to approximately 5mm (1, 2). The female now becomes receptive to a male but is not in estrus as it exists in other mammals. Once the follicles have enlarged to 5 mm, they stabilize and remain so for 10–12 days or until copulation initiates further maturation of one or more follicles. Spontaneous ovulation has been reported, but it is not usual. In alpacas, serial observations of the ovary via laparoscopy revealed that the follicles grow rapidly (10). A follicle reaches maturity (8–12 mm) in approximately 3–5 days. Follicles may remain in this state for 10–12 days. If coitus occurs during this time, ovulation may occur. If not, the follicle regresses, but at the same time a follicle on the opposite ovary matures, providing a constant follicular wave for at least 30–36 days (10).

Early studies had described ovulation as taking place at 26 hours after stimulus, but in those studies, the stimulus was human chorionic gonadotrophin (HCG), not copulation (38, 55, 62, 122, 123). In more recent, detailed studies carried out in alpacas, it was found that only 60% of the females had ovulated at 48–72 hours. A few individuals failed to ovulate (10). Knowledge of the variations in ovulation time, post-coitus, is important in breeding management.

The receptive female llama will accept repeated breeding by the male for periods varying for hours to days, presumably associated with the time of ovulation. An unreceptive female demonstrates unwillingness by refusing to become recumbent, running away from the male, and, if he persists, spewing stomach contents at him.

Following ovulation, a corpus luteum (CL) forms, similar to that seen in other livestock species (38, 45, 72, 78, 79). The maximum size of the CL is approximately 16 mm (8, 137, 142). If conception occurs, the CL persists until late in pregnancy, being necessary to maintain pregnancy until the last 2 months of gestation, but the precise time for cessation of the CL function is unknown (142). Presumably, in lamoids, the placenta is not a good source of progesterone, as it is in some livestock species. Detailed studies to verify these suppositions have not yet been conducted.

If conception does not occur, the CL enlarges to its maximum size in 7–10 days and then regresses. During this short period, the follicles on the ovaries decrease in size to 3 or 4 mm. As the CL regresses, the follicles increase, returning to the normal 8–12 mm size by 18–21 days postovulation. Once again the female becomes receptive to a male and will remain in this state until copulation and ovulation occur, the more rare spontaneous ovulation occurs, or the ovarian quiescent state ensues (possibly seasonally).

The camelid ovarian cycle is unique. There is no luteal cycle, per se, nor is there a period of estrus with behavioral receptivity based on periodic surges of estrogen activity. Hormone levels, correlated with the lamoid ovarian cycle, are less precisely known than in livestock species. A good deal of work has been done to establish progesterone levels in order to diagnose pregnancy. Less is known about estrogen and androgen levels, and little is known of follicle stimulating hormone (FSH) and luteinizing hormone (LH) levels.

PREGNANCY. The ovarian bursa completely encases the ovary so that transport of the ovum to the oviduct is easily accomplished; in livestock species, the ovum reaches the ampulla (midportion) of the uterine tube within 2 hours, where fertilization takes place and the zygote begins the cleavage process. The zygote remains in the uterine tube for 3–6 days in livestock species. South American researchers have indicated that the alpaca zygote reaches the uterus in 3 days.

Once the zygote reaches the uterus, it will implant in the right or left horn. Over 95% of successful llama and alpaca pregnancies have been implanted in the left horn. Other studies have indicated that 99–100% of pregnancies implant in the left horn (53, 59, 60, 62, 63). Since there is an equal distribution of CL in both the right and the left ovary, and with each ovary encased within a bursa, this means that the ovum and subsequent zygote from the right ovary must migrate from the right horn to the left horn or be absorbed (59, 60, 62, 63).

The precise time of fetal membrane attachment to the uterine mucosa in lamoids is unknown, but extrapolating from data accumulated from studies in livestock species, it is assumed that the developing zygote is free in the uterus for approximately 30 days. Bravo (7) did not find a firm attachment of alpaca embryos to the uterus at 30 days. At 60 days, the placenta had developed a vascular network. Full attachment to the uterine mucosa, with the embryo receiving nourishment from the dam via the attached placenta, is completed by approximately 60–90 days.

Early embryonic death occurs more frequently in alpacas and llamas than in livestock species (9, 53–55, 63). Estimates of 30–50% losses of embryos prior to 90 days have been reported. The precise cause of early embryonic death is unknown, but failure of the right horn to maintain a suitable environment for the conceptus, hormonal deficiencies, or chromosomal aberrations may be factors. Infections have not been identified as abortiofacients in lamoids.

Fetal development proceeds in lamoids as it does in other livestock species. Prenatal growth in alpacas has been described (7). It was found that 85% of fetal weight was gained after 210 days gestation. The usual length of gestation ranges from 335 to 360 days (12, 81, 121), with the occasional female carrying the fetus for over a year. Gestations as long as 13 months have been reported; however, the author has dealt with a number of female llamas suspected of pregnancies of over a year, only to ultimately find a discrepancy in breeding dates. Twinning is rare (134, 146).

The growth of the fetus is illustrated in Figures 17.22 and 17.23. The crown-rump length progresses uniformly, with an increase in rate during the last 3 months.

Fetal Membranes (28, 68, 90, 94, 98, 99, 116, 135).

Placentation of camelids has been classified as diffuse and epitheliochorial, similar to that of the mare and sow. However, camelid fetal membranes are unique. Early embryonic development of the fetal membranes, from the blastocyst stage to attachment to the uterus, is not unusual. Between 70 and 90 days, the surface of the chorion becomes dotted with numerous half-circular, domed projections that fit into corresponding depressions in the uterine mucosa (Figs. 17.24, 17.25). At 20X, a capillary network may be seen on the surface of the domed placentomas. The attachment is tenuous, and the chorion may be peeled from the mucosa with no resistance.

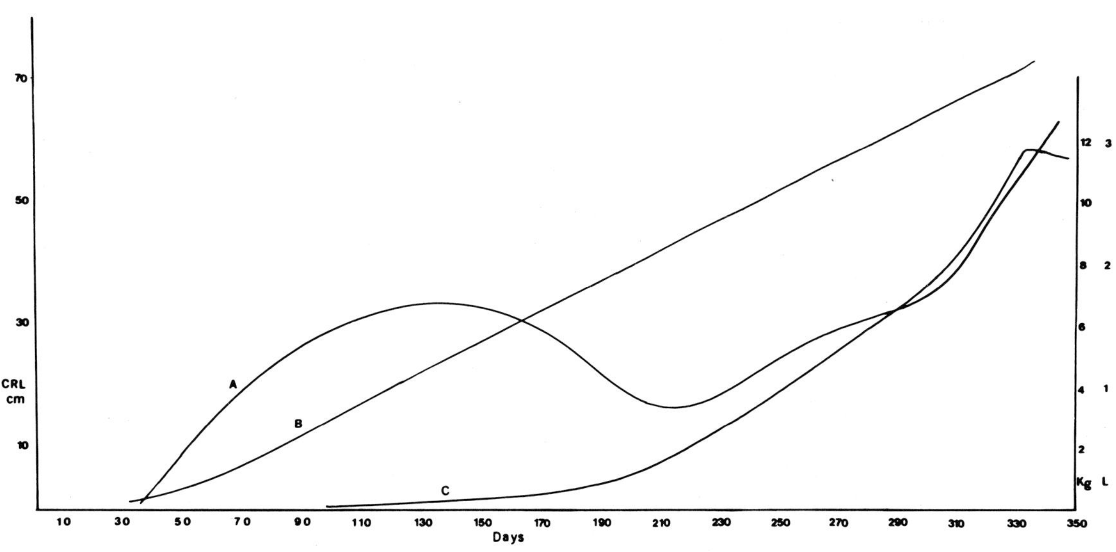

17.22 Fetal growth curve of llama and fluid volume: **(A)** amniotic fluid volume, **(B)** crown-rump length, **(C)** fetal weight.

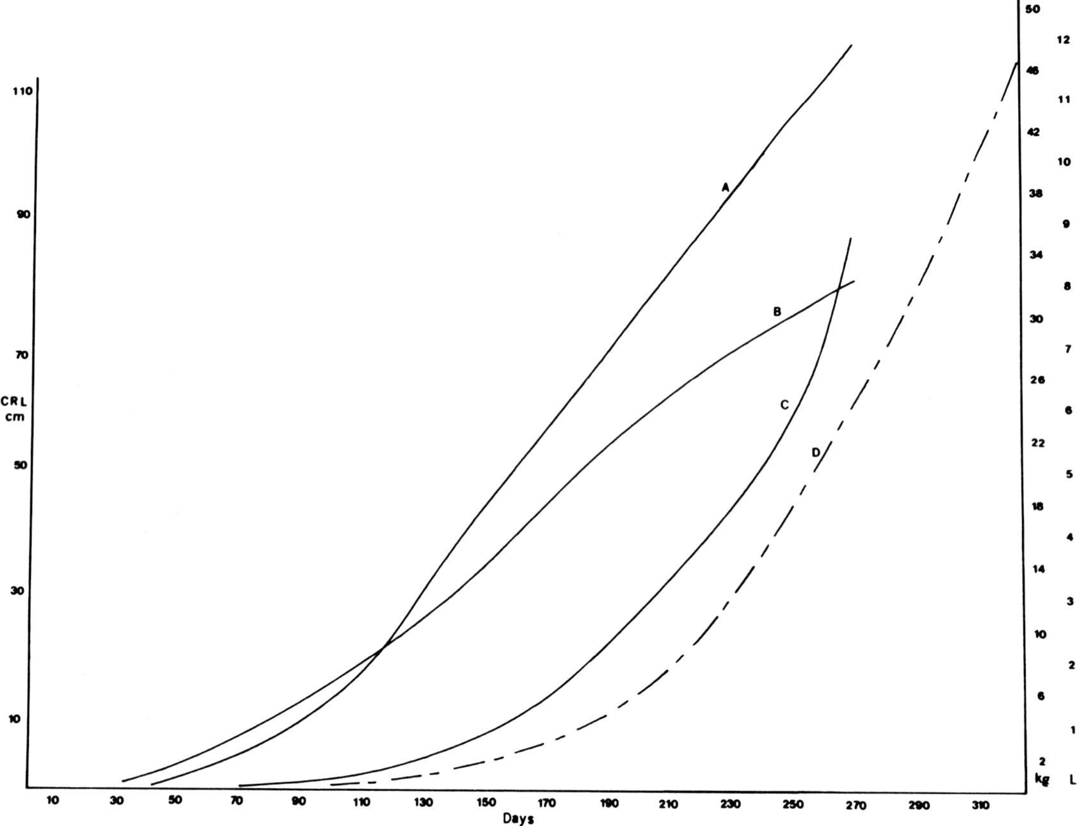

17.23 Fetal growth curves: **(A)** bovine crown-rump length, **(B)** bovine amniotic fluid volume, **(C)** bovine fetal weight, **(D)** equine fetal weight.

At this stage, the embryo is encased within an amniotic vesicle that is free-floating within the allantochorion, attached to the allantois by the umbilical cord and vessels (Fig. 17.26). This relationship is maintained until the last 2 months of the gestation (14).

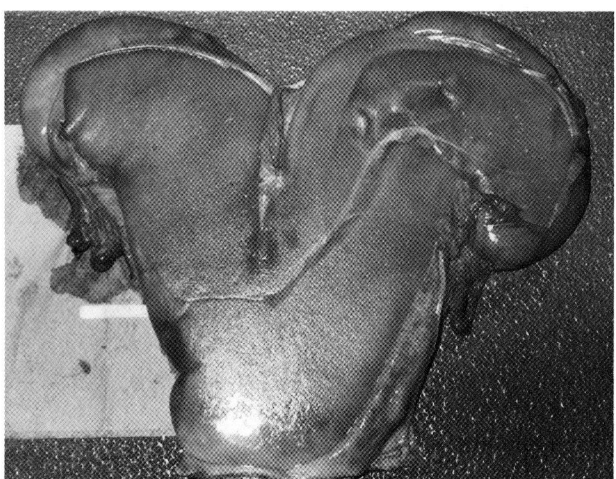

17.24 Llama placenta, in situ, approximately 4-month gestation.

The allantochorion contains the fetal vascular supply. The surface of the chorion gradually changes from the domed placentoma to a multifolded papilla. It appears that each dome elongates, producing folds that expand to provide a greater surface area. The tip of each tuft is larger than the neck. If the placentoma be-

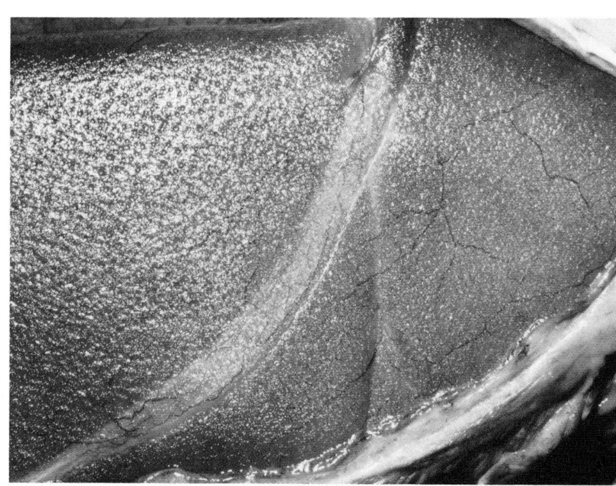

17.25 Surface of a llama chorion at 4-month gestation.

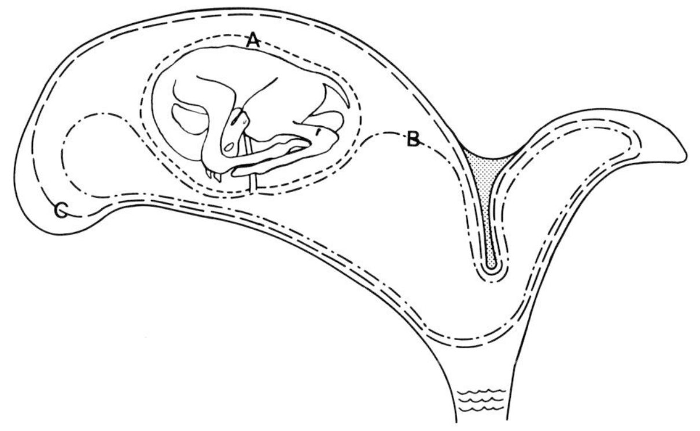

17.26 Diagram of early lamoid placenta: **(A)** amnion, **(B)** allantois, **(C)** chorion.

comes edematous as a result of disease, it looks like a miniature mushroom. The papillae fit into corresponding crypts in the uterine mucosa.

The papillae vary in size and shape, but generally the base is smaller than the tip. They may be columnar, rectangular, or shaped like an inverted cone and are 0.25–1.5 mm long. The density of the papillae is greatest in the patches, but a few papillae are found in the interspaces.

On visual inspection, reddish, irregularly shaped patches occupy most of the surface of the chorion, with lighter colored interspaces (Fig. 17.27). The surface appears to be a roughened, undulating membrane grossly, but when viewed through a dissecting microscope at 20X, hundreds of multifolded papillae per square centimeter may be seen. Patches of papillae are most dense on the greater curvature and toward the center of the crescent-shaped placenta. The tips of the placenta have lighter patchiness, and a strip 2–3 cm wide, extending the length of the lesser curvature in juxtaposition to the large vessels of the allantochorion, is nearly devoid of papillae. A branching pattern of vessels may be traced from the large vessels arising from the lesser curvature of the placenta to each patch of papillae.

The most unique characteristic of the camelid fetal membranes is the development of an extra membrane of fetal epidermal origin. This membrane was described in the dromedary camel 10 years ago (98, 99) but was not described in SACs until 1988 (68).

The epidermal membrane (EM) is an opaque whitish membrane, approximately 1–2 mm thick, covering the surface of the fetal body, head, neck, and limbs at near full term. The EM is attached to the neonate at the mucocutaneous junctions such as at the lips, nostrils, eyelids, ears, anus, vulva, and prepuce (Fig. 17.28). The EM is also attached at the junction of the skin and footpad, coronet of the nail, and at the umbilicus (Fig. 17.29). Since the EM does not cover the nostrils or the mouth, there is little danger of suffocation postpartum if the membranes are not immediately removed from the neonate.

The EM is friable and easily torn or brushed from the surface of the neonate with only slight friction. Even with little movement or abrasion, it dries out and withers away soon after parturition. This is in contrast to the amnion of most mammals, which may completely envelop the nose and mouth, causing suffocation of a weak, nonstruggling neonate. Histologically, the EM consists of a layer of stratified squamous epithelial cells lying next to the fetus and an outer keratinized

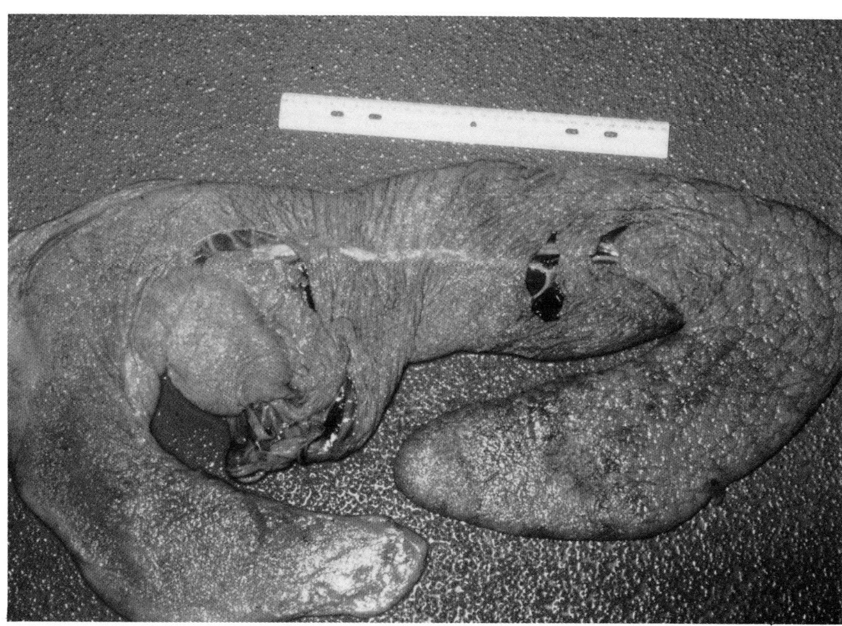

17.27 Full-term llama placenta, chorion outside.

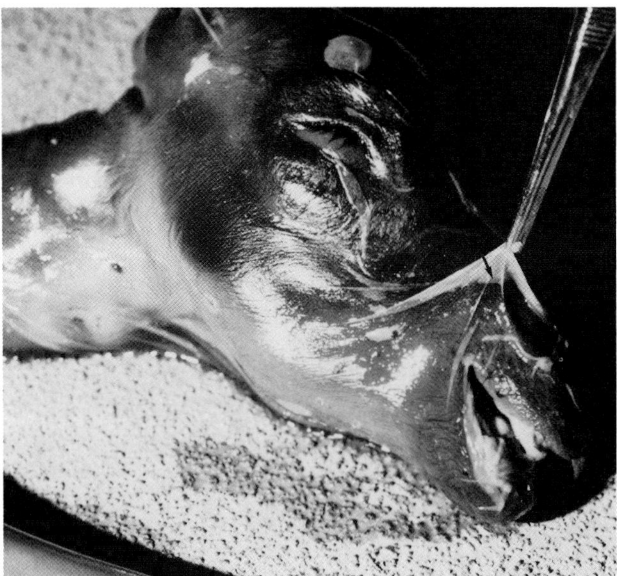

17.28 Epidermal membrane attached to the nostrils, eyelids, and lips.

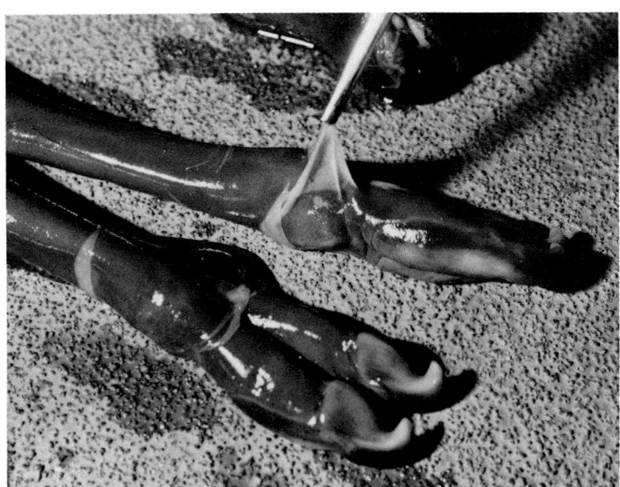

17.29 Epidermal membrane attached to pads and nails.

layer with indistinct cell outlines and no nuclei (100). The fetus is usually delivered with the EM intact. However, if parturition is prolonged, with erratic or intense labor, or if manual assistance is necessary, the EM will split and disintegrate.

The precise function of the EM is unknown. The fetuses of noncamelid placental mammals float freely in the amniotic fluid. In the later stages of gestation in camelids, the EM separates the skin from the amniotic fluid. Since all of the camelid body orifices are unaffected by the EM, excretory products from the digestive tract of the fetus are discharged into the amniotic sac, as in other mammals.

The amniotic fluid of the llama remains watery throughout gestation, as does that of the camel, producing a slippery surface on the EM that facilitates delivery (101). In contrast, the amniotic fluid of the mare and cow becomes mucoid toward the end of gestation, which also lubricates the fetus and facilitates delivery.

The EM originates from the epidermis of the fetus. The precise embryology of the membrane is not known in lamoids, but the time of its development has been studied in the camel (100). Microscopic changes could be identified with a fetal crown-rump length (CRL) of 17 cm, or approximately midgestation. Gross appearance of the membrane did not occur until just before the development of the hair, which seemed to elevate the membrane away from the skin surface (100). In llamas, the EM has not been observed grossly until the last 2 months of gestation. Prior to this time, aborted fetuses have been surrounded by the amnion, which had not become adherent to the chorion.

At full term, the llama fetus is situated within the pregnant horn and the body of the uterus (Figs. 17.30, 17.31). The amniotic sac extends to the tip of the pregnant horn and occupies all the space not occupied by the allantoic sac. The amnion may be easily peeled from the fetal side of the chorion. The chorionic attachment to the allantois is more secure. Figure 17.32 is an electron microscopic picture of the placentome. There is a minimal amount of fluid in the amniotic sac.

The allantoic sac extends into the pregnant horn, though not to its tip, and occupies all of the space in the nonpregnant horn. One or more hippomanes (allantoic calculi) are present in the allantoic sac, varying in size from 1 × 1 × 1.5 cm to 1 × 2 × 5 cm and weighing from 2 to 10 g (Fig. 17.33).

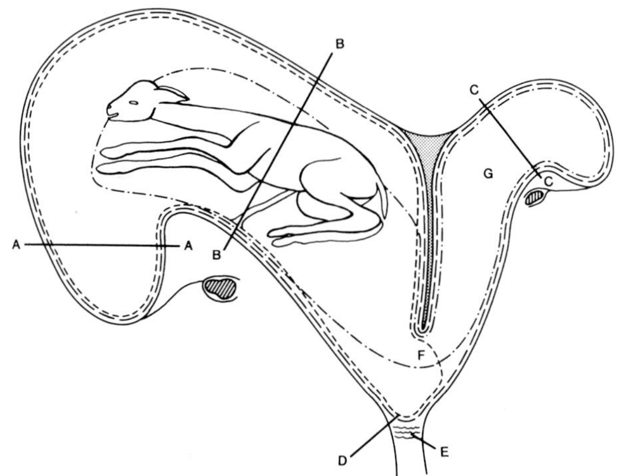

17.30 Diagram of full-term llama placenta: **(AA, BB, CC)** cross section (see Fig. 17.31), **(D)** site of amniochorion dehiscence, **(E)** cervix, **(F)** body of uterus, **(G)** nonpregnant horn.

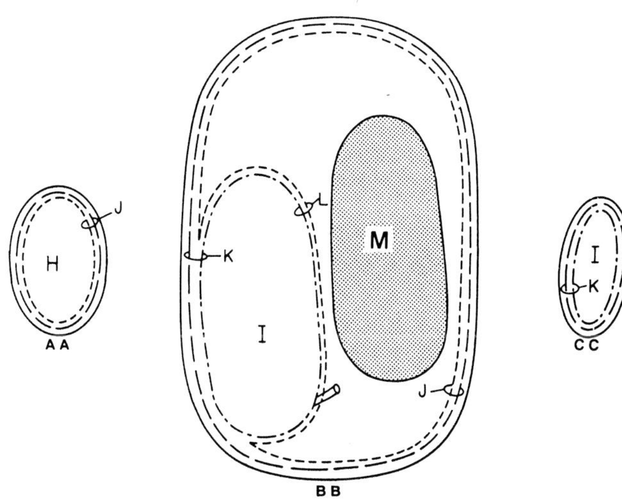

17.31 Diagram of cross section of full-term fetal membranes: **AA**, **BB**, and **CC** correspond to locations from Figure 17.30, **(H)** amniotic cavity, **(I)** allantoic cavity, **(J)** amniochorion, **(K)** allantochorion, **(L)** amnioallantois, **(M)** fetus covered with epidermal membrane.

Pregnancy Determination (21, 65, 86). Methods used to determine pregnancy in lamoids include behavior, progesterone analysis, rectal palpation, ballottement, and ultrasonography.

Behavior. Usually, a mature, nonpregnant female will accept mating by a breeding male. In South America, refusal of the advances of the male by a female is considered to be a positive diagnosis of pregnancy. Refusal may be a good preliminary indication of pregnancy, but many factors may modify this behavior, and for the llama owner or manager in North America, additional information must be obtained to verify pregnancy. Certain pathologic conditions simulate pregnancy (pyometra, retained CL, mummified fetus).

Breeding strategies that continually leave a male with females may foster development of a male that ignores even receptive females. Also, the male and one or more females may simply be incompatible.

An extremely aggressive male may overpower a timid female and force copulation, even though the female is pregnant. There is some danger if this should happen, since the male inserts the penis through the cervix and even into the horns of the uterus during copulation. Physical entry into the uterus after 90 days may traumatize the developing fetal membranes or introduce infection into the uterus. In either case, abortion may ensue.

Progesterone Analysis (65). Serum progesterone analysis has been promoted as the definitive method for pregnancy determination in llamas. While it is true that elevated levels of progesterone indicate the presence of a CL, this is not always confirmation of pregnancy. If this fact is kept in mind, progesterone levels may be useful as a management tool, not only for determining pregnancy, but also for evaluating various types of infertility problems.

Radioimmunoassay (RIA) and enzyme immunoassay (EIA) are standard analytic techniques for deter-

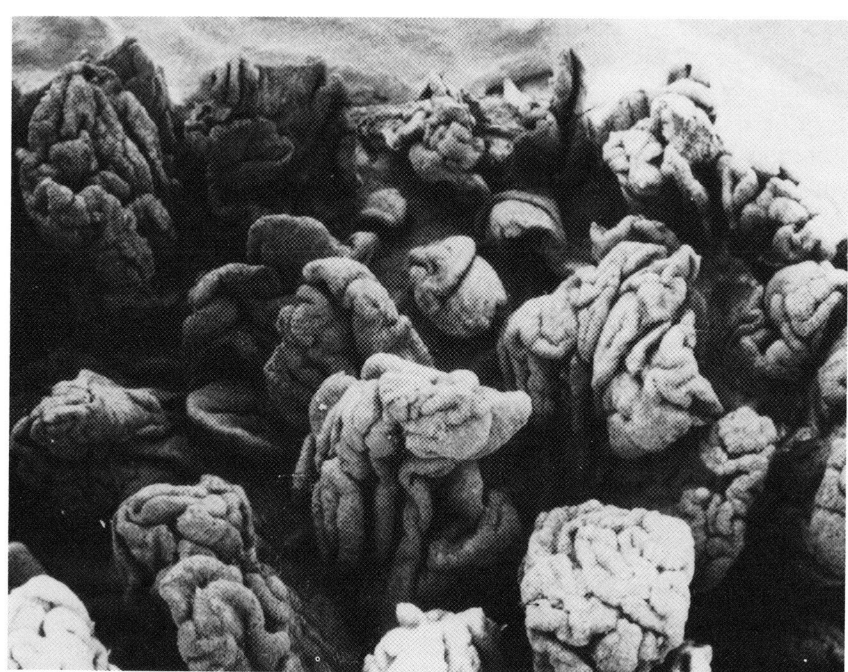

17.32 Scanning electron microscope picture of the endometrial face of the chorion in a full-term llama placenta. (Magnification 0.025 KX)

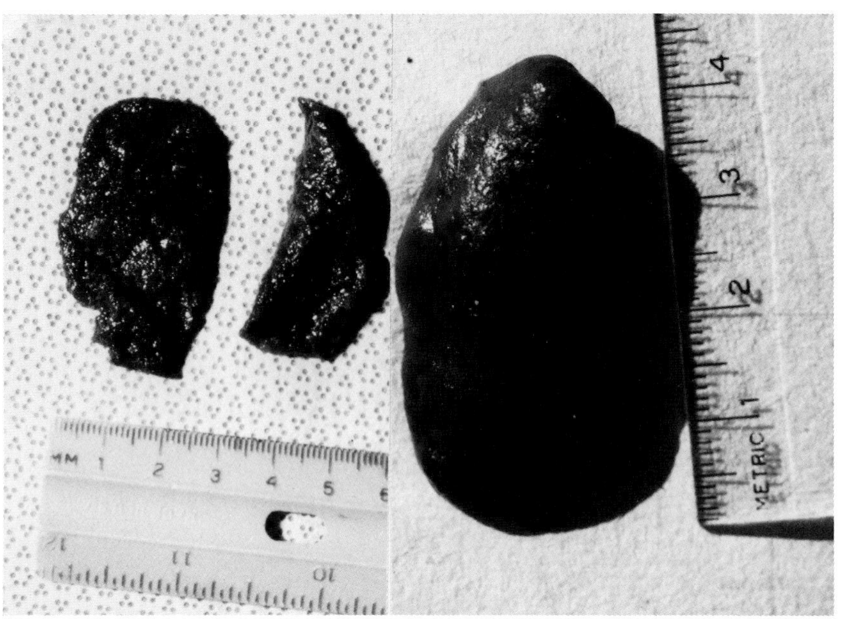

17.33 Hippomanes from llama allantoic cavity.

mination of progesterone levels. There is some variation between laboratories, but as long as results are consistent and the same laboratory is used for all determinations, this should not cause great concern.

Some laboratories using RIA report that levels of 2 ng/ml are indicative of the presence of the CL. Higher levels, 5–8 ng/ml, have been reported but do not correlate with better maintenance of the CL. A different laboratory may use 1 ng/ml as the cutoff point. It should be noted that cases of successful pregnancies have been reported in which progesterone levels were less than 0.5 ng/ml. At the other extreme, progesterone levels of over 2 ng/ml have resulted from a retained CL, with no fetus present.

Rectal Palpation **(19).** Rectal palpation has been the method of pregnancy determination in horses and cattle for decades. The general relationship of pelvic organs is illustrated in Figure 17.34. The smaller size of llamas and alpacas makes rectal palpation more difficult, but it is a valid technique and may be done safely if certain precautions are observed.

Adequate restraint is a prerequisite for rectal palpation and ultrasound examination. Several different types of chutes prevent side-to-side motion of the animal (see Chap. 3). Some llamas will lie down when subjected to an unpleasant situation, others constantly alternate between lying down and jumping up. The latter behavior makes examination difficult and dangerous. Some clinicians prefer to perform llama rectal examination with the animal in sternal recumbency, since abdominal pressure pushes the pelvic viscera into a more accessible location. To assure continued recumbency, it may be necessary to sedate the llama with 0.15 mg/kg xylazine intravenously.

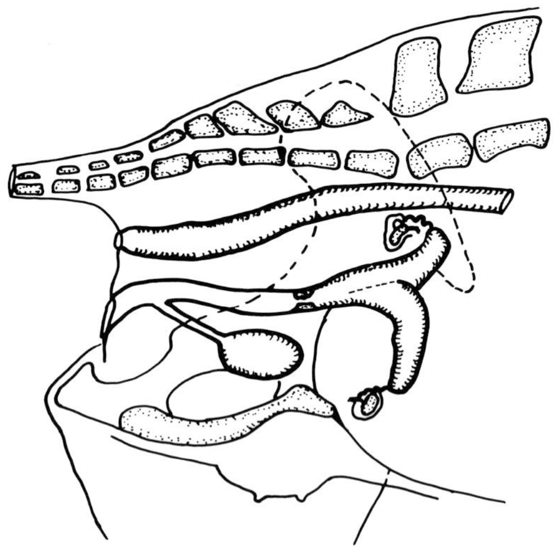

17.34 General relationship of pelvic organs in a lamoid female.

Persons with large hands (glove size larger than 8) or with large forearms will find it difficult to examine any except the largest animals. Adequate lubrication is the key to success. Fecal pellets should be gently removed from the rectum and methyl cellulose or other lubricants instilled into the rectum with an irrigation-tipped 60 ml syringe or dose syringe. The rectum should be slowly dilated, with the hand held in a cone position, palm facing dorsally. More lubricant should be added as needed.

Some examiners find it helpful to use a lubricant

containing xylocaine to diminish mucosal irritation and reflex straining. Commercial xylocaine lubricants are available, but a less expensive mixture may be prepared by mixing 10 ml injectable 2% xylocaine with 100 ml methyl cellulose.

The anus may be the most restrictive site in the examination process. The anal epithelium may tear slightly during dilation. Excessive anal tone may be diminished by epidural anesthesia (see Chap. 5). Xylocaine (1–2 ml, 2%) will provide adequate relaxation of the sphincter but will not prevent peristaltic activity in the rectum. While a rectal examination using epidural anesthesia was being conducted, the female contracted the rectum around the author's wrist. The spasm did not subside for about 10 minutes. Nothing could be done except wait, because any vigorous attempt to withdraw the hand would have split the rectal wall.

Lamoids are not as susceptible to rectal trauma as the mare but are more sensitive than the cow. See Chapter 6 for a discussion of rectal laceration.

The cranial half of the uterine horns diverge at approximately 180 degrees from each other (Fig. 17.14). Judicious palpation will allow measurement and evaluation of the horns and the ovaries. It is important to remember that the ovaries are encased within an ovarian bursa, which may hinder evaluation. The relaxed ovary is ventral to the broad ligament. Retraction of the uterine horn aids in delivery of the ovary for palpation.

Examiners familiar with rectal palpation of the pregnant mare or cow may find slight differences in the uterine tone of a llama. The amniotic vesicle is not as taut, thus the bulge in the uterine horn is less pronounced. Even at 60–90 days, the uterus has been described as "doughy," which in a mare or cow, would be suggestive of pyometra.

Pregnancy of a primiparous female may be determined by rectal palpation at 30 days by experienced llama palpaters, relying on a unilateral increase in the diameter of the pregnant horn. In multiparous females, the left horn is usually larger than the right. If determination is to be limited to a single examination, it is preferable to examine at 40–45 days, at which time the pregnant horn should be 7–8 cm in diameter (palm width). See Table 17.2 for approximate size of the uterine horn at various stages of pregnancy. Beyond 90 days, the uterus will be positioned cranial and ventral to the brim of the pelvis, making it difficult to reach the uterus for evaluation. After 8 months, the fetus may be accessible for palpation.

Information such as inability to palpate the uterus, flattened taut vagina, and firm cervix may be suggestive of pregnancy but not conclusive evidence. There are too many congenital anomalies that produce mucometria to rely on vague information, especially when examining a nulliparous female. The middle uterine artery develops fremitus during the last trimester of pregnancy, but this is not used routinely for pregnancy evaluation or differentiation between pregnancy and pyometra, as it is in the bovine. It is not possible to slip the fetal membranes in llamas. The relative quantity of placental fluids is much less in lamoids than in other livestock species. Some have even made the mistake of concluding the presence of a mummified fetus because of the lack of fluids.

Determination of the age of the fetus via rectal palpation is difficult after 90 days. This is also true late in pregnancy, when various parts of the body and limbs may be palpable. Notice from Figure 17.22 that increases in the CRL is gradual, even during the last trimester, while the body weight increases exponentially during the last 2 months.

Ballottement. External signs of pregnancy may be lacking in female llamas. Udder development may be minimal, especially in a nulliparous female. The body contour changes in most females, but the fiber coat tends to mask changes. As late as 8 months, the fetus weighs only 3.5 kg. By 10–11 months, the fetus may be balloted from the right side. Compartment one of the stomach occupies the entire left side of the abdomen, so the pregnant uterus is diverted to the right side. Ballottement is carried out as in cattle. A clenched fist is pressed up against the abdominal wall and a short vigorous push is exerted while the fist is held in place. If the female is pregnant, the push will cause the fetus to bounce away from the push, being cushioned in the fetal fluids, but it then drifts back and bumps the fist. The procedure should be repeated at a number of locations on the right side before the conclusion is reached that the female is not pregnant.

Ultrasonography. The use of ultrasound techniques for evaluation of the tubular reproductive tract and the ovaries has added a new dimension to veterinary medicine. The rapid improvements in technology in this field parallel those of the computer industry. Units that were state of the art when this chapter was written will probably be outmoded when the book is published. Units are currently available that allow the transducer to be carried into the rectum and manipulated by the hand of the palpater. This is the most desirable method to use on pregnancies of less than 120 days.

More sophisticated units allow transabdominal evaluations, which are more applicable for pregnancy determination later in the gestation period. In one instance, repeated rectal palpation and rectal ultrasound evaluation led a clinician to conclude that a female was not pregnant, and he was ready to institute hormonal therapy. A last examination using the transabdominal approach detected a fetal heart beat in the abdomen, ventral to the stomach.

Conclusions. All of the techniques described in this section have application for pregnancy determination in lamoids. None of the procedures are 100% accurate, and some may be limited to certain stages of pregnancy and to individual examiners of limited size. It is likely that employment of more than one system will be necessary to provide optimum management of a breeding herd of lamoids.

PARTURITION (15). Trying to predict the imminence of parturition is fraught with frustration. Though the abdomen enlarges, growth may be hidden by the heavy fiber coat of many llamas and alpacas. Field biologists are able to assess pregnancy in guanacos and vicuñas by body contour, but these wild camelids lack the thick fiber coat of the alpaca and llama.[2]

Pregnant females within a month of parturition change behavior and appear restless and uncomfortable, with more frequent sniffing at the dung pile and possibly more voiding. Some females develop ventral edema, but this is not the problem that it is in mares and cows. Udder development is not necessarily correlated with nearness of parturition. The udder of a primiparous female may show little or no development until after parturition. The udder of a multiparous female usually enlarges 2–3 weeks before delivery, and the nipples may swell 3–4 days before delivery. Wax may form on the end of the teat, but its absence is not evidence that parturition is not imminent.

Normal parturition is initiated by hormonal changes and is divided into three stages. *Stage one* begins with cervical relaxation and uterine contractions that propel the fetus toward the pelvis, dilating the cervix. This stage may last from 2 to 6 hours and tends to be longer in primiparous females. The signs of stage one include slight discomfort, excessive vocalization (humming), and repeated defecation and urination.

Stage two is the expulsion of the fetus. The amniochorion may dehisce within the birth canal, or the chorion only may dehisce and the amnion protrude through the vulva as a fluid-filled sac. In either case, a little fluid is expelled, usually dripping from the vulva. It is possible that the fluid-filled sac may be a pouch of the epidermal membrane, pushed ahead of the fetus. At this stage the perineum will begin to protrude.

The most common normal presentation is cranial longitudinal, with a dorsosacral position and the head lying dorsal to the extended limbs (Fig. 17.35). A slight variant of this may occur, with the limbs positioned over the top of the head (Fig. 17.36). The posterior longitudinal presentation, dorsosacral position with the hind limbs extended, is also normal but much less common (Fig. 17.37). The risk to the life of the fetus is greater in a caudal presentation dystocia because of the danger of occlusion of the umbilical vessels as a result of stretching or pressure.

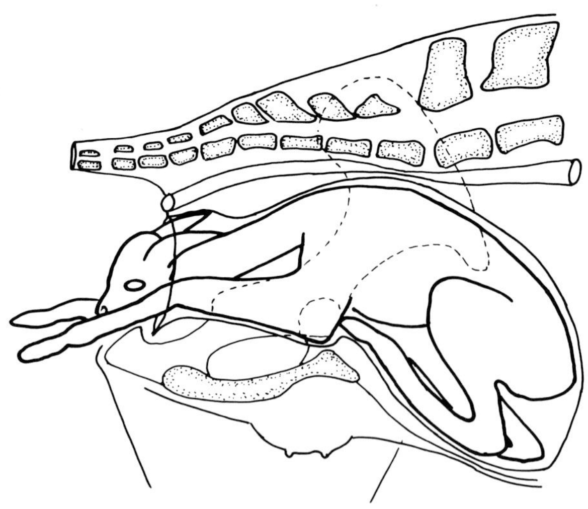

17.35 Normal llama delivery, cranial presentation, dorsosacral position.

Uterine contractions initially occur every 10 minutes, increasing in frequency and intensity as expulsion progresses. At this stage, the female is definitely uncomfortable. She may lie down and rise repeatedly, lie on her side, or even roll. If the fetus has been partially delivered, it may be traumatized by such actions. The

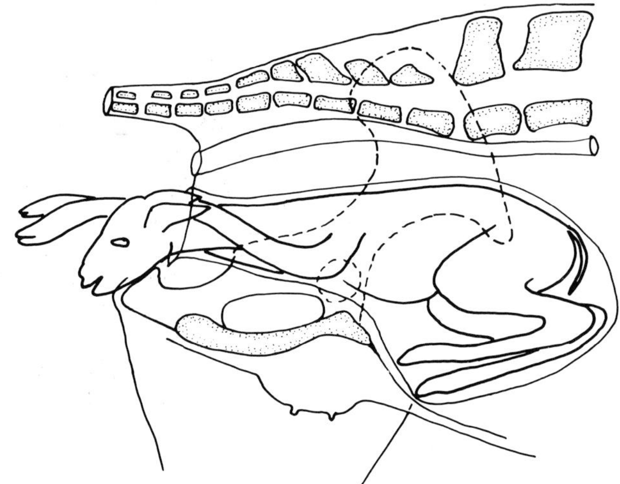

17.36 Normal llama delivery, only with legs above the head.

2. W. L. Franklin, personal communication.

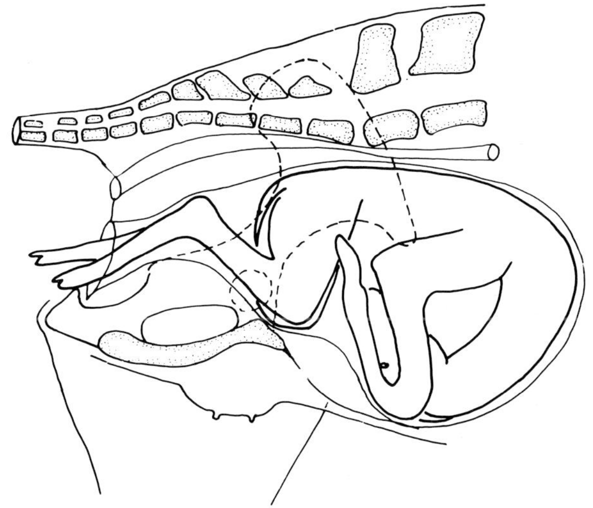

17.37 Normal but uncommon llama delivery, caudal presentation, dorsosacral position.

female may look back at her side, vocalize, and exhibit other signs of colic. In an uncomplicated parturition, the unassisted female should deliver the fetus within 45–60 minutes after fluid first appears at the vulva.

The majority of females deliver the fetus while in the standing position. In observations made on alpaca parturition in Peru, 65–73% of the fetuses were delivered while the female was standing. An additional 20–24% were delivered from sternal recumbency and 7–12% while the female was lying on her side.

The umbilical cord usually ruptures 15–20 cm from the abdomen. Maternal care is minimal. The mother will not attempt to remove the epidermal membrane or lick the cria to dry it. There is usually nose-to-nose touching, with humming that supposedly functions to establish the mother-cria bond.

The majority of births take place during daylight hours, with the preponderance occurring in the morning (71). However, llamas in North America have been known to give birth at night. They seem to have the ability to regulate parturition as a voluntary activity. Too much attention and excitement may actually delay parturition.

The neonate should struggle to its feet within an hour or two and start exploring the mother to find a nipple.

Stage three of parturition is expulsion of the placenta. The epitheliochorial placentation releases readily, and delivery of the placenta should occur within 2 hours. Retention of the placenta is rare in lamoids. Dystocia or uterine inertia predisposes retention of the placenta. Failure to expel the placenta by 6 hours should be considered abnormal, but at this point the only recommended therapy is the administration of oxytocin (20–30 units intramuscularly). If a segment of the placenta is protruding from the vulva, it should be grasped gently by a gloved hand and slight tension applied. Frequently, the membranes will be sitting loosely in the vagina and the body of the uterus, and a slight tug is all that is needed to effect delivery.

It has never been necessary to manually separate the placenta from the uterine mucosa. If the placenta has not delivered by 12 hours, the use of the same protocols as for dealing with the problem in a mare are recommended.

The lamoid placenta is crescent shaped (Fig. 17.28). In the majority of cases, the membranes will be reddish in color, with the chorion on the outside. In a few instances, the placenta will be turned inside out, with the amnion exposed, and have a whitish, glistening surface. Each placenta should be inspected to determine the presence of the two tips, a good indication of complete expulsion.

The average llama placenta, exclusive of fluids, weighs approximately 3 kg (range 0.74–1.44 kg). The greater curvature measures 196–280 cm (77–110 in.) and the concave curvature measures 96–210 cm (40–83 in.).

POSTPARTUM COMPLICATIONS (82)

Failure to Deliver the Placenta. This has already been discussed.

Prolapse of the Uterus and Vagina. See Chapter 6.

Too vigorous pulling on the placenta immediately after delivery of the fetus may evert the uterus. Replacement of the uterus at this time is easily accomplished.

Uterine Infection. Metritis is rare except in cases of dystocia in which trauma has been inflicted by manipulations. A few cases have been associated with the obese female, postpartum.

Postpartum Hemorrhage. Hemorrhage can arise only from lacerations of the uterus or vagina. A persistent flow of blood should be investigated immediately (see Chap. 6).

Uterine Tear. See Chapter 6.

Agalactia. Lactation failure following parturition is common in llamas (see also Chaps. 10 and 21). The problem is seen more often in primiparous females, but it also occurs in multiparous females. Lactation in lamoids is presumably controlled by the same systems as in other livestock species. If the fetus is delivered prematurely, hormonal preparation of the mammary gland to begin secretion may not have been completed.

Inadequate milk let down may be a factor. Placement of the neonate in the nursing position may stimulate the dam to allow milk let down, or administration of intramuscular oxytocin in repeated doses of 20 units every 2 hours is appropriate therapy. Both actions should be accompanied by gentle massage of the udder with warm water and stripping milk from the teats. A careful watch of the baby is necessary to assure that sufficient milk is being consumed. Otherwise, the cria must be supplemented or orphaned until an adequate milk flow has been established.

Rejection of the Cria. Fortunately, rejection of the cria is extremely rare in lamoids; in fact, female alpacas and llamas may accept other crias. In one zoo herd, a particular female would accept every cria in the herd long after its own mother had weaned it. Vicuñas and guanacos will not accept any cria other than their own.[3]

Involution of the Uterus. Discharge from the vulva postpartum (lochia) is scanty and is usually absent after 6–8 days. Postpartum involution of the uterus occurs rapidly in lamoids. In a study conducted with alpacas, the average weight of the uterus was 883 g 24 hours after parturition, with the pregnant horn being approximately 15 cm in diameter (143). Ten days postpartum, the uterus weighed only 155 g and the pregnant horn was 3.5 cm and in 20 days, 83 g and 3 cm, respectively. Such a rapid involution is necessary to maintain a 12-month birthing interval. Female llamas will accept copulation within 2–3 days postpartum, but the uterus is not involuted and it is not desirable that breeding take place until 10–20 days following parturition.

A male may attempt to copulate with a female when she is recumbent and parturition is imminent.

OBSTETRIC PROCEDURES (85, 120, 140). Dystocia refers to any parturition that is more prolonged than expected. Breeders report a low prevalence of dystocia in llamas as contrasted with sheep and cattle. In observations of large numbers of animals in Peru, it was determined that the prevalence of dystocia in alpacas was less than 2.4% and that the entire parturition process in the alpaca should be completed within 3.5 hours (140). Causes of dystocia may be related to fetal or maternal factors (Table 17.3).

Malposition. The factors that orient the fetus to the normal parturient presentation and position are unknown, as are those factors that cause malpositioning. Several malpositions are described and illustrated.

Table 17.3. Causes of fetal and maternal dystocia

Fetal	Maternal
Malposition	Uterine torsion
Congenital defects	Uterine inertia
Schistosomus reflexus	Failure of cervix to dilate
Ankylosis of major joints	Malformed pelvis
Hydrocephalus	Stenosis of the vagina
Edema and maceration of fetus	

The most common malposition is cranial longitudinal presentation in the dorsosacral position, with the limbs extended but the head and neck flexed backward to the side (Fig. 17.38). Others include (1) cranial longitudinal presentation, dorsosacral position, with the head and one limb extended but one limb retained (Fig. 17.39); (2) cranial longitudinal presentation, dorsosac-

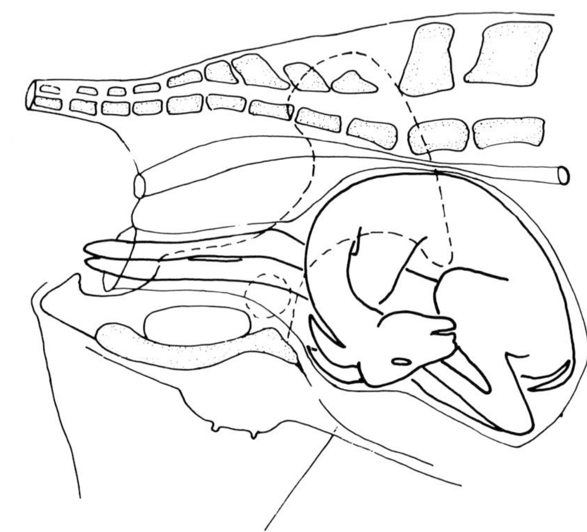

17.38 Lamoid dystocia, cranial presentation, dorsosacral position, with head retained to one side.

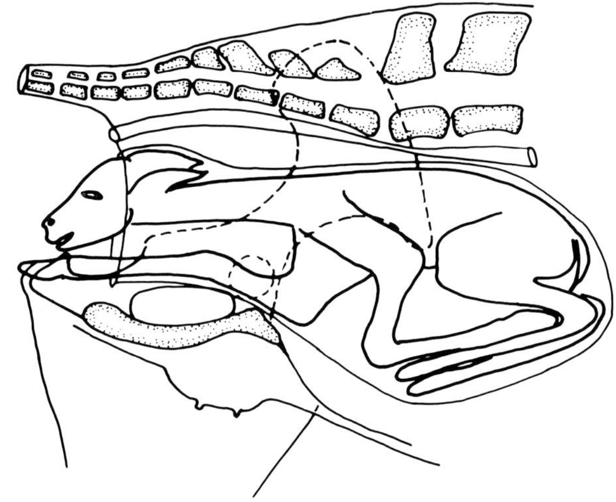

17.39 Lamoid dystocia, cranial presentation, dorsosacral position, one limb retained.

3. W. L. Franklin, personal communication.

ral position, with one limb extended but the head and one limb retained (Fig. 17.40); (3) cranial longitudinal presentation, dorsosacral position, with the limbs extended but the head retained between the limbs (Fig. 17.41); (4) cranial longitudinal presentation, dorsosacral position, with the head extended but both limbs retained (Fig. 17.42); (5) cranial longitudinal presentation, dorsosacral position, with both limbs and head retained (Fig. 17.43); (6) caudal longitudinal presentation, dorsosacral position, with the limbs retained (breech presentation) (Fig. 17.44).

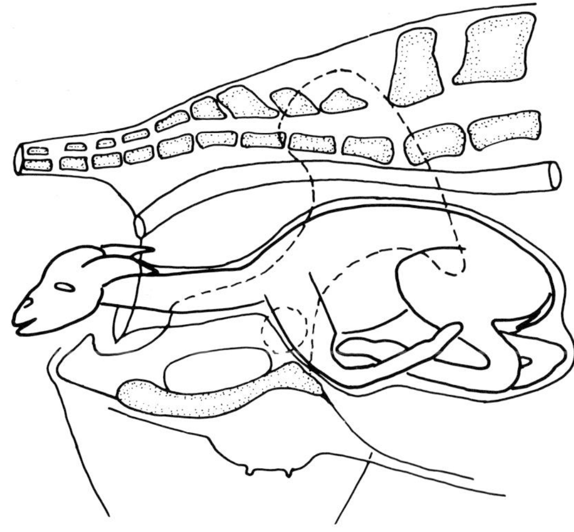

17.42 Lamoid dystocia, cranial presentation, dorsosacral position, both forelimbs retained.

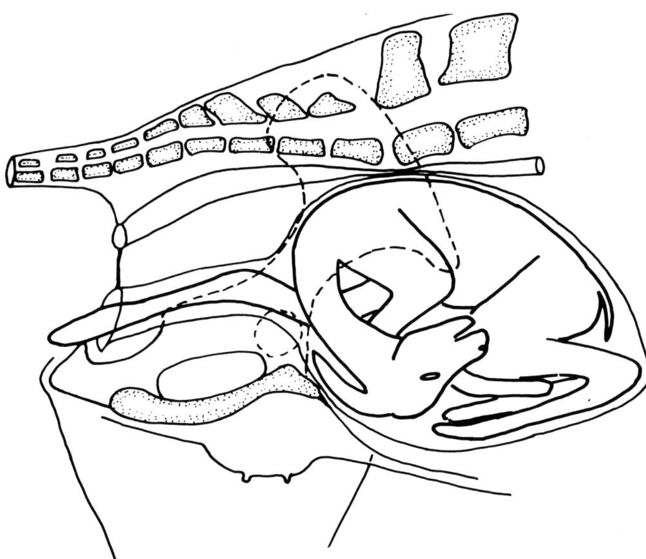

17.40 Lamoid dystocia, cranial presentation, dorsosacral position, head and forelimb retained.

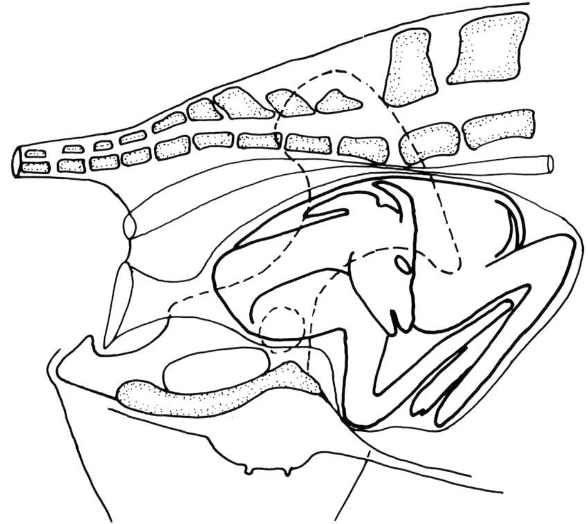

17.43 Lamoid dystocia, cranial presentation, dorsosacral position, head and both forelimbs retained.

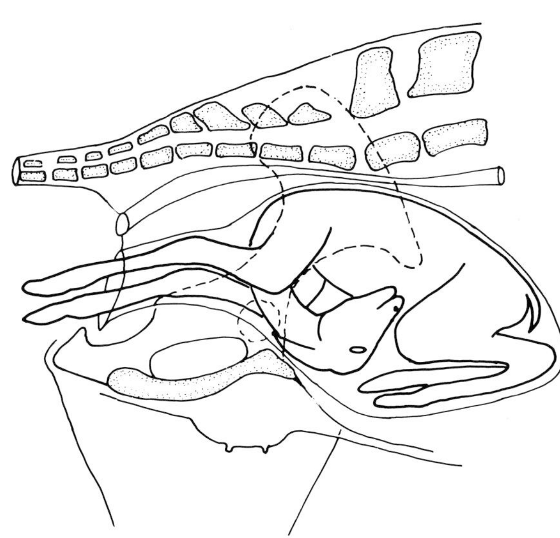

17.41 Lamoid dystocia, cranial presentation, dorsosacral position, head retained between legs.

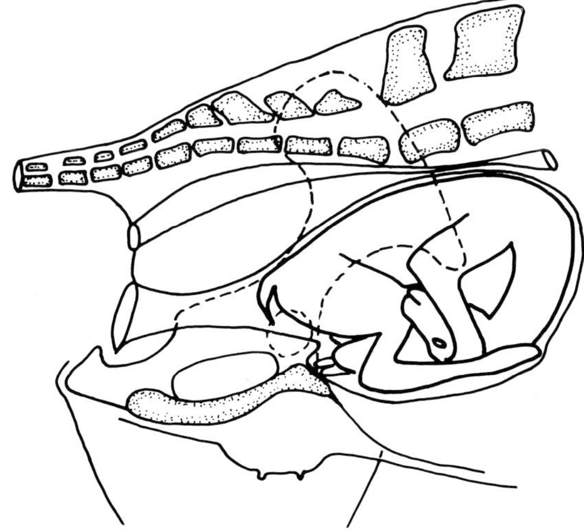

17.44 Lamoid dystocia, caudal presentation, dorsosacral position, hind limbs retained (breech).

Other less common dystocias are cranial longitudinal presentation, dorsopubic position, with head and forelimbs extended (Fig. 17.45) and transverse ventral presentation, dorsoilial position, with all four limbs and the head extended (Fig. 17.46).

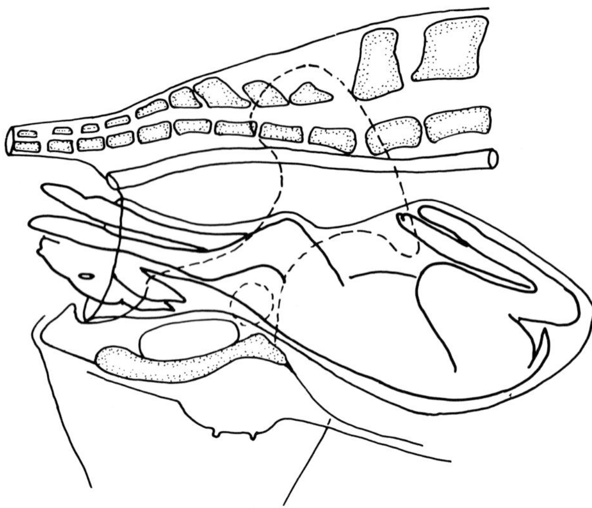

17.45 Lamoid dystocia, cranial presentation, sacropubic position, head and forelimbs extended.

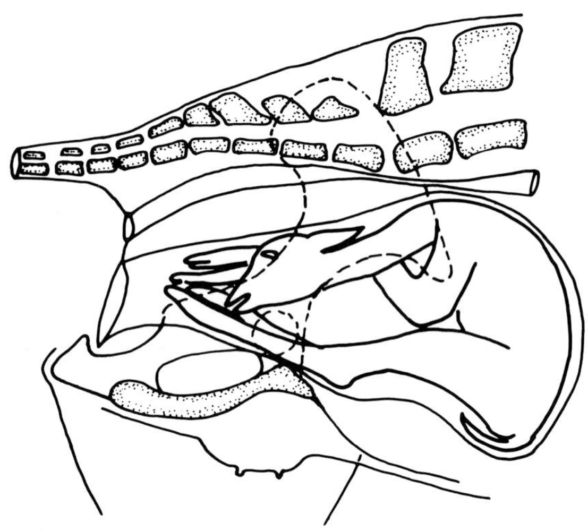

17.46 Lamoid dystocia, transverse presentation, dorsoilial position, four limbs and head extended.

Manipulation of Dystocias (114, 119, 147). Space does not permit detailed discussions of obstetric procedures. The reader is referred to a standard veterinary obstetrics textbook (120). A few unique facts should be kept in mind. Lamoids are small and there is little room for manipulation, even by a person with small arms and hands. It may be necessary to draft the smallest person available to perform any necessary internal manipulation, under appropriate direction. If manipulation by a large person is essential, epidural anesthesia should be administered to provide analgesia; additional relaxation may be produced with butorphanol (see Chap. 5).

The limiting dimensions of the birth canal are not at the pelvic inlet but rather at the level of the caudal end of the sacrum and the ischiatic spines of the ilia (Figs. 17.47–17.50). Figures 17.47 and 17.49 also illustrate a cranial view of the pelvic inlet with variable dimensions in a ratio as represented by the measurements of one adult female weighing approximately 140 kg. The vertical distance was 11 cm, width 10.5 cm, and the diagonal 12 cm. Figures 17.48 and 17.50 are a caudal view that show the relationship of the ischia ilia and sacrum. The vertical distance is 12.5 cm, the narrowest width 8.5 cm, and the diagonal 14 cm.

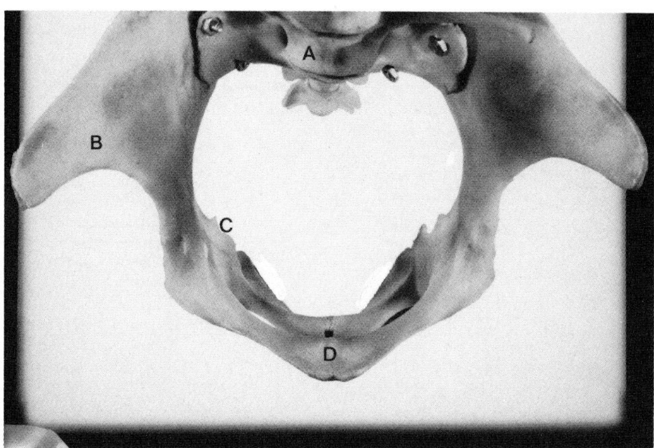

17.47 Female llama pelvis, cranial view: **(A)** sacrum, **(B)** ilium, **(C)** ischiatic spine, **(D)** pubis.

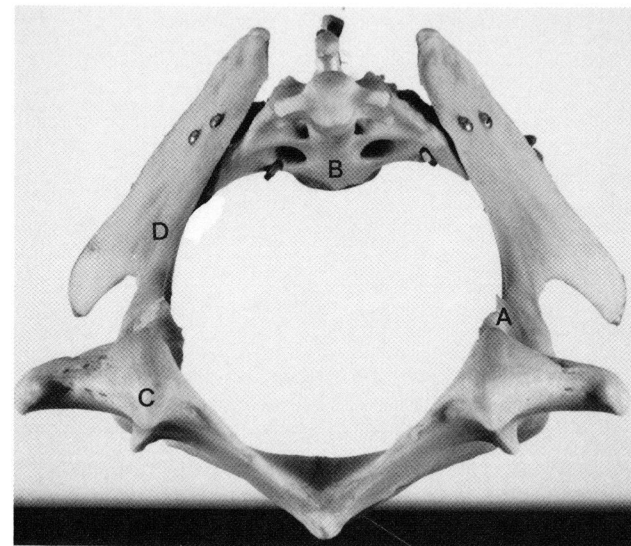

17.48 Female llama pelvis, caudal view: **(A)** ischiatic spine, **(B)** sacrum, **(C)** ischium, **(D)** ilium.

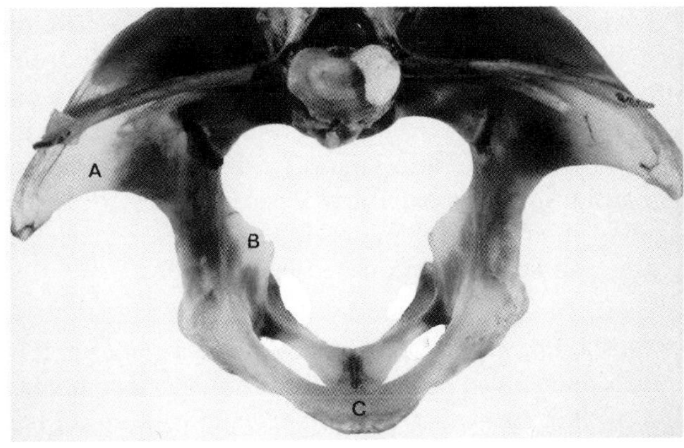

17.49 Male llama pelvis, cranial view: (A) ilium, (B) ischiatic spine, (C) pubis.

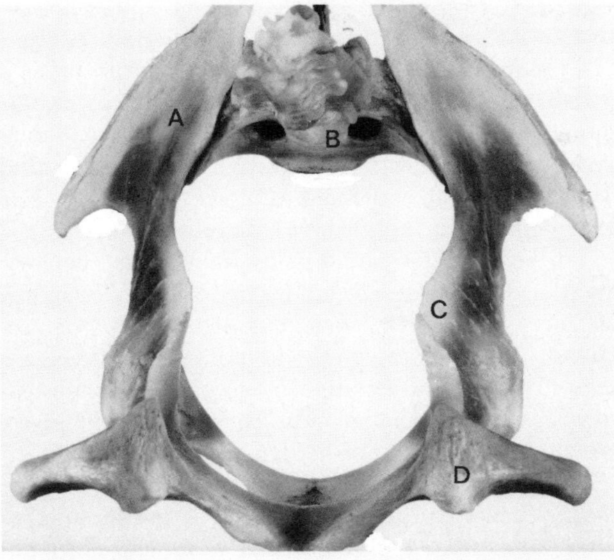

17.50 Male llama pelvis, caudal view: (A) ilium, (B) sacrum, (C) ischiatic spine, (D) ischium.

Some ligamentous relaxation may occur at the time of parturition to allow the sacrum to tilt up slightly, but it is not likely that there will be any give in the width. The author has noted that the ischiatic spines may be so close that the hand must be inserted in a vertical plane to pass this anatomic obstruction.

Amniotic fluid is scanty, and if the epidermal membrane has been rubbed off by manipulation, lubrication will be needed to facilitate delivery. Soap is contraindicated, since it is irritating to the mucosa and dissolves surface-protecting oils. Methylcellulose is excellent.

In most livestock species, the fetus is likely to impact at the hips. In the llama, the shoulder girdle is more likely to impact. From a normal delivery presentation and position, before the shoulders reach the pelvic canal, it is helpful to twist the fetus 45 degrees and gently pull on one leg at a time. The adult pelvic girdle is basically a vertical rectangle, with the greatest cross-sectional dimension on the diagonal.

The use of obstetric chains is not warranted. Usually, only manual grasping is necessary. If repulsion is necessary, a clean, disinfected light-weight nylon cord may be secured to a limb to allow later access to the limb.

If the hips lock, the fetus should be repelled and twisted on its longitudinal axis 45–90 degrees before traction is applied dorsally. The fetal pelvis is wider than it is deep, and the twist will serve to coincide the fetal pelvis with the greatest vertical dimension of the dam's pelvic girdle. Other manipulations are similar to those recommended in cattle and sheep dystocias.

Any of the caudal presentations carry more risk of fetal death with prolonged delivery. The umbilical circulation is quickly compromised because of the caudal position of the umbilicus on the abdomen. It is wise to advise any client who is conducting preliminary obstetric examinations that caudal presentations usually require professional assistance and should be considered emergencies.

Delivery from the caudal presentation must be quick and efficient. There must be adequate lubrication, and the cervix must be fully dilated before traction is applied. If the clinician feels that more than 10 minutes will elapse before the fetus can be delivered, a cesarian section may be preferable.

Many dystocias caused by congenital anomalies required delivery by cesarian section, or, in the hands of a skilled operator, fetotomy may be performed.

Maternal Dystocia. *Uterine torsion* occurs in llamas and alpacas. The causes are unknown. The torsion may be in either direction. Ranges of 90–360 degrees rotation in the vagina have been reported. Rectal examination, manual vaginal examination, or a vaginal speculum examination will identify the problem. The primary clinical sign of torsion is prolonged stage one parturition. The cervix may partially dilate, but relaxation cannot be completed because of mechanical inhibition.

The management of uterine torsion will depend on the degree of rotation, the size of the female, and the distress experienced by the female. Rolling the female while pressing against the uterus through the wall of the abdomen with fists or a board may be of help in some cases. Some degree of sedation may be necessary. The torsion may be corrected by the female herself through such colicky manuevers as getting up and down or rolling. One alpaca became upset while being restrained in a chute, reared up, and fell over backward. After she scrambled to her feet, reexamination showed that the torsion had been corrected.[4] Manual maneuvers should not be continued for more than 10–15 minutes. If the torsion persists longer than this, a cesarian section may be necessary to save the life of the fetus and the dam. Uterine rupture is a possible sequel to torsion.

Uterine inertia is usually caused by prolonged, unproductive effort during stage one or two of parturition. Following correction of malpositioning, neither uterine nor abdominal contractions will continue if the female is exhausted. In such cases, though delivery will be more difficult without the assistance of contractions, it is unwise to administer oxytocin until after the fetus is delivered.

Failure of the cervix to dilate is difficult to differentiate from false labor. A small female carrying a large fetus may experience colicky signs during the last month of pregnancy, caused by partial obstruction of the digestive tract by the massive uterus. The relaxation of the cervix is under hormonal control, which may be abnormal. Good breeding records, careful observations, and a physical examination are necessary to precisely identify this problem.

Prostaglandins ($PGF_{2\alpha}$) are the trigger for cervical relaxation and may be administered subcutaneously at a dose of 15–25 mg total dose. However, if a mistake has been made in the breeding date, this drug will cause abortion. Relaxation occurs 24–72 hours following the administration of $PGF_{2\alpha}$. If the llama is showing signs of stage one, it may be necessary to manually dilate the cervix.

Pelvic stenosis may be caused by abscesses, tumors, or healed but malaligned fractures. A cesarian section may be necessary to relieve the dystocia prior to correction of the basic disorder.

PREGNANCY TERMINATION (36). The termination of pregnancy in lamoids may be indicated for the same reasons as in other livestock. Accidental mating is the most common indication, but suspected prolonged gestation may be considered sufficient reason for the induction of parturition. No studies have been conducted to determine the optimum method for pregnancy termination in the llama, but principles developed for other livestock may be applicable (36).

Early Gestation. Two major methods have been recommended to induce abortion. After the impregnated ovum has reached the uterine horn, presumably after 3–4 days, uterine irrigation with 25 ml 2% lugols iodine solution, 250 mg of tetracycline in 25 ml saline, or 25 ml 70% ethyl alcohol are effective in destroying the ovum and flushing it from the uterus.

Alternatively, $PGF_{2\alpha}$ (lutalyse), at a total dose of 15 mg, may be administered once intramuscularly from 6 to 100 days following copulation. The 6-day lag allows time for the CL to begin formation. If prostaglandins are administered to llamas or alpacas, they should be constantly observed for at least an hour to detect reaction. Should the llama become dyspneic or colicky, oxygen should be administered immediately.

Midgestation. In cattle, after 150 days gestation it is recommended to induce abortion with a combination of dexamethasone and prostaglandin. A suggested dose for a llama would be 15 mg dexamethasone and 15 mg lutalyse, administered intramuscularly. Abortion should occur within 72 hours.

Late Gestation. The primary indication for late gestation termination or induction of parturition is a female suspected of prolonged gestation. The female should always be examined for pregnancy before induction is begun. Clients have been embarrassed to find that the female they thought to be showing all the signs of impending parturition was just getting fat.

A veterinarian should be cautious about acquiescing to a client's desire to induce parturition. Numerous instances of incorrect breeding dates have been reported. Futhermore, valid 13-month gestations are known. Prolonged gestation, as recognized in holstein cows, is not known in lamoids. The fetus does not overgrow the ability of a normal female to deliver it.

Either dexamethasone or prostaglandins may be used to induce parturition. A dose of 10 mg dexamethasone, administered intramuscularly, should effect delivery in 48–72 hours. In cattle, retained placenta is common following dexamethasone usage. No information is available for lamoids. Lutalyse, at a dose of 15 mg, may be used, with no concern about retained placenta. Again, parturition should take place within 72 hours.

INFERTILITY

Female

Early breeding management strategies for alpacas and llamas in Peru yielded only approximately 50% live births. The strategy used was similar to that recommended for management of sheep. The reproductive physiology of lamoids is unique, not at all like sheep, and sheep methods were not successful with lamoids. While management of llama and alpaca herds and the individual animal has markedly improved fertility rates, numerous problems remain to be solved. Data are

4. P. Miller, personal communication.

sorely lacking on the precise causes of infertility in both males and females.

North American experiences with therapy and management are equally limited. A detailed discourse on these matters would lack factual foundation and simply be an extrapolation from knowledge of cattle, horses, sheep, and goats. Therefore, this discussion will only outline what is known about infertility in llamas and suggest some approaches to the problems.

ETIOLOGY (76). Congenital defects (5) account for much infertility of the female llama and alpaca. This is a fact both in North America and in the Andes. In one study in Peru, in over 10% of the females examined at slaughter, one or more anomalies were seen that could compromise fertility (137). Buyers should be encouraged to require prepurchase examinations of breeder animals if they are old enough that such an examination may be conducted. Otherwise, a written agreement relative to congenital anomalies should be part of the buyer-seller contract.

Following is a list of the anomalies that have been seen or reported in the female llama and alpaca reproductive tract: ovarian aplasia, ovarian hypoplasia, tubular hypoplasia, segmental aplasia (oviduct, uterine horn, cervix, vagina), persistent hymen, uterus unicornis, double cervix, and intersex. See Chapter 22 for a full discussion.

Hormonal defects are suspected, but as yet no good study of normal hormonal cycles other than progesterone have been undertaken. Therefore, it is not possible to compare or evaluate levels to determine whether or not they may be abnormal. Some females fail to ovulate or refuse to accept copulation. These are both under hormonal control. Failure to maintain a CL has been recognized as a clinical entity, and progesterone implants are being used to support pregnancy, with some reported successes.

Physical abnormalities should be noted. A horizontal vulva (shelving) may be seen in old, emaciated, or poorly conformed females. The labia may lack tone. Nothing is really known as to how or whether these may contribute to infertility. They are of concern in the mare or cow.

Inflammation of the reproductive tract includes vaginitis, cervicitis, metritis, endometritis, and pyometra. True venereal diseases are rare in lamoids. Brucellosis has been reported in South America but not in North America (see Chap. 7). The normal flora of the vagina and uterus is not known. Numerous species of bacteria have been cultured from infertile females, but Koch's postulates have not been demonstrated (11, 97). Perhaps, as in other females, the organisms are opportunistic pathogens. It should be kept in mind that in about one-third of the infertile females cultured, samples show no bacterial growth. This may be either accurate or a result of technique error. In the author's clinic, acute and peracute metritis is usually associated with a hemolytic *Escherichia coli* infection. *Corynebacterium pyogenes* is the second most prevalent organism cultured.

INFERTILITY EXAMINATION. It is vitally important that systematic, thorough examinations be conducted and that detailed records be kept. It is only through such records that it will be possible to amass sufficient data to serve as a sound basis for rational evaluation. Table 17.4 is a suggested check list.

The examination should be preceded by a detailed history. Unfortunately, infertile females are frequently shifted from one owner to another, often without the new owner being aware of the problem. Females with no ovaries have been "guaranteed" to have had two or three babies.

The vaginal examination may be conducted using a heifer glass vaginal speculum (2.5 cm outside diameter, 25 cm long). Specula that are constructed for use in goats are too short to reach the cervix (15 cm). In larger and multiparous females, a standard equine glass or cardboard speculum may be used, but it is longer than necessary (4 cm in diameter, 25 cm long). A piece of polyvinyl chloride plastic pipe of suitable diameter may be smoothed off on the end or fired and used as a speculum after sterilization. The female llama has no estrous period, with relaxation of the cervix. Refer to the dimensions of the reproductive tract to estimate distances to various structures.

It is possible, in multiparous females examined by small-handed people, to manually palpate the vagina after suitable cleansing and gloving. Rectal palpation is a valid and necessary procedure for evaluation of the reproductive tract. It can be done safely on all but the smallest females and virginal alpacas. Obesity greatly restricts movement in the pelvic canal and may preclude an adequate examination. A detailed description of rectal palpation has been given previously. It is unfortunate, but some owners have been swayed by exaggerated rumors of the dangers of rectal palpation and will not allow such an examination to be made. It may then be impossible to evaluate an infertile female and recommend a course of action.

Ultrasonography is a valuable aid, not only for pregnancy diagnosis, but also for conducting the infertility examination. No reports of detailed findings have yet appeared in the literature, but this is in the offing.

Uterine cytology (115), endometrial cultures, and sensitivities are vital for selection of proper therapy for metritis. An equine uterine culture swab (Tiegland) is

Table 17.4. Llama reproduction examination—female

Identification

Date ________

Name ________ Age ________ Owner ________

ISIS No. ________, Llama Registry No. ________

Color

Body ________ Neck ________

Head ________ Legs ________

History

Previous pregnancies—0, 1, 2, 3, 4

Live births—0, 1, 2, 3, 4

Abortions—0, 1, 2, 3

Breeding dates during past 6 months ________

Number of males used ________

Fertility of male—known ________ unknown ________

Response to male, past 2 months ________

Previous medical problems ________

Previous fertility treatments and response ________

Fertility rate of the herd ________

Rectal examination

Cervix diameter ________ cm, length ________ cm

Cervix tone ________

Right horn

Diameter ________ cm, length ________ cm

Left horn

Diameter ________ cm, length ________ cm

Consistency ________

Right ovary ________ × ________ × ________ cm

Left ovary ________ × ________ × ________ cm

structures present

Pregnant ________ yes, ________ no, ________ months

Vaginal examination

Vulva

Conformation ________

Discharge ________

Hymen ________

Vaginal mucosa

Color ________ Exudation ________

Cervical os

Cytology ________

Exudation ________

Cervical culture ________

Uterine culture ________

Uterine cytology ________

Uterine biopsy ________

Hormone assay

Progesterone ________ ng/dl

Ultrasound evaluation ________

Other diagnostic procedures—laparoscopy, laparotomy ________

Conclusions ________

recommended. It is useless, in fact misleading, to obtain a culture from the vagina or external os of the cervix. It is difficult to thread a tube through the cervix, but by gentle persistence it can be done. The cervix never relaxes to allow easy access.

Two approaches may be used. A small-handed person may enter the vagina with a gloved hand. A finger should be used to locate the cervical os and begin dilatation. The tube should be inserted alongside the arm, up to the finger, and gently pushed forward with periodic changes of direction to move over the rings. In another method, a short vaginal speculum is pressed around the os of the cervix. The culture tube is inserted through the os and the manipulation continued by visual contact, or the speculum may be withdrawn and allowed to rest on the tube while the other hand is inserted into the rectum to grasp the cervix and aid in the threading process. There is usually insufficient room for both a speculum in the vagina and an arm in the rectum.

Cultures should be interpreted in relation to the cytology. If no inflammatory cells or discharge is present, the organism cultured may not be a pathogen.

Endometrial Biopsy. The histologic evaluation of the uterine mucosa has become a standard diagnostic technique in mares and cows suffering from infertility. Much less experience has been gained in llamas, but some generalizations can be made. The technique is similar to passing the swab for a culture. The tip of the biopsy forceps must be threaded through the cervix and, with a hand in the rectum to fix the uterus, a snip of tissue may be pinched off the mucosa. Some of the larger equine forceps have jaws that may be too large for a llama, and injudicious use may penetrate the uterine wall. Cultures can be obtained from the biopsy tissue before placing it in fixative.

Each clinician should be consistent in the general location from which the specimen is collected. Unless a uterine mass must be biopsied directly, the lateral wall of the left horn is an appropriate location.

The uterine mucosa consists of an epithelial layer of tall columnar cells and a connective tissue layer containing the glands. The density of the connective tissue is greater and the number of glands in the mucosa much less in a llama than in a mare, leading to misinterpretation by inexperienced pathologists. Other lesions of inflammation are similar in both species.

Pigmented macrophages have been observed in the endometrium. This may be suggestive of abortion, parturition, or other causes of hemorrhage, as it is in mares (115). Fibrosis of the uterine glands is an unfavorable lesion. Since llamas do not cycle as most mammals, a variable histologic picture associated with stages of the estrous cycle cannot be described.

Laparoscopy (77, 144). Laparoscopy has been used effectively in experimental work to document ovarian activity during various stages of the reproductive cycle. In Peru, the technique used is to physically restrain the animal in dorsal recumbency on a special table that tilts the animal into a semivertical position with the head down. Local anesthesia is used, and two 1 cm incisions made cranial to the udder. The fiberoptic scope is inserted through one incision and a forceps for tissue manipulation through the other. Clear visualization of the ovaries requires that the ovarian bursa be gently lifted from the ovary.

Passive regurgitation was not observed in the Peruvian studies, but the animals had been fasted for 18 hours (144). The procedure can be completed in 3–5 minutes.

It is also possible to visualize the ovaries via a right-flank approach, with the animal in a standing position.

In the male, intraabdominal vasectomy may also be done using laparoscopy. For more details on laparoscopy techniques, see Harrison and Wildt (77).

Hormone Analysis. Progesterone levels have been used extensively to determine pregnancy in llamas, but it should be reiterated that positive levels indicate only the presence of a CL. Repeated or periodic progesterone samples may be of help in evaluating certain infertility problems such as recurrent early embryonic death. Levels of progesterone have been detected in milk and in urine.[5] Studies of other hormones associated with the reproductive process are sorely needed.

ARTIFICIAL INSEMINATION AND EMBRYO TRANSFER. Both artificial insemination and embryo transfer have been done, but the techniques are not perfected (42, 49, 51, 70, 137, 152).

TREATMENT OF INFERTILITY AND METRITIS. The techniques currently being used to treat infertile mares and cows are being applied to llamas. Statistics are not available as to the efficacy of various therapies.

Sexual rest is an important management tool. Animals that have experienced any difficulty with parturition should be given at least 30 days for optimal uterine involution before being exposed to a male.

Various hormones have been administered to livestock and horses to correct deficiencies based on actual measurement of hormone levels or on the basis of clinical signs and palpation examination. No baselines have been established in llamas for most of the hormones, so hormone therapy must be based on extrapolation from

5. J. Paul-Murphy, personal communication, 1987.

regimens for other species. Before these drugs are prescribed, it is important to be certain that the basic reproduction cycle of lamoids is understood. Caution in dosages of the hormones is important.

Discussion of therapy for metritis usually includes a list of antibiotics that have proven useful. Such a list would be inappropriate for lamoids, because no consistency of therapy has been established. Clinicians in different regions of North America are administering the antibiotics they use in mares or cows, and none of the data have been correlated to determine efficacy.

The trend is to minimize the use of uterine flushes with disinfectants or antimicrobials, but rather to use physiologic saline to thoroughly wash out all exudate. One of the newer therapeutic regimens is to flush the uterus as described and finish with a uterine infusion of llama plasma.

FERTILITY EXAMINATION OF THE MALE. A fertility examination should begin with a complete history and a thorough physical examination to identify problems that may preclude breeding, such as arthritis, or that may inhibit mounting and copulation. In the fertility examination, the use of a chart such as that illustrated in Table 17.5 will facilitate completeness. The individual should be identified by registration number (the number should be seen) or by color and markings.

An examination for breeding soundness varies somewhat according to the age of the animal and the reason for the examination. An examination for sale of a breeding male should encompass a complete set of parameters. The examination of a weanling or yearling as a potential breeding male must, of necessity, be limited. The examination of a male with identified or suspected fertility problems is complex.

Breeding males may also be examined for insurance purposes. The veterinarian must ascertain whether the insurance is for mortality only or if the client has contracted for breeding assurance, in which case much more detail is required in the way of examination and evaluation.

History is vital. Has the male bred previously? Has breeding resulted in living babies? Is he aggressive or shy? Is he intimidated by dominant females? What is the status of his libido? It would be desirable to see the male actually breeding a female, but most of the history must be obtained by judicious questioning of the owner. The owner may or may not have been able to determine whether or not the male has made penetration.

A thorough examination of the male reproductive organs should be conducted, including evaluation of the testicles for size and consistency. The testes should be measured. In Peru, studies demonstrated that male alpacas with normal-sized testicles (4.8 × 3.2 cm) produced 30% more offspring than males with small testicles (3 × 1.9 cm) (141).

The epididymis should be palpated. Measurements of the penis can be made only with the penis extruded from the prepuce. This requires tranquilization or anesthesia. Some information may be obtained by palpation through the skin. Rectal palpation should enable examination of the accessory sex glands.

Semen Collection (20, 41, 50, 80, 83, 151). A complete fertility examination must include semen evaluation. This is difficult in lamoids, since no method has been effective in collecting semen from every animal. Various techniques have been tried, both in Peru and in North America. Peruvian researchers have placed a sponge in the vagina of a receptive female. However, if semen deposition is actually through the cervix, this technique cannot be successful. They concluded that it was not useful.

Artificial vaginas have been employed to collect semen from stallions, bulls, rams, and alpaca males. Since males must be trained to use the dummy female, this method is applicable only for research projects.

Electroejaculation has been of limited effectiveness. The male must be sedated and even lightly anesthetized. Various types of ejaculators have been used. The exact power, pulse frequency, and duration needed have not been established. In the author's clinic, a variable-voltage bovine unit has been used, attached to a three-longitudinal electrode ram probe. Before proceeding, the feces should be removed from the rectum. The technician must be prepared to collect semen at this point and also when the probe is inserted, since either stimulation may cause premature ejaculation. It is most desirable to manually extrude the penis from the prepuce prior to any rectal stimulation, so that semen may be collected from the penis rather than from the prepuce.

Stimulation should begin with low power and pulses at 5-second intervals. As erection occurs, the power and duration of sustaining the pulse may be increased. Urine flow may complicate collection. The semen should be collected in warmed tubes (a number of tubes should be ready to collect different fractions). The semen should be handled and evaluated as for semen from other livestock species.

A less invasive method of semen collection has been borrowed from wildlife biologists, who have collected semen from other exotic species. The technique utilizes a human condom as an intravaginal sac. Not every male will cooperate and breed a female prepared for such a collection, but the method is being studied

Table 17.5. Llama reproduction examination—male

Identification Date ________

Name ________ Age ________ Owner ________

ISIS No. ________, Llama Registry No. ________

Color

Body ________ Neck ________

Head ________ Legs ________

History

Born at present ranch—yes ________, no ________

Age at time of purchase ________

Pastured or housed alone—yes ________, no ________

Number and sex of other animals in the group ________

History	Prior to purchase	After purchase
Number of crias sired	1, 2, 3, 4, 5, +	1, 2, 3, 4, 5, +
Number of females bred	1, 2, 3, 4, 5, +	1, 2, 3, 4, 5, +
Age at time of first breeding	1, 2, 3, 4, 5	1, 2, 3, 4, 5

Physical examination

General body condition Good ________, thin ________, fat ________

Conformation faults ________

Testicles ________

Right ________ × ________ × ________ cm

Left ________ × ________ × ________ cm

Consistency ________ firm ________ soft ________ hard ________

Nodules ________ Other ________

Epididymus ________

Abnormalities ________ Cryptorchid—yes ________ no ________

Penis

Length ________ cm, diameter ________ mm

Abnormalities

Preputial adhesions ________, curvature ________

Semen evaluation

Volume ________ ml, color ________

pH ________, density ________

Concentration ________ million/ml

Motility ________

Live/dead ________%

Abnormal forms ________

Behavior

Hand reared—yes ________, no ________

Aggressive to people—yes ________, no ________

Precopulatory behavior

Aggressive ________, timid ________

Copulatory behavior

Proper position—yes ________, no ________

Penetration—yes ________, no ________

and shows promise to be the most efficient and least invasive of the available methods of semen collection in llamas and alpacas (80).

Items required to carry out this method of semen collection include a condom (select one that is nonspermacidal, nonlubricated, and has a reservoir tip); rubber sheeting of the type used as a dental dam; rubber cement (Weldwood); super glue; a plastic rod or tubing, 1 × 60 cm (3/8 × 24 in.); and stainless steel ball bearings, 1 cm (3/8 in.) in diameter.

The rubber sheeting should be cut into 15 cm (6 in.) squares, with a slit in the center about 4 cm long. The condom should be unrolled and pushed through the slit, then fixed to the rubber sheet with rubber cement and allowed to dry thoroughly for an hour or so. A ball bearing is placed in the tip of the condom to aid in positioning and retention within the vagina. Likewise, the plastic rod is used to stretch the condom and aid in its insertion into the vagina. The condom should be rinsed with sterile physiologic saline just prior to insertion and then lubricated on the outside with a nonspermicidal lubricant.

The female is prepared by wrapping the tail and thoroughly cleaning and drying the perineal area. The condom should be inserted into the vagina until the rubber sheet lies against the vulva. The sheet should be glued to the perineum with spots of super glue at each corner. Following insertion, the plastic tube should be carefully removed. This can be facilitated if the tube is blown into to dilate the vagina and condom slightly during withdrawal. The opening into the condom should be lightly lubricated. Johnson recommends that the normal odors of the perineum be collected by wiping the perineum with a gauze sponge prior to gluing the sheet and condom in place and wiping the gauze over the sheet prior to the breeding.

A check should be made to ascertain that intromission is accomplished and to help the male direct the penis or shift position. Once the male has finished, the sheet may be gently pulled from the perineum and the apparatus carefully withdrawn.

Semen Evaluation. The semen of the llama is translucent to whitish crystalline in color and is quite viscous. The pH is neutral to slightly alkaline. It is difficult to evaluate semen volume, since ejaculation is prolonged and it cannot be determined when it is finished. Peruvian studies in the alpaca list volume ranges of 0.2–6.6 ml (41), but when semen is collected with an electroejaculator, the operator's persistence and continued collection of fluid from the accessory glands may increase the volume but lower the concentration of sperm.

The concentration of sperm in the semen is highly variable and cannot be used as a criterion for evaluating fertility (93). In the few cases where concentration of sperm has been determined, the range has been from 1000 to 255,000/μl. Using an artificial vagina with conditioned males, as much as 12.5 ml of semen has been collected, having a concentration of 600,000/μl.

The shape and size of the sperm have been detailed previously. Sperm morphology is a valid criterion for evaluation of fertility. Morphologic defects include coiled and bent tails, separated heads, proximal and distal cytoplasmic droplets, and acrosomal defects. Lamoid erythrocytes are ovoid and, if present in semen, may be confused with separated sperm heads since they are both about the same size. Statistics are unavailable on the desirable ratio of normal to abnormal sperm, but in a fertile male, 70% of the sperm should be normal (80).

The morphology of the sperm should be evaluated at 1000X. It may be necessary to dilute the semen to separate the sperm, which can be done during the staining process by mixing the sperm with a larger volume of stain A prior to making the smear. A variety of stains may be used (120, 124).

Evaluation of the motility of lamoid sperm in the viscid semen may be misleading. Lamoid spermatozoa are much slower than those of rams or bulls because of the thick seminal fluid. It is imperative that the semen be maintained at a constant temperature of 37°C from the time of collection until motility is evaluated, otherwise motility should not be considered in the fertility examination.

Llama semen has been successfully frozen in a glycerol–egg yolk buffer (74).

Male Infertility (25)

ETIOLOGY. Little investigation has been carried out to delineate the various causes of infertility in male lamoids. Congenital defects are some obvious causes and include such conditions as cryptorchidism, ectopic testicle, hypogonadism, persistent frenulum, prepucial adhesion, small penis, curvature of the penis, and intersex (137).

HYPERTHERMIA. Lamoids evolved in cool to cold climates and are adapted to such conditions. They are not heat tolerant and have not developed mechanisms to deal with excess heat, unlike their camel kin. When kept in hot, humid climates, especially if unshorn as they usually are in North America, body temperatures may elevate to 40.5°C (105°F). No specific studies have been conducted, but breeders have reported that some males are not fertile during the hot summer months.

Similar problems may develop in males that are febrile from an infectious disease or that are recumbent for prolonged periods from injury. The ventrum of lamoids is the thermal window, and a recumbent animal has no way to readily dissipate heat.

HYDROCELE. See Chapter 6 for a discussion of this condition. The author has seen two llamas with scrotal hydrocele. In one case, the cause was an abscess at the external inguinal ring, obstructing fluid flow into the peritoneal cavity. In the other case, the etiology was not determined. Sterile, normal fluid was contained between the visceral and parietal tunics. There was no evidence of an inflammatory response. Ultrasonic examination confirmed the presence of nonpurulent fluid.

Surgery (a type used in human males for hydrocele) was performed on one llama. Strict surgical asepsis was maintained. The tunica vaginalis communis was incised and folded off the testicle. Excess tunic was removed, and the tunic was then sutured back to itself behind the epididymis. Thus the tunic sac was obliterated, and any fluid produced was absorbed from the scrotal subcutaneous tissue and drained via the scrotal veins. The scrotal skin was closed with simple interrupted sutures. This male died of other complications before any benefits of the surgery could be evaluated.

TRAUMA. The prepuce, scrotum, and testicles may be traumatized during aggressive intermale encounters. The wounds should be managed as are any other lacerations (see Chap. 6). Unattended lacerations of the prepuce may result in posthitis and, ultimately, stenosis and phimosis (inability to extrude the penis).

A previously successful breeding male began to fail to complete copulation. He chased the females and assumed his usual breeding position, but at the time intromission should have occurred, progress stopped and he arose and left. Upon examination, it was observed that a stricture prevented full extension of the penis. Attempts to forcibly extrude the penis elicited a pain response, even though the llama was sedated. This male exhibited a strong libido, but as erection had become painful, he simply quit.

Another source of trauma to the penis is entangling fibers from the female's perineal region. North American llama owners are reluctant to clip fleece from their animals, but the perineal area of all breeding females should be clipped sufficiently to preclude fibers from obstructing copulatory efforts. One or two caught fibers may lacerate the glans and cause balanitis. If fibers wrap around the glans and become twisted, ischemic necrosis may occur.

Prepubertal adhesions may persist into adulthood. Stenoses of the prepuce are serious impediments to successful breeding; surgical correction is usually necessary. Standard techniques used on bulls have been successfully employed in llamas and may include multiple triangular release reconstruction surgery or removal of circumferential collar and resuturing of the preputial mucosa. Infectious diseases of the male reproductive system are either rare or have not been reported. Brucellosis, *Brucella melitensis,* has been reported in South America but not in North America. Trichomoniasis and campylobacteriosis are unknown. No specific abscesses have been observed in the testicle. Infections are frequently a sequel to lacerations and severe contusions.

HORMONAL DEFICIENCIES. Hypogonadism is likely to result in low levels of testosterone, but little is known about normal levels in male lamoids. Certainly, some males lack libido, but whether this is caused by a hormonal defect or is a behavioral defect is unknown.

BEHAVIORAL ABNORMALITIES. Males may be overly timid or hyperaggressive. Such behaviors may be inherited, as in other livestock species, or may be developed. A young male, just starting to breed, may be intimidated by an aggressive female. The major known behavioral anomaly is that of the human-imprinted (rogue) male (see Chap. 3). Such behavior does not make the male infertile, but it may preclude his usefulness as a breeding male because of the danger to humans who must handle him.

REFERENCES

1. Acosta, R. L. 1960a. (Induction of follicular growth and ovulation in young alpacas) Induccion del crecimiento folicular y de la ovulacion en alpacas jovenes. B.S. tesis, Fac. Med. Vet. Univ. Nac. Mayor San Marcos (Lima).

2. ______. 1960b. (Induction of follicular growth and ovulation in young alpacas) Induccion del crecimiento folicular ye de la ovulacion en alpacas jovenes (sum). Vet. Zootec. (Lima) 12(32):10.

3. Asdell, S. A. 1946. Patterns of Mammalian Reproduction. Ithaca, N.Y.: Comstock.

4. Baptidanova, Y. P., et al. 1975. Comparative morphology of the intrauterine development in Tylopoda and Artiodactyla-Ruminantia. Z. Obsch. Biol. 36(5):664–69.

5. Benirschke, K. 1967. Sterility and fertility of interspecific mammalian hybrids. In K. Benirschke, ed. Comparative Aspects of Reproductive Failure. New York: Springer, pp. 218–34.

6. Brandt, J. F. 1841. (Report on the knowledge of the morphology of the female organs of llamas) Beitraege zur Kenntnis des Baues der inneren Weichteile des Lamas. Mem. Acad. Sci. (St. Petersburg) 6:1–78.

7. Bravo, W. M., and Sumar, J. K. 1981. (Fetal growth

in alpacas) Desarralo fetal de la alpaca. Proc. 4th Conv. Int. Camelidos Sudam., Punte Arenas, Chile, pp. 14–15.

8. ______. 1984. Some anatomical parameters of the reproductive tract in alpacas. Resumenes Invest., Univ. Nac. Mayor San Marcos (Lima).

9. ______. 1985a. (Factors affecting fertility in alpacas) Factores que determinar fertilidad en alpacas. Proc. 5th Conv. Int. Camelidos Sudam., Cuzco, Peru, p. 4.

10. ______. 1985b. (Ovarian follicular activity in the alpaca) Actividad folicular del ovario de la alpaca. Proc. 5th Conv. Int. Camelidos Sudam., Cuzco, Peru, p. 7.

11. Brenea P., L. E. 1956. (Contributions to the bacterial study of infectious diseases of alpacas) Contribucion al estudio bacteriologico de los enfermedades infecciosas de los alpacas (metritis, mastitis). B.S. tesis, Fac. Med. Vet. Univ. Nac. Mayor San Marcos (Lima).

12. Brown, C. E. 1936. Rearing wild animals in captivity, and gestation periods. J. Mammal. 17:10–13.

13. Bucher, F. 1968. (Care and breeding of vicuña in the Zurich zoo) Haltung und Zucht von Vikunjas (*Vicugna vicugna*) im Zuericher Zoo. Zool. Gart. 36:153–59.

14. Bustinza M., J. 1961. (Macro and microscopic study of the placentation of the alpaca) Estudio macro y microscopico de la placentacion de la alpaca *Lama pacos*. B.S. tesis, Fac. Med. Vet. Univ. Nac. Mayor San Marcos (Lima).

15. Bustinza M., J., Gallegos, M., and Santos, M. A. 1970a. (Observations on the delivery of alpaca) Observaciones del parto de alpaca. Proc. 1st Conv. Camelidos Sudam. (Auquenidos), Puno, Peru, pp. 153–55.

16. Bustinza M., J., Matusita, A., and Gallegos, M. 1970b. (Contribution to the embryologic pattern of the alpaca) Contribucion al patron embriologico de la alpaca. Proc. 1st Conv. Camelidos Sudam. (Auquenidos), Puno, Peru, pp. 148–49.

17. ______. 1970c. (Multiple gestation in alpacas) La gestacion multiple en las alpacas. Proc. 1st Conv. Camelidos Sudam. (Auquenidos), Puno, Peru, pp. 150–52.

18. Caballero V., E. C. 1968. (Arterial system of the genital organs of the female alpaca) Sistema arterial de los organos genitales de la alpaca hembra. B.S. tesis, Fac. Med. Vet. Univ. Nac. Mayor San Marcos (Lima).

19. Calderon, W. 1968. (Diagnosis of pregnancy by rectal palpation in alpacas) Diagnostico de prenez por el metodo de palpacion rectal en alpacas. Bol. Extraordinario 3:35–39.

20. Calderon, W., Sumar, K., and Franco E. 1965. (Advances in the artificial insemination of alpacas) Advances en la inseminacion artifical de las alpacas. Rev. Fac. Med. Vet. (Lima) 22:19–35.

21. Calderon, W., Novoa, C., and Franco, E. 1970. (Examination of the alpaca for pregnancy) Examen de la prenez en la alpaca. Bol. Extraordinario 4:43–48.

22. Calle Escobar, R. 1972. (Breeding and improvement of alpacas) Crianza y mejoramiento de alpacas. Peru Minist. Agric. Univ. Nac. Agrar. Bol. 19:1–66.

23. Campos Grace, K. 1965. (Comparative study of the vaginal cytology in alpacas with actual and false pregnancy) Estudio comparativo de la imagen citologia vaginal en alpacas con prenez verdadera y pseudo prenez. B.S. tesis, Fac. Med. Vet. Univ. Nac. Mayor San Marcos (Lima) pp. 1–48.

24. Cardozo, A. 1967. (Preliminary information on anestrus in llamas) Informe preliminar sobre anestro en llamas. Segundas J. Agron., La Paz, Bolivia, pp. 1–9.

25. Carreras, M., and Pacheco, E. 1970. (Testicular biopsy in alpacas) Biopsia testicular en alpacas. Proc. 1st Conv. Camelidos Sudam. (Auquenidos), Puno, Peru, pp. 101–3.

26. Casas P., H. 1962. (Histologic aspects of the testicle of the alpaca) Aspectos histologicos del testiculo de la alpaca, *Lama pacos*. B.S. tesis, Fac. Med. Vet. Univ. Nac. Mayor San Marcos (Lima), pp. 1–21.

27. Casas P., J. H., San Martin, F. M., and Copaira, A. M. 1963–66. (Histological aspects of the testicle of the alpaca) Aspectos histologicos del testiculo de la alpaca, *Lama pacos*. Rev. Fac. Med. Vet. (Lima) 18–20:223–38.

28. Cevallos, E., and Montalvo, C. 1983. (Histology of the placenta of the alpaca) Histologia de la placenta de la alpaca. Resumenes Proyectos Invest. Realizados (Lima) 1:22–23.

29. Chaman, E. 1960. (Vaginal cytology before/after ovulation in alpacas in heat) Imagen citologia vaginal antes y despues de la ovulacion en las alpacas en celo. B.S. tesis, Fac. Med. Vet. Univ. Nac. Mayor San Marcos (Lima), pp. 1–31.

30. ______. 1960b. (Vaginal cytology before and after ovulation in alpacas in heat) Imagen citologia vaginal antes y despues de la ovulacion en las alpacas en celo (sum). Vet. Zootec. 12(32):13.

31. Collazos V., G. D. 1972. (Study of the superficial drainage of the penis and prepuce of the alpaca) Estudio de la irrigacion superficial del pene y prepucio de la alpaca, *Lama pacos*. B.S. tesis, Fac. Med. Vet. Univ. Nac. Mayor San Marcos (Lima), pp. 1–20.

32. Condorena, N., and Fernandez-Baca, S. 1972. (Relation between frequency of services and fertility in the alpaca) Relacion entre frecuencia de servicos y fertilidad en la alpaca. Rev. Invest. Agropecu. 1(1):11–19.

33. Condorena, N., and Franco, L. E. 1970. (Sexual behavior in the alpaca with controlled breeding of 24 hours) Conducta sexual de la alpaca en empadres controlados de 24 horas. Bol. Extraordinario 4:49–52.

34. Condorena, A. N., and Velasco, N. J. 1978. (Comparison of two mating systems in the alpaca) Comparacion de dos sistemas de empadre en la alpaca. Mem. Asoc. Latinoam. Prod. Anim. 13:159–60.

35. Delhon, G., Zuckerberg, C., von Lawzewitsch, I., Larrieu, E., Oporto, R., and Bigaztti, R. 1983. (Cytological study of the testicle of the guanaco) Estudio citologico de las gonadas de guanaco *Lama guanicoe*, macho, en las estudios prepuperales, sexualmente maduros y seniles. Rev. Fac. Cienc. Vet. 1(1):47–60.

36. Drost, M. 1986. Elective termination of pregnancy. In J. Howard, ed. Current Veterinary Therapy: Food Animal Practice, 2nd ed. Philadlephia: W. B. Saunders, pp. 797–98.

37. England, B. G., Cardozo, A. G., and Foote, W. C. 1969a. A review of the physiology of reproduction in the New World camelidae. Int. Zoo Yearb. 9:104–10.

38. England, B. G., Foote, W. C., Matthews, D. H.,

Cardozo, A. G., and Rira, S. 1969b. Ovulation and corpus luteum function in the llama, *Lama glama*. J. Endocrinol. 45:505–13.

39. England, B. G., Foote, W. C., Cardozo, A. G., Matthews, D. H., and Riera, S. 1971. Estrous and mating behavior in the llama (*Lama glama*). Anim. Behav. 19(4):722–26.

40. Engle, E. T. 1926. The copulation plug and accessory genital glands of mammals. J. Mammal. 7:119.

41. Fernandez-Baca, S. 1964. (Some considerations of methods of semen collection on alpacas) Algunas consideraciones sobre los metodos de coleccion del semen de la alpacas. An. 2nd Congr. Nac. Med. Vet. Zootec., Lima, Peru, pp. 188–90.

42. ______. 1966. (Artificial insemination in alpacas and vicuñas) Inseminacion artificial en alpacas y vicuñas. Bol. Extraordinario 1:104–5.

43. ______. 1967. (Some aspects of reproduction in the alpaca) Algunos aspectos de la reproduccion de la alpaca. Bol. Extraordinario 2:62–65.

44. ______. 1968. (Sexual behavior of the alpaca in breeding at Campo) Conducta sexual de la alpaca (*Lama pacos*) en Emparde a Campo. Mem. Asoc. Latinoam. Prod. Anim. Mex. 3:7–20.

45. ______. 1970a. Luteal function and the nature of reproductive failures in the alpaca. Ph.D. diss., Cornell Univ., pp. 1–173.

46. ______. 1970b. (Reproduction in the alpaca) La reproduccion en la alpaca. Proc. 1st Conv. Camelidos Sudam. (Auquenidos), Puno, Peru, pp. 139–43.

47. ______. 1970c. (Studies on reproduction in alpacas) Estudios sobre la reproduccion en la alpaca, *Lama pacos*. Bol. Extraordinario 4:33–42.

48. ______. 1971. (The alpaca—reproduction and breeding) La alpaca—reproduccion y crianza. Bol. Divulg. 7:1–41.

49. ______. 1972. Artificial insemination in the breeding of alpacas and vicuñas, Gainesville, Fl. 6th Conf. Anim. Prod. Health. FAO Work. Pap. 4.

50. Fernandez-Baca, S., and Calderon V., W. 1963–66. (Methods of collection of semen of the alpaca) Metodos de coleccion de semen de la alpaca. Rev. Fac. Med. Vet. (Lima) 18–20:13–26.

51. Fernandez-Baca, S., and Novoa, C. 1969. (First trial of artificial insemination in alpaca with vicuña semen) Primeraensayo de inseminacion artificial en alpacas, *Lama pacos* con semen de vicuña, *Vicugna vicugna*. Rev. Fac. Med. Vet. (Lima) 22:9–18.

52. Fernandez-Baca, S., Gallegos, M., Novoa, C., and Moro, M. 1968. (Some aspects that should be considered to increase the fertility in the alpaca) Aspectos que deben tomarse en cuenia para incrementar la fertilidad de las alpacas. Bol. Extraordinario 3:42–45.

53. Fernandez-Baca, S. E., Hansel, W., and Novoa, C. 1970a. Corpus luteum function in the alpaca. Biol. Reprod. 3(2):252–61.

54. ______. 1970b. Embryonic mortality in the alpaca. Biol. Reprod. 3(2):243–51.

55. Fernandez-Baca, S. E., Madden, D. H., and Novoa, C. 1970c. Effect of different mating stimuli on induction of ovulation in the alpaca. J. Reprod. Fertil. 22(2):261–67.

56. Fernandez-Baca, S., Novoa, C., and Sumar J. 1971. (Seasonal variations in reproduction of alpacas) Variaciones estationales de la reproduction en la alpaca. Mem. Asoc. Latinoam. Prod. Anim. 6:158.

57. ______. 1972a. (Reproductive activity in the alpaca maintained separate from the male) Actividad reproductiva en la alpaca mantenida enseparacion del macho. Mem. Asoc. Latinoam. Prod. Anim. 7:7–18.

58. Fernandez-Baca, S., Sumar, J., and Novoa, C. 1972b. (Male sexual behavior when females are changed) Comportamiento sexual de la alpaca macho frente a la renovacion de las hembras. Rev. Invest. Pecu. 1(2):115–28.

59. Fernandez-Baca S., Sumar, J., Novoa, C., and Leyva, V. 1973a. Localization of the corpus luteum and the location of the embryo in the alpaca) Localizacion del cuerpo luteo y la ubicacion del embrion en la alpaca. Cuarta, Reun. Latinoam. Prod. Anim., Guadalajara, Mexico, G-55, pp. 15–19.

60. ______. 1973b. (Relationship between the location of the corpus luteum and that of the embryo in the alpaca) Relacion entre le ubicacion del cuerpos luteo y la localizacion del embrion en la alpaca. Rev. Invest. Pecu. 2(2):131–35.

61. Fernandez-Baca, S., Novoa, C., Sumar, J., Condorena, N., Leyva, V., and Franco, E. 1974. (Reproduction systems of alpacas) Sistema de empadre de las alpacas. Bol. Divulg. 15:129–38.

62. Fernandez-Baca, S., Sumar, J., and Novoa, C. 1976. (Functional activity of the ovary and uterine horn in alpacas) Actividad funcional del ovario y cuerno uterino en la alpaca. Mem. Asoc. Latinoam. Prod. Anim. 11:70.

63. Fernandez-Baca, S., Hansel, W., Saatman, R., Sumar, J., and Novoa, C. 1979. Differential luteolytic effects of right and left uterine horns in the alpaca. Biol. Reprod. 20(3):586–95.

64. Flores F., R. F. 1970. (Histologic study of the testicle of alpacas with apparent inability to reproduce) Estudio histologico del testiculo de alpacas aparentemente inaptas para la reproduccion. B.S. tesis, Fac. Med. Vet. Univ. Nac. Mayor San Marcos (Lima), pp. 1–29.

65. Foote, W. C. 1982. Determination of pregnancy in the llama—progesterone analysis. Llama World 1(2):18.

66. Foote, W. C., and Cardoza, A. 1968. (Ovarian function and uterine involution in the llama) Funcion ovarica y uterina (involucion) en la llama, *Lama glama*. Mem. Segunda Asoc. Latinoam. Prod. Anim., Lima, Peru 3:186.

67. Foote, W. C., England, B. G., and Wilde, M. E. 1968. Llama reproduction: A South American problem. Utah Sci. 29(2):43–45.

68. Fowler, M. E., and Olander, H. 1988. The fetal membranes of the llama, *Lama glama*. J. Am. Vet. Med. Assoc. (Submitted)

69. Franco E., L. L., Sumar, J. K., and Varela, M. H. 1981. (Ejaculation of the alpaca) Ejaculacion en alpacas. Proc. 4th Conv. Int. Camelidos Sudam., Punte Arenas, Chile, p. 4.

70. Francoeur, R. T. 1972. Artificial insemination for

species in danger (buffalo, alpaca, antelopes). Oryx 11(5):364–66.

71. Franklin, W. L. 1982. Biology, ecology and relationship to man of the South American camelids. In M. A. Mares and H. H. Genoways, eds. Mammalian Biology in South America. Linesville, Pa.: Pymatuning Laboratory of Ecology, Univ. of Pittsburgh Spec. Publ. 6, pp. 457–89.

72. Fuertes, Q. J. 1961. (Formation of the corpus luteum and observation on the endometrium of young alpacas during the first days of pregnancy) Formacion del cuerpo luteo y algunas observaciones en el endometrio de alpacas jovenes durante los primeros dias de la gestacion. B.S. tesis, Fac. Med. Vet. Univ. Nac. Mayor San Marcos (Lima), pp. 1–37.

73. Gonzalez, S. 1968. (Fertility of alpacas on a ranch in the department of Puno according to age) Fertilidad de las alpacas de una hacienda del departamento de Puno de acuendo con la edad. Bol. Extraordinario 3:40.

74. Graham, E. F., Schmell, M. K. L., Eversen, B. K., and Nelson, D. S. 1978. Semen preservation in nondomestic mammals. Symp. Zool. Soc. Lond. 43:153–73.

75. Guildbride, P. D. L., and Moro, M. 1965. Mating behavior in alpacas. Q. Rev. Vet. Inst. Trop. High Altitude Res. (Oct–Dec):8.

76. Hamerton, A. E. 1941. Report on the deaths occurring in the society's gardens during 1939–40. Proc. Zool. Soc. Lond. 111:151.

77. Harrison, R. M., and Wildt, D. E., eds. 1980. Animal Laparoscopy. Baltimore: Williams & Wilkins.

78. Iniquez, R. L. 1969. (Length of life of the corpus luteum and its influence in the reproductive canal) Largo de vida del cuerpos luteo y su influencia en al canal reproductivio. B.S. tesis, Fac. Cienc. Agon., Univ. Mayor San Simon, Cochabamba, Bolivia, pp. 1–54.

79. Iniquez, R. L., and Cardozo, A. 1968. (Length of life of the corpus luteum in llamas and its influence on the reproductive canal) Largo de vida del cuerpos luteo en llamas y su influencia en el canal reproductivo. Mem. Segunda Asoc. Latinoam. Prod. Anim., Lima, Peru 3:186.

80. Johnson, L. 1988. Semen collection. In Llama Reproduction. Proc. South American Camelid short course, Colorado State Univ., p. 14.

81. Kenneth, J. H. 1947. Gestation periods. Edinburgh Imp. Bur. Anim. Breed. Genet.

82. Kraft, H. 1968. (Birth of a llama and eclampsia of the newborn) Geburt eines Lamas und Eklampsie des Neugeborenen. Berl. Munch. Tieraerztl. Wochenschr. 13:228–29.

83. Kubicek, J. 1974. (Semen collection in the alpaca through a urethral fistula) Samenentnahme beim Alpaka durch eine Harnrohrenfistel. Z. Tierz. Zuechtungsbiol. 90(4):335–51.

84. de Lamo, D. A., and Defosse, A. 1984. (Anesthesia for prolonged surgical intervention of guanacos in captivity) Anestesia para intervenciones quirurgicos prolongados de guanacos en captividad. Vet. Argent. 1:44–47.

85. Lang, E. M. 1945. (Embryotomy in a guanaco in a zoo) Geburtshilfe im Zoologischen Garten. Zool. Gart. 14:29–32.

86. Lantz, R. K., and Kerstetter, H. 1983. Female progesterone—important indicator. 3 L llama (18):13–14.

87. Larrieu, E. J., Oporto, N. R., and Bigatti, R. O. 1984. (Reproduction of South American camelids in Argentina) La Reproduccion de los camelidos Sudamericanos en Argentina. Vet. Argent. 1(9):875–80.

88. Larrieu, E. J., Bigatti, R. O., and Oporto, N. R. 1985. (Sanitary aspects of South American camelids in Argentina) Sanidad en camelidos Sudamericanos en Argentina. Vet. Argent. 2(20):931–34.

89. Leupold, J. 1967. The new world tylopoda: Guanaco, alpaca, and llama breeding. DTW 74(16):414–17. German

90. Levina, M. V. 1960. A type of adaptive variability in the amniotic epithelium of certain mammals (alpaca). Biol. Sci. [Transl.] 120:990–92.

91. Leyva, W., and Sumar, J. 1981. (Evaluation of body weight to breeding and about the reproductive capacity of female alpacas at one year of age) Evaluacion del peso corporal al empadre sobre la capacidad reproductiva de hembras alpacas de un ano de edad. Proc. 4th Conv. Int. Camelidos Sudam., Punta Arenas, Chile.

92. McIntosh, W. C. 1930. General notes on the anatomy of the female llama. Anatomy (Lond.) 1(64):353–62.

93. Merilan, C. P., Sikes, J. D., Read, B. W., Boever, W. J., and Knox, D. 1979. Comparative characteristics of spermatoza and semen from a Bactrian camel, dromedary camel and llama. J. Zoo Anim. Med. 10:22–25.

94. Meschia, G., et al. 1960. Observations on the oxygen supply to the foetal llama. Q. J. Exp. Physiol. 45(3):284–91.

95. Milligan, S. R. 1982. Induced ovulation in mammals. Oxf. Rev. Reprod. Biol. 4:1–46.

96. Mogrovejo, S. D. 1952. (Studies of the semen of the alpaca) Estudios del semen de la alpaca. B.S. tesis, Fac. Med. Vet. Univ. Nac. Mayor San Marcos (Lima).

97. Moro, S. M., and Samame, H. 1964. (Microbiologic aspects in the infertility of alpacas) Aspectos microbiologicos en la infertilidad de las alpacas. An. 2nd Congr. Nac. Vet. Zootec., Lima, pp. 190–91.

98. Morton, W. R. M. 1960. The full-term fetal membranes of some camelidae. Anat. Rec. 136:247.

99. ______. 1961. Observations on the full-term foetal membranes of three members of the camelidae. J. Anat. 95(2):200–209.

100. Musa, B. E. 1977. A new epidermal membrane associated with the foetus of the camel, *Camelus dromedarius.* Zentralbl. Veterinaermed. Anat. Histol. Embryol. 6:355–58.

101. Musa, B. E., and Abu Sineina, M. E. 1976. Studies on the allantoic fluids of the camel, *Camelus dromedarius.* Acta Vet. (Beograd.) 26(3):107–14.

102. Navarro A., L. F. 1971. (Study of the peripheral spinal innervation of the external genitalia of the male alpaca) Estudio de la inervacion espinal periferica de los genitales externos de la alpaca macho *Lama pacos.* B.S. tesis, Fac. Med. Vet. Univ. Nac. Mayor San Marcos (Lima), pp. 1–27.

103. Neuville, E., and Neuville, H. 1914. (The penis and its glands in llamas and dromedary) Du penis et du gland du lama et du dromedaire. C.R. Soc. Biol. (Seance).

104. Novoa, C. 1967. Reproduction in camelidae. M.S.

thesis, College of North Wales, Bangor.

105. ______. 1970. Reproduction in camelidae—A review. J. Reprod. Fertil. 22:3–20.

106. Novoa, C. A., and Sumar, J. 1958. (In vivo collection of ova and tests on embryo transfer in alpacas) Coleccion de huevos in vivo y ensayos de transferencia en alpacas. Bol. Extraordinario 3:31–34.

107. Novoa, C., Sumar, J., and Franco, E. 1970. (Complementary mating of female alpacas) Empadre complementario de hembras alpacas vacias. Bol. Extraordinario 4:53–59.

108. Novoa, C., Fernandez-Baca, S., Sumar, J., and Leyva, V. 1972. (Puberty in alpacas) Pubertad en la alpaca. Rev. Invest. Pecu. 1(1):29–35.

109. Novoa, C., Sumar, J., Leyva, V., and Fernandez-Baca, S. 1973. (Increased reproduction in alpacas in commercial operations with the method of alternate use of males in breeding) Incremento reproductivo en alpacas de explotaciones comerciales mediante metodo de empadre alternado. Rev. Invest. Pecu. 2(2):191–93.

110. Pacheco Ibanez, O. 1968. (Testicular biopsy in alpacas) Biopsia testicular en alpacas. B.S. tesis, Fac. Med. Vet. Univ. Nac. Tec. Altiplano (Puno), pp. 1–54.

111. Padedes Laos, J. 1965. (Effects of equine chorionic gonadotrophins on the uterus of young alpacas) Efectos de la gonadotropina serica equina sobre los uteros de alpacas jovenes. B.S. tesis, Fac. Med. Vet. Univ. Nac. Mayor San Marcos (Lima), pp. 1–35.

112. Palomino M., H. 1962. (Spermogram and sperm dimensions in the alpaca) Espermogram y dimensiones de los espermatozoides de la alpaca. B.S. tesis, Fac. Med. Vet. Univ. Nac. Mayor San Marcos (Lima).

113. Palomino M., H., and Torres R., D. 1968. (Microscopic and macroscopic aspects of the ovary and uterus of alpacas during the 8–44 days of gestation) Aspectos macro y microscopico del ovario y utero de alpacas durante la gestacion 8–44 dia. Rev. Fac. Med. Vet. (Lima) 22:36–53.

114. Patterson, K. 1982. Dystocia. Llama World 1(1):4–7.

115. Powers, B. 1987. Uterine biopsy in llamas. Proc. South American Camelid short course, Colorado State Univ.

116. Prystowsky, H. 1960. In C. A. Villee, ed. The Placenta and Fetal Membranes. Baltimore: Williams & Wilkins, pp. 1–159.

117. Raedeke, K. 1977. The reproductive ecology of guanaco (*Lama guanicoe*) in Southern Chile. Proc. 57th Annu. Meet. Am. Soc. Mammal., Michigan State Univ.

118. Ramos R., M. A. 1975. (Serum testosterone levels in male alpacas at sea level) Niveles de testosterona serica en alpacas machos al nivel del mar. B.S. tesis, Fac. Med. Vet. Univ. Nac. Mayor San Marcos (Lima).

119. Ritscher, D., Linke, K., Carlt, D., and Shroeder, K. 1977. (Report on dystocia in zoo animals) Beitrag zur Geburthshilfe bei Zootieren. Int. Symp. Erkr. Zootiere 19:371–81.

120. Roberts, S. J. 1971. Veterinary Obstetrics and Genital Disease, 3rd ed. Ithaca, N.Y.: Published by author.

121. Rode, P. 1936. (Duration of gestation in wild mammals after C. E. Brown, comparison with results of G. Jennsion) Les Durees de gestation des mammiferes sauvages d'apres C.E. Brown, Comparison avec les resultats de G. Jennison. Mammalia 1:26–28.

122. Rodriquez, R. 1959. (Ovulation in alpacas) Ovulacion en las alpacas. B.S. tesis, Fac. Med. Vet. Univ. Nac. Mayor San Marcos (Lima), pp. 1–21.

123. ______. 1959. (Ovulation in alpacas) Ovulacion en las alpacas (sum) Vet. Zootec. 11(28):17.

124. Rosenberg, G., ed. 1979. Clinical Examination of Cattle. (English ed. transl. by Roy Mack). Berlin: Paul Parey.

125. Ruiz, R. L. 1970. (Testicular biopsy in alpacas using the Vim-Silverman biopsy needle) Biopsia testicular en alpaca mediante el uso de la aguja de Vim-Silverman. B.S. tesis, Fac. Med. Vet. Univ. Nac. Mayor San Marcos (Lima), pp. 1–22.

126. Sambraus, H. H. 1975. (Choice of a sexual partner in male domestic livestock) Sexual Partnerwahl mannlicher Haustiere. Tieraerztl. Umschau 30(11):535–43.

127. San Martin, M. 1962. (Physiology of reproduction of alpacas) Fisiologia de la reproduccion de las alpacas. Symp. Probl. Ganad. Peru, Ind. Grafica, pp. 113–21.

128. San Martin, M., Vega, E., and Gonzalez, S. C. 1960. (Mitogenic activity and primordial states of oogenesis in the ovary of alpacas. Possible primary or secondary gonadotrophins) Actividad mitogenica y estadios precoces de la oogenesis en el ovario de alpacas. Posibles efectos primarios o secundarios de las gonadatropinas. Rev. Fac. Med. Vet. (Lima) 15:3–16.

129. San Martin, M., Copaira, M., Zuniga, J., Rodriquez, R., Bustinza, G., and Acosta, L. 1968. Aspects of reproduction in the alpaca, *Lama pacos*. J. Reprod. Fertil. 16(3):395–99.

130. Sato S., A., Valencia L., R. A., and Montoya O., L. 1986. (Anatomic revision of the reproductive apparatus of the alpaca female) Revision anatomica del aparato reproductor de la alpaca hembra (*Lama pacos*). Rev. Camelidos Sudam. 2:26–29.

131. Schmidt, C. R. 1973. Breeding season and notes on some other aspects of reproduction in captive camelids. Int. Zoo Yearb. 13:387–90.

132. Silva, C. H. 1960. (Vaginal cytology pre and post-ovulation in alpacas in heat) Imagen citologia vaginal antes y despues de la ovulacion en las alpacas en celo. B.S. tesis, Fac. Med. Vet. Univ. Nac. Mayor San Marcos (Lima).

133. Steklenev, E. P. 1968. (Anatomical morphological characters and physiology functions of the oviducts in the genera *Lama* and *Camelus*). 4th Congr. Reprod. Artif. Insemination, Paris.

134. ______. 1968. Anatomic morphological peculiarities of the structure and physiological function of fallopian tubes of camelids. An. 6th Int. Congr. Reprod. Artif. Insemination, Inst. Nat. Rech. Agron. 1:71–74.

135. Steven, D. H., Burton, G. J., Sumar, J., and Nathaniels, P. W. 1980. Ultrastructural observations on the placenta of the alpaca, *Lama pacos*. Placenta 1(1):21–32.

136. Sumar, J. 1980. (Twins in the alpaca) Gestacion gemelar en la alpaca. Rev. Invest. Pecu. 5(1):58–60.

137. ______. 1983. Studies on reproductive pathology in alpacas. Dep. Obstetrics Gynaecology, Fac. Vet. Med., Uppsala, Sweden.

138. ______. 1984. (Reproductive physiology of the al-

paca) Fisiologia reproductiva de la alpaca. Bol. Cient. (La-Raya) 1.

139. ______. 1985a. Reproductive physiology in South American camelids. In R. B. Land and D. E. Robinson, eds. Genetics of Reproduction in Sheep. London: Butterworth.

140. ______. 1985b. (Some aspects of obstetrics of the alpaca) Algunos aspectos obstetricos de la alpaca. Bol. Tec. 2.

141. Sumar, J., and Bravo, W. 1986. Fertility of female alpacas based on the size of testicles of breeding males. 7th Annu. Rep. CRSP, Univ. of California, Davis.

142. Sumar, J., and Leyva, V. 1981. (Role of the corpus luteum in the maintenance of pregnancy in the alpaca) Rol del cuerpo luteo en el mantenimiento de la prenez en la alpaca. Proc. 4th Conv. Int. Camelidos Sudam., Punto Arenas, Chile.

143. Sumar, J., Novoa, C., and Fernandez-Baca, S. 1972. (Reproductive physiology, postpartum in the alpaca) Fisiologia reproductiva post-partum en la alpaca. Rev. Invest. Pecu. 1(1):21–27.

144. Sumar, J., Bravo, W., and Leyva, V. 1981. (Endoscopy in alpacas and llamas) Observacions de ovario in situ. Proc. 4th Conv. Int. Camelidos Sudam., Punta Arenas, Chile.

145. Thibault, C. 1973. Sperm transport and storage in vertebrates. J. Reprod. Fertil. [Suppl.] 18:39–53.

146. Tillman, A. 1978. Twin llamas born alive. Llama Newsl. 1:3–4.

147. Torrey, S. 1978. Normal and abnormal deliveries. Llama Newsl. 1:3–4.

148. ______. 1980. Llama reproduction, some notes on the literature. Llama Newsl. 6:3–4.

149. Vander Vliet, W. L., and Hafez, E. S. E. 1974. Survival and aging of spermatozoa: A review. Am. J. Obstet. Gynecol. 118 (7):1006–15.

150. Vilca, L. M. A. 1975. (Endometrial alterations in alpacas in the first post service and its relation to the functionality of the corpus luteum) Alteraciones endometriales en alpacas, *Lama pacos* en el primer post servicio y su relacion con la funcionalidad del cuerpo luteo. B.S. tesis, Fac. Med. Vet. Univ. Nac. Mayor San Marcos (Lima).

151. Watson, P. F. 1978. A review of techniques of semen collection in mammals. Symp. Zool. Soc. Lond. 43:97–126.

152. Wiepz, D. W., and Chapman, R. J. 1985. Nonsurgical embryo transfer and live birth in a llama. Theriogenology 24:251–57.

18 Urinary System

ANATOMY

Kidney

The kidneys are nonlobulated, shaped like those of a sheep (11). Both kidneys are the same size (approximately 5 × 9 cm) and fixed in the dorsal abdominal area. The left kidney is located ventral to the transverse processes of the 5th to 7th lumbar vertebrae. The right kidney is located slightly more cranial, being beneath the 4th to 6th transverse processes of the lumbar vertebrae. Kidney weight varies from 120 to 170 g in llamas weighing from 74 to 120 kg (1).

Ureters and Bladder

These structures are not unique.

Urethra

The male urethra is described in Chapter 17. A dorsally situated urethral diverticulum at the ischial arch prevents passage of an urethral catheter into the bladder (8). The female urethra is large, with the external orifice located at the ventral border between the vagina and vulva. A ventral diverticulum at the external orifice makes female urethral catheterization difficult, but not impossible (see Chap. 4).

CHARACTERISTICS OF LAMOID URINE (1–5, 9, 10)

The urine of 138 alpacas maintained at an elevation of 4200 m was analyzed in Peru (Table 18.1) (2, 3). In general, there was insignificant variation with age, sex, or physiologic state except for ketones. Acetoacetic acid was detected in 42% of the nonpregnant alpacas and in 100% of the pregnant alpacas. Acetone was detected in only 2% of the nonpregnant alpacas but in 88% of the pregnant alpacas. The significance of urinary ketones is unknown, since no clinical ketosis has been reported in lamoids.

Urea is excreted by adult alpacas at 6.08 g/L urine (9). Urea excretion is slightly higher in young as compared to adult animals, and in pregnant animals, higher yet (10). In general, alpacas have higher rates of urea excretion than any other animal besides humans. The amount of ammonia excreted (0.13 g/L) does not vary with age or sex (9).

Urine collected from normal llamas in California had similar characteristics to that of the alpacas (Table

Table 18.1. Normal lamoid urinalysis

Parameters	Alpacas kept at 4200 m (n = 138)	Llamas kept at sea level (n = 15)
Volume (L/24 hr)	0.125–3.8 (1.06)	
Color	Clear, yellow-amber	Clear, light yellow-amber
Specific gravity	1.010–1.048 (1.021)	1.013–1.048 (1.023)
pH	Alkaline 94%, acidic 2%	7–8.5
Protein	Negative	Negative (12), 1+ (3)
Glucose	Negative	Negative (10), 1–3+ (5)
Ketones	50% positive 1+	Negative (6), trace – 1+ (9)
Urobilinogen	52% positive 1+	Negative (13), 2–3+ (2)
Bilirubinogen	45% positive 1+	Negative
Indican	45% positive	
Blood	Negative	Negative
Sediments	Triple phosphates common, ammonium urate rare	Calcium oxalate common in alkaline urine, uric acid rare

18.1). Table 18.2 provides data for selected urinary tract diseases.

DIAGNOSTIC PROCEDURES

Urinary tract diseases are diagnosed by a combination of clinical signs, urinalysis, serum biochemistry, hemogram, and special procedures such as renal angiography, radiography, ultrasonography, and cystoscopy in the female. An elevated serum urea nitrogen (SUN) level may simply be a reflection of anorexia and is seen as an ancillary finding in many sick llamas. An elevated SUN associated with an elevated creatinine is significant. Renal function tests as commonly used in dogs and cats are not employed in lamoids.

Urine may be collected as a free catch during urination at a communal dung heap, by urethral catheterization in the female, and by cystocentesis in both the female and the male by fixing the bladder per rectum and inserting a 10–15 cm (4–6 in.), 18 gauge needle on the midline just cranial to the pubis. The area is surgically prepared, and in the male the penis and prepuce are pushed laterally to allow the midline insertion of the needle.

Percutaneous renal biopsy may be accomplished by guiding the needle with ultrasonography or fluoroscopy.

URINATION BEHAVIOR

Lamoids are communal dung pile users for both defecation and urination. With stimulation to void, both male and female lamoids seek out a dung pile. At the approach, the animal will sniff the pile and, if satisfied, will turn around and assume a squatting position, with the hind legs spread apart and brought forward under the body. Defecation usually occurs first, followed immediately by urination. A llama or alpaca will usually urinate two to four times a day, but while carrying a heavy load in the wilderness may urinate only upon arising in the morning and again in the evening.

A llama may refuse to urinate while being transported. This must be considered when a llama is trailered into a clinic. If the bladder is distended with urine, any restraint method employing bands around the body may cause rupture of the bladder if the animal should struggle (see Chap. 6). Likewise, proceed with caution when conducting a rectal examination on an animal having a distended bladder; rupture of the bladder has occurred from application of too much pressure. A newly hospitalized llama may refuse to urinate or defecate for a few hours if on a concrete or wooden floor. The animal should be moved to a lawn or dirt area to give it a chance to void before concluding that there is oliguria or no passage of feces.

Dysuria is characterized by abnormal posture at the dung pile or by straining as if to urinate, but with urine dribbling or no urine flow. It may be difficult to differentiate dysuria from tenesmus.

DISEASES

Congenital renal agenesis and persistent urachus are discussed in Chapter 22. Urolithiasis and rupture of the bladder are discussed in Chapter 6 (7). Primary infectious diseases of the urinary system are discussed in Chapter 7 and include leptospirosis, clostridial diseases, anthrax, coccidioidomycosis, tuberculosis, and septicemia. There are no reported parasitic diseases of the lamoid urinary system.

The prevalence of primary nephrosis or nephritis is low in the author's practice, but other clinicians have reported this as a frequent cause of death. Secondary nephritis may be more common. Insufficient numbers of cases have been studied clinically and at necropsy to categorize nephritis (glomerulonephritis, interstitial nephritis, pyelonephritis), as is done in other species. Iatrogenic toxicity from the administration of gentamicin has accounted for the majority of primary nephrosis cases in the author's practice.

Table 18.2. Urinalysis in selected diseases

	Dehydration	Urinary tract hemorrhage	Chronic nephritis	Cystitis
Gross appearance	Clear	Clear	Clear	Cloudy to hemorrhagic
Specific gravity	↑	↑	↓	↑
Refractive index	↑ ±	↑	↓	↑
Protein	0	+1–4	+1–2	+1–4
Color	Yellowish-amber	Reddish	Yellowish	White to reddish
Glucose	0	+1	+1–2	0–+1
Ketones	0	0	0–+1	0
Cells	±	± RbC	0–+1	Neutrophils-epithelial
Bacteria	0	0	0–+1	++

Renal Failure

Reduced blood supply to the kidneys causes a prerenal failure. This usually occurs with peripheral hypotension, most often caused by shock. Damage to the glomeruli or tubules causes malfunction in varying degrees according to the insult the tissue sustains.

NEPHROSIS. Nephrosis is a degenerative disorder of either the glomeruli or tubules and may be caused by endotoxemia, renal ischemia, or nephrotoxic agents (oak tannins, oxalates, ethylene glycol, lead, arsenic, aminoglycoside antibiotics, myoglobin, hemoglobin). Renal ischemia is associated with shock and may be exacerbated by general anesthesia. In horses and dogs, surgical manipulation of the abdominal viscera results in a reflex decreased blood flow to the kidneys. A similar phenomenon may occur in lamoids. Partial or complete vascular occlusion to a segment of the intestine results in a buildup of endotoxins in the lumen. If the obstruction is corrected surgically, endotoxic shock and hypotension may occur as a result of the rapid absorption of endotoxins once circulation is restored. The animal may die from the direct effects of the shock or develop renal failure from renal ischemia.

Severe, prolonged dehydration, as may occur with diarrheal diseases, may predispose to ischemic nephrosis. Excessive quantities of myoglobin and hemoglobin in the urine produce degeneration of the kidney tubules. Myoglobinuria may be seen following crushing injuries or violent struggling or be associated with white muscle disease. Hematuria or hemoglobinuria may be observed in renal trauma (automobile accident), copper poisoning, blood transfusion reactions, severe burns, neoplasia, dicoumarol poisoning, urolithiasis, or urethral catheterization; or they may be associated with infectious diseases (cystitis, pyelonephritis, urethritis, prostatitis, septicemia).

NEPHRITIS. Inflammatory lesions of the kidneys are usually caused by infectious agents, which may produce focal or diffuse glomerulonephritis, interstitial nephritis, pyelonephritis, or embolic nephritis.

CLINICAL SIGNS OF RENAL FAILURE. Acute renal failure is characterized by oliguria or anuria if the urinary tract is obstructed. Early in the course of renal failure, the urine is highly concentrated. Later, there may be polyuria and polydypsia, with granular epithelial casts in the urine sediment. The urine may become acidic, with elevated levels of SUN and creatinine.

Some of the foregoing signs may be seen in chronic renal disease, accompanied by anorexia, weight loss, depression, straining, and mild anemia. A low-grade fever of 40–41°C (104–106°F) may be seen with suppurative nephritis. The urine may contain bacteria, leukocytes, blood, and elevated levels of protein. Concentration of the urine varies, as does the quantity of urine produced, but usually the concentration is low and the volume output is high.

Uremia is the terminal syndrome of renal failure and is characterized by anorexia, weight loss, depression, muscular weakness, muscular tremors, dyspnea, oliguria, albuminuria, hyperemic mucous membranes, uremic odor from the breath, tachycardia from dehydration, recumbency, coma, and death.

TREATMENT. Acute renal failure must be treated early and intensively to avoid permanent damage to the glomeruli and tubules. The animal must be carefully rehydrated to overcome renal hypotension, renal ischemia, and oliguria. Urine production should be monitored to assure that the kidneys are able to function. Furosemide (0.5–1 mg/kg) may be given intramuscularly twice daily to cause diuresis. However, furosemide will be ineffective if tubular nephrosis is severe. Any electrolyte imbalance must be corrected and administration of fluids continued until the animal is able to drink adequate quantities of water.

Appropriate parenteral antibiotics are indicated for infectious nephritis and may prevent secondary infection in nephrosis. Once the animal is stabilized and eating, protein intake should be minimized by offering grass hay.

Cystitis and Urethritis

Cystitis and urethritis are more common in the female because of a shorter urethra and the possibility of retrograde invasion by opportunistic bacteria. Cystitis and ureterolithiasis traumatize the mucous membrane, predisposing to infection. In one female llama with segmental agenesis of the vagina, repeated breeding by a male resulted in penetration of the urethra by the penis and traumatic urethritis. Bladder paresis and urine stagnation predispose to cystitis. One case of a tumor of the bladder has been reported to have caused cystitis.

CLINICAL SIGNS. Urination is painful and frequent, with only small quantities of urine produced. The urine may contain blood, leukocytes, bacteria, and excessive numbers of epithelial cells in the sediment.

DIAGNOSIS. Clinical signs and urinalysis usually suffice to confirm this diagnosis. Urine should be cultured and a sensitivity test performed.

TREATMENT. Diuresis and appropriate parenteral antibiotic therapy for 10–14 days are usually successful.

Obstruction of Urinary Tract

See Chapter 6.

Posthitis

Posthitis is an inflammation of the prepuce.

ETIOLOGY. No specific infectious diseases cause this condition in lamoids, as in sheep. Trauma, caused by biting during aggressive male interaction, is the usual cause. The laceration may be minimal or severe.

CLINICAL SIGNS. Lacerations are evident. Heat, swelling, exudation, and dysuria may also be observed (Fig. 18.1). The swelling may obstruct urine flow.

TREATMENT. Recent lacerations may be cleansed, debrided, and sutured. Infected wounds should be treated locally by application of disinfectants (povidone-iodine) and alternating hot and cold packs to disperse the edematous inflammatory response. Parenteral, broad-spectrum antibiotics may be administered.

REFERENCES

1. Becker, E. L., Schilling, J. A., and Harvey, R. B. 1955. Renal function and electrolytes in the llama. Am. J. Physiol. 183:307–8.

2. Cardenas C., W. 1959. (Contribution to the study of the urine of alpacas. Some physiologic variations) Contribucion al estudio de la orina de la alpaca. Algunas variaciones fisiologicas. Tesis, Fac. Med. Vet. Univ. Nac. Mayor San Marcos (Lima).

3. Cardenas C., W., and Vallenas P., A. P. 1959. (Contributions to the study of the urine of alpacas) Contribucion al estudio de la orina de la alpaca. Rev. Fac. Med. Vet. (Lima) 13–14:89–105.

4. Engelhardt, W. 1978. (Renal urea excretion and renal concentration capacity of llama [*Lama glama*] on protein-poor diet) Renale Harnstoffexcretion und renal Konzentrierungsfahigkeit beim Lama (*Lama glama*) bei proteinarmen Diaten. Diss., Hohenheim Univ. West Germany.

5. Engelhardt, W., and Engelhardt, W. von. 1976. Diminished renal urea excretion in the llama at reduced food intake. In Tracer Studies on Non-Protein Nitrogen for Ruminants. Vienna: International Atomic Energy Agency, pp. 61–62.

6. Hammerton, A. E. 1934. Report on the deaths occurring in the society's gardens during 1933. Proc. Zool. Soc. Lond., p. 389.

7. Kock, M. D., and Fowler, M. E. 1982. Urolithiasis in a three-month-old llama. J. Am. Vet. Med. Assoc. 181:1411.

8. Timm, K. I., and Watrous, B. J. 1988. Urethral recess in two male llamas. J. Am. Vet. Med. Assoc. 192(7):937–38.

9. Vallenas, A. 1959. (Contribution to the study of the urine of alpacas) Contribucional estudio de la orina de la alpaca. Rev. Fac. Med. Vet. (Lima) 12(14):80–105.

10. ______. 1960. (Urea in the urine of the alpaca) La urea en la orina de alpaca. Rev. Fac. Med. Vet. (Lima) 15:113–23.

11. Villavicencio, M., and Villafuerte, J. A. 1972. (Macro and microscopic study of the kidney of the alpaca) Estudio macro y microscopico del rinon de alpaca, *Lama pacos*. Tesis, Fac. Med. Vet. Univ. Nac. Tec. Altiplano (Puno), pp. 1–68.

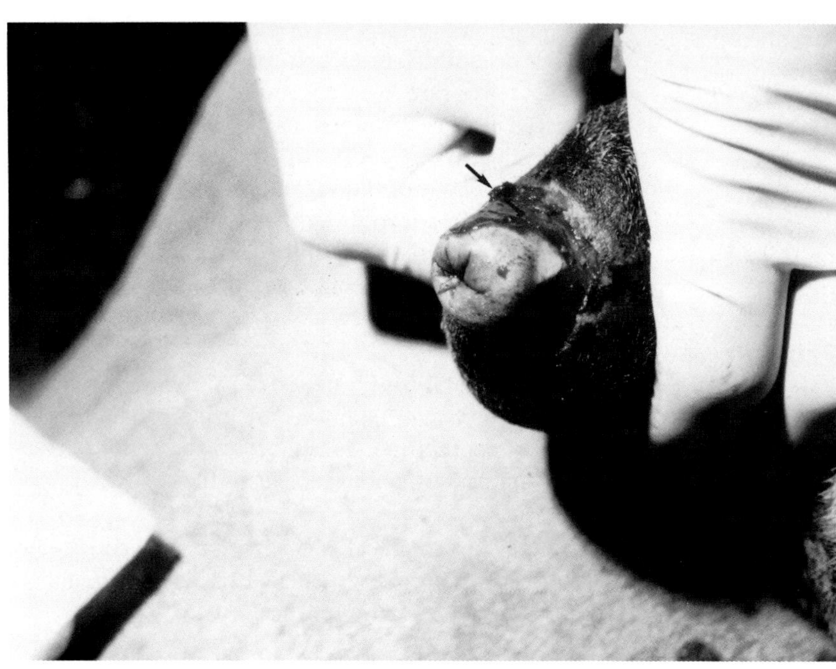

18.1 Posthitis in a llama.

19 Organs of Special Sense

EYE

Anatomy (8)

Lamoids have large, expressive eyes, with long eyelashes. The pupil is horizontally oblong, and this shape is accentuated by the corpora nigra located on the dorsal and ventral borders of the iris (Fig. 19.1). The cornea and lens resemble those of other ungulates. Vascularity of the chorioretina is pronounced and similar to that of the bovine. The vessels converge on the optic disc, which is located in the medial ventral position. There is no fovea.

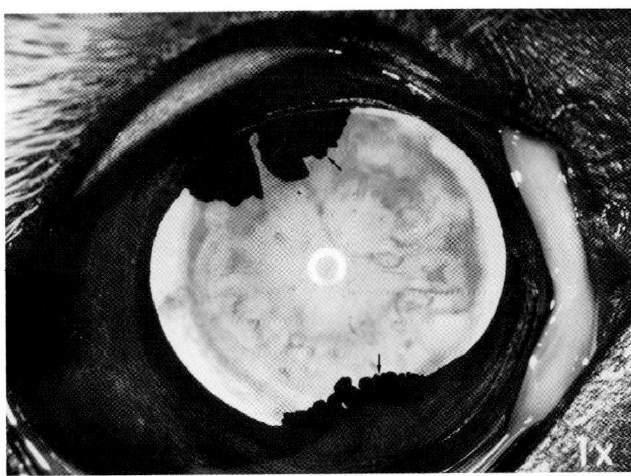

19.1 Granula iridica (corpora nigrum) of a llama.

Lamoids are diurnal and have no need for a tapetum to intensify light. The red eyeshine seen under intense light at night, or from a photoflash, is a reflection of the fundus.

The nasolacrimal duct originates as paired canaliculi connecting the punctae on the upper and lower eyelids, approximately 5 mm from the medial commissure to the lacrimal sac (Fig. 19.2). The duct traverses the osseous lacrimal canal in close association with the osseous canal of the infraorbital nerve (Fig. 19.3) and exits within the nares near the mucocutaneous junction, approximately 1 cm dorsal from the floor of the nostril (see Fig. 13.1). The orifice is approximately 2–3 mm in diameter.

Ophthalmic Diagnostic Procedures

Ophthalmic examinations on lamoids are carried out in a similar manner to those performed on other

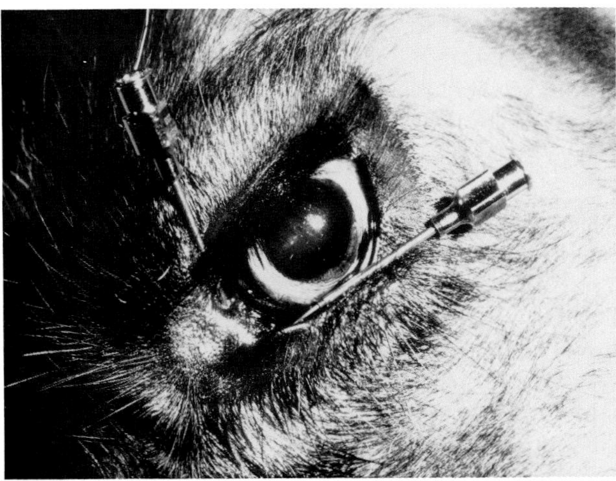

19.2 Cannulae in the nasolacrimal ducts.

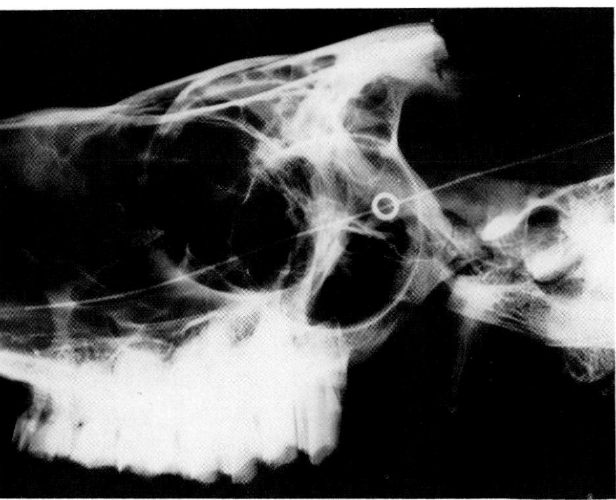

19:3 Lateral radiograph of a radiopaque cannula in the nasolacrimal duct illustrating the relationship to the roots of the maxillary cheek teeth.

domestic large animals (9). Reflexes, such as pupillary and palpebral, are similar. Reflection of the conjunctival mucous membranes is more difficult than in the horse but easier than in the cow.

Diseases

Infectious diseases involving the eye are discussed in Chapter 7 and include aspergillosis, moraxellosis (3), and equine herpes virus type 1. Parasitic diseases are discussed in Chapter 8 and include *Thelazia californiensis* and various species of flies that are attracted to lacrimal secretions. Congenital eye anomalies are discussed in Chapter 22 and include agenesis of the eyelids, microphthalmia, cataracts (1), blindness, apigmentation of the iris (glass eye), and cyclopian.

The eyelids and cornea are subject to contusion, abrasion, laceration, ulceration, and foreign body penetration. The diagnosis and management of these conditions are similar to the procedures employed when dealing with similar problems in an equine or bovine eye. Treatment should be begun immediately and carried out intensively to avoid loss of vision and, perhaps, loss of an eye (2, 7).

A method that has been found useful in treating ocular conditions requiring intensive, repeated medication in llamas is the insertion of an indwelling catheter into the nasal orifice of the nasolacrimal duct. Insert the catheter gently until the llama blinks, indicating the cornea or conjunctiva has been touched. Then withdraw the catheter 1–2 cm. Anchor the catheter in place by affixing tape to the catheter and suturing the tape to the skin near the nostril. The eyelids are then sutured closed to protect the cornea from light and repeated movement of the conjunctiva over the cornea. Medication can then be instilled into the conjunctival sac, as required, without stressing the llama.

It is beyond the scope of this book to delve into the intricacies of diagnosis and therapy of ocular diseases. Detailed discussions of cattle ocular diseases are found in Whitley and Moore (9).

Obstruction of the nasolacrimal duct has been observed and diagnosed. The etiology may be a temporary plug of mucus or swelling of the duct from inflammation. Prolonged inflammation may result in fibrosis and permanent occlusion of the duct. Clinical signs are epiphora, with or without concomitant conjunctivitis. The nasolacrimal duct may be cannulated with a 1 mm catheter at the nasal orifice or with a 22 gauge lacrimal irrigation needle at the eyelid. The duct may then be flushed with normal saline to establish patency. Alternatively, a fluorescein dye may be instilled into the eye and observations made to see if and when the dye appears at the nasal orifice.

EAR

Anatomy (4–6)

The external pinna is elongated and highly mobile (Fig. 19.4). The ears are expressive of health and emotional state. The auditory canal is located on the lateral aspect of the annular cartilage of the pinna. The cochleal eminence is easily mistaken for the ear canal when inserting an otoscope cone.

The osseous ear canal enters the petrous temporal bone immediately ventral to the zygomatic process of the temporal bone (5). In the adult, the canal is directed slightly rostrad and ventrad. At a depth of 1.8 cm, the canal bends ventrally at an angle of approximately 120° in a percentage of llamas (Fig. 19.5) and continues on for a distance of 1 cm. The irregularly shaped tympanic membrane is located on the medial side of the distal canal (Fig. 19.5) and is approximately 0.8 cm in diameter.

The canal is essentially straight in a neonate. Apparently, the external auditory canal is partially composed of cartilage in the neonate and ossifies at an unknown later time. The osseous ear canal is extremely narrow in the llama. The inside diameter of the external orifice, measured from the skeletal preparation of a large

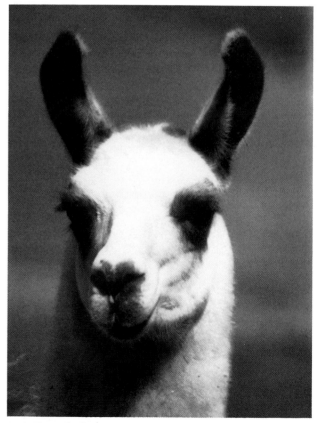

19.4 Ears of a llama.

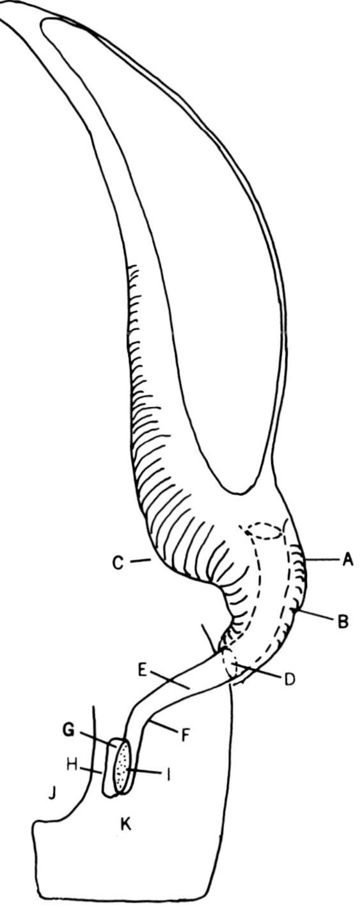

19:5 Diagram of the relationship of the pinna, external ear canal, tympanic membrane, and middle ear: **(A)** lateral side of the left pinna, **(B)** anular cartilage of the pinna, **(C)** conchal eminence, **(D)** external orifice of, **(E)** osseous ear canal, **(F)** bend of canal, **(G)** middle ear, **(H)** inner ear, **(I)** tympanic membrane, **(J)** cranial cavity, **(K)** tympanic bulla.

male, was 6 mm, narrowing to 4 mm at the bend. Addition of the epithelial lining further restricts canal size.

It is not possible to view the tympanic membrane in approximately 50% of adult llamas because of the bend and narrowness of the external ear canal. Edema and inflammation of the canal also obstruct viewing. The tympanic bulla is large and extensively honeycombed, but there is no fundic cavity (Fig. 19.6). The inner ear lies between the middle ear and the cranial cavity.

Diagnostic Procedures

An unsedated llama is reluctant to allow even a casual examination of the ear. Deep examination of the canal is virtually impossible without anesthesia. If exudate oozes from the ear, it is important to exclude the presence of foreign bodies (grass awns) or ticks. Radiographic examination will demonstrate sclerosis of the tympanic bulla of the petrous temporal bones (Fig. 19.6). Clinical evaluation of cranial nerve deficits in llamas is the same as in other mammals.

Diseases

LACERATIONS. Lacerations of the pinna are common in adult males because of intermale aggression. If the event causing the laceration is observed and immediate attention can be given, such wounds may be cleansed, debrided, and sutured with reasonable success. Lacerations of the poll may transect the ear muscles, preventing motor control of the pinna. Every effort should be made to realign severed ends of the muscles of the pinna.

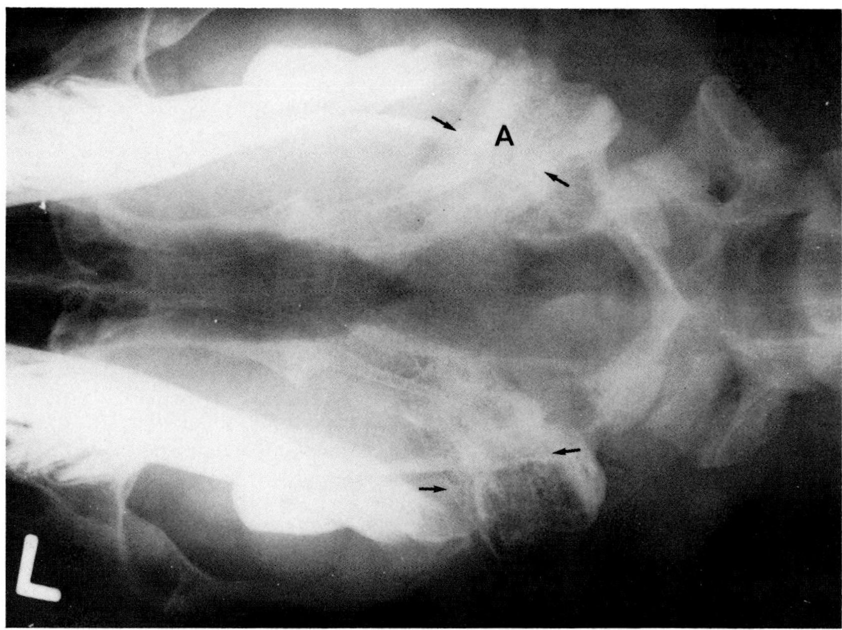

19.6 Dorsoventral radiograph of the skull with sclerosis of the tympanic bulla: **(A)** affected bulla.

OTITIS EXTERNA

Etiology. Inflammatory lesions of the external ear canal are common, but the cause of the inflammation is not always readily apparent. The spinose ear tick, *Otobius megninii,* may be a regional problem (see Chap. 8). Grass awns may lodge in the canal and scarify the epithelium, providing a portal of entry for opportunistic pathogens.

Clinical Signs. The signs of otitis externa are head shaking, scratching the ear with a hind foot or against a post or barn, head tilt, peculiar positioning of the pinna, and exudation from the external ear canal.

Diagnosis. Diagnosis is based on clinical signs and a thorough physical examination of the outer ear canal following cleansing of the ear and removal of all debris and ear wax. The epithelial surface may be hyperemic and ulcerated. Cultures taken from the external ear canal are not likely to be helpful, since the normal flora may harbor many opportunistic pathogens.

Treatment. The external ear canal should be cleansed and irrigated with povidone-iodine solution twice daily, followed by instillation of a broad-spectrum antibiotic ointment.

OTITIS MEDIA AND INTERNA

Etiology. Infection of deeper structures is usually a direct extension of infection in the external ear canal. Grass awns may also penetrate the tympanic membrane and initiate infection.

Clinical Signs. Otitis media is usually associated with facial nerve paralysis (Figs. 19.7, 19.8) (see also Chap. 20) and Horner's syndrome (5). The cardinal signs of Horner's syndrome are slight ptosis of the upper eyelid, inability of the pupil on the affected side to dilate in subdued light, and the nictitating membrane pushing out over the bulb as a result of retraction of the bulb deeper into the orbit, which makes the eye appear to be smaller (microphthalmia). This syndrome, plus facial paralysis, is virtually pathognomonic evidence of a lesion in the middle ear, because the sympathetic fibers involved in Horner's syndrome are in juxtaposition to the facial nerve only near the middle ear.

MISCELLANEOUS CONDITIONS. Congenital diseases of the ear include agenesis of the pinna, shortened pinna, and floppy pinna (see Chap. 22). In the neonate, a temporary floppy pinna may be the result of premature birth. This condition corrects itself as the cartilage strengthens with growth.

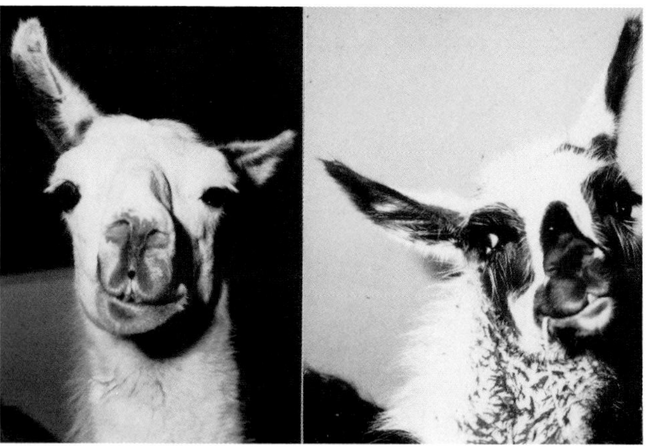

19.7 Facial paralysis.

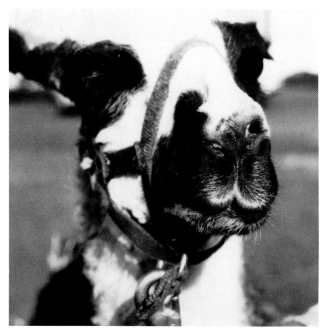

19.8 Chronic facial paralysis with lip pulled back toward the affected side.

The most common noninfectious, nonparasitic disease is frostbite (see Chap. 9).

REFERENCES

1. Barrie, K. P., Jacobson, E., and Peiffer, R. L., Jr. 1978. Unilateral cataract with lens coloboma and bilateral corneal edema in a guanaco. J. Am. Vet. Med. Assoc. 173:1251–52.

2. Bistner, S. 1986. Basic ophthalmic therapeutics. In J. L. Howard, ed. Current Veterinary Therapy: Food Animal Practice, 2nd ed. Philadelphia: W. B. Saunders, pp. 824–28.

3. Brightman, A. H., McLaughlin, S. A., and Brumley, V. 1981. Keratoconjunctivitis in a llama (*Staphylococcus aureus, Moraxella liquefaciens*). Vet. Med. Small Anim. Clin. 76(12):1776–77.

4. Fleischer, G. 1973. Studies of the skeleton of the auditory organs of mammals including humans. Saeugetierkd. Mitt. 21(2):131–239.

5. Fowler, M. E., and Gillespie, D. 1985. Middle and inner ear infection in llamas. J. Zoo Anim. Med. 16:9–15.

6. Herre, W. 1953. (Studies of the skeleton of the middle ear in wild and domestic animals forming the genus *Lama*) Studien am Skelet des Mitteloheres wilder und Domestizierten formen der Gattung *Lama.* Acta Anat. 19:271–89.

7. Murphy, J. M. 1983. Administration of ocular therapy. In N. E. Robinson, ed. Current Therapy in Equine Medicine. Philadelphia: W. B. Saunders, pp. 378–82.

8. Sevilla Cordova, J. A. 1973. (Muscles of the eyelids and ocular globe of the alpaca) Musculos de los parpados y del globo ocular de la alpaca, *Lama pacos.* Tesis, Fac. Med. Vet. Univ. Nac. Mayor San Marcos (Lima), pp. 1–23.

9. Whitley, R. D., and Moore, C. P. 1986. Ocular diagnostic techniques in food animals. In J. L. Howard, ed. Current Veterinary Therapy: Food Animal Practice, 2nd ed. Philadelphia: W. B. Saunders, pp. 819–24.

20

Nervous System

ANATOMY

No comprehensive treatises on the anatomy of the nervous system of any of the camelids have been published. A few references are to be found in the periodic literature, and anatomic subjects are popular as theses for students (2, 5, 7–14, 16, 18–21, 23–26). Unfortunately, South American theses are not readily accessible. Most papers deal with the specific nerves of a limited region of the body or of the brain.

The general morphology of the brain of lamoids does not differ from other domestic ungulates, nor does the basic distribution of peripheral nerves (12, 22, 26). The location of nerves that are important in surgical procedures have been discussed in the appropriate section. The spinal cord terminates at the midsacral region (Fig. 20.1).

DIAGNOSIS

Clinical diagnosis of neural function should follow the same pattern as for other domestic animals. The neurologic examination is used to establish the presence and location of a neural lesion(s), and diagnostic procedures are used to determine the cause of the lesion(s). The neurologic examination is similar to that for cattle and sheep, although llamas tend to respond more slowly to many of the stimuli. Special procedures include radiography, fluoroscopy, and myelography for evaluation of compression of the spinal cord or brain. Cerebrospinal fluid may be obtained from the occipitoatlantal space or the lumbosacral space (see Chap. 4).

All of the new sophisticated techniques for evaluating neural function are applicable to and have been performed on lamoids. Computed tomography, muscle and nerve biopsies, and the various electrodiagnostic procedures (electromyography, nerve conduction velocities, evoked potentials) will be particularly useful when normal values have been established.

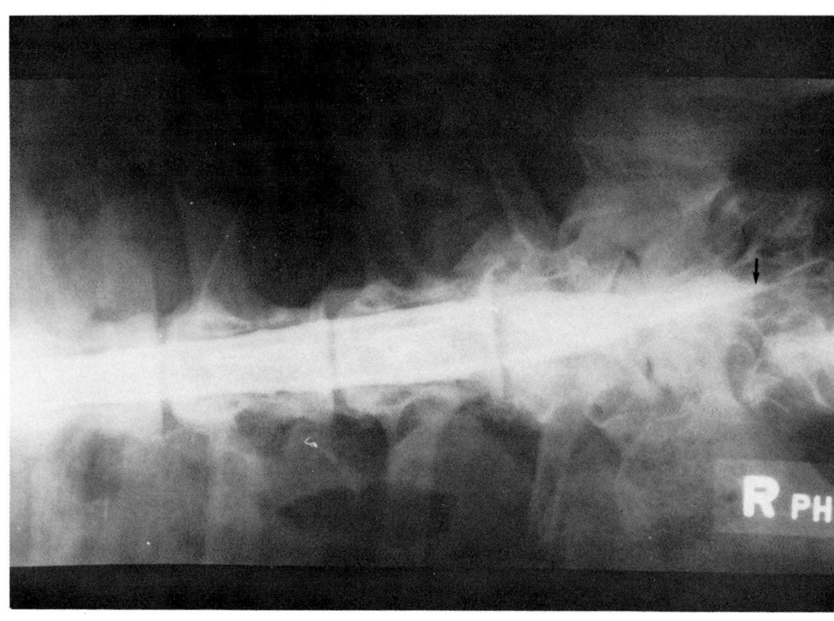

20.1 Dorsoventral radiograph of the terminal spinal cord with contrast media in the subarachnoid space. The meninges terminate at the midsacral region.

DISEASES

Congenital Diseases

Hydrocephalus is the most frequently seen congenital deformity of the nervous system. The cause is unknown. Internal hydrocephalus (dilatation of the lateral ventricles) in a llama was reported to be caused by partial stenosis of the cerebral aqueduct (3). Clinical signs included inability to stand, constant adduction of the right front leg, wry neck to the left, erect ears pulled to the left, and a domed forehead. At necropsy, bilaterally symmetric dilatation of the lateral ventricles of the cerebrum was seen. The brain seemed to expand upon removal of the calvarium. A large cardiac ventricular septal defect was also noted (3).

A definitive diagnosis of hydrocephalus is not easily made on the basis of clinical signs unless there is gross enlargement of the head. Many normal llama and, especially, alpaca neonates have a slightly domed forehead. Doming may be exaggerated when deformities of the facial bones occur. Plain film radiography may be of little assistance in diagnosis. Computerized tomography is the quickest and most accurate method for diagnosing hydrocephalus.

Congenital disorders affecting the spinal cord may be primary, such as meningocele or myelomeningocele associated with spina bifida, or the spinal cord may be affected secondarily by compression from vertebral anomalies such as hemivertebrae (see Chap. 22).

Infectious Diseases

Infectious diseases involving the central nervous system are discussed in Chapter 7. These include rabies, facial paralysis from middle ear infection, neural abscesses, and Borna disease (1).

Parasitic Diseases

Parasitic diseases involving the nervous system include tick paralysis, toxoplasmosis, and meningeal worm (see Chap. 8).

Noninfectious Diseases

Spinal cord neuronal degeneration causing ataxia, paresis, and paralysis has been reported in llamas (15). Similar degeneration has been diagnosed in the author's clinic. Although a definitive etiologic diagnosis has not yet been determined, copper deficiency is suspected (see Chap. 2).

TRAUMA. Concussion and contusion of the brain have resulted from kicks by horses and from running into solid objects when agitated or frightened. Laceration of peripheral nerves may occur with laceration of the skin and muscles or internally from sharp fragments of bone fractures. Nerves may be incised or contused during surgical procedures. One llama lost motor control of the lower lip following trephine removal of a cheek tooth. Temporary loss of motor or sensory function may occur from direct contusion of a nerve or from pressure on a nerve from an edematous or inflammatory lesion.

Partial radial paralysis may be a sequel to prolonged lateral recumbency during anesthesia if the forelimb is not pulled forward properly or is not padded (Fig. 20.2). Hot packs over the humerus may hasten reduction of the contusion, and the lower limb should be padded or wrapped to prevent abrasion of the fetlock during recuperation.

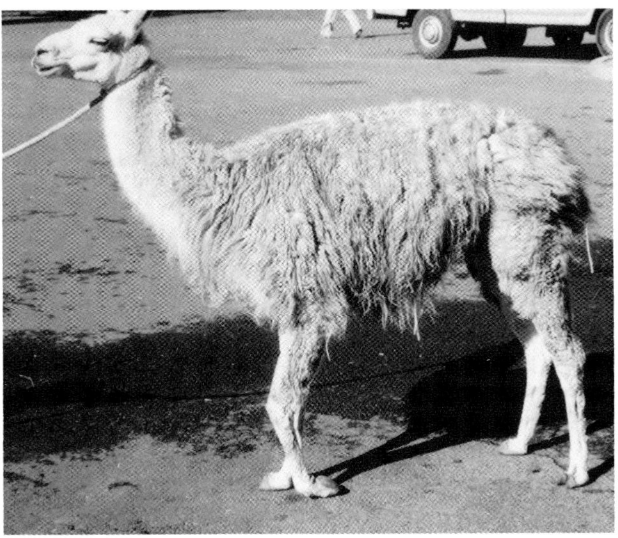

20.2 Postsurgical radial nerve paralysis.

SPINAL INJURY. Injury to the spinal cord usually follows vertebral fractures or luxations. The cervical cord of one male llama was transected by a fracture of cervical vertebra 2. The llama was attempting to return to a group of females from which he had been separated and ran headlong into a fence. For a discussion of other vertebral fractures, see Chapters 6 and 11.

LLAMA DOWNER SYNDROME. Ailing llamas may be reluctant to rise from sternal recumbency. In many instances, the animal may be physically unable to rise. It is difficult to establish whether the nervous system, muscular system, skeletal system, or a metabolic disorder is the cause. Neither ketosis nor postparturient hypocalcemia have been reported in lamoids. Electrolyte imbalance or uremia may contribute to malaise and depression.

Prolonged recumbency in a lamoid is hazardous because covering the ventral abdomen impairs thermoregulation. A moderate fever frequently accompanies the downer syndrome.

There may be many ultimate causes for the downer syndrome. A thorough physical examination is necessary to exclude the obvious, but some cases defy diagnosis and therapy.

CRANIAL NERVE DYSFUNCTION. Published clinical reports of cranial nerve (CN) dysfunction in lamoids have involved only 2 of the 12 CNs, (6, 17). Space does not permit nor is sufficient information available to provide a detailed discussion of CN dysfunction. An abbreviated review is provided.

Etiology. Cranial nerve dysfunction may arise within the brain from meningoencephalitis (listeriosis, toxoplasmosis, rabies), toxins (botulism), neoplasia, contusion, or concussion. Peripheral CNs may be traumatized from basilar skull fractures and inflammatory lesions in the areas traversed by the nerves. Facial nerve paralysis is a prime example of this. A llama developed multiple CN dysfunction (CN V–XII) following an extensive mycotic infection of the caudal nasal cavity and nasopharynx.

A blow to the throat may result in fracture of the hyoid apparatus and subsequent hypoglossal nerve paralysis. Excessive tension on the tongue during endotracheal intubation or dental surgery may cause temporary paralysis of the tongue as a result of stretching of the hypoglossal nerve. Other causes of CN dysfunction include any space-occupying lesion (hematoma, abscess, tumor) in the vicinity of a nerve.

Clinical Signs Associated with Individual Nerves

CN I (olfactory)—loss of sense of smell.

CN II (optic)—blindness. Optic nerve degeneration and retinal degeneration has followed infection with equine herpes type I virus in llamas and alpacas.

CN III (oculomotor)—this nerve, as well as CN IV and VI, innervates the muscles of the globe. Various eye position abnormalities occur, depending on the species. Nothing is known of the specific positional problems associated with paralysis of these nerves in lamoids.

CN IV (trochlear)—see CN III.

CN V (trigeminal)—dropped jaw that cannot be closed, difficult prehension, food in the oral cavity.

CN VI (abducent)—see CN III.

CN VII (facial)—see detailed discussion in Chapter 19.

CN VIII (vestibulocochlear, acoustic)—loss of hearing and equilibrium.

CN IX (glossopharyngeal)—paralysis of soft palate, pharynx, and cervical esophagus.

CN X (vagus)—laryngeal muscle paralysis and, potentially, vague autonomic dysfunction due to loss of parasympathetic input to the viscera, particularly with bilateral vagal lesions.

CN XI (spinal accessory)—paralysis of portions of the brachiocephalicus, sternocephalicus, and trapezius muscles.

CN XII (hypoglossal)—paralysis of muscles of the tongue. Interferes with deglutition, prehension, and mastication.

Diagnosis. Diagnosis requires detailed neurologic evaluation.

Treatment. The primary cause must be eliminated, if possible. Antiinflammatory agents, antimicrobials, and supportive treatment are indicated. Prognosis for recovery of cranial nerve function depends on the cause and severity of the lesion as well as prompt diagnosis and appropriate therapy.

FACIAL NERVE PARALYSIS

Etiology. The clinical syndrome associated with facial nerve paralysis in llamas is known, and a detailed discussion follows. The facial nucleus may be damaged by intracranial lesions as already described, but, more often, the nerve becomes involved in an extension of otitis media and interna as the facial nerve passes through the facial canal in the petrosal bone and emerges through the stylomastoid foramen (4). Individual branches of the nerve may be traumatized by blows to the face, space-occupying lesions (hematoma, abscess, tumor), lacerations (bites, surgical incisions), edema or cellulitis from snake bite, direct trauma from prolonged pulling against a halter (training and trailering accidents), or lying in lateral recumbency on a surgery table without adequate padding of the head. Trauma to the zygomatic arch may involve only the auriculopalpebral branch of the nerve, in which case, only the ear and eyelid muscles are involved.

Clinical Signs. The facial nerve supplies motor function to all the muscles of facial expression (ear, eyelids, nose, cheek, lips, and caudal portion of the digastric muscle) (4). Loss of function results in unilateral or bilateral ear drooping and inability to position the ear (see Fig. 19.7). This is a dramatic sign in llamas, since the ears are so expressive. In unilateral dysfunction, the nose is pulled toward the unaffected side (see Fig. 19.7). In cases of chronic facial paralysis, the paralyzed muscles atrophy. This may result in the nose being pulled back toward the affected side, complicating a differential diagnosis (see Fig. 19.8). The lips on the affected side may droop, allowing saliva to drip. Feed may also fall from the lips, because the llama cannot move feed into the teeth for chewing and subsequent swallowing. The nostril on the affected side fails to dilate symmetrically with the opposite nostril upon inspiration.

Paresis of eyelid muscles results in failure of closure of the palpebral fissure and excessive drying of the cornea, progressing to corneal ulceration. In one such case, eventually the eye had to be enucleated.

Head shaking or scratching at the ear with a hind foot may be seen. An exudate may be present in the affected ear, but not always.

Diagnosis. Diagnosis is usually based on clinical signs. The external ear canal should be examined for exudation and foreign bodies. This usually necessitates sedation for a thorough examination. Sclerosis of the tympanic bulla may be evident on a radiograph (see Fig. 19.6).

Treatment. In cases of trauma, administration of antiinflammatory agents is indicated along with hot packs to restore circulation and encourage drainage of edema. Space-occupying lesions should be dealt with as appropriate. Culture and sensitivity tests should be done to aid in appropriate antibiotic therapy.

Otitis media is treated with broad-spectrum antibiotics (gentamicin sulfate 1 mg/kg three times daily) and irrigation of the external ear canal with dilute povidone-iodine solution.

REFERENCES

1. Altmann, D., Kronberger, H., Schueppel, K. F., Lippmann, R., and Altmann, I. 1976. (Enzootic meningioencephalomyelitis simplex in New-world tylopods and equines) Bornasche Krankheit bei Neuwelttylopoden und Equiden. Verhandlungsber. 18th Int. Symp. Erkr. Zootiere, Innsbruck 18:127–32.

2. Arlamowska-Palider, A. 1973. Morphology of the sacral plexus in some artiodactylous animals. Folia Morphol. 32(1):11–17.

3. Brown, R. J. 1973. Hydrocephalus in a newborn llama. J. Wildl. Dis. 9:146–47.

4. DeLahunta, A. 1977. Veterinary Neuroanatomy and Clinical Neurology. Philadelphia: W. B. Saunders.

5. Demmel, U. 1980. (Branches of the vagus nerves in the neck of alpaca, *Lama guanacoe pacos*) Die Halsaeste des Nervus vagus beim Alpaka, *Lama guanacoe pacos.* Acta Zool. 61(3):141–46.

6. Fowler, M. E., and Gillespie, D. 1985. Middle and inner ear infections in llamas. J. Zoo Anim. Med. 16:9–15.

7. Hecker, A., Andermann, E., and Rodin, E. A. 1972. Splitting automatism in temporal lobe seizures. Electroencephalgr. Clin. Neurophysiol. 33(4):453–54. (Reference to spitting in llama)

8. Herre, W., and Thiede, U. 1965. (Studies on the brains of South American tylopods) Studien an Gehirnen Sudamerikanischer Tylopoden. Zool. Jahresber. Anat. 82:155–76.

9. Howell, A. B., and Straus, W. L. 1934. Note on the spinal accessory nerve of long-necked ungulates (llama). Proc. Zool. Soc. Lond., pt. 1, pp. 29–32.

10. Kajava, Y. 1912. (The vagus nerve and the origin of the aortic arch in the llama.) Die Kehlkopfnerven und die Arterienbogenderivate beim Lama. Anat. Anzeiger 40:265–79.

11. Kian T., O. T. 1974. (Morphological aspects of the cerebellum of the alpaca) Aspecto morphologicos del cerebelo de la alpaca (*Lama pacos*). Tesis, Fac. Med. Vet. Univ. Nac. Mayor San Marcos (Lima).

12. Kitsutani O., G. 1978. (Peripheral innervation of the upper arm and shoulder of the alpaca) Inervacion periferica de los segmentos hombro y brazo de la alpaca (*Lama pacos*). Tesis, Fac. Med. Vet. Univ. Nac. Mayor San Marcos (Lima).

13. Kruska, D. 1980. (Changes of brain size in mammals caused by domestication) Domestikationsbedingte Hirngrossenanderungen bei Saugetieren. Z. Zool. Syst. Evol. 18(3):161–95.

14. Matusita, A., and Vargus, A. 1970. (Cerebellum of the alpaca as a contribution to the study of the neuroanatomy of alpaca) Cerebelo de alpaca como una contribucion al estudio de la neuroanatomica de alpaca. Primera Conv. Camelidos Sudam. (Auquenidos), Puno, Peru, pp. 63–64.

15. Palmer, A. C., Blakemore, W. F., O'Sullivan, B., Ashton, D. G., and Schoot, W. A. 1980. Ataxia and spinal cord degeneration in llama, wildebeeste and camel. Vet. Rec. 107(1):10–11.

16. Puschner, H. 1971. (Abnormal axonal swellings in the nucleus gracilis of animals with no neurological signs) Eigenartige Axonschwellungen im Nucleus Gracilis bei neurologisch Unauffalligen Tieren. Zentralbl. Veterinaermed. [A] 18(5):365–72.

17. Rebhun, W. C., Jenkins, D. H., Riis, R. C., Dill, S. G., Dubovi, E. J., and Torres, A. 1988. An epizootic of blindness and encephalitis associated with a herpes virus indistinguishable from equine herpes virus I in a herd of alpacas and llamas. J. Am. Vet Med. Assoc. 192(7):953–56.

18. Reperant, J. 1971. Comparative morphology of the encephalon and the endocranial mold among the present-day tylopoda mammals, Artiodactyla. Bull. Mus. Natl. Hist. Nat. Zool. 4:185–322.

19. Sato Sato, A., and McFarland, L. Z. 1970. (Descriptive anatomical study of the cerebral hemispheres of the alpaca) Estudio anatomico descriptivo de los hemisferios cerebrales de la alpaca (*Lama pacos*). Bol. Extraordinario 4:116–27.

20. Sato Sato, A., and Tobaru O., T. K. 1976. (On the morphology of the cerebellum of the alpaca) Aspectos morfologicos del cerebelo de la alpaca (*Lama pacos*). Zentralbl. Veterinaermed. [C] 5(2):105–12.

21. Sato Sato, A., Guzman, J., and Nunez, Q. 1968. (Preliminary studies on the measurements of some organs of the alpaca) Estudio preliminar sobre las medidas de algunos organos de la alpaca (*Lama pacos*). Rev. Fac. Med. Vet. Lima 22:61–69.

22. Schumacher, S. von. 1906. (On the vagus nerve in the llama and vicuña) Ueber die Kehlkopfnerven beim Lama (*Au-*

chenia lama) und Vicunna (*Auchenia vicunna*). Anat. Anzeiger 28:156–60.

23. Trevino, G. S., and Alden, C. L. 1972. Mucocytes in the brain of a llama: A case report. J. Wildl. Dis. 8:359–64.

24. Vargas Caceres, A. 1969. (Contributions to the macro and microscopic description of the cerebellum of the alpaca) Contribucion a la descripcion macro y microscopica del cerebelo de la alpaca (*Lama pacos*). Tesis, Fac. Med. Vet. Univ. Nac. Tec. Altiplano (Puno), pp. 1–29.

25. Welker, W. I., Adrian, H. O., Lifshitz, W., Kaulen, R., Caviedes, E., and Gutman, W. 1976. Somatic sensory cortex of llama (*Lama glama*). Brain Behav. Evol. 13(4):284–93.

26. Yoshima Watanabe, A. 1976. (Descriptive anatomical study of the brachial plexus of the alpaca) Estudio anatomo descriptivo del pleto braquial en la alpaca, *Lama pacos.* B.S. tesis, Prog. Acad. Med. Vet. Univ. Nac. Mayor San Marcos (Lima).

21 Neonatology

CHARACTERISTICS OF THE NORMAL LLAMA NEONATE

The Spanish word for a baby lamoid is "cria" (birth to weaning), and it is the designation most often used for baby lamoids by North American owners as well. The term is used in this book.

The birth weight of a thoroughly dried llama cria varies from 8 to 18 kg (18–40 lb). Birth weight is determined by genetic factors, size of the mother, degree of maturity, and the nutrition of the dam during gestation. The neonate is not likely to gain weight during the first 3 days of life; in fact, it may lose up to 0.5 kg (1 lb). Greater weight loss than this may indicate dehydration or lack of milk intake. After the first few days, weight gain should be about 250 g (0.5 lb) per day for the first 2 weeks and 0.5 kg (1 lb) after that.

The neonate is usually covered by a thin, semitransparent epidermal membrane (see Chap. 17) that is attached at all the mucocutaneous junctions, at the coronets of the nails, and at the umbilicus. This membrane does not completely encircle the cria and is not as likely to obstruct the nostrils as is the amnion, though folds of the epidermal membrane may slip over a nostril. The lamoid fetus is not encased in the amniotic membrane at normal birth.

The lamoid mother does not lick the cria to dry it, nor does she nudge or otherwise stimulate the cria to arise. The mother may nuzzle the cria and vocalize with a humming sound. Some llama owners call this "kissing," and relate it to bonding between mother and baby.

The cria immediately begins to struggle, attempting to get up. A normal cria is able to stand, albeit unsteadily, within an hour and will immediately attempt to make contact with the mother. Directional instincts may be poor initially, but the cria will soon locate the udder and begin nursing.

Little has been written on llama and alpaca nursing behavior. In a study of a few animals, first nursing occurred at about 1 hour (10). The suckling posture is described as reverse parallel, with the cria standing at the side of the mother, its tail directed toward the mother's head. Nursing may be stimulated, if the cria is standing, by tickling its tail. Frequency of nursing varies with the age of the cria. During the first 10 days of life, it will nurse two to three times per hour during the daylight. Up to a month of age, nursing frequency may be twice per hour.

The time elapsed at each nursing episode varies from 5 seconds to 3 minutes, but the majority of episodes last less than 30 seconds. The newborn cria will spend about 5% of its time nursing; this will drop to about 3.5% by the age of 1 month. Llama crias begin nibbling at hay or grass at 10–14 days. As the intake of solid food increases, nursing episodes and time spent nursing decrease (10).

The body temperature of the recent newborn should be the same as that of the dam, 37.7–38.9°C (100–102°F). Once the cria has stabilized to the ambient environment, body temperature may fluctuate more in a cria than in an adult and may rise to 39.2°C (102.5°F) normally. The heart rate varies from 60 to 90 beats per minute and the respiratory rate from 10 to 30 breaths per minute. Lamoids are obligate nasal breathers, so any upper respiratory obstruction will cause dyspnea.

The umbilical cord ruptures during parturition anywhere along its length, from 5 to 30 cm (2–12 in.). The eyelids are open and the incisor teeth are erupted.

IMMEDIATE CARE OF THE NEWBORN

Llama owners vary greatly in the care given to the neonate. Some allow the entire process to proceed naturally, while others wish to be present at each delivery, assisting in the parturition and lavishing care on the cria. The weather may have a significant bearing on whether or not special care must be given, but with the high value of llamas and alpacas, it is logical to give maximum care in all cases. The following instructions are based on the owner/manager or veterinarian being present at the time of parturition.

Make certain that the cria is breathing and clear the airways. Epidermal membranes may be removed from the muzzle by gentle rubbing with a towel. Insert a finger into the mouth to remove any collected mucus. The stimulus of the finger in the mouth may initiate a nursing reflex or stimulate the cria to move. Suction is the most satisfactory method for removal of excess fluids from the nostrils and mouth, but in a field situation, the cria can be held upside down for a few seconds or gently swung in an arc to develop mild centrifugal action to clear the passageways. Lamoids have long necks and long legs, so care must be taken to avoid traumatizing the head. It may be advisable to grasp both a hind and foreleg before spinning.

If the cria has still not begun to breathe, artificial respiration must be initiated. The most beneficial method is mouth to nose resuscitation, since the lamoid is an obligate nasal breather. Chest massage and compression are also useful. In a hospital situation, administration of oxygen via a nasal tube or endotracheal intubation is appropriate. Also examine the mucous membranes of the mouth and check for capillary refill time to ascertain the status of circulation.

The umbilical stump should be cleaned, shortened to less than 20 cm (8 in.), and dipped in 2–7% tincture of iodine (Fig. 21.1). Avoid smearing iodine on the skin, since it is caustic and will cause dermatitis. The plastic case for a 20 ml syringe or a plastic 35 mm film container is satisfactory as a dipping cup. The cria should be dried thoroughly with towels and accurately weighed.

The foregoing procedures may be carried out in the presence of most llama mothers. Rarely are they aggressive, especially if eye contact is avoided. Once initial care has been completed, it is best to leave the mother and cria undisturbed to establish bonding and nursing.

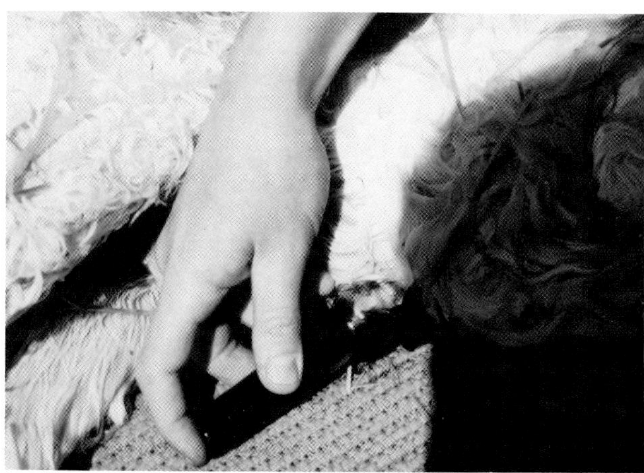

21.1 Applying iodine to the umbilical cord.

In a herd or pasture situation, a good deal of socialization occurs, with other females gathering to nose the newborn (6, 10). Some owners prefer to isolate mother and newborn for a few hours in a cleanly strawed stall to minimize distractions for both mother and cria. This is a must for the disinterested mother.

Although human interference should be limited to essentials, the cria should be kept under constant observation to note when it can stand and when it begins nursing and for how long. If the cria has not nursed by 6 hours following birth, intervention is necessary.

The udder should be palpated for subsequent comparison, since udder development may be quite small at the time of parturition, especially in primiparous females. Some females produce the same type of "waxing" as is seen in the mare. Each teat of the mother should be cleared of the waxy plug at the tip, but avoid expressing more than necessary.

It is neither necessary nor desirable to give an enema to every lamoid neonate. The cria should be observed for passage of the meconium, which usually occurs within 18–24 hours. Failure of passage of the meconium in a nursing cria by 24 hours, especially if straining is evident, may indicate administration of an enema. Warm water (200–500 ml) may be given via a bulb syringe, emptied fleet enema container, enema can, or water bottle system. Avoid rigid tubing, and be gentle with the insertion.

PREMATURITY

Intensive care of the premature infant has become commonplace in humans, horses, cattle, and companion animals. No studies have been reported on the characteristics of a premature lamoid cria, but sufficient observations have been made to establish certain factors, which, combined with extrapolation from known care for other premature ungulates, may save the life of a premature cria. Prematurity may be determined on the basis of birth weight, length of gestation, observable characteristics of the neonate, and laboratory analysis of blood. There is considerable variation in the length of gestation of llamas and alpacas (330–360 days, with an occasional pregnancy continuing for over a year). Such variation makes it difficult to establish prematurity on the basis of the age of the fetus. Furthermore, an accurate breeding date is sometimes difficult to establish. When pasture breeding is practiced, unobserved early embryonic death may be followed by breeding within a few days. The degree of maturity should not be based entirely on the number of days in the uterus. Foals born at full term, with known breeding dates, have nevertheless shown signs of immaturity.

Unusually low body weight is the most evident characteristic of lack of maturity. Generally, if the cria weighs less than 8 kg (18 lb), there should be concern; if it weighs less than 7 kg (15 lb), some degree of prematurity should be assumed. However, an absolute weight cannot be considered as sole determinant. For instance, if the expected delivery weight of a mature fetus is 16 kg (35 lb), a cria delivered at 11 kg (25 lb) may be immature.

Observable Signs of Prematurity

Premature crias are weak and unable to stand or hold the head up to nurse. Overextension of the fetlocks, from tendon and ligament immaturity, causes the cria to walk on the fetlocks. The sucking reflex may be weak or entirely absent, especially in the early premature cria.

Premature crias have floppy ears, a result of immaturity of the aural cartilage (Fig. 21.2). However, not all tipped or floppy ears are caused by prematurity; genetic factors may also be involved. An immature fiber coat has a silky feel, especially over the back and rear quarters. The eyelids may be stuck together in crias that are a month or more premature.

The rubbery covering over the ungulate hoof is also present on the lamoid fetal nail (Fig. 21.3). In a mature cria, the rubbery mass is removed from the toe within 6–12 hours as the cria struggles to stand and take its first steps. The covering persists for 1–2 days in premature crias.

The epidermal membrane is thin, friable, and easily rubbed off a full-term fetus within a few hours after birth. In the premature cria, the membrane is thicker, and remnants may cling for 24 hours.

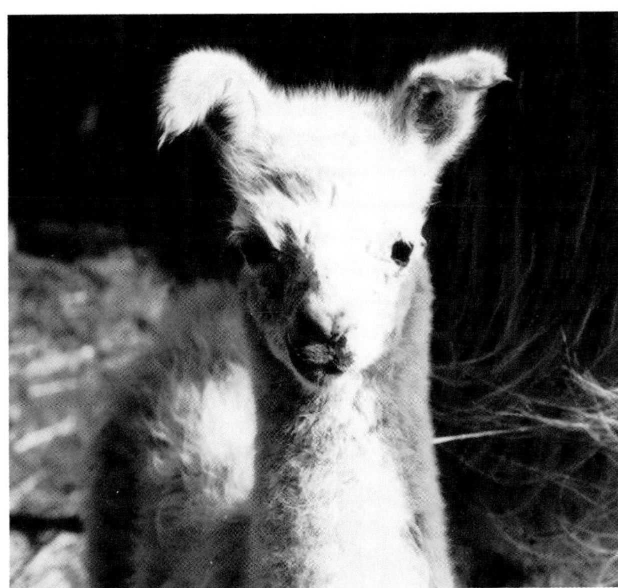

21.2 Floppy ears of a premature cria.

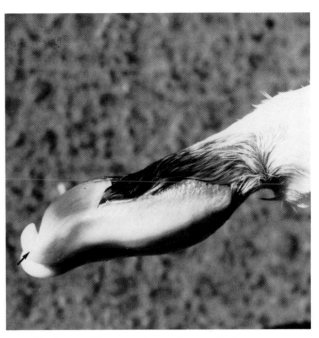

21.3 Persistent rubbery covering on the toenail of a premature cria.

The incisor teeth have erupted in the normal, full-term fetus (Fig. 21.4). Failure of these teeth to erupt for days or weeks after birth is a primary indication of prematurity.

Bradypnea (less than 10/min) is common in the premature cria. There is an absolute hypercapnia, but this fails to initiate respiratory effort, and PaO_2 is low. Although pulmonary surfactants have not been studied in lamoids, it is assumed that conditions present within the alveoli of the llama lung are similar to those of foals, calves, and humans and that the absence of surfactants in the premature cria decreases oxygen transfer across the alveolar membrane.

Metabolic Defects in Premature Crias

All neonates are hypoglycemic at birth and for a few hours thereafter. Premature crias remain hypoglycemic and lack the energy to stand or nurse. The premature cria has poor thermoregulatory ability and is thus at great risk of hypothermia. The body temperature of a cria suspected to be premature must be carefully monitored. Leukopenia, caused by an absolute neutropenia, is characteristic of prematurity. The immature adrenal cortex is unable to respond to adrenocorticotrophic hormone stimulation to produce cortisol and deal with stress.

The intestinal mucosa of the premature cria is not prepared for absorption of immunoglobulin (Ig) macromolecules, so even though colostrum is administered via

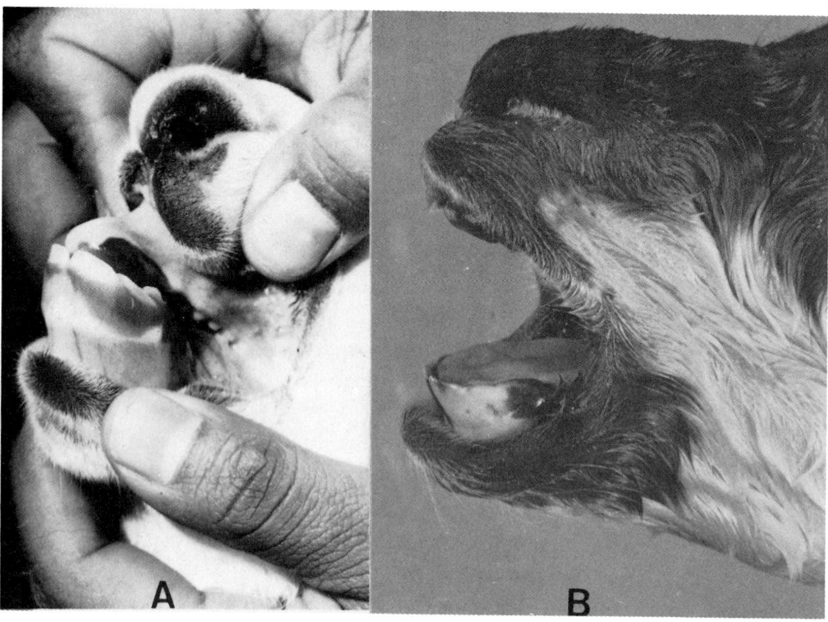

21.4 Cria incisors: **(A)** normally erupted incisors of a day-old llama cria, **(B)** incisors not erupted in a premature cria.

stomach tube, there may be a failure of passive transfer of Igs. This is an extremely important factor, necessitating parenteral administration of plasma to avoid mortality from neonatal infections.

Premature foals have incomplete formation of the carpal and tarsal bones, predisposing to angular limb deformities. This phenomenon has not been investigated in premature lamoids, but it warrants consideration, since angular limb deformities are common in llamas and alpacas.

It is important to recognize that the fully mature cria may exhibit one or more of the characteristics of immaturity. The overall morphology and activity of the cria must be evaluated on an individual basis. Intrauterine septicemia may simulate many of the signs of prematurity, as may congenital heart defects. A neonatal maladjustment syndrome has been reported in foals wherein the foal fails to adapt to extrauterine life, even though fully mature. This situation has not been reported in lamoids but should be considered.

Prematurity is life threatening. Prompt diagnosis and intensive care is mandatory. The veterinarian should work closely with clients to educate them on early recognition so that prompt, effective remedial action may be taken.

LACTATION

Milk production is vital to the life of the neonate. See Chapter 10 for a detailed discussion on the anatomy and physiology of lactation and milk composition.

Agalactia is a common postpartum disorder and may be temporary or permanent. The etiology of agalactia may be as simple as failure of milk letdown because of lack of oxytocin stimulation, or it may be the result of lack of development of the glandular tissue or patency of one or more teats. Other causes of agalactia or dysgalactia in livestock include hyperthermia, toxemia, mastitis, pain (lameness, arthritis), digestive upsets, ergot ingestion, genetic factors, hormonal failures, and stress. If parturition is premature, glandular tissue will lack maturity. The degree of immaturity will depend on the stage of prematurity. Mastitis may destroy glandular tissue in one or more quarters. Mastitis is more likely to occur in a multiparous female, but it is possible in a primiparous female.

Failure of milk letdown may be treated by stimulation of the udder with a warm water bath and massage or by intramuscular injection of oxytocin (30–40 units per animal), repeated at 3- to 4-hour intervals if necessary. Oxytocin, or any other drug, will not increase milk secretion in a gland that is nonfunctional.

Failure of the cria to obtain milk may also be brought about by weakness or anatomic inability of the cria to nurse. The female may be a poor mother and refuse to stand still for the cria. Pain caused by mastitis, udder edema, or simple engorgement with milk may cause the female to prevent the cria from nursing.

A primiparous female may abandon the cria, but this is rare. Abandonment may result from anxiety or turmoil at the time of parturition, which prevents proper bonding. Owners should be aware that unnecessary interference at parturition may be detrimental, particularly in a primiparous female. If the cria is weak or septicemic and does not respond properly, the female may lose interest and wander back to the herd and a more social situation.

Most llama and alpaca females are good mothers. In fact, they may allow nursing by crias other than their own (wild lamoids will not allow crias other than their own to nurse). This provides the owner with an option for cross fostering if this becomes necessary. An interesting side light to this situation is that females may inadvertently switch babies. One parentage verification study indicated that a given female could not be the mother of the cria she was nursing. Subsequent investigation determined that on this ranch, females of similar appearance gave birth to similar looking crias at approximately the same time. It was deduced that somehow they had switched crias. The owners of these animals had sold one pair before the switch was discovered.

The first 2 days are crucial to the life of the neonate. Adequate observation and examination of the udder should be made to ensure that lactation is taking place and that the cria is ingesting colostrum and milk. Twice-daily weighing of the cria may be indicated. Numerous crias have been lost because owners failed to recognize that the cria had not obtained vital milk.

Milk production will normally increase over the first few days of birth. Some females do not begin milk production for 3–4 days after parturition. This may have serious consequences for the cria, since it will be deprived of colostrum and nourishment until intestinal absorption of the Igs is no longer possible. Suitable milk replacement must be provided for such crias, and failure of passive transfer of antibodies must be dealt with as described later. In these cases, the female should not be pronounced as incapable of milk production too quickly. A few days of intensive work with the female and cria may relieve a manager from untold hours of labor in hand rearing a cria.

Another problem associated with lactation occurs when the cria must be orphaned for the first few days of life because of prematurity, environmental conditions, infection, or injury. In such a situation, the wise owner will milk the female to maintain milk production. This milk may be used to feed the cria and, more importantly, it may then be possible to reunite mother and cria. Owners have reported success after as long as 10 days of separation.

TRANSFER OF IMMUNOGLOBULIN THROUGH COLOSTRUM

Lamoids have an epitheliochorial placentation and as a result, in common with other ungulate species, obtain passive protection from Igs via intestinal absorption of macromolecules in colostrum. Failure to ingest colostrum during the first 24 hours of life is probably the most important predisposing cause of mortality in lamoid neonates. In Peru, serum IgG concentrations of dying alpaca crias was significantly lower than those crias that lived (1, 2). Colostral intake serves two purposes: (1) a source of Igs for absorption into the circulatory system across the intestinal mucosa and (2) local effects, protecting the mucosa against endotoxins and microorganisms. The first requires ingestion within 24 hours of birth, while the second will benefit the animal for a number of days and is brought about by local action of the specific Igs, nonspecific complement, transferrins, and lactoferrins (7).

The suggested composition of lamoid and camel colostrum is provided in Table 10.3. Alpaca colostrum is said to have the consistency of condensed milk. In contrast to bovine colostrum, alpaca and llama colostrum is low in fat (0.7%) but high in protein. Camel colostrum is similar to lamoid colostrum in fat percentage, but it is white and watery in contrast to the thick and creamy colostrum of cattle (see Chap. 10). The high protein content of colostrum is the result of the presence of Igs.

Production of Immunoglobulins

In the cow, preparation of the mammary gland for colostrum production begins about 5 weeks prepartum. The stimulus is probably rising estrogen levels. Special receptors on the epithelial cells of the mammary gland selectively bind serum Ig, which is, in turn, taken into the cell and ultimately transported to the lumen and hence the colostrum (7). Factors that influence the amount of Igs in bovine colostrum are:

1. Failure to allow the mammary gland to make preparation for colostrum production. This may result if the previous cria is allowed to continue to nurse for a year or if the female serves as a wet nurse for multiple crias.
2. Such genetic factors as breed differences.
3. Multiparous cows produce more and higher quality colostrum than uniparous cows.
4. Energy-deficient diets result in a decrease in the volume of colostrum produced but do not alter the composition.
5. Ig content of the first milking is double that of the second milking, and content is halved with each succeeding milking (7).
6. Premilking dissipates IgG.
7. Leakage of colostrum from an engorged udder.
8. Administration of long-acting corticosteroids over a period of 9–19 days to induce parturition.
9. Premature birth.
10. Prenatal mastitis.
11. Immune status of the female prior to parturition.

Absorption of Immunoglobulins

Colostral proteins are absorbed in the distal small intestine. Igs of milk deposited in compartment one (C-1) of the stomach will be delayed, or Ig may be denatured before it ever reaches the small intestine. A number of other macromolecules may be absorbed along with Igs, including alkaline phosphatase and G glutamyltransferase. Elevated levels of the two enzymes in the neonate may not be indicative of a disease state (7).

In cattle, a number of behavioral factors modify the ultimate levels of Igs in the circulation of the calf. Mothering has a beneficial effect, with higher levels attained when the calf is kept with the mother and allowed to nurse freely, as contrasted with calves allowed to nurse periodically but kept separate from the dam. Lowest of all are levels reached in bottle-fed calves, even though given equal or greater volumes of true, first-milk colostrum (7).

It is not known how these factors affect lamoids. Even though the llama female does not lick the cria as does a cow with her calf, a bonding and nursing response nevertheless occurs. Other factors that may affect lamoid immune response follow. Cold weather decreases cria vigor and hence overall colostral intake and absorption. Heat stress likewise inhibits Ig absorption efficiency (7). A cria delivered following a dystocia is not likely to have a depressed Ig uptake, but one delivered by cesarean section will. Such animals must be watched carefully.

Absorption is directly related to the amount of Igs ingested. There seems to be better absorption from a first ingestion with a higher concentration of Ig than from the same total quantity of Ig in a larger volume of milk (7).

Using experience from calf-rearing as a guide, crias deprived of all colostrum are at risk of dying from colisepticemia within 3–4 days of birth. If some Ig has been absorbed, the risk of disease is still great but will occur later in the form of diarrheas, pneumonia, or chronic polyarthritis. If the dam had not been vaccinated against nor exposed to a specific pathogen, the cria remains at risk from that pathogen. Even crias absorbing adequate Igs may succumb to an overwhelming infection.

No studies have been conducted in lamoids to determine the exact time sequence of passage of macromolecules across the intestinal mucosa and closure of intestinal permeability to colostral Ig. Extrapolating from studies in calves, if no ingestion of colostrum or milk occurs, there would be a spontaneous closure to absorption 24 hours postpartum. Closure begins at approximately 12 hours. Early ingestion of colostrum causes a more rapid closure (12).

FAILURE OF PASSIVE TRANSFER (FPT) OF IMMUNOGLOBULINS

The llama neonate, as is true with other domestic animals, is born with incompletely developed immunodefense mechanisms. Although leukocyte populations are well developed at birth, they have not received any antigenic stimulation. Maximum lymphoid development in the spleen and intestine will not have occurred (7). A few days are required before the immune system is primed and Ig production is possible.

Detection of FPT

Even with intense management of calves, it is thought that 10–30% of the calves are hypo- or agammaglobulinemic as a result of failure of passive transfer of Ig (FPT). This is of significance in neonatal morbidity and mortality (12). Veterinarians dealing with llamas must assume this to be true in lamoids also and act accordingly.

Early recognition of FPT is crucial to the well-being of the cria. A history of no ingestion of colostrum during the first 24 hours would be prima facie evidence of FPT, but this may not always be known. The cria may have appeared to nurse without obtaining colostrum for reasons enumerated in the agalactia discussion. Also, the amount of colostrum intake is important.

Single radial immunodiffusion is the most specific laboratory test to determine the level of Ig in calves and foals. Other reliable methods include refractometer measurement of total protein, serum electrophoresis, zinc sulfate turbidity, and zinc sulfite precipitation. All of these methods have been used in lamoids, but, except for total protein evaluation and electrophoresis, the results have been equivocal. Electrophoresis is good but time consuming, and action must be taken prior to obtaining results. This leaves total protein evaluation as the only practical test available, but one that has not yet been evaluated sufficiently. Total protein levels of less than 5 g/dl are suggestive of FPT. Levels between 5 and 6 g/dl are equivocal, and levels over 6 g/dl indicate probable successful passage of Ig.

The management of FPT depends on the stage at which one becomes involved. Involvement at parturition is the ideal situation. If the cria has failed to nurse by 6 hours, an attempt should be made to offer it colostrum obtained directly from the mother or llama or goat colostrum that has been stored frozen. Mare and cow colostrum has been used, but goats are more likely to have been immunized for the diseases of most concern in lamoids. Furthermore, goat colostrum and milk composition is most nearly like that of lamoids (see Table 10.3). It will be virtually impossible to milk sufficient colostrum from the postparturient female to supply the needs of the cria. It will probably be more satisfactory to rely on frozen goat colostrum. However, the source of the colostrum must be scrutinized. The desired colostrum is the first-drawn milk only. Many livestock people operate on the principle that since the milk is not normal for up to 72 hours after parturition, all fluid withdrawn during that time is colostrum. Unless it is specified that only first-drawn milk is to be used, suitable colostrum may not be supplied. Furthermore, it is important to determine that the herd is free of disease and that the colostrum is collected and stored under sanitary conditions.

If a cria has a poor sucking response, it is much safer to intubate until the cria gains strength (9, 10). If it is bottle fed, the bottle should be held level, even with the head, not above it, to avoid aspiration (Fig. 21.5). The hole in the nipple used for a weak baby should be tiny, then enlarged with a cross cut as strength is gained. A human baby nipple or a lamb nipple with a cross cut, rather than a round hole for an orifice, is recommended for feeding the cria. Offer 120 ml (4 oz), or as much as the cria will take, every 2–3 hours up to 24 hours or until the cria is able to stand and nurse on its own.

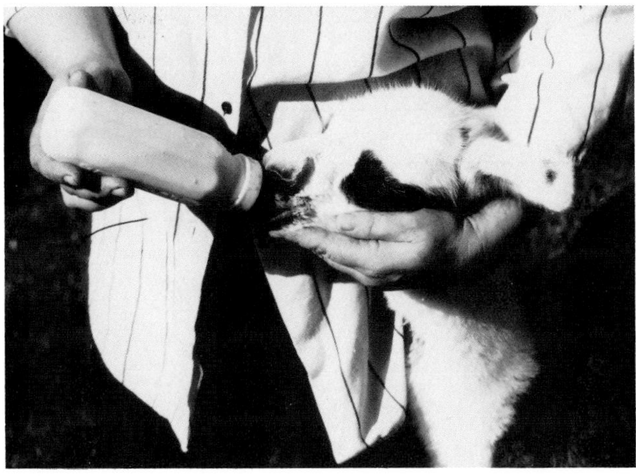

21.5 Bottle position for feeding an orphan llama.

If the cria refuses or is unable to suckle an artificial nipple, it is necessary to intubate the cria. Intubation is easily carried out by straddling the recumbent cria in a kneeling position. Many different tubes and methods are available to administer colostrum.

A tube with a 10–13 mm outside diameter (24 French) and an end port, not a blind tip,[1] is recommended. Larger tubes may cause interference with cardiac function. The tube should be lubricated with water. Hold the head in a semiflexed position to insert the tube into the mouth. No speculum is necessary. Gently push the tube to the pharynx and allow the cria to swallow it. Palpate the left cervical region for esophageal placement and continue insertion only to the thoracic inlet. Fluid traversing the thoracic esophagus may cause reflex closure of the esophageal groove and shunting of the colostrum to C-3 of the stomach, where it belongs. *Do not* insert the tube into the stomach, since this will ensure placement of the colostrum into C-1 one of the stomach. Milk in C-1 will ferment, contributing to digestive upset.

The first tube feeding should be given by 12 hours postpartum in the amount of approximately 1% of the body weight, 112 ml (4 oz) for a 11.34 kg (25 lb) cria. Repeat the tube feeding every 2 hours until 6% of the body weight is reached. The stomach capacity of most mammals is 25–50 ml/kg of the animal's body weight. For a 11.34 kg llama cria, this would amount to 280–560 ml, but it is undesirable to use the higher volumes until the stomach has expanded and is prepared to accept such amounts. Otherwise, the fluid may back up and spill into C-1 or, worse, cause regurgitation with the attendant risk of aspiration. Intubation should be repeated at 15 and 20 hours if necessary.

If 24 hours have elapsed since birth, it must be assumed that the intestine is refractory to absorption of Igs. At this time, the only recourse is to administer blood, plasma or serum, preferably obtained from the dam. Blood typing is in its infancy in lamoids, but erythrocyte factors are known and plasma is preferable, at a volume of 10–20 ml/kg body weight. Since no studies have been conducted to determine the most suitable volume for lamoids, extrapolations have been made from livestock studies. For a 11.34 kg (25 lb) cria, the recommended volume is 120–240 ml. Plasma may be administered intravenously, intramuscularly, or subcutaneously. However, the volume is quite high for the latter two, and even with dispersal in a number of sites, the cria will experience distress and possibly lameness for a few days. The preferred technique is to give plasma intravenously.

It should be noted that plasma can be given orally prior to intestinal closure, but it should also be understood that prematurity may preclude any intestinal absorption of Ig. Parenteral administration of plasma should always be used for any cria suspected to be premature.

In a herd of zoo llamas, one female allowed nursing by many of the crias, which essentially kept her in constant milk production. Any cria born to such a female would be at risk of FPT because the mammary gland may not have been stimulated to produce colostrum.

In a neonate of 48–72 hours with FPT, there is great risk of infection, and suitable antibiotic and other sup-

1. Harris flush tube, K 45, 24 French; Pharmaseal Toa Alta, Puerto Rico 00758.

portive therapy should be provided. Hypothermia contributes to cria weakness and poor colostrum absorption. It is necessary to ensure that the body temperature is appropriate before giving colostrum.

The neonate is always hypoglycemic before nursing (Table 21.1) and requires carbohydrate to cope with early extrauterine life. The elevated levels of lactose in lamoid colostrum meet this need. A colostrum-deprived cria should be given an intravenous infusion of a 10% dextrose solution (20 ml/kg body weight) to overcome postnatal hypoglycemia and stimulate activity to nurse.

A variety of methods have been used to freeze and store colostrum. Some place 2–4 oz in small plastic freezer bags. Others pour colostrum into an ice cube tray for freezing. Each cube is approximately 1 oz. After freezing, the cubes are packaged in a plastic bag for storage. Cubes or plastic packets are removed from the freezer and thawed as required. Colostrum should not be thawed in a microwave oven.

CARING FOR THE ORPHANED LAMOID

The cria may be orphaned at birth as a result of rejection by the mother, disease, injury or death of the mother, or from a variety of the factors previously discussed in this chapter. Successful rearing of an orphan lamoid is an art (4, 5). Certain individuals within the llama industry have made tremendous contributions to the knowledge of the rearing of orphans (3, 4). Their experience and expertise should be sought when faced with the challenge of long-term hand feeding. However, the veterinarian should be able to deal with short-term problems and make recommendations of how to deal with FPT and neonatal infections.

Some basic information follows. Llamas will rarely learn to drink milk from a bucket. Many crias will refuse to allow supplementation of mother's milk by nursing on a bottle, seeming to desire one or the other. There are exceptions, but it requires much patience to succeed. If the female is slow in coming into lactation, it may be necessary to supplement by intubation rather than bottle feeding. It is important not to overfeed, or the cria will have no stimulus to attempt nursing.

Orphans will tolerate well a variety of llama milk substitutes, including lamb milk replacer, cows milk, or goat milk. If milk is selected, experienced orphan rearers recommend the use of goat milk because it is the most nearly like llama milk. Furthermore, goat milk fat is naturally homogenized and more easily digested than the larger fat globules of the milk of other species.

Table 21.1. Postnatal serum chemistry values

Parameter	Precolostrum ingestion	Postcolostrum ingestion	< 1 month	Weanling
Glucose (mg/dl)	52.8–92.7	154–288	93–287	107–158
Blood urea nitrogen (mg/dl)	30.9–42.5	19.9–25	9–22	11–29
Total protein (g/dl)	4.71–5.34	5.92–7.31	3.7–6.7	5.1–10.3
Albumin (g/dl)	3.63–4.15	3.11–4.02	2.3–4.3	3.3–4.6
Globulin (g/dl)	0.96–1.33	2.1–3.1	0.7–2.9	1.1–2.9
A:G ratio	2.9–4.27	0.91–1.88		
Calcium (g/dl)	10.4–11.7	10.6–12.2	9.3–10.8	8.6–11
Phosphorus	5.7–7	4.9–8.6	7–11.2	5.1–10.3
Magnesium (mg/dl)	2.1–3.8	2.7–3.4		
Sodium (m mol/L)	149–154	148–153	148–156	149–155
Potassium (m mol/L)	4.4–7.9	4.2–7	4.6–5.9	4.3–7.4
Chloride (m mol/L)	108–122	107–118	100–117	102–114
SGOT (IU/L)	34.9–52.3	63.9–104.4	162–503	234–600
CPK (IU/L)	64.5–154	14.7–117.3	9–49	11–49
Creatinine (mg/dl)	5.1	1.75	1–3.5	1.2–2.7

Note: Data on pre- and postcolostrum by L. W. Johnson, personal communication.

Table 21.2. Postnatal hematology

	Precolostrum ingestion	24 hours postcolostrum	< 1 month of age	Weanling
PCV (%)	35.6–40.4	32.5–35.7	23–35	25–44
Hb (g/dl)	15.1–16.7	13.2–15.1	10–15	11.2–19.6
Total protein (g/dl)	5.03–5.5	6.16–7	4.7–6.1	5–7.2
Leukocytes (1/μl)	13,050–23,583	10,942–18,758	6,800–17,200	8,000–23,900
Bands	rare	0–2,480	0–880	0–107
Neutrophils	10,041–20,230	7,094–14,210	4,416–13,416	2,560–17,064
Lymphocytes	604–3,424	1,756–4,052	1,760–4,818	3,048–12,412
Monocytes	450–963	151–725	105–1,464	80–1,659
Eosinophils	0–1,650	64–690	0–630	0–3,042

Note: Pre- and postcolostrum data by L. W. Johnson, personal communication.

The artificial milk most often chosen is one of the commercial lamb milk replacers (see Table 10.3). By diluting the replacer at 1:6, the composition is close to that of mature llama milk. Artificial foal milk has a much higher lactose content and may cause osmotic diarrhea.

Lamoids, like other ungulates, will consume approximately 10% of their body weight in milk daily for the first couple of months. For the 11.34 kg (25 lb) neonate, this amounts to 1100 ml (40 oz). To feed that much fluid, 5 oz must be ingested every 2 hours from 6:00 A.M. to 8:00 P.M. Lamoids start to eat solid food at 2–3 weeks of age, and milk consumption decreases as solid food ingestion increases.

The lamoid neonate will nurse two to three times per hour in a normal situation. The orphan should be offered food at least every 2 hours for the first few days. The interval can be increased to 3–4 hours after a week, as long as the cria is able to consume the extra volume necessary to meet daily requirements.

Since llamas are generally not active at night, offering milk to the orphan during the hours of darkness may not be necessary, as long as sufficient volume is ingested during the day. Scrupulous cleanliness must be practiced with all utensils used for preparation and administration of milk for an orphan.

NEONATAL DISEASES (8, 11)

Neonatal septicemia has been discussed in Chapter 7. The congenital/hereditary diseases are discussed in Chapter 22 or in the appropriate organ system discussion. Defects that should be considered include choanal atresia, atresia ani and atresia coli, persistent urachus, and cardiac anomalies. Acquired conditions include urethral obstruction, ruptured bladder, and retained meconium, all of which are discussed in appropriate sections.

WEANING

Most llama crias wean themselves by 6 months of age. A few will persist in nursing for over a year if the female will tolerate it. Some females may kick the cria away at 4–5 months. However, in these instances, the amount of milk consumption may be negligible and the nursing has become a behavioral pattern. In vicuñas, the crias are weaned at approximately 6 months and expelled from the herd at 9–12 months. Guanacos have a slightly different weaning pattern, and yearlings may still be found with the mother while a cria of the year is nursing.

If a cria has converted to pasture and hay, there is little advantage to continued nursing after 6 months, and there may be a decided disadvantage to the female if she is pregnant again. Some owners wean at 5 months, and this is entirely satisfactory if the cria is well adapted. Orphaned crias may be able to make it on their own at 2 months of age, but there will be less risk of stunting if the nursing period can be prolonged.

IMMUNOPROPHYLAXIS

The most protective regimen for the lamoid cria is to make certain that the dam is immunized at least 2 months prior to parturition and that a booster vaccination is given 4–6 weeks before parturition. This regimen will ensure maximum production of specific Igs in the colostrum.

It is well recognized that the immune system of the neonate lacks maturity and that the neonate may not be able to respond to vaccination at an early age. Nonetheless, veterinarians with sheep experience recognize that enterotoxemia extracts a high toll in lambs that are not vaccinated by 2 weeks of age. Knowledge of clostridial diseases in lamoids in North America is meager, but prudence dictates that vaccinations should be administered within the first month of life and boostered a month later and again at weaning.

The specific vaccine recommended will be dependent upon the region and prevalence of diseases in local cattle, sheep, and goats. Basically, it is recommended that *Clostridium perfringens* type C and D toxoids and *C. tetani* toxoid be given. It is also appropriate to use multiple clostridial toxoids such as 7-way toxoids. Vaccines for other diseases may better be administered shortly before weaning. If leptospirosis is a problem in the area, a multiple serovar bacterin should be given. In rabies-endemic areas, a killed rabies vaccine should be given, and anthrax spore bacterins are indicated in certain areas. Crias should be given only one-fourth to one-half the dose of anthrax spore vaccine recommended for the adult (see Chap. 7).

REFERENCES

1. Garmendia, A. E., and McGuire, T. C. 1987. Mechanisms and isotypes involved in passive immunoglobulin transfer to the newborn alpaca. Am. J. Vet. Res. 48:1465–71.

2. Garmendia, A. E., Palmer, G. H., DeMartini, J. C., and McGuire, T. C. 1987. Failure of passive immunoglobulin transfer: A major determinant of mortality in newborn alpacas. Am. J. Vet. Res. 48:1472–76.

3. Herriges, S. 1981a. Caring for newborn llamas. Llama Newsl. 7:1–3.

4. ______. 1981b. Baby llamas—caring for the newborn. 3L Llama 9:1–4.

5. Jacobi, E. F. 1958. (Bottle feeding a young guanaco) Guanaco baby aan de fles. Artis (March-April) 6:193–97.

6. Kraft, H. 1957. (The behavior of the newborn and mother in camels) Das Verhalten von Muttertier and Neugeborenen bei Cameliden. Saeugtierkd. Mitt. 5:175–76.

7. Naylor, J. M. 1986. Colostrum and passive immunity in food producing animals. In J. L. Howard, ed. Current Veterinary Therapy: Food Animal Practice, 2nd ed. Philadelphia: W. B. Saunders, pp. 99–105.

8. Palza Perez, F. R. 1971. (The percent natality and mortality and successfully reared young at weaning in alpacas during the last 10 years at model ranches) Porcentaje de natalidad, mortaliday y crias logradas al destete en alpacas durate los ultimos diez anos en la granja modelo de Auquenidos La Raya y la Hacienda Picotani. Tesis, Fac. Med. Vet. Univ. Nac. Tec. Altiplano (Puno), pp. 1–50.

9. Pilters, H. 1954. (Investigations of inborn behavior in tylopods with special consideration of the New World forms) Untersuchungen ueber angeborene Verhaltensweisen bei Tylopoden, unter besonderer Beruecksichtigung der neuweltlichen Formen. Z. Tierpsycol. 11(2):213–303.

10. Prescott, J. 1981. Suckling behaviour of llamas (*Lama glama glama*) and Chapman's zebra (*Equus burchelli antiquorum*) in captivity. Appl. Anim. Ethol. 7(3):293–99.

11. Rath, E. 1953. (Diseases of newborn sheep and alpacas in the Puno) Enfermedades de los recien naciodos en ovinos y auquenidos en el Departamento de Puno y su atencion. Gac. Vet. (Lima) 1.

12. Stott, G. H., Marx, D. B., Menefee, B. E., and Nightengale, G. T. 1979. Colostral immunoglobulin transfer in calves. I. Period of absorption. J. Dairy Sci. 62:1632–38.

22

Congenital/ Hereditary Conditions

CONGENITAL PROBLEMS of llamas and alpacas are common. Veterinarians providing service to owners/breeders should give these problems special attention. Misconceptions and misunderstanding are prevalent. Unfortunately, little factual information is available to guide a breeder in managing a breeding program. Yet, much is known about similar or identical conditions in livestock. While direct extrapolation to lamoids is unacceptable, the principles of herd management are the same for all ungulates.

Though not all congenital conditions are of equal importance, clients should be advised of the presence of any defect and provided with information on the potential impact on breeding and performance. It is then the responsibility of the client to determine the disposition of the animal.

This chapter will survey the entire problem of congenital anomalies. Information will be presented as to various causes of such anomalies, and special attention will be focused on potential hereditary conditions. Since reported information is sparse, veterinarians should participate in the information-gathering process. Keeping detailed records is vital to obtaining crucial information for the benefit of the llama/alpaca industry as well as to offer protection to the veterinarian in the event that the animal is sold or defects affect a future breeding program. It is important to properly identify the animal and, if possible, obtain information on genealogy.

TERMINOLOGY

Various terms used to describe certain conditions are often erroneously used interchangeably by breeders and veterinarians, creating confusion. A *congenital* condition is present at the time of birth. Unfortunately, some congenital defects may not be readily apparent at the time of birth. In humans and livestock, certain biochemical defects may not be visible until later in life. Conformation characteristics may not become apparent until after the cria has grown. Yet in these instances, the foundation for the characteristic is present at the time of birth.

A *hereditary* condition is genetically transmitted from parent to offspring. The manifestation of the condition may be present at the time of birth or develop subsequently. The term *genetic* is frequently used interchangeably with hereditary, but they are not synonymous. Certain genetic disorders may cause serious defects in a single individual, but the disorder will not be passed on to subsequent generations. However, though certain types of intersex may be in this category, reproduction may be impossible because of the nature of the defects.

Embryogenesis is a complex, marvelously integrated process. The wonder is that the majority of offspring are normal. Many factors may influence the well-being of the fetus, and numerous agents other than genetic factors may disrupt organogenesis. The science of *teratology* ("monster" in Greek) deals with overall birth defects. A *teratogen* is any agent that causes abnormal development of the fetus. The furor over testing drugs that might be prescribed for pregnant females was spawned by the thalidomide disaster of the 1970s. Both physical and chemical effects on the fetus were known before that time, but now an entire discipline of medicine and biology deals with such topics. *Teratogenesis* is the process by which teratogens exert their effect.

CAMELID GENETICS

All camelids have a diploid chromosome number of 74 (1, 3, 36, 48). Fertile hybrids have been produced between all four species of South American camelids (SACs) (19). In theory, hybrids are also possible between camels and SACs, since the karyotypes of all the camelids are identical.

There are three pairs of submetacentric autosomes and 33 pairs of acrocentric autosomal chromosomes. The X chromosome is the largest submetacentric chromosome and the Y chromosome is a very small acrocentric chromosome. Some confusion over the classification of camelid chromosomes has arisen among investigators, perhaps because of variations in staining procedures and evaluation at different phases of meiosis (3). Chromosome banding patterns and nucleolus organizer regions have also been identified, but a complete discussion of karyology is beyond the scope of this book.

TERATOGENESIS

Etiology

The causes of congenital/hereditary defects are manifold (Table 22.1). Genetic factors will be discussed at length, and the effects of infectious diseases deserve special mention. Although no specific congenital defects caused by infectious agents have been reported, it seems likely that they occur. Consider a few examples from other species.

A number of virus infections are teratogenic in humans, cattle, sheep, goats, swine, cats, and ferrets. The ultimate effects on the fetus are determined by the species involved, the strain of the virus, and the stage of pregnancy at the time of exposure to the teratogen. Bovine virus diarrhea virus (BVDV) has caused cerebellar dysplasia, ocular defects, inferior brachygnathia, alopecia, internal hydrocephalus, and impaired immunologic competence in calves and lambs (32).

Blue tongue virus (BTV) has been shown experimentally to cause central nervous system defects and arthrogryposis in lambs. Exposure of pregnant heifers to BTV resulted in abortion, arthrogryposis, prognathia, and a "dummy-calf" syndrome (32). It is important to note that modified live virus (MLV) BTV vaccines may also exert teratogenic effects on the fetus of the pregnant ewe. The use of any MLV vaccine in any species other than those for which the vaccine was prepared is hazardous.

Table 22.1. Etiology of birth defects

Genetic
Mutant genes
Familial characteristics
Chromosomal aberrations
Infectious agents damaging fetus
Physical effects on the fetus
Trauma
Hyperthermia
Irradiation
Chemical
Drugs
Poisonous plants
Malnutrition
Excesses
Deficiencies

Both hog cholera virus and swine influenza virus are teratogenic. Feline panleukopenia virus (FPLV) causes cerebellar hypoplasia in kittens and ferrets (32). It is interesting that mature ferrets are refractory to overt infection with FPLV, yet teratogenesis occurs. In humans, examples of teratogenesis include congenital syphilitic blindness and congenital deafness from prenatal infection with German measles virus.

Chemically induced teratogenesis is being intensively studied in humans, livestock, and laboratory animals. No chemically induced teratogenic defects have been identified in lamoids. However, such effects are known to occur in all other species studied, so it should be expected that chemical teratogenesis will ultimately be identified in lamoids. Some congenital defects identified in lamoids are known to be chemical teratogen–induced in other livestock species. It should be pointed out that these defects are also known to be inherited traits in one or more species (Table 22.2). Veterinarians should investigate both possibilities when congenital deformities occur.

Table 22.2. Congenital conditions in lamoids and their inheritability in other domestic animals and humans

Condition	Bovine	Equine	Ovine	Caprine	Porcine	Canine	Feline	Human
Skeletal								
Ankylosis, carpus		U						
Angular limb deformity								
Carpal valgus		S	S					Y
Carpal varus			U					
Femorotibial valgus								
Metacarpophalangeal valgus								
Arthrogryposis	Y	Y	Y		Y			Y
Femur, shortened							Y	
Hemivertebra	S				Y	U		
Spinal agenesis								
Metacarpal, shortening						U	Y	
Patella, medial luxation						Y		Y
Polydactyly	Y	U	Y	Y	S	Y	Y	Y
Scoliosis	U		U					Y
Syndactyly	Y		U		U	Y		Y
Tail, agenesis			U		U	U	Y	
Talus, vertical								
Tendon contracture								Y
Carpus			U					
Stifle			U					
Head/face								
Cerebellar hypoplasia	Y	S	S		U	S	Y	Y
Choanal atresia								Y
Cyclopia	U	U	U	U	U		U	U
Encephalomeningocele			U				U	U

Table 22.2. ***(continued)***

Condition	Bovine	Equine	Ovine	Caprine	Porcine	Canine	Feline	Human
Facial bones								
Agenesis								
Lateral deviation		U						
Hydrocephalus, internal[a]		U	U		S	Y	Y	Y
Mandible								
Brachygnathia	Y	Y	Y	Y	U	Y		
Micrognathia			Y		U			
Prognathia	Y		U			Y		Y
Maxilla								
Brachygnathia					U	Y		
Prognathia		Y				Y		Y
Nares, agenesis								
Nasal passages, stenosis						U		
Palate								
Agenesis								
Palatoschisis (cleft)	Y	U	Y		U		Y	Y
Teeth, retention of deciduous								
Reproductive system								
Cervix								
Agenesis								
Double	Y							
Fallopian tubes, segmental agenesis	Y				U			Y
Hymen, imperforate	S				U			Y
Intersex, pseudohermaphrodite	U	Y	Y	Y	Y	U	U	U
Ovary								
Agenesis	Y						U	Y
Hypoplasia	Y						U	
Penis								
Corkscrew	U							U
Curvature								
Hypoplasia	U	U						U
Persistent frenulum	Y				U			
Testes								
Cryptorchidism	Y	Y	Y	Y	Y	Y	U	Y
Cystic structures								
Ectopic	Y						U	
Hypoplasia	Y		Y				U	Y
Twinning	Y	Y	Y	Y				Y
Uterus	Y				U		U	
Segmental agenesis								
Unicornis								
Vagina, segmental agenesis	Y		U				U	Y
Digestive system								
Atresia ani	Y	U	Y		Y			Y
Atresia coli	U	U						Y
Megaesophagus		U				S	S	
Pyloric stenosis								
Cardiovascular								
Atrial septal defect		U			U	U	U	U
Aortic arch, persistent, right[b]		U				Y	U	
Ductus arteriosus, patent		U			U	Y	S	Y
Portocaval shunt								
Tetralogy of Fallot	U	U				Y	U	U
Transposition of great vessels		U			U		U	
Ventricular septal defect	Y	U	Y		U	Y	U	U
Eye								
Blindness, cause not determined	U					Y		
Cataract[c]	Y	Y				Y	Y	Y
Ectropion		U				U		
Entropion	Y	U	Y		U	U	U	Y
Eyelid, hypogenesis							U	Y
Iris, nonpigmented (glass)	Y	U			Y	Y	U	
Miscellaneous								
Dwarfism	Y	Y	Y	Y	Y	U		Y
Ears, short				Y	S			
Hernia								
Diaphragmatic		U	U		S	Y	Y	Y
Inguinal	U	U			Y	U	U	
Umbilical[d]	Y	Y	Y		Y	Y	Y	U
Renal agenesis	U	U	U	U	U	S	U	Y
Polythelia, supernumerary teats		Y					U	Y
Teat agenesis								
Toenails, crooked	Y	Y	Y		Y			
Urachus, patent	U		U		U		U	

Sources: Bovine, Leipold et al. 1983; equine, Huston et al. 1977; ovine, Dennis and Leipold 1979, Saperstein et al. 1975; caprine, Leipold and Dennis, 1984; porcine, Huston et al. 1978; canine, Erickson et al. 1977; feline, Saperstein et al. 1976; human, Elsas and Priest 1979, McKusick 1986.

[a]Brown 1973.

[b]Kolaczkowski and Soboncinski 1971.

[c]Ingram and Sigler 1983.

[d]Fowler 1987.

Note: Y = inheritance confirmed; S = inheritence suspected; U = occurs but etiology unknown; blank = no information.

Some general principles should be understood: (1) The degree of susceptibility to the effects of a teratogen is determined by the genotype of the animal. Not all species are equally affected. (2) The teratogen, to affect the fetus, must pass through the placenta in the metabolically active form. (3) The nature of the deformity is dose dependent. High doses of a certain teratogen at a critical time result in resorption. Slightly lower levels result in dead, deformed fetuses, still lower levels in living, deformed fetuses, and at the lowest levels in normal, live offspring. (4) The fetus must be exposed to the teratogen at a specific period during gestation. Knowledge of embryology and, especially, the time and sequence of organogenesis is fundamental to understanding teratogenesis. (5) Chemically dissimilar teratogens may produce identical effects on the fetus.

Poisonous plant ingestion by a pregnant lamoid is an ever-present hazard to the fetus (26, 27). Lamoids are fastidious in their eating habits, rarely consuming large amounts of strange plants, but they do investigate and try new plants. A low-dose intake may be a saving factor in lamoids. Table 22.3 lists plants known to produce teratogenic defects in livestock.

The presence of a birth defect is vivid and alarming to the breeder. However, of perhaps even greater importance are the effects that chemical agents may have on the reproductive process without obvious outward expression. Teratogens may have a direct effect on ova or spermatozoa, causing infertility. High doses early in gestation may cause fetal death with resorption or undetected abortion. Lethal effects may be the result of maternal ingestion early in gestation, even though fetal death occurs late in gestation or postpartum. Nonlethal effects may either prevent reproduction or allow reproduction of constitutionally unsound individuals that may be highly susceptible to other diseases.

HEREDITARY TRAITS

Hundreds of anatomic and physiologic traits are passed from parents to offspring by gene pairing (29, 32). Over 400 gene loci have been mapped on human chromosomes (8, 35), but only 19 in cattle (33), 16 in sheep (42), 11 in horses (23), and 5 in pigs (24).

Fiber coat color inheritance in llamas and alpacas has received attention by both South American (18) and North American (20, 49, 50) investigators, but definitive genetic studies have not been conducted and reported. A detailed discussion of coat color determination is beyond the scope of this book.

Body conformation is also an inherited characteristic. This topic will be discussed more fully later.

Chromosomal Aberration

A number of chromosomal abnormalities have been reported in domestic animals. These defects occur during meiosis and include fusion of chromosomes, translocations of segments of chromosomes, loss of a segment, and other changes (22). The expression of the defect is determined by whether or not the change occurred on an autosomal pair or one of the sex chromosomes. Chromosomal aberrations may affect a single individual or be perpetuated as inherited characteristics. Chromosomal aberrations may be identified by a combination of family pedigree analysis, identification of interspecific somatic cell hybrids, and cytogenetic studies, including karyotyping and various banding staining.

Genetic studies have been developed to the stage of highly technical, submolecular/biochemical complexities that are far beyond the scope of this work. Lamoid inheritance is still in the descriptive stage. Although most of the congenital defects reported in lamoids are known to be inherited in one or more species of other domestic animals or humans, it is important to recognize that

Table 22.3. Plants with known teratogenic effects in livestock

Plant name		Species affected	Stage of gestation involved (days)	Type of defect
Scientific	Common			
Astragalus spp. *Oxytropis* spp.	Locoweed	Cattle, sheep	1–100	Flexure of carpus, abortion
Conium maculatum	Poison hemlock	Cattle	40–70	Arthrogryposis
Datura stramonium	Jimson weed	Swine	60–120	Arthrogryposis
Leucaena leucocephala	Koa haole, lead tree	Swine, rats		Fetal resorption, polypodia
Lupinus spp.	Lupine, blue bonnet	Cattle	40–70	Arthrogryposis, scoliosis, cleft palate
Nicotiana tobaccum	Tobacco	Swine, rats		Twisted limbs, dorsal flexure of hind limb digits
Sorghum vulgare	Sudan grass	Horses		Carpal ankylosis
Trachymene cyanantha	Wild parsnip	Sheep		Crooked legs
Veratrum californicum	False hellebore, corn lily	Sheep	14	Cyclopia

many may also be produced by other etiologic agents, as listed in Table 22.1. In fact, such defects as arthrogryposis are more likely to be caused by exposure of the dam to a toxic substance at a crucial time during gestation than by genetic damage.

Nonetheless, prudent llama/alpaca breeders and veterinarians should consider the prevalence of certain defects in particular lamoid blood lines and in multiple environmental situations. A veterinarian should not be dogmatic, but should educate and assist.

Detection of Inherited Traits (22, 30, 38)

The detection of an inherited trait is dependent upon the mode of inheritance. If a characteristic is dominant, one of the parents will be phenotypically positive and, generally, at least 50% of its offspring will express the phenotype. However, even though a characteristic may be dominant, environmental or genetic factors may affect the degree of expression of a phenotype.

The majority of inherited defects are recessive, and both parents must contribute the gene in order for the offspring to exhibit the trait. Recessive traits may be simple, in which only one gene is involved, or multifactorial, which complicates expression and detection in a population.

A carrier male and female will produce 75% phenotypically normal offspring, but 50% of their offspring will be carriers. Veterinarians dealing with suspected inherited traits in lamoids should discuss this thoroughly with owners.

The diagnosis of an inherited trait is a laborious, costly, time-consuming process. Familial repetition is the most important data necessary, and this requires detailed genealogy of both normal and abnormal offspring. Statistical evaluation of familial data is frequently required.

The ultimate evaluation is based on breeding trials. No such trials have been reported for lamoids, but lamoid owners may consider the studies conducted in artificial insemination (AI) establishments for cattle. Table 22.4 provides a listing of the number of matings required to exclude carrier status of a male for a simple recessive defect.

Table 22.4. Number of matings required to exclude carrier status of a male lamoid for a simple recessive defect

	Probability of error	
	5%	1%
Male mated to females that are		
Homozygous aa	5	7
Heterozygous Aa	11	16
Mixed—50% Aa, 50% AA	23	35

Source: Modified from Hamori 1983, p. 47.

Breeding in such numbers is possible in an AI stud, where selected sires can be test mated with specifically purchased cows known to be homozygous or heterozygous carriers, but this is difficult or impossible on the working ranch. Another method is to test breed sires on daughters, because if heterozygosity is suspected, at least 50% of the male's daughters should also be heterozygous. This method requires 23 matings to detect a recessive gene in the male.

It is both expensive and time consuming to conduct such test breedings in a male, and it is impossible to test breed a female to detect a recessive carrier state. Reversing the sex status of animals in Table 22.4, if the female were mated to (aa) males, 5 births would be required, and if bred to (Aa) males, 11 births. Such proof is not likely to be forthcoming in lamoids.

Since detection of the carrier state of a simple recessive trait in lamoids by breeding trials is unlikely, other methods must be used to identify and eliminate carrier animals from a breeding program. This may be possible using information and practices developed in cattle and sheep breeding.

Consider a hypothetical simple recessive trait (Table 22.5). Homozygous (AA) individuals are completely free of the trait and homozygous (aa) individuals express the phenotype. While heterozygous (Aa) individuals do not express the phenotype, they may not be as healthy as an (AA) individual in performance characteristics such as milk production, fertility, growth, mothering ability, and disease resistance, all factors that may be evaluated in livestock.

Table 22.5. Expected expression of a phenotype among the offspring of parents having a recessive trait

AA	×	Aa	=	0
Aa	×	Aa	=	25%
Aa	×	aa	=	50%
aa	×	aa	=	100%

Source: Modified from Hamori 1983.
Note: AA = homozygous (free from trait); Aa = heterozygous (carrier); aa = homozygous (affected).

Furthermore, in livestock, a number of biochemical defects such as afibrinogenemia may be measured in the laboratory. Aa individuals for this trait show an intermediate level of fibrinogen that can be detected by serum analysis.

The problem in the llama/alpaca industry is that no biochemical defects are known; in fact, basal blood parameters are just beginning to be reported. Neither have standards been established for milk production, growth, mothering ability, etc. Nonetheless, these standards can be developed. The llama/alpaca industry is in its infancy in North America. It is important that responsible breeders begin to use the basic principles of animal breeding developed with livestock.

Cytogenetic studies should be carried out and karyotypes and banding staining be done. Detailed, sophisticated biochemical standards must be established.

BREEDING MANAGEMENT SYSTEMS

It is inappropriate to discuss all of the various breeding management systems in a medical text such as this. Since some of the systems have profound influence on the prevalence of congenital defects, veterinarians and breeders would be well advised to consult contemporary books on the subject (30). *Inbreeding* is a mating system in which the progeny produced by parents are more closely related than the average of the population from which they come. Father-daughter, brother-sister, grandfather-granddaughter, and other close relationship breedings have been carried out with llamas both intentionally and unknowingly. The parentage of some llamas is unknown, and only recently has it become possible to verify parentage in lamoids as is routinely done in cattle and horses (17, 49). This will be discussed later. *Linebreeding* is a form of inbreeding in which an attempt is made to concentrate the inheritance of some one ancestor or ancestral line in a herd.

Inbreeding increases homozygosity and is used in livestock breeding to strengthen a given characteristic. Unfortunately, it can also concentrate undesirable traits. Inbreeding is a technique that should be practiced only by highly skilled and experienced breeders who are willing to cull (not sell) individuals exhibiting undesirable traits.

In general, inbreeding is followed by a decline in traits closely related to physical fitness such as fertility, mothering ability, viability, and growth rate (41). Detailed records were kept on a herd of inbred dorcas gazelles, *Antidorcas gazellei,* at a zoo. As the inbreeding coefficient increased, so did the neonatal mortality rate. The calves died of inanition, weakness, white muscle disease, and a variety of other infectious and noninfectious diseases. The neonates lost their "coping" ability (41). Llama/alpaca breeders should be fully cognizant of the ramifications of the practice of inbreeding.

CONGENITAL CONDITIONS

Table 22.2 lists congenital conditions that have been identified by the author (13, 14), reported in the literature (5, 21, 31, 51), or reported by personal communications. The inheritability of similar conditions in humans and other animal species is indicated. The reader is again reminded that these conditions may have other than hereditary causes. Some of the conditions will be discussed in detail because of their importance to the llama/alpaca industry. Others are simply listed. It may be valuable to attach this table to a clipboard near physical examination forms to be reviewed prior to conducting a health and soundness examination for prepurchase, insurance, or evaluation for breeding soundness.

Skeletal Defects

ANGULAR LIMB DEFORMITY. Conformation of the limbs in association with the body is an inherited trait in all animals. There seems to be a high prevalence of crooked legs in llamas and alpacas. Carpal valgus is most prevalent (12), but carpal varus, metacarpal phalangeal valgus, and femorotibial valgus have also been seen. Similar defects of the long bones of horses and livestock have been reported.

Although there is evidence that some forms of angular limb deformity are familial (12), all types should not be placed in the same etiologic and diagnostic category. Nutrition is thought to be a factor in some, trauma in others, while in many cases the true cause is unknown. This is also true in the horse.

In carpal valgus, the prominent sign is inward bowing of one or both carpi (Figs. 22.1, 22.2). When the defect is allowed to progress, the carpi overlap each other when the animal is standing still. Abrasions at the medial aspect of the carpi may be noted from the trauma of knocking the carpi against one another when walking. In one individual, the deviation was so severe that the legs were actually crossed, though when viewed from the front, the legs appeared to be straight because hair hid the crossed upper forearm and arm. Outward bowing of the carpi is more rare (Fig. 22.3). Bowing of the fetlock has been seen (Fig. 22.4).

Carpal valgus may be present at birth, but an evaluation should be delayed for a month to allow normal straightening to occur. The degree of deviation may develop at 2–6 months of age and progressively become more severe, up to 15 months of age. However, even in cases of development a few months after birth, a spontaneous correction of the deviation may occur.

Radiographs should be taken to evaluate the carpus and contiguous long bones. The ulnar physis is approximately 3–5 cm proximal to the radial physis. The ulnar epiphysis extends distally along the lateral radius and attenuates as it becomes a part of the radial epiphysis. Radiographs and anatomic preparations show no physical separation of these two epiphyses in the majority of individuals. However, the author has examined some animals with separated epiphyses.

Variable radiographic changes may be observed in

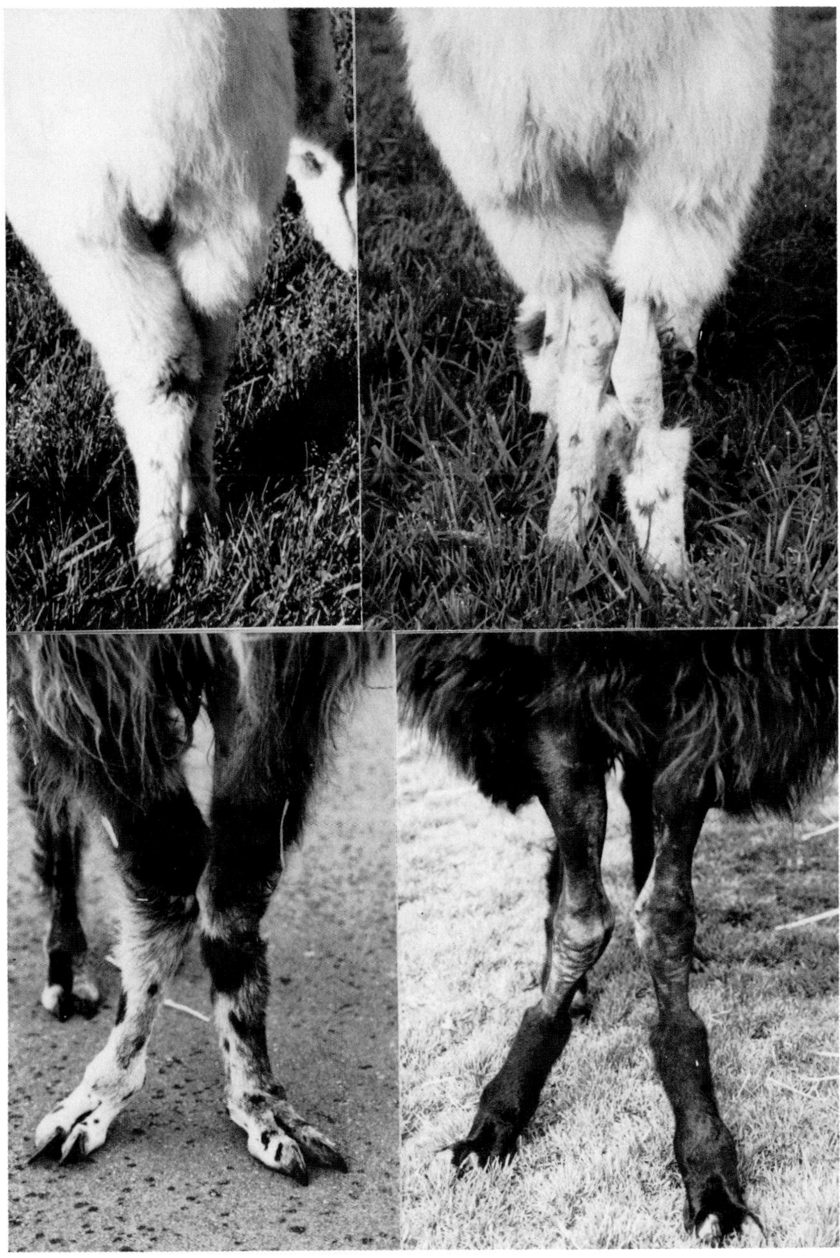

22.1 Carpal valgus.

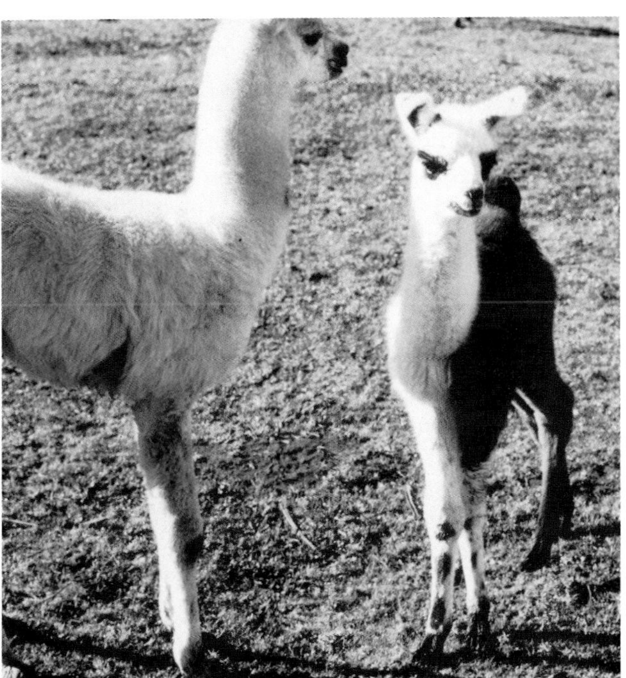

22.2 Carpal valgus in a neonate.

the carpal region. Lesions of metabolic bone disease are rarely observed. Inflammation of the radial physis, characterized by flaring and widening of the physis, may be caused by trauma.

The typical radiographic lesion of carpal valgus is a wedge-shaped radial epiphysis, with the base of the wedge on the medial aspect of the carpus. The width of the radial physis is variable, but the ulnar physis is flared, doubly cupped in shape, with hyperplasia of the distal ulna (Fig. 22.5) (12).

The pathogenesis of carpal valgus appears to be a cessation of growth at the ulnar physis on the lateral aspect of the limb, allowing continued growth of the medial radial physis, producing inward bowing of the limb at the carpus.

The surgical management of angular limb deformity is discussed in Chapter 6. Tubular splints may be applied to the limbs of young animals (less than 2 months of age)

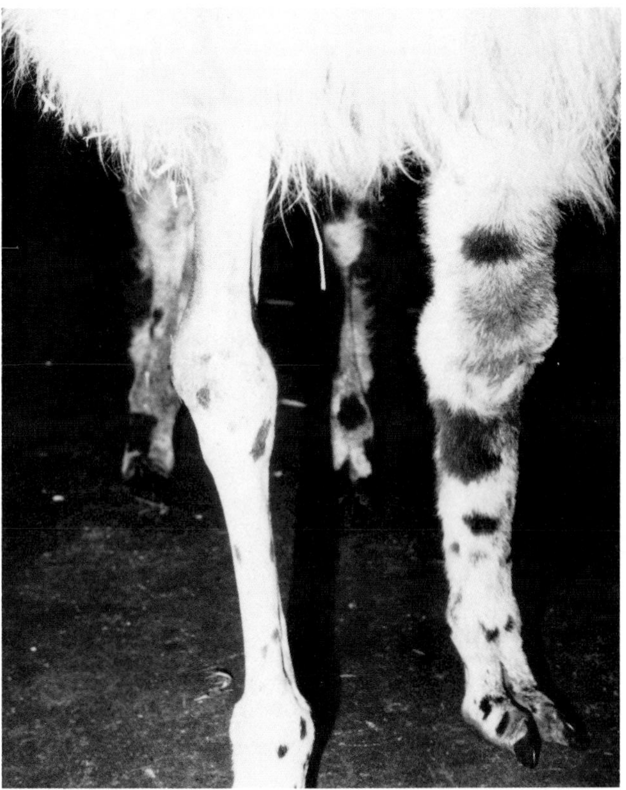

22.3 Carpal varus (outward bow).

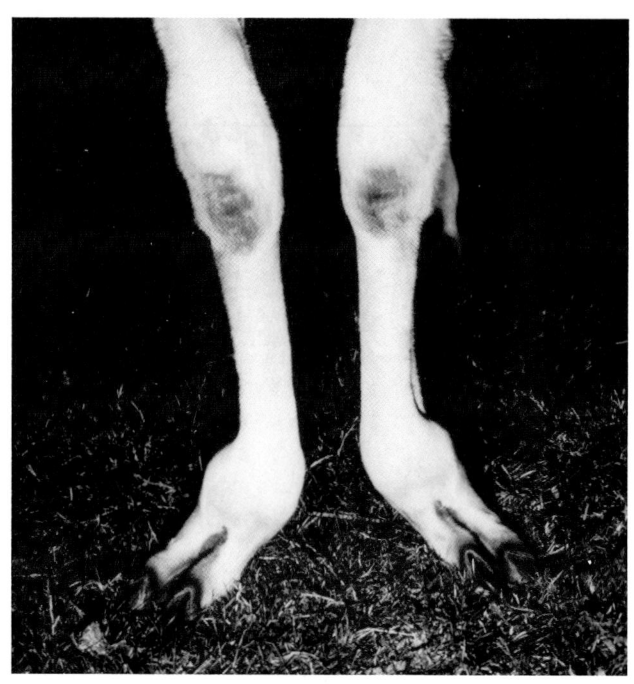

22.4 Angular deformity of fetlock.

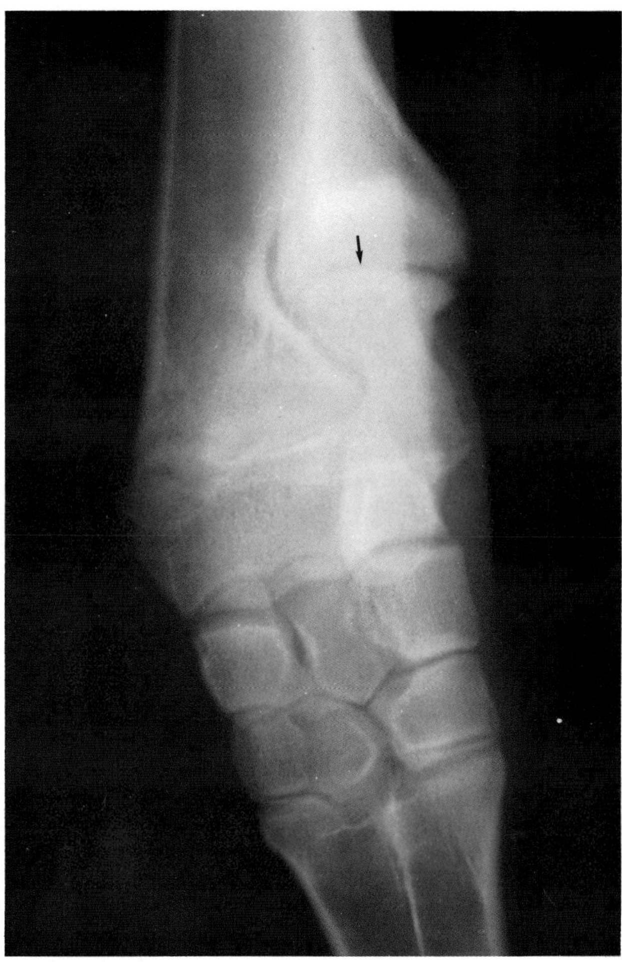

22.5 Dorsopalmar radiograph of a llama with carpal valgus.

with mild deviation. It is unlikely that any appreciable straightening of the limb will occur after the animal is 15 months of age, though the physis may not be entirely closed until 3 years of age.

ARTHROGRYPOSIS. Arthrogryposis is congenital, persistent flexure or contracture of a joint. The bones of the joint are malformed, and their relationship to contiguous bones is distorted to the extent that it is difficult to identify the bones or the joint with radiography. Arthrogryposis may be uni- or bilateral, with single or multiple joints involved. In llamas, the elbow and carpus have been most frequently affected (Fig. 22.6), but other joints are also affected (Figs. 22.7, 22.8). Arthrogryposis is frequently present in the neonate with multiple congenital defects (polydactyly, carpal tendon contracture, choanal atresia).

The cause of arthrogryposis in lamoids is unknown. In livestock, teratogens are frequently involved (Table 22.3). Affected crias are unable to stand. It is impossible

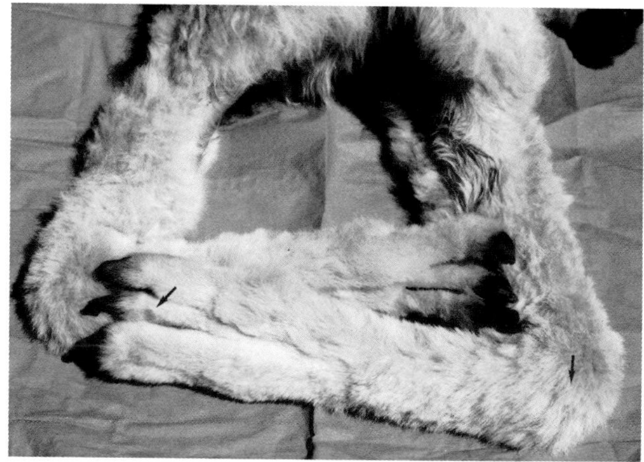

22.6 Carpal arthrogryposis and polydactyly.

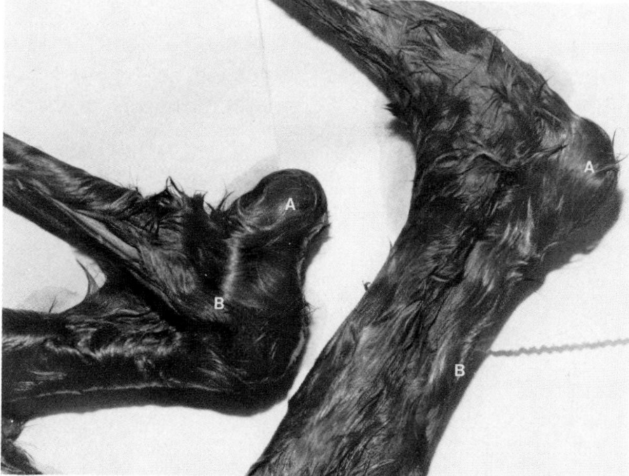

22.7 Tarsal arthrogryposis in a stillborn, full-term llama fetus.

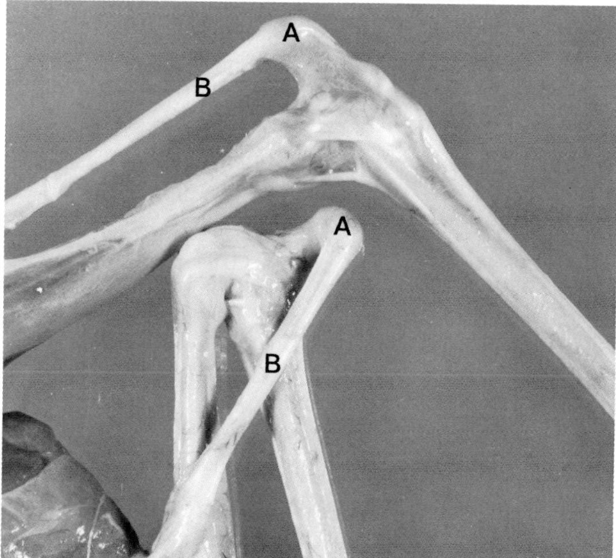

22.8 Tarsal arthrogryposis: **(A)** tuber calcis, **(B)** tendon of gastrocnemius.

to straighten the limb. The distal segment of the limb may be pointed in any direction or rotated 180 degrees. The joint is usually swollen, but not from the accumulation of synovia.

The diagnosis of multiple joint arthrogryposis is obvious, but it should be differentiated from tendon contracture, in which the bones of the joint are usually properly formed. Trauma should be considered when a single joint is involved.

Surgical correction of arthrogryposis is usually impossible. Euthanasia should be recommended.

SHORTENING OF LONG BONES. Unilateral shortening of the femur and metacarpus have been reported in lamoids. The cause is unknown. The animal may compensate and be used as a pet, depending on the degree of shortening.

LUXATION OF THE PATELLA. The author has dealt with two cases of congenital bilateral medial luxation of the patella in llamas. Others have also observed lateral luxation. Full medial luxation causes the cria to stand in a crouched position (Fig. 22.9). The stifle joint is thickened, and the patella is palpated in the medial position rather than in the dorsal groove of the femur. It is impossible to manipulate the patella to the normal position.

Upward fixation of the patella is an acquired condition in older llamas (see Chap. 6). A predisposition may be a congenital conformational weakness (straight rear limbs and laxity of the tendons and ligaments). The

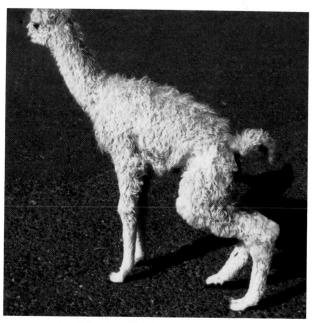

22.9 Bilateral medial patellar luxation in a llama neonate.

mechanisms for upward fixation in a llama is different than in a horse. The distal patella ligament is a sheet of tendinous tissue rather than one, two, or three discrete ligaments. With laxity of the tibiopatellar and femoropatellar ligaments, the patella may lodge at the dorsal tip of either the medial or lateral ridge of the trochlea.

The prognosis for medial luxation is unfavorable. Surgery was partially effective in one cria, in which the patella was firmly bound medially by shortened collateral patellar ligaments. These attachments were severed, and the crest of the tibia, on which the major mass of the distal patellar ligament was inserted, was relocated more laterally and secured to the tibia with lag screws. The trochlear groove was deepened to provide a better channel for the patella. These are standard procedures, developed for dogs with a similar luxation.

HEMIVERTEBRA. Hemivertebra refers to partial agenesis of one or more of the vertebrae. Spina bifida is the ultimate manifestation of this defect. Malformation of the spinal cord is usually associated with spina bifida. No confirmed cases have been reported in lamoids, but hemivertebra of the 4th cervical (C-4) vertebra has been diagnosed in association with subluxation of the cervical vertebrae and spinal cord trauma in a juvenile alpaca.

Clinical signs included ataxia and falling when attempting to avoid capture for restraint. The ataxia was exacerbated by restraint, particularly if the head and neck were manipulated. The diagnosis was confirmed by radiography and myelography. The body of C-7 was only partially formed. There was a marked subluxation between C-6 and C-7 (Fig. 22.10). In the dorsoventral projection, the articular facets were missing, allowing even greater instability (Fig. 22.11). The stenosis of the neural canal was confirmed by contrast myelography administered via the lumbosacral space.

The anatomic defect was easily identified at necropsy. The spinal cord was flattened at the region of the subluxation, and neuronal degeneration was observed histologically.

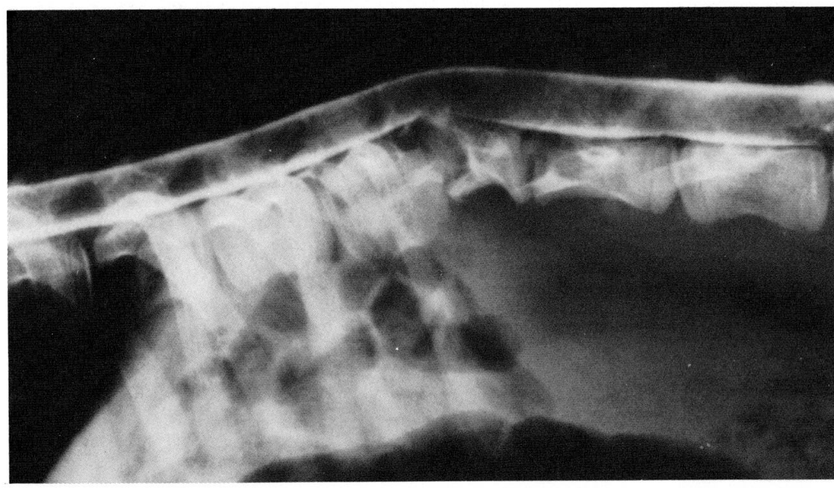

22.10 Lateral radiograph of hemivertebrae of the 1st lumbar vertebrae in a llama neonate. Spinal cord compression is noted by contrast myelography. (Photo courtesy Dr. Richard Cambre, Denver)

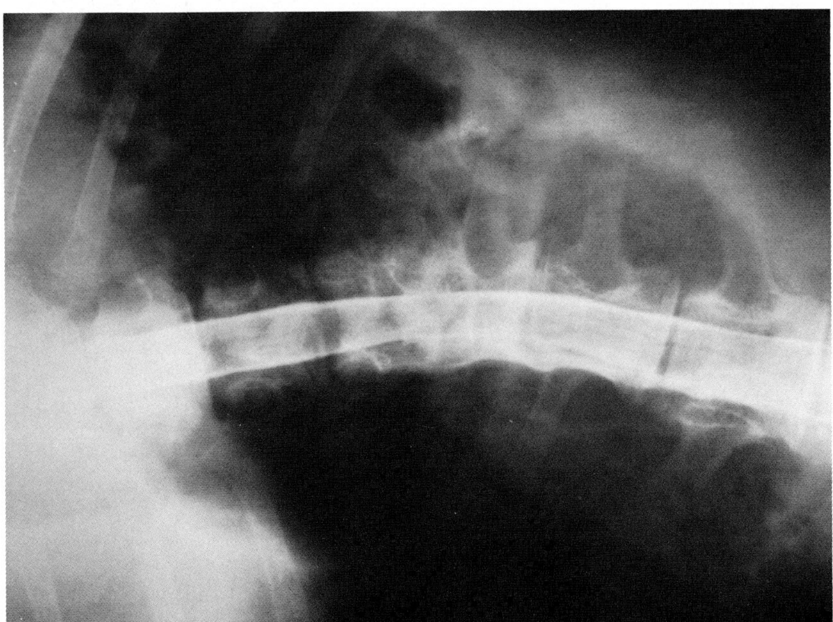

22.11 Dorsoventral radiograph of hemivertebrae of the 1st lumbar vertebrae in a llama neonate. (Photo courtesy Dr. Richard Cambre, Denver)

POLYDACTYLY/SYNDACTYLY. Polydactylism is a common congenital defect in llamas (47). From one to three accessory digits may occur on one or all four limbs (Fig. 22.12). Fusion of two normal digits (syndactyly) is less common (Fig. 22.13). Both conditions have been identified as inherited traits in cattle, dogs, and humans. The conditions are evident on clinical examination. The degree of development of the accessory digits varies, but it may be complete, with a full complement of tendons, ligaments, and bones, including metacarpals and metatarsals. Polydactyly is frequently seen in multiple-anomaly situations.

Accessory digits may be removed surgically to allow use of the animal as a pet, but prudent breeding practice should exclude such an animal from further breeding.

SCOLIOSIS. Various forms of curvature of the spinal column occur as isolated incidents (Fig. 22.14). The etiology is unknown. Wry neck may be trauma induced

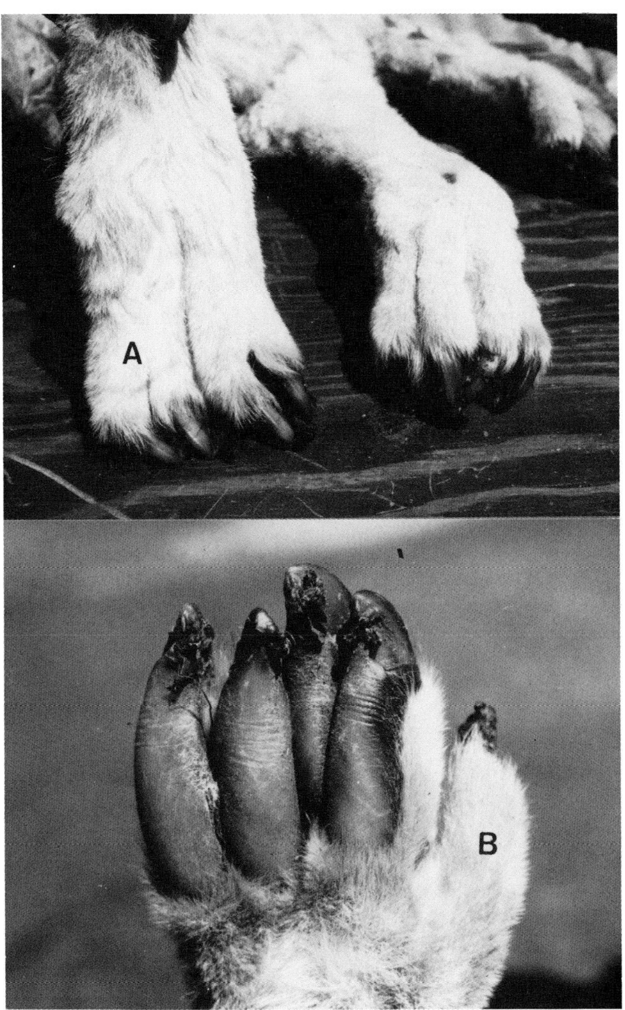

22.12 (A) Polypodia, (B) polydactyly.

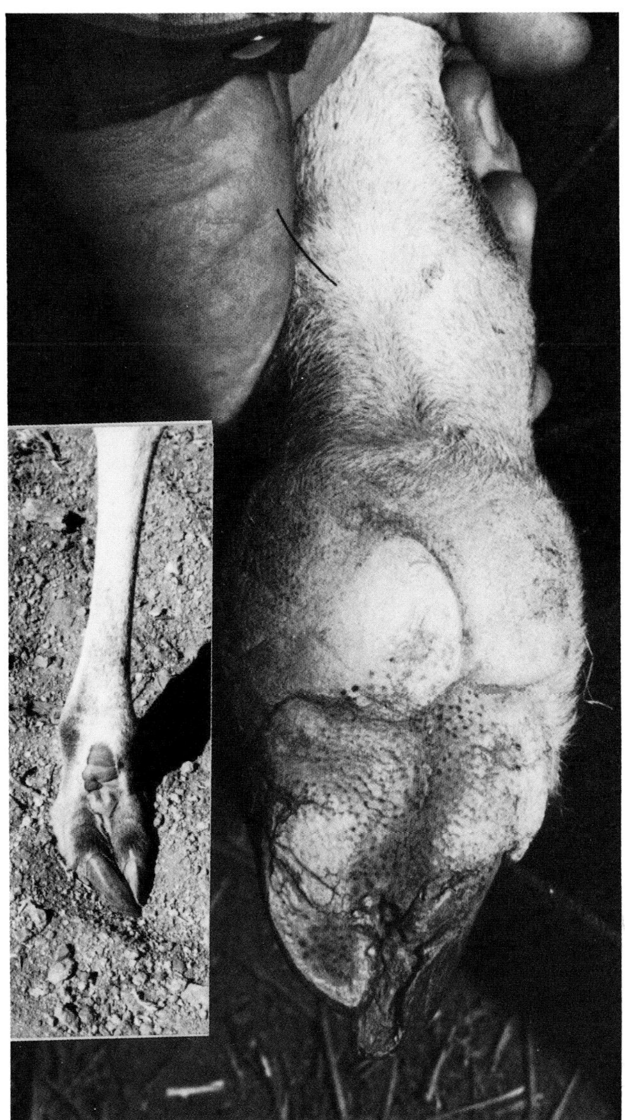

22.13 Syndactyly.

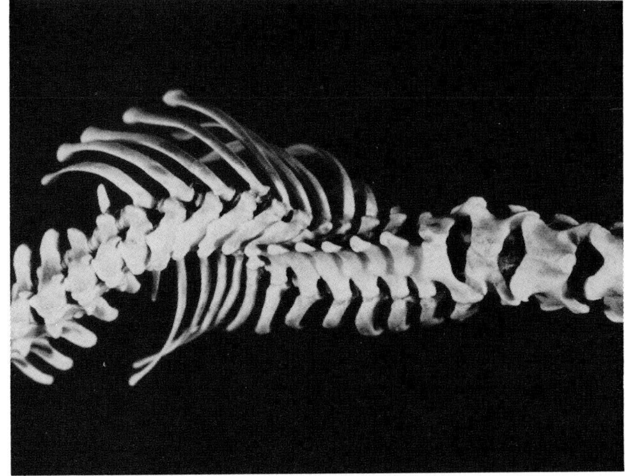

22.14 Scoliosis.

from overzealous traction during dystocia. In true congenital scoliosis, changes that indicate permanent distortion of the vertebrae may be seen on radiography.

LUXATION OF THE TIBIOTARSAL BONE. Bilateral luxation of the tibiotarsal bone was diagnosed in a 7-month-old female llama. Based on the history provided and interpretation of radiographs, it appeared that this condition was congenital. In another llama, a unilateral luxation of the tibiotarsal bone was thought to be traumatic in origin.

In a llama suffering from luxation, the tibiotarsal bone lies in a horizontal rather than a vertical position, and the articular grooves of the tibia articulate with the caudal aspect of the tibiotarsal bone rather than the trochlea (Fig. 22.15). Externally, the cranial surface of the tarsus bulges where the tibiotarsal bone projects forward. Movement of the tarsus is restricted, causing a mechanical lameness.

The condition in llamas is similar to congenital convex pes valgus (congenital vertical talus, congenital flat foot, teratologic dislocation of the talonavicular joint) in human infants (46). The etiology in human infants is unknown, but it is thought to be genetic. Peculiar fetal positioning within the uterus has also been considered. Surgical realignment and pinning of the tibiotarsus may correct the defect in human infants but has not been performed in llamas.

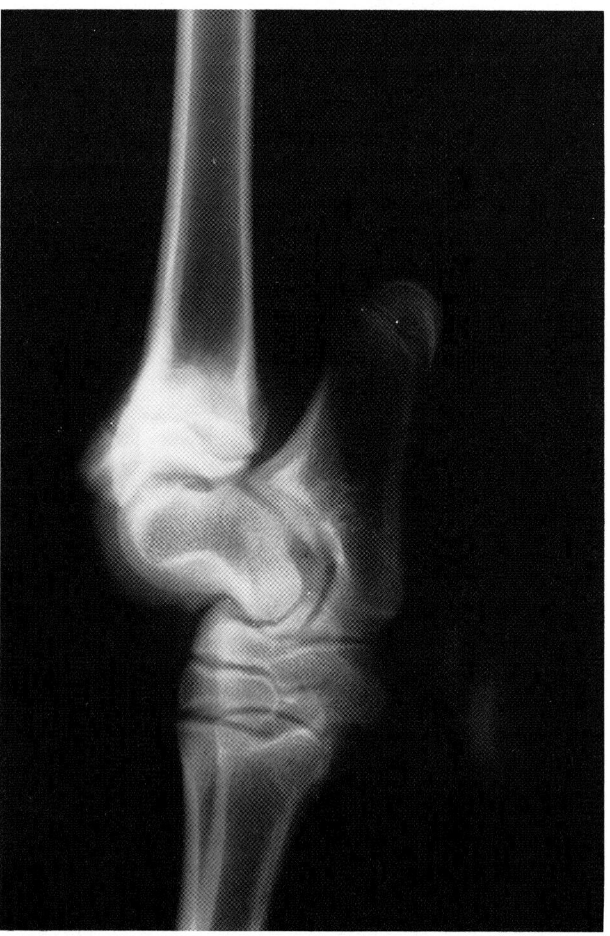

22.15 Lateral radiograph of tibiotarsal bone luxation. Compare with Figure 11.31.

Face and Head Defects

CRANIOFACIAL DYSGENESIS. A number of congenital defects of the face, nasal cavity, and pharynx (Table 22.2) may be lethal because of the obligate nasal breathing of the cria. The precise relationship between the various defects is unknown. The embryologic development of the nasopharyngeal region is complex, yet it seems logical that these conditions may be the result of interference with development at a particular time.

The least evident defect may be stenosis of the nasal passages. Choanal atresia is common and may consist of a membranous or osseous partition between the nasal and pharyngeal cavities (Fig. 22.16) (11). Agenesis of the facial bones causes variable shortening of the face and muzzle (Fig. 22.17) and accentuates the doming of the forehead that may be mistaken as a hydrocephalic condition. In extreme cases, agenesis of the facial bones, along with other tissue dysgenesis, may result in cyclopia. The nares may be totally occluded (Fig. 22.17).

The etiology of lamoid facial dysgenesis is unknown. Teratogens are known to produce similar congenital defects in sheep. A familial relationship is known in humans with choanal atresia (9).

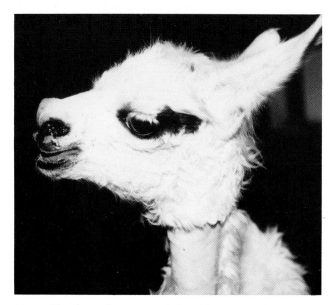

22.16 Flared-nostril, open-mouth breathing characteristic of choanal atresia.

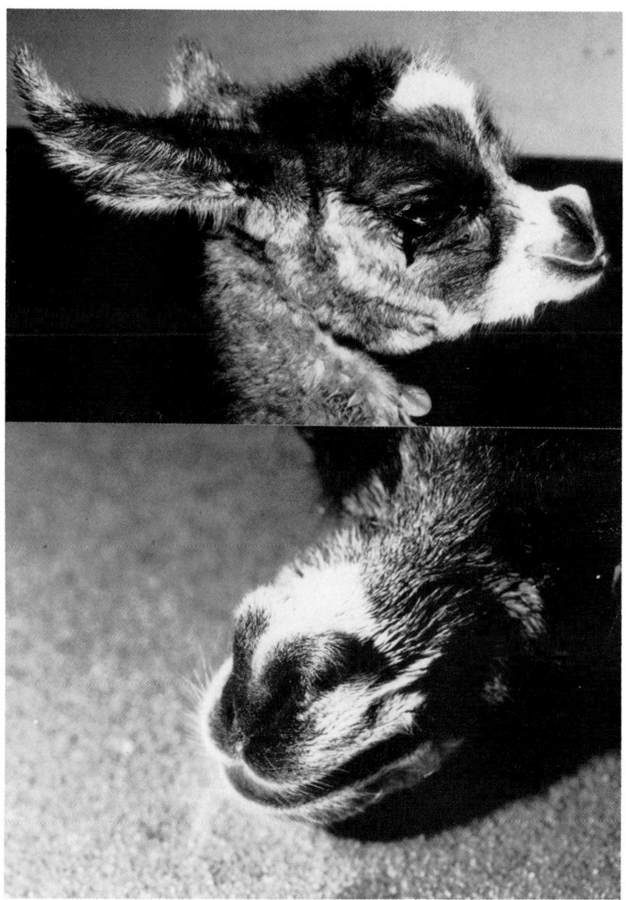

22.17 Choanal atresia with deformed face and nostril agenesis.

Clinical signs vary with the nature of the defect. All produce some impairment of respiration. Complete occlusion of the nasal passageways causes a characteristic breathing pattern in the cria. On inspiration, the mouth is opened slightly and filled with air. Then the lips are slightly closed, while air continues to be sucked into the mouth, ballooning the cheeks. The lips close tightly and the cheeks compress to force air around the elongated soft palate, which is positioned ventral to the epiglottal cartilage. With expiration, air is forced out of the larynx into the oropharynx, and complete exhalation requires further effort to push the air around the soft palate and out the mouth.

An affected cria stands with the head extended, since this position restricts air flow the least. Also, from the extended head position it may be possible for the soft palate to flip dorsal to the epiglottal cartilage, allowing free flow of air into the trachea. During this time, breathing is more normal.

Restricted expiratory air flow entraps excessive air in the pharynx, which may, in turn, be swallowed, causing tympanites. Affected crias not only have difficulty breathing but find it almost impossible to nurse. The time required to obtain sufficient oxygen to sustain life precludes time for swallowing milk. Aspiration pneumonia is a common sequel. Affected crias are known to chew at and ingest fiber from the mother. Numerous hairballs have been observed in compartment one of the stomach at necropsy.

Nasopharyngeal obstruction may be partial or complete and uni- or bilateral. Some affected animals are not detected as neonates but have respiratory deficiencies as an adult. Such conditions are difficult to differentiate from acquired chronic respiratory diseases.

Definitive diagnosis of these conditions may require radiographs. In a neonate with suspected choanal atresia, a 5 mm catheter should be inserted intranasally. The head should be maintained in an elevated position to prevent back flow of the medium from the nostril; 10 ml of a contrast medium (hypaque) should be deposited into the nasal cavity, followed by immediate exposure of both a lateral and a dorsoventral view (Figs. 22.18, 22.19). Both nasal cavities should be evaluated.

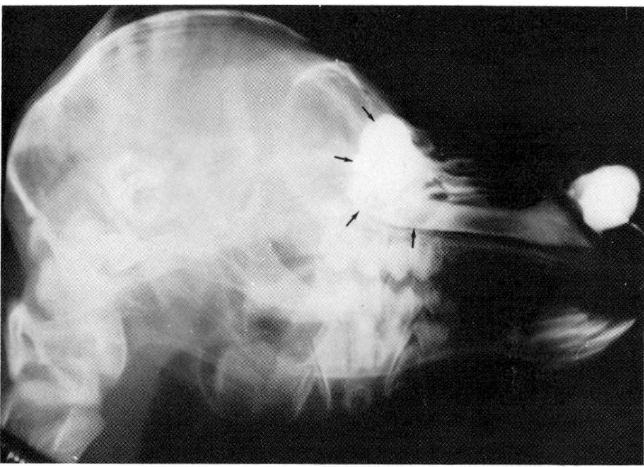

22.18 Lateral radiograph of choanal atresia, radiopaque liquid instilled into nostril.

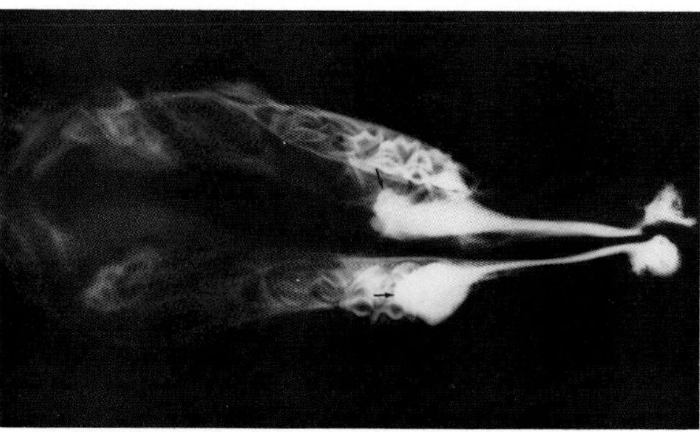

22.19 Dorsoventral radiograph of choanal atresia, radiopaque liquid instilled into nostril.

The prognosis for the life of a cria with choanal atresia is unfavorable. Surgery has been performed in an attempt to salvage a cria as a pet, but results have been poor (see Chap. 6). Euthanasia is a humane alternative.

JAW DYSGENESIS. The most common congenital disorders of llamas/alpacas involve malformations of the mandible or maxilla (Figs. 22.20–22.25). This is a significant problem within the industry. Overgrowth and protrusion of the incisors are considered by some to be normal, yet the teeth are cut off to improve appearance. Though alpacas have continuously growing incisors, with proper alignment, the teeth are naturally worn off and overgrowth does not occur. There is little question that the various forms of shortening or elongation of the jaws are hereditary. Genetic transmission is known in other livestock, pets, and humans (Table 22.2). Peruvian investigators have reported on genetic transmission in llamas and alpacas (4, 49).

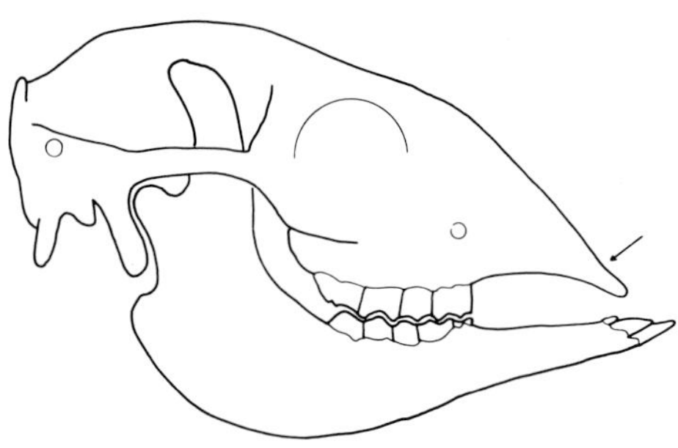

22.23 Diagram of superior brachygnathism in a neonate, which may prevent nursing.

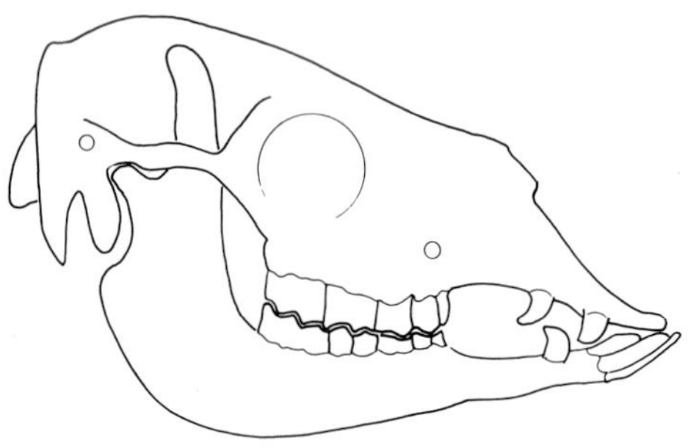

22.20 Diagram of normal jaw relationships.

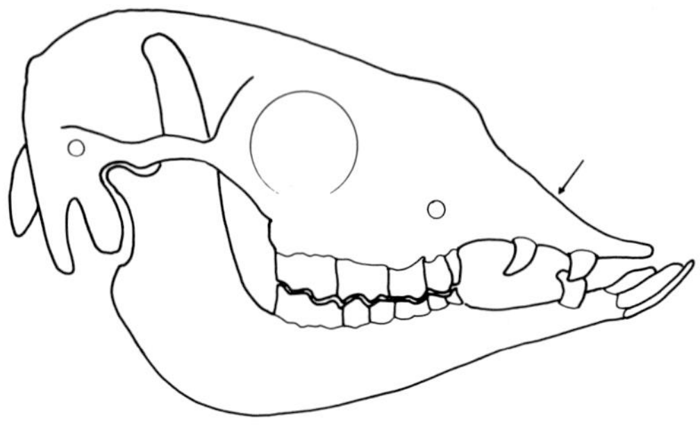

22.24 Diagram of superior brachygnathism in an adult male llama.

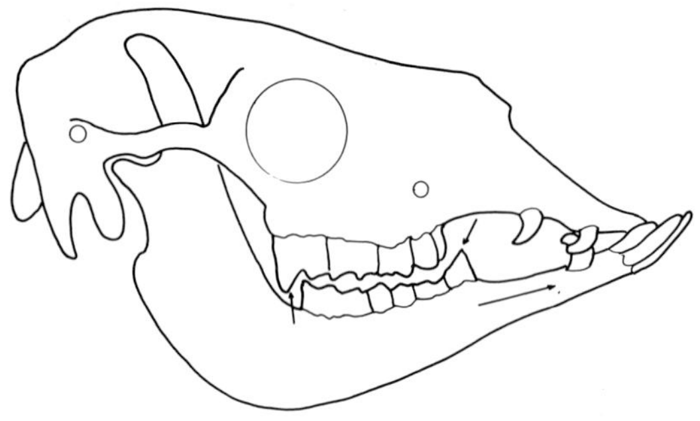

22.21 Diagram of jaw deformity, elongated mandible.

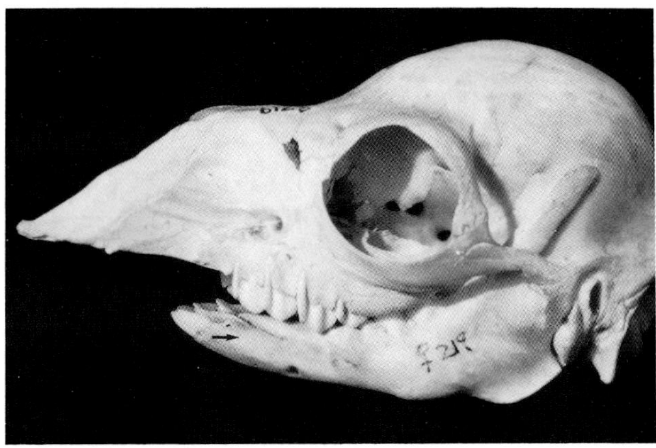

22.22 Mandibular hypogenesis in an alpaca.

Retention of deciduous incisors is common, and a familial tendency is suspected in llamas, but the precise etiology is unknown (Fig. 22.26). Other skull defects are illustrated in Figures 22.27–22.29.

DYSGENESIS OF THE PALATE. Palatal defects of lamoids have involved both the hard and soft palate, including clefting or complete absence (Fig. 22.30). Cleft palate does not seem to be a part of the choanal atresia/facial deformity syndrome. The etiology is unknown. Clinical signs may be present at birth, with milk flowing from the nostrils while the cria nurses. With a small cleft, signs may not be evident until solid food ingestion begins and food particles enter the nasal cavity, producing a rhinitis (Fig. 22.31). A nasal exudate that contains food particles is highly suggestive of a cleft, which may be confirmed by examination of the oral cavity. A laryngoscope may aid in visualizing the extent of the defect.

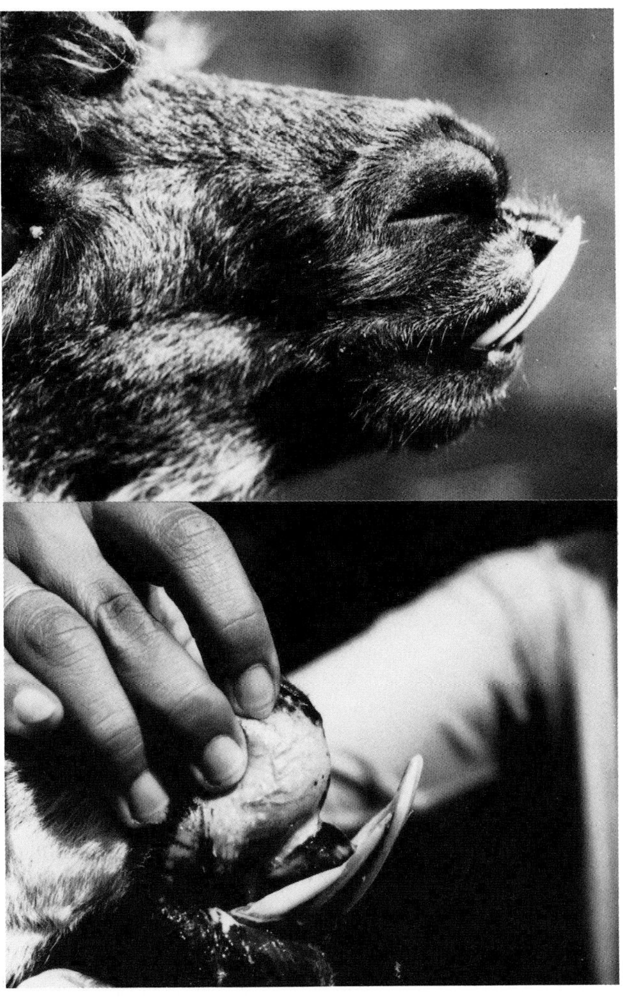

22.25 Superior brachygnathism in an alpaca.

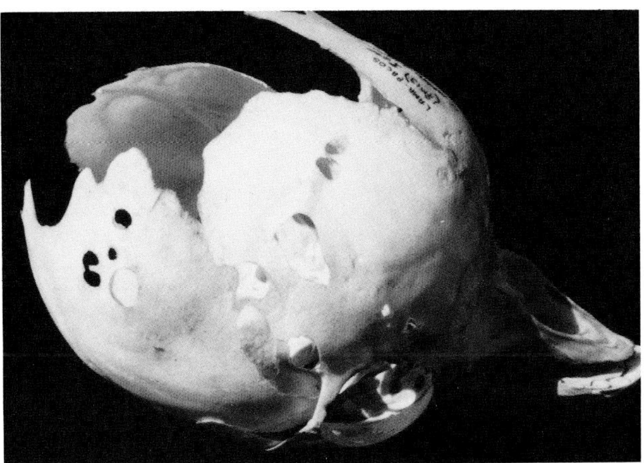

22.27 Hydrocephalic skull from an alpaca.

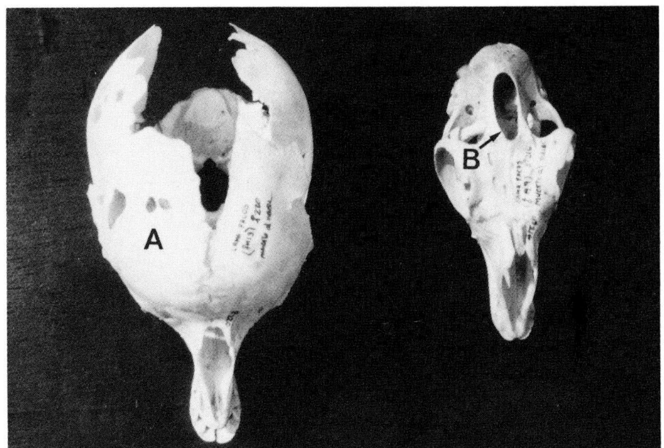

22.28 Alpaca skull deformities: (A) hydrocephalus, (B) cerebromeningiocele.

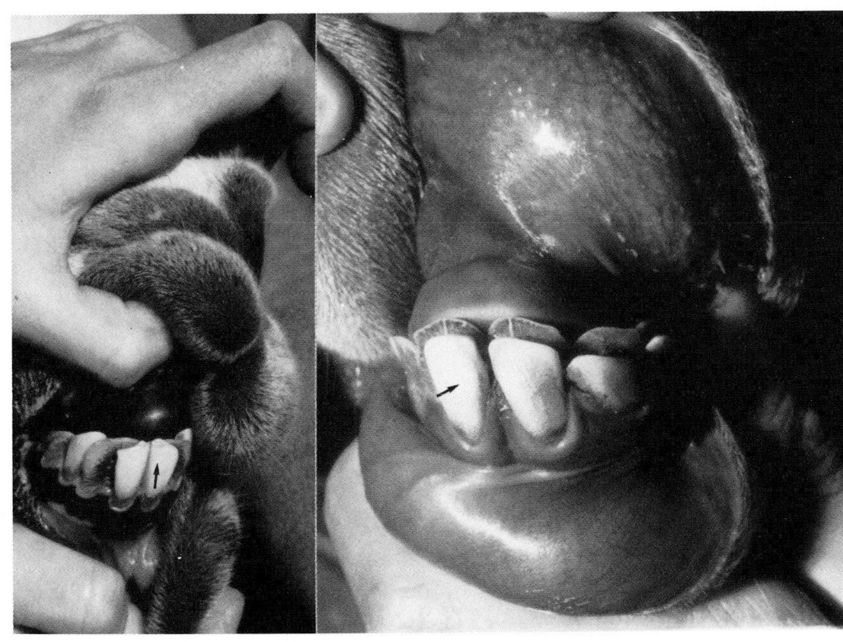

22.26 Retained deciduous incisors on labial side.

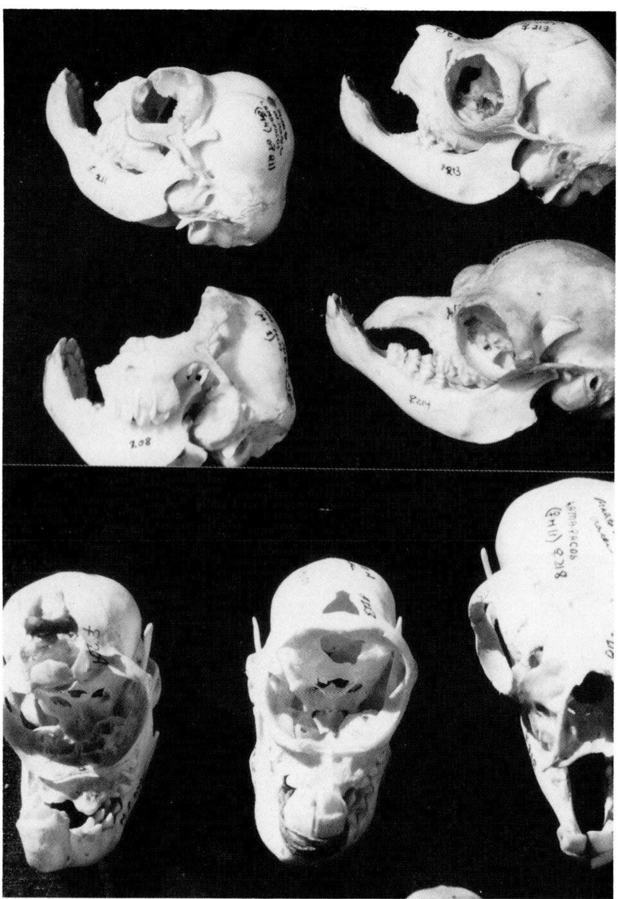

22.29 Skull deformities in alpacas.

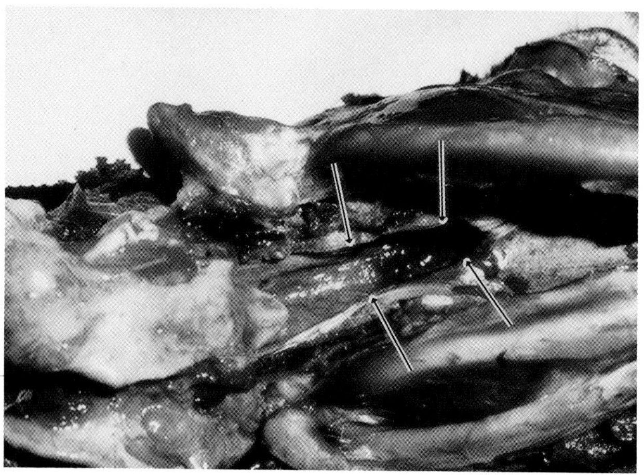

22.30 Cleft palate in a llama neonate.

Surgical correction of cleft palate has not been reported. Feeding management is likely to provide only temporary relief, and euthanasia should be recommended.

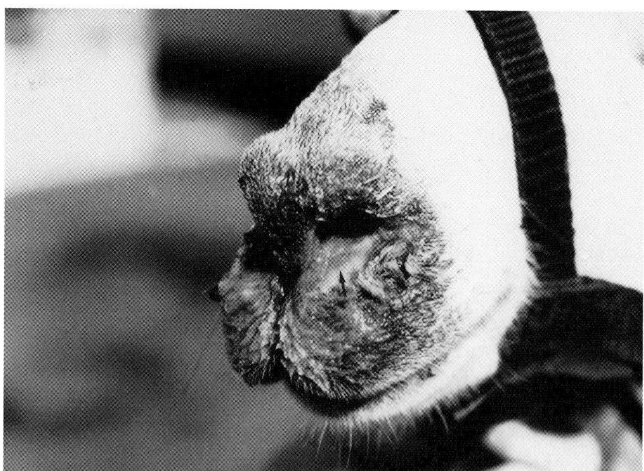

22.31 Nasal exudate containing feed particles, characteristic of cleft palate.

Reproductive System Defects

Much has been written about congenital/hereditary defects of the reproductive system of llamas and alpacas. Many of the defects seriously impair or prevent reproductive performance. The prevalence of reproductive defects in both North and South America is alarming. In one study in Peru, as many as 10% of the animals had one or more defects (45). Veterinarians should be aware of the scope of the problem (Table 22.2) and consider these conditions on any soundness or infertility examination.

HYPOGENESIS/AGENESIS OF REPRODUCTIVE ORGANS. Failure of development, particularly of female reproductive organs, is often seen. The etiology is unknown in lamoids, but genetic transmission has been reported in cattle and humans (Table 22.2). The major clinical sign is infertility, although pregnancy is possible in some cases, such as uterus unicornis (Fig. 22.32).

Segmental agenesis of the tubular genital tract of the female is common. Stenosis or occlusion of the tract may occur at any location from the oviduct to the hymen. Unilateral agenesis of an oviduct may never be detected. Agenesis within the uterus or vagina prevents outflow of uterine secretions, resulting in accumulation of fluid (mucometria) and dilatation of the segments of the tract cranial to the agenesis (Fig. 22.33).

The dilated uterus may be mistaken for pregnancy on rectal palpation. The fluid may be milky to slightly reddish in color and have the consistency of skim milk. The fluid is sterile unless organisms have been introduced by diagnostic manipulations. It is difficult to differentiate mucometria from placental fluids on palpation, but it is

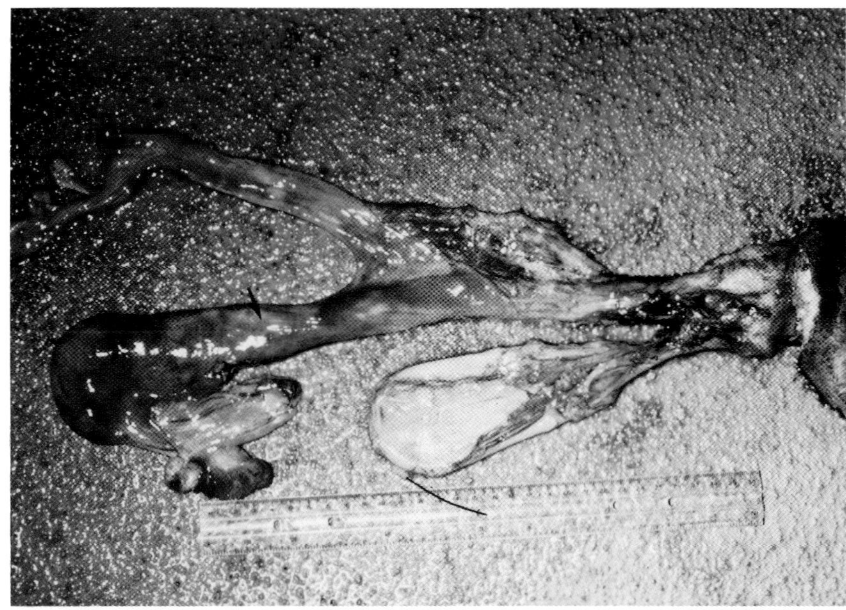

22.32 Uterus unicornis.

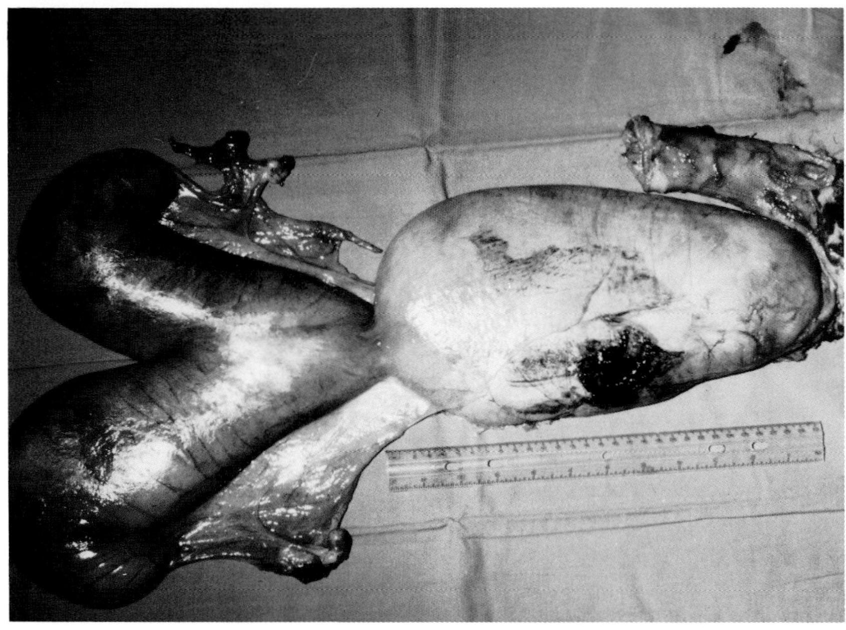

22.33 Mucometria caused by segmental agenesis of the vagina.

easy to differentiate it from pyometra on ultrasonography. Exudates caused by pyometra have a flocculent appearance, while mucometria and placental fluids are homogeneously clear.

The diagnosis of segmental agenesis involves a combination of rectal palpation, ultrasonography, examination with a vaginal speculum, aspiration of fluid, and visualization at laparotomy or laparoscopy, depending on the location of the lesion. See Chapter 17 for discussion of the normal anatomy of the reproductive system.

Uncorrected tubular agenesis precludes pregnancy except for uterus unicornis and unilateral oviduct agenesis. The veterinarian may be asked to open the tract, especially if the occlusion is at the level of the hymen or caudal vagina. Such surgery is possible, but the client should be advised of the likelihood that this condition is hereditary and that such an animal should not be used for breeding. Furthermore, depending on the length of time that the mucometria has been present, damage to the uterine mucosa may be irreparable. Ovariohysterectomy may be indicated to allow use of the female for fiber production, as a pet, or as a packer (see Chap. 6).

Ovarian hypogenesis and agenesis also occur (Fig. 22.34).

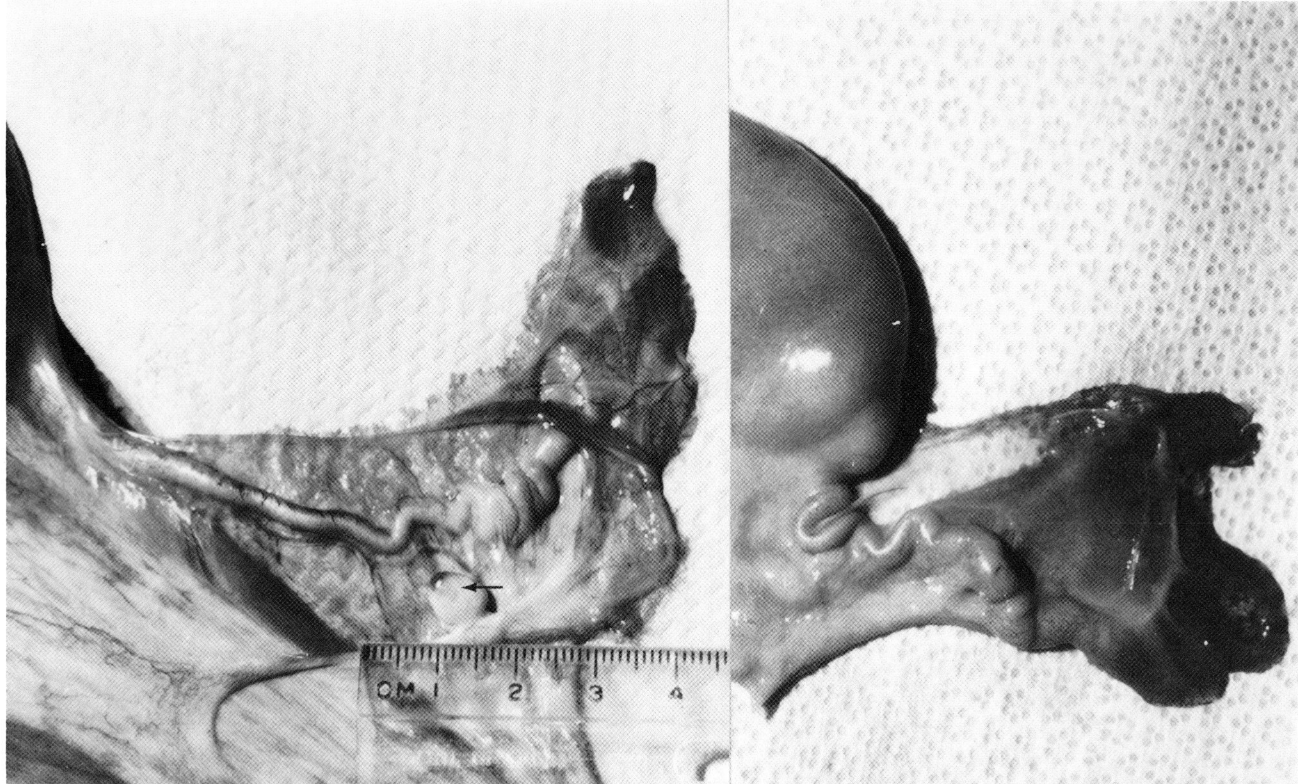

22.34 Ovarian dysgenesis: (left) hypogenesis, (right) agenesis.

INTERSEX. An intersex is any animal in which there is ambiguity in the structure of the gonads, reproductive tract, or external genitalia (39). Various forms of intersex are known to occur in lamoids. Anatomic variations are numerous, and clinical manifestations vary according to the hormone levels involved.

There are four stages of development of the male and female sexual organs (34): (1) chromosomal sex, as determined by the X and Y chromosomes at the time of fertilization, (2) gonadal sex, which occurs as the ovary and testis develop from the undifferentiated embryo gonad, (3) somatic sex, as other sexual organs develop, and (4) psychic sex, as the animal develops male or female behavior patterns.

A definition of terms follows (39). A *pseudohermaphrodite* has the gonads of one sex but an alteration in one or more of the other criteria of sex identification. A *true hermaphrodite* has both ovarian and testicular tissue, with intermediate external genitalia. A *lateral hermaphrodite* has an ovary on one side and a testicle on the other. A *unilateral hermaphrodite* has an ovotestis on one side and either an ovary or a testicle on the other. A *bilateral hermaphrodite* has ovotestes on both sides.

The embryologic anatomy of genital organs is complex and confusing, but basic understanding is necessary for a consideration of the topic (Table 22.6) (34). Gonadal development begins with a swelling called the genital ridge, which forms on the Wolffian body in the dorsal abdomen. The testicle and ovary develop from the genital ridge. Initially, the gonad is indifferent, with a medulla and cortex. The medulla is the potential male portion and the cortex the potential female portion. The Wolffian body is attached to the cloaca by the Wolffian duct, which will become the vas deferens and the epididymis in the male.

As sexual differentiation takes place in the female, the Mullerian duct develops, which eventually becomes the uterus, vagina, oviduct, and fimbria of the oviduct. The Wolffian duct disappears, but vestigial structures may persist, which are called the epoophoron, paroophoron, and Gartner's duct.

The etiology of intersex in lamoids is unknown, but certain forms are known to be genetically transmitted in all livestock species (Table 22.6). Intersexes may also result from hormonal defects. Genital development may fail at any of three stages (34).

First, distributions of sex chromosomes during meiosis or even mitotic division may result in sex chromosome aneuploidy in gametes. Fragments of sex chromosomes or autosomes bearing sex-influencing genes may be abnormally distributed as a result of partial or complete deletion or translocation in chiasma formation.

Table 22.6. Homologies of male and female reproductive systems

Undifferentiate stage	Male	Female
Internal genitalia		
Gonad	Testis	Ovary
Mesonephric tubules (Wolffian body)	Vas deferens Paradidymus (rudiment)	Epoophoron Paroophoron
Mesonephric duct (Wolffian duct)	Epididymus Vas deferens Ejaculatory duct	Duct part of epoophoron (Gartner's duct)
Mullerian duct	Appendage of testis (rudiment)	Fimbria of oviduct
	Prostatic utricle (uterus masculinus)	Uterus Vagina (all or part)
Urogenital sinus	Prostatic, membranous and cavernous urethra	Urethra vestibule, vagina in part
	Bulbourethral glands	Vestibular gland
	Prostate	Paraurethral gland
External genitalia		
Genital tubercle	Glans penis Corpus penis	Glans clitoris Corpus clitoris
Urethral fold	Raphe of scrotum and penis	Labia minor
Labioscrotal swelling	Scrotum	Labia majora

Second, gonadal morphogenesis may be disturbed because of abnormal corticomedullary relationships on the genital ridge. Third, secondary and accessory genital structures may develop abnormally under the influence of an irregular endocrine environment or as a result of teratogenic factors.

The clinical manifestations of intersex are highly variable. Behavioral patterns may be altered, and the external genitalia may appear as intermediates from expected morphology. A female pseudohermaphrodite llama had an enlarged clitoris, with the cartilaginous projection normally seen on the glans penis (Fig. 22.35). Her tubular organs were normal, based on rectal palpation and digital vaginal examination. It was not possible to insert a vaginal speculum past the hymen, but a finger could explore as far as the finger could reach. The ovaries were not located. This female mounted other females, attempting to force them into recumbency. This is normal male behavior, but it has also been seen in normal females.

The definitive diagnosis of intersex is difficult. The ultimate diagnosis is based on gonadal histology, but other clues include the appearance of external genitalia, morphology of the reproductive ducts, altered karyotype, and hormone analysis. The female pseudohermaphrodite described above had a normal karyotype but

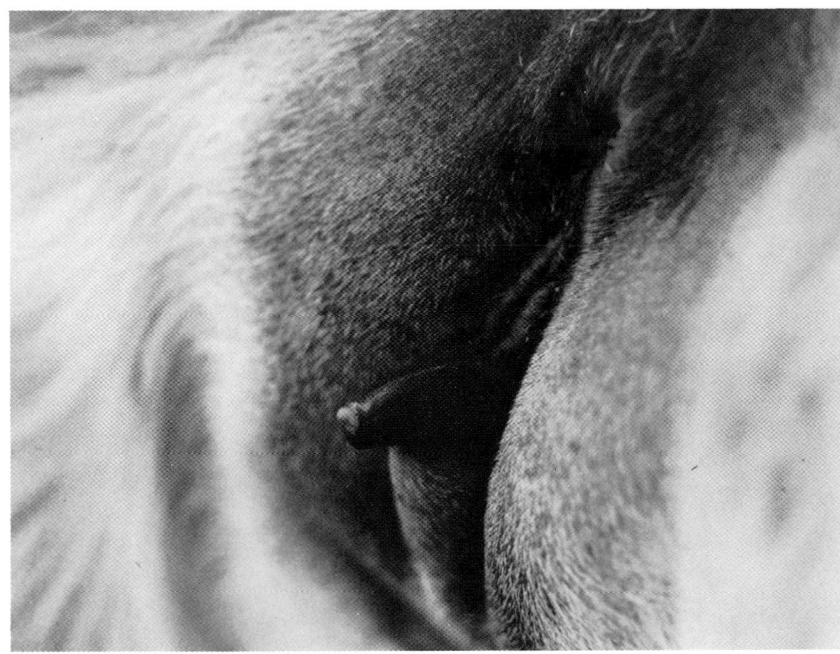

22.35 Female pseudohermaphrodite.

significantly altered testosterone levels. The female's estrogen level was 6.2 pg/ml, progesterone 0.1 ng/ml, and testosterone 325 pg/ml. The basal estrogen level of the domestic female mammal is usually less than 10 pg/ml. If there is any follicular activity, the levels are over 10. A level of 6.2 pg/ml estrogen in the female llama indicated no follicular activity. A progesterone level of 0.1 ng/ml is basal.

A testosterone level of 325 pg/ml is approximately 10 times normal for a female. A cow would have 10–15 pg/ml and a mare 25–40 pg/ml as basal testosterone. The level in this female llama was approximately what would be expected in a cryptorchid stallion (200–500 pg/ml).

Any of a long list of hereditary defects of male livestock species warrant exclusion of the individual from breeding (22). Such congenital defects of male lamoids include testicular hypoplasia (Fig. 22.36), cryptorchidism, testicular cysts, penile hypoplasia, persistence of the penile frenulum, and curvature of the penis. It should be recommended to llama clients that such defects also warrant exclusion of males for breeding.

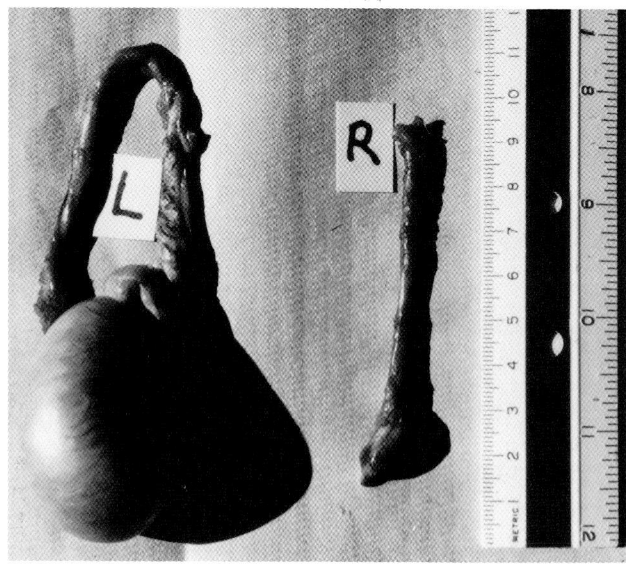

22.36 Testicular hypogenesis (R), normal (L).

Digestive Tract Defects

Atresia ani and *atresia coli* are known to occur in lamoids. The etiology is unknown. In cattle, atresia coli has been associated with excessive pressure exerted during rectal palpation (33). *Megaesophagus* may be either congenital or acquired (see Chap. 13). The etiology is unknown.

Cardiovascular Defects

Cardiovascular defects are seen sporadically in most animal species. None are unique to lamoids (Table 22.2). Ventricular septal defect (VSD) (Fig. 22.37) is relatively common in llamas and may occur singly or associated with other cardiovascular or congenital defects.

Clinical signs may be limited to auscultation of a holosystolic murmur or be accompanied by cyanosis and exercise intolerance. The author is aware of an adult llama with VSD that lives a normal life. The presence of

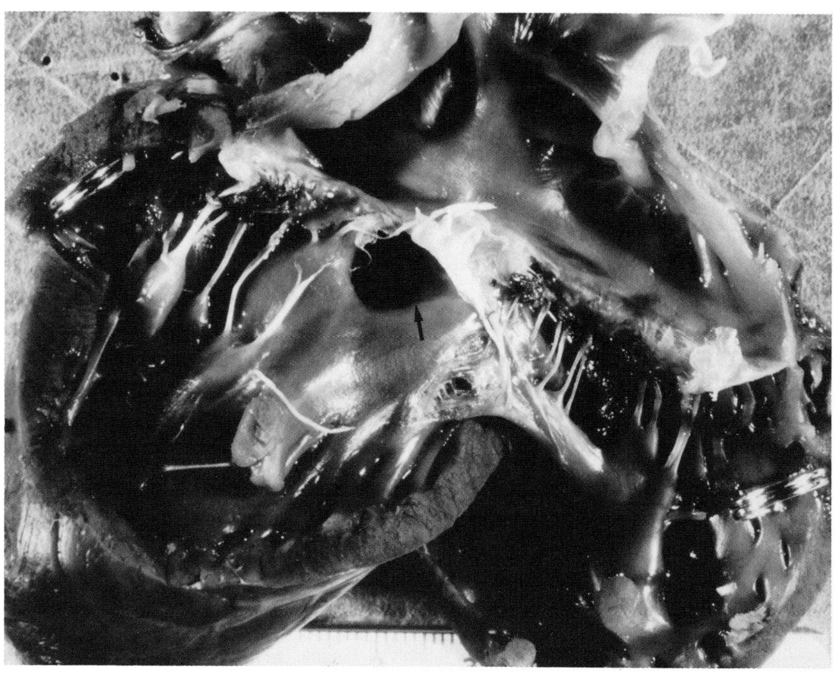

22.37 Ventricular septal defect.

a murmur is a frequent, perhaps normal, clinical finding in the newborn. The murmur should disappear by 1 week of age. Transposition of the great vessels is rare (Figs. 22.38, 22.39) and would be lethal shortly after birth unless accompanied by ventricular or atrial septal defect.

The diagnosis of VSD should be suspected with the presence of a murmur but can be definitively diagnosed with ultrasonography. Other cardiovascular defects may be diagnosed only though radiography, fluoroscopy, or angiography.

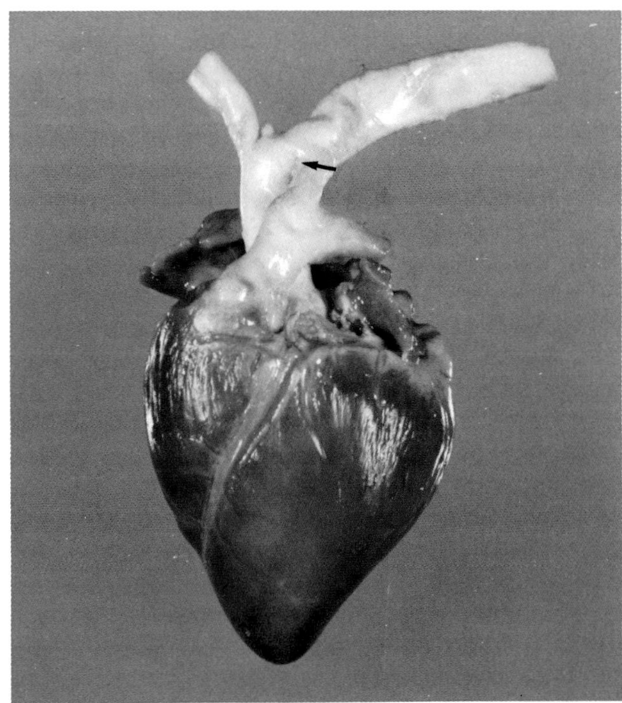

22.39 Normal crossover of aorta and pulmonary artery in a llama neonate.

Miscellaneous Defects

Many other defects are listed in Table 22.2. Similar defects have been reported in other livestock, pets, and humans. One other defect that is worthy of special mention is crooked toenails (see Figs. 10.13, 10.14). Overgrown nails and crookedness are a common clinical entity. Some nails grow crooked despite judicious and regular nail trimming. Crooked hoofs and nails are known to be genetically transmitted in cattle, horses, sheep, and pigs. Selection of breeding stock should include a consideration of sound feet and legs.

Nonanatomic Defects

A discussion of congenital/hereditary defects would be incomplete without mention of physiologic characteristics that have a genetic basis. None of these are known inherited traits in lamoids, but they are so important in livestock that mention should be made here. Consider the following: milk production, mothering ability, disease resistance, growth rate, thermoregulatory adaptability, feed utilization, birth weight, semen quality, neonatal mortality, fertility, early embryonic death, and resistance to neoplasia.

Conformation

Conformation traits are inherited. This does not mean that every cria will have the conformation traits of

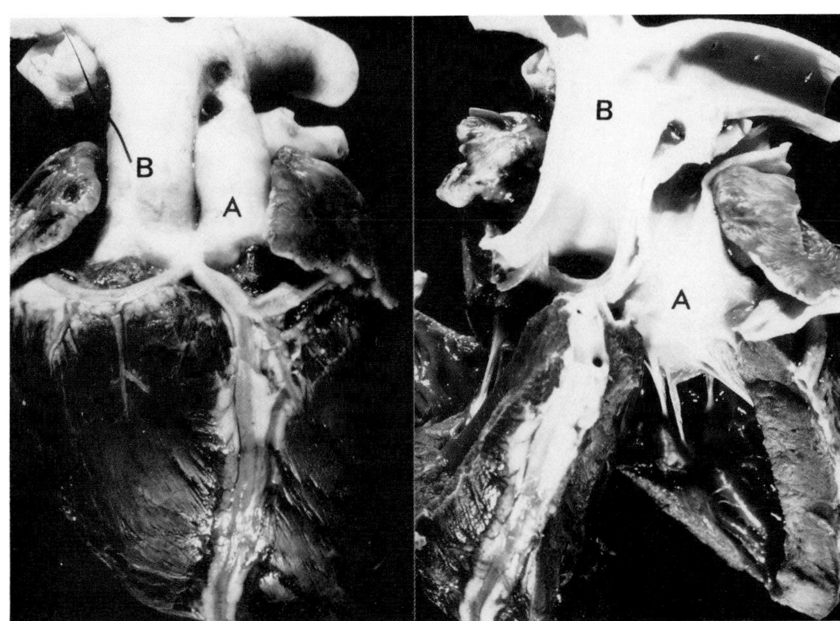

22.38 Transposition of the aorta and pulmonary artery: **(A)** pulmonary artery, **(B)** aorta.

either the sire or dam, because environment and nutrition may modify the expression of genetic predisposition to a given trait. Some owners have had a tendency to emphasize fiber coat quality and quantity over conformation. This may be a mistake.

No breed standards have been established for alpaca or llama conformation. However, the general principles of form, function, and balance apply to all animals. The following discussion describes basic llama conformation as it relates to camelid gaits and anatomy. The terminology is that used in describing horse and livestock conformation (16).

Conformation is the proportionate shape or contour of an animal. It is the appropriate arrangement of body parts for assembly into the whole animal (balance). To understand form and function, it is necessary to understand the *gaits* of lamoids (6, 52). Camelids have three natural gaits: the walk, pace, and gallop. The pace is not unique to camelids but is used by camelids as the medium-speed gait. The pace is physically demanding, and certain anatomic modifications make this an efficient gait for camelids.

Natural pacers have relatively long legs, with each limb being longer than the trunk, allowing the animal to develop a long stride. The forward part of the thorax is narrow, permitting the upper forelimb to freely move forward and back. Also, in camelids, the attachment of the hind limb to the pelvis is narrow, and the abdomen is less rounded than in other livestock species, allowing the hind limb freer motion. Camelid limbs are also set more closely to the midline than in other species, eliminating some of the side to side rolling that occurs when the center of body gravity is changed with each stride.

Basically, the pace is an unstable gait because lateral stability is decreased. The pace is designed to permit an animal to move swiftly over open country. The unique foot of the camelid may be an adaptation to increase the stability of the animal for the pacing gait. All other two-toed ungulates have ligaments that tie the digits together. Camelids have a splay-toed foot (not to be confused with splay footed) that spreads and provides a strong base of support. This, combined with the padded foot, makes the camelid one of the more surefooted ungulates.

The diagram in Figure 11.1 illustrates the basic relationships of the lamoid skeleton. There are significant differences in the angulation of certain joints compared with those of the horse or cow.

Many conformational faults may be seen in the neonate. Owners are frequently alarmed to see a calf-kneed cria walking on its fetlocks. Judgment should be reserved until the cria is a few weeks of age to give tendons and ligaments opportunity to strengthen.

FORELIMB, SIDE VIEW. Normal stance is illustrated in Figure 22.40. Stance behind the vertical (camped back in front) and in front of the vertical (camped forward or camped out in front) are also shown in Figure 22.40. Balance is impaired in either situation. Some animals show little angulation of the joints (straight legged or post legged) (Fig. 22.41). Conversely, too much angulation, especially of the shoulder, weakens the limb (Fig. 22.42).

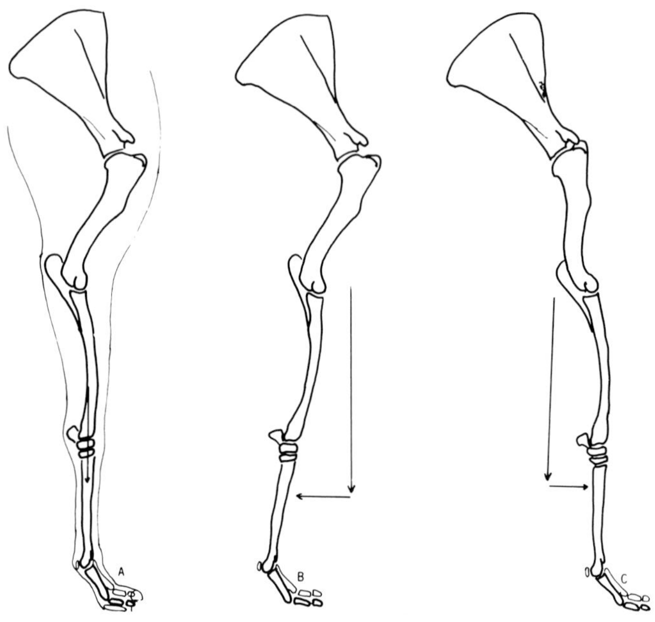

22.40 Forelimb, lateral view: **(A)** normal, **(B)** camped behind, **(C)** camped forward.

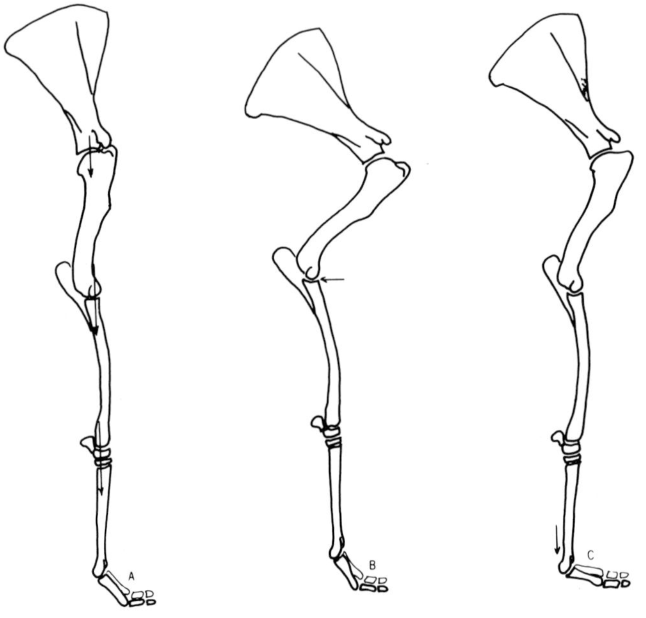

22.41 Forelimb, lateral view: **(A)** straight or post leg, **(B)** excessive angulation of shoulder, **(C)** hyperextension of the fetlock.

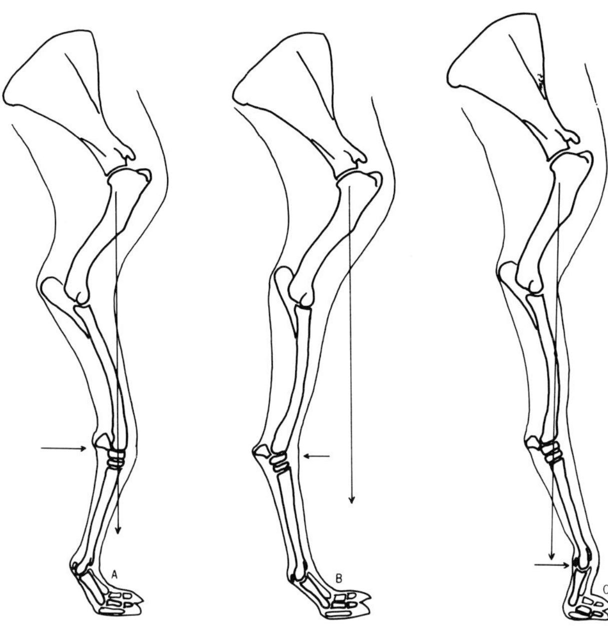

22.42 Forelimb, lateral view: (A) buck-knee, (B) calf-knee, (C) contracted flexor tendons of fetlock.

The carpus may be bowed forward (buck-knee) or backward (calf-knee) (Figs. 22.42–22.43). Calf-knee is the more serious of the two. Figures 22.42–22.44 illustrate a condition called "down in the fetlock" or "weak pastern." Normally, phalanx one (P-1) is semivertical, with approximately a 45–50 degree angle with the ground. P-2 and P-3 lie horizontally within the foot.

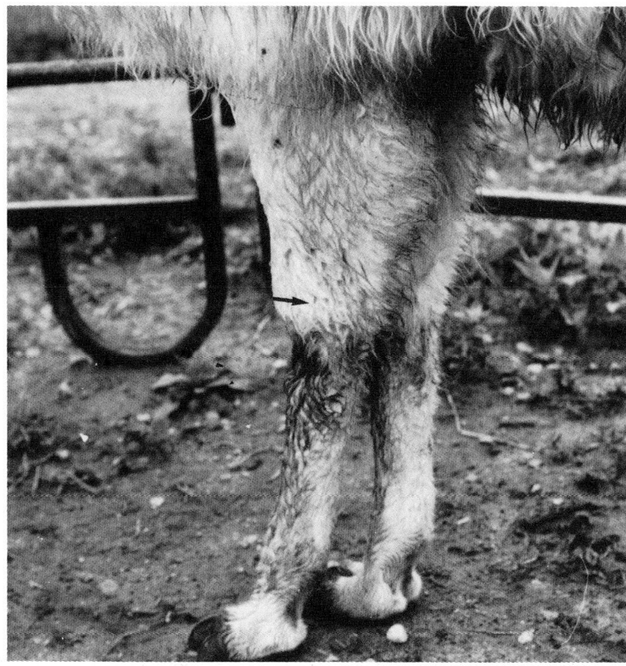

22.43 Calf-knee.

Dropped fetlock may be a specific congenital defect, or it may be acquired from trauma or deterioration of the ligamentous support from prolonged weight bearing if the opposite limb is incapacitated for a long time. Congenital weakness would be suspected with bilateral or quadrilateral involvement.

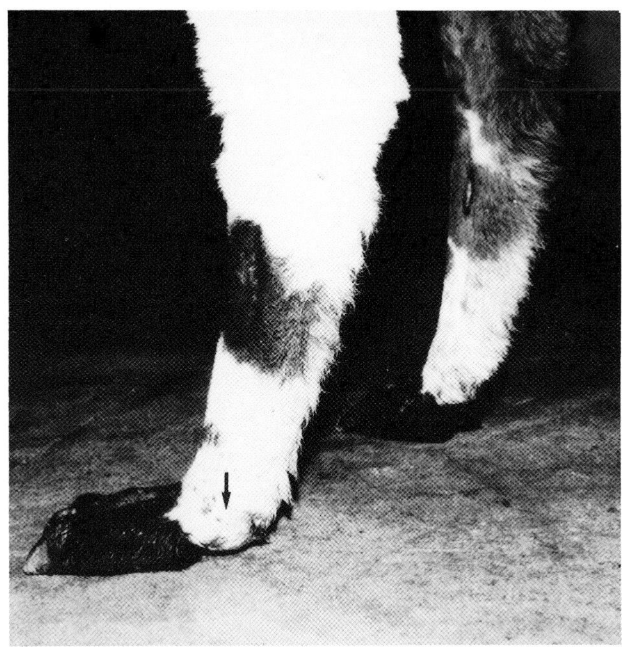

22.44 Hyperextension of fetlock.

The angulation of the pastern and the fibroelastic digital cushion of the foot provide the most important cushions for the limb.

FORELIMB, FRONT VIEW. The limbs of llamas are closer to the midline than in most other domestic animals for reasons described earlier, but faults include base narrow and base wide (Figs. 22.45, 22.46). Angular limb deformity, discussed previously, and angulation of the carpus (Figs. 22.1–3, 22.47) and fetlock (Figs. 22.4, 22.48) have been seen.

HIND LIMB, SIDE VIEW. Normal, camped behind, and camped forward are illustrated in Figure 22.49. Many domestic lamoids have a tendency to stand slightly sickle hocked (Figs. 22.50, 22.51); however, the overall stance of the rear limb is straighter than that of the horse or cow. The rear limb may be too straight (post leg) (Fig. 22.50) or have excessive angulation (Fig. 22.50, 22.51). Fetlock, pastern, and foot faults occur on the rear limbs also.

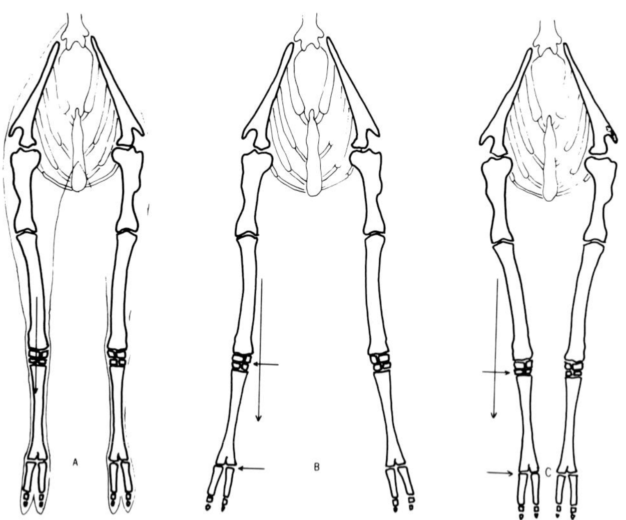

22.45 Forelimb, front view: **(A)** normal, **(B)** base wide, **(C)** base narrow.

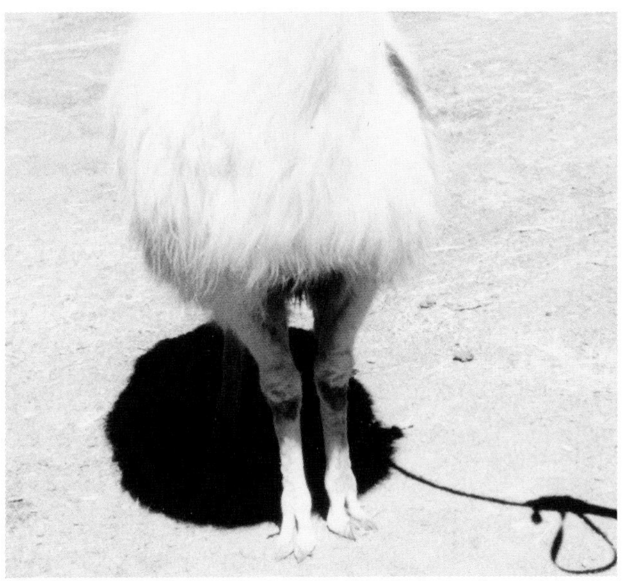

22.46 Base-narrow stance.

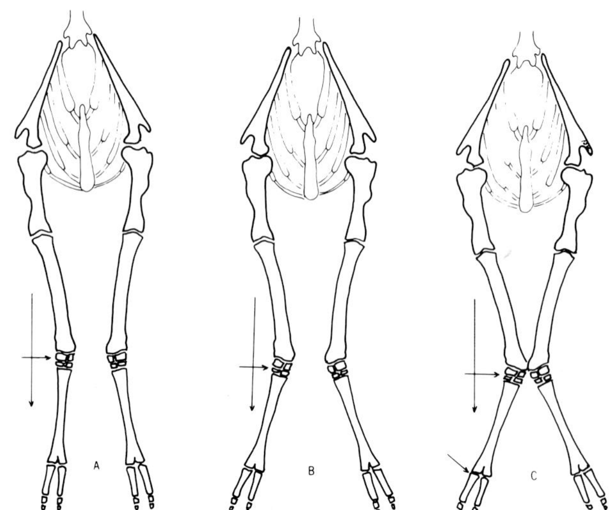

22.47 Angular limb deformity: **(A–C)** degrees of carpal valgus.

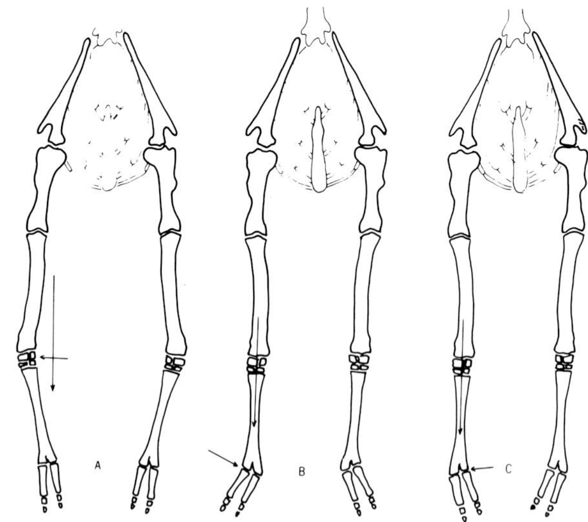

22.48 Forelimb, front view: **(A)** carpal varus, **(B)** angular deformity of fetlock (splayed), **(C)** angular deformity of fetlock (pigeon-toes).

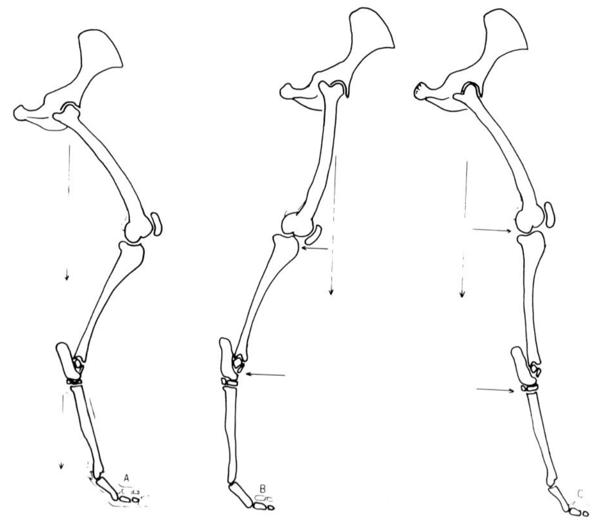

22.49 Hind limb, lateral view: **(A)** normal, **(B)** camped behind, **(C)** camped forward.

HIND LIMB, REAR VIEW. The llama may stand base wide or base narrow (Fig. 22.52). If the hocks are too close together (a common fault), it is called "cow-hocked" (Fig. 22.53). Long bone angular limb deformities of the hind limbs are rare.

MISCELLANEOUS CONFORMATION FAULTS. Llamas may have an excessively narrow chest, barrel chest, sway back (lordosis), camel back (kyphosis), variable set of the neck and tail, small head, or large head. Conformational faults and defects of the head were discussed previously. Other congenital conditions are illustrated in Figures 22.54–22.57.

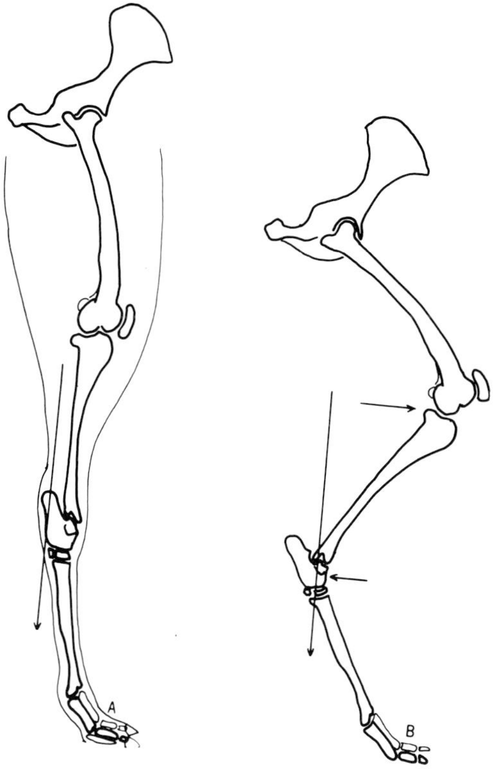

22.50 Hind limb, lateral view: (A) straight-leg, (B) excessive angulation (sickle-hock).

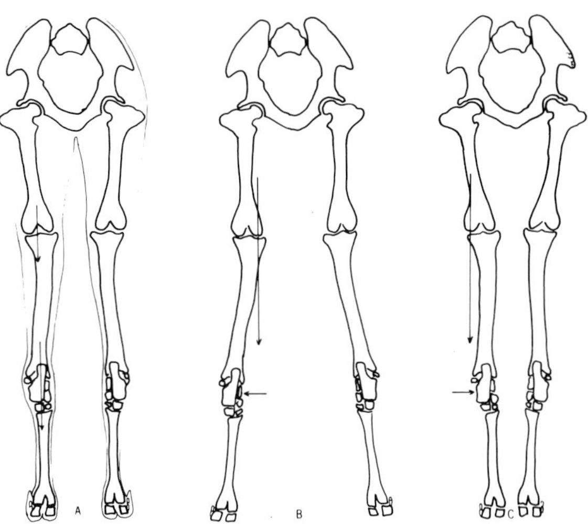

22.52 Hind limb, rear view: (A) normal, (B) base wide, (C) base narrow.

BLOOD TYPING AND PARENTAGE VERIFICATION

Blood typing was first applied to solve problems of mismatched blood transfusions in humans and later to solve problems of disputed paternity. In the late 1920s, systematic studies of blood groups in cattle were undertaken, which led to a wide use of blood-typing tests to verify the accuracy of pedigrees in registered cattle. Similar studies have been carried out in other domestic animals, but blood typing to date has been most successfully applied to cattle and horses. Both cattle and horse breed

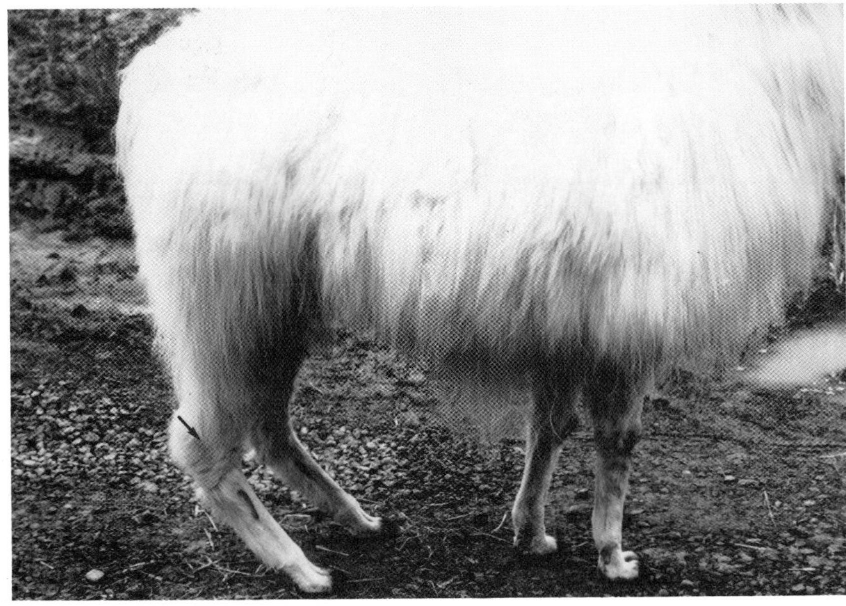

22.51 Sickle-hock.

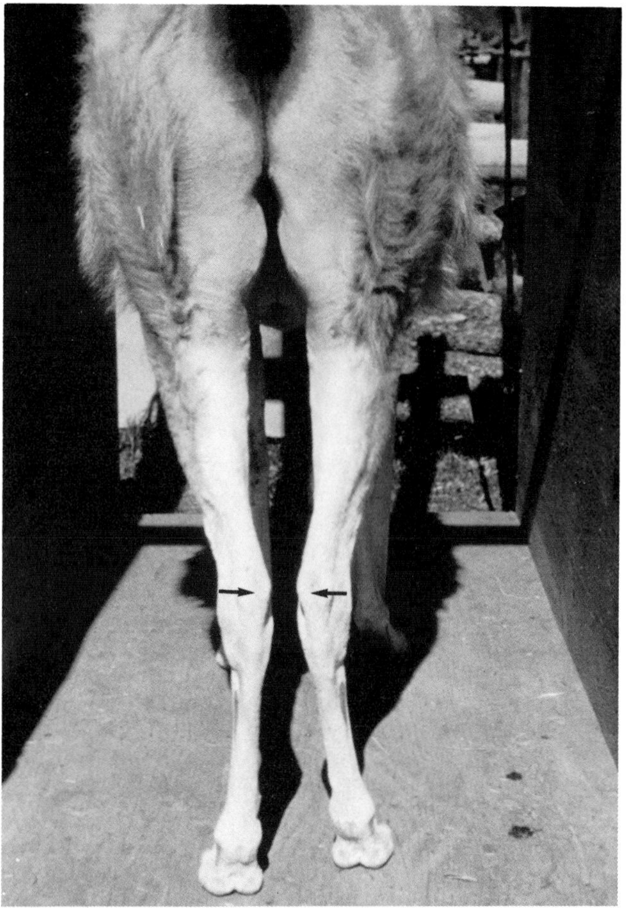

22.53 Cow-hock.

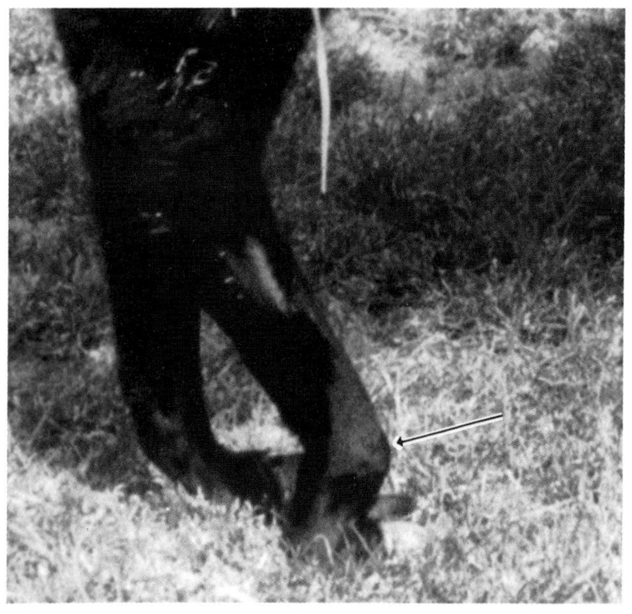

22.54 Contracted flexor tendon, flexing the fetlock.

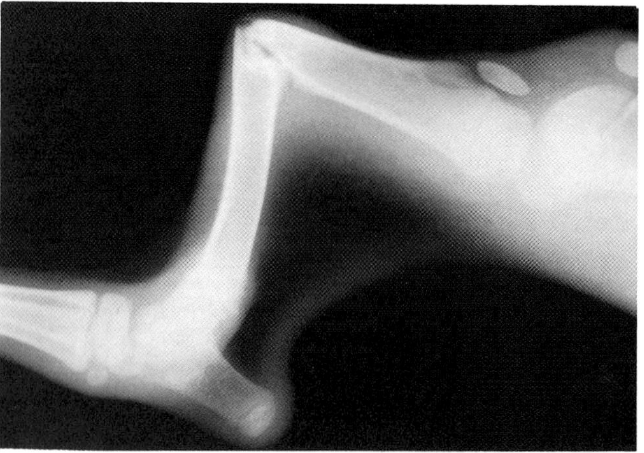

22.55 Contracted tendon of the gastrocnemius muscle, resulting in tibial fracture in the fetus.

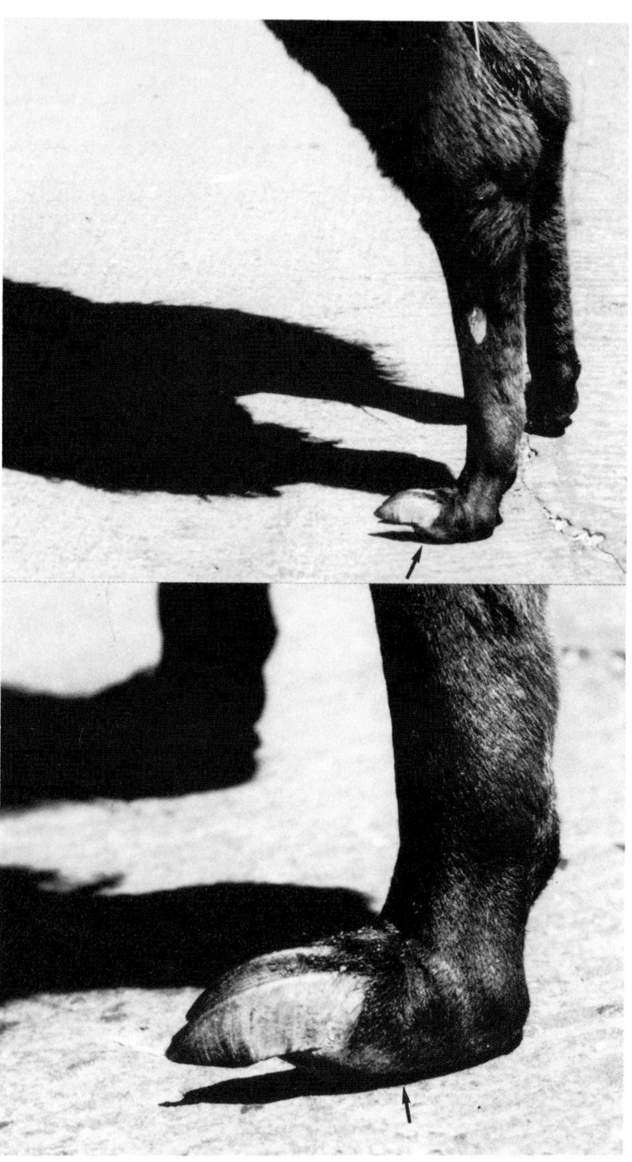

22.56 Hyperextension of the pastern.

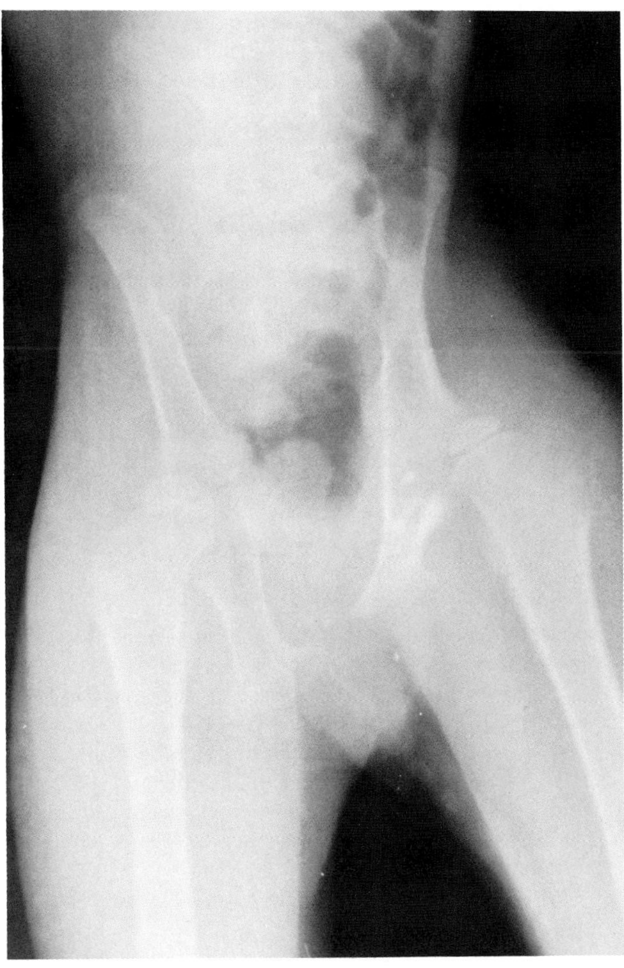

22.57 Hypogenesis of llama pelvis.

registries have developed intensive blood-typing programs designed to keep pedigree errors to a minimum among registered animals (17, 37, 40).

Basic studies of blood group factors, protein variation, and enzyme patterns have now been conducted in llamas (17, 40). Sufficient variation among individuals has been found to validate the use of blood-typing tests for parentage verification. Specific blood group antibodies are harvested from immunized llamas and prepared in the laboratory for serologic testing against the blood of animals being tested. To date, five erythrocyte factor systems have been identified: A-B, C-no C (-), D-(-), E-(-), and F-(-). The A-B, C, and D systems have been tested on over 100 sire, dam, and offspring trios. The E and F systems have been tested on fewer animals. The phenotypic distribution of blood group factors in llamas and alpacas is noted in Figures 22.58–22.60.

Electrophoresis studies, using polyacrylamide gel sheets, have resulted in the identification of two protein systems. Transferrin proteins are found in the serum and are responsible for the transport of iron in the body.

	Red Blood Cell Type	Llamas N=179	Alpacas N=60
AB LOCUS			
	AA	35	49
	AB	90	11
	BB	54	0
C(-) LOCUS			
	CC	177	60
	(-)(-)	2	0
D(-) LOCUS			
	DD	61	2
	(-)(-)	118	54
E(-) LOCUS			
	EE	8N=87	0
	(-)(-)	79	60
F(-) LOCUS			
	FF	4 N=41	1
	(-)(-)	37	59

22.58 Phenotypic distribution of blood group factors in llamas and alpacas.

	RBC FACTORS			
	AB System	C System	Trans.	Postalb.
CRIA	BB	C	I,X	B,K
DAM	AB	C	R,X	B,K
MALE 1	AB	C	I,I	E,K
MALE 2	AA	C	L,U	H,K

MALE 2 IS EXCLUDED FROM BEING THE SIRE BECAUSE THE CRIA HAS NO A BLOOD FACTOR OR L OR U TRANSFERRIN

22.59 Two males as potential sires based on a limited number of factors.

	RBC FACTORS			
	AB System	C System	Trans.	Postalb.
CRIA	BB	C	I,X	B,K
DAM	BB	C	I,R	E,K
POSSIBLE SIRE	AA	C	I,X	H,K

THE MALE IS EXCLUDED AS THE SIRE BECAUSE THE CRIA HAS NO B RED CELL FACTOR OR H POSTALBUMIN PROTEIN

22.60 Parent exclusion based on a limited number of factors.

Eleven transferrin variants have been observed and given letter designations D, F, I, K, L, O, R, T, U, X, and Z.

Postalbumins are proteins of unknown function, but four variants have been found to date and named B, E, K, and N.

The identification of specific enzymes is commonly used in genetic studies. Screening tests have been conducted for numerous enzyme systems in llamas, but the only systems showing promise, to date, are catalase (CAT), glucose phosphate isomerase (GPI), and phosphorogluconate dehydrogenase (PGD). CAT is present in the erythrocyte and functions to remove peroxide ions formed during normal cell metabolism. Two variants have been identified in llama blood by starch gel electrophoresis and named F and S.

Three variants of GPI (F, I, and S) have been found in llamas, but only F and I in alpacas. Two variants of PGD (F and S) have been found in llamas and alpacas. The variations in these enzymes were recognized late in the study and have not been extensively tested.

No variation was found in hemoglobin and albumin proteins and the enzyme phosphoglucomutase.

Parentage verification is accomplished by comparing the blood types of an offspring with those of its alleged sire and dam. If the blood types of the offspring can be accounted for on the basis of the types present in the parents, the parents qualify (Figs. 22.59, 22.60). All parentage cases are based on the principle of genetic exclusion. This means that the burden of proof rests in showing that a certain animal cannot be a parent of the animal in question. When a parentage is said to qualify, it can only be assumed that such is correct. No test exists that proves parentage; rather, blood-typing tests disprove parentage.

Lamoid blood typing and parentage verification are in their infancy. Other applications closely allied to the genetic transmission of blood group factors and protein and enzyme systems include cross matching for blood transfusion, hybrid identification (35), and genetic diversity studies. Work on these uses is continuing.

REFERENCES

1. Benirschke, K. 1967. Sterility and fertility of interspecific mammalian hybrids. In K. Benirschke, ed. Comparative Aspects of Reproductive Failure. New York: Springer, pp. 218–34.

2. Brown, R. J. 1973. Hydrocephalus in a newborn llama. J. Wildl. Dis. 9:146–47.

3. Bunch, T. D., Foote, W. C., and Maciulis, A. 1985. Chromosome banding pattern homologies and NORs for the Bactrian camel, guanaco and the llama. J. Hered. 76:115–18.

4. Bustinza C., V., and Jahuira H., F. 1985. (Frequency of genetic defects and their productivity implications in the exploitation of alpaca rearing in the Department of Puno) Frecuencia de defectos geneficos y sus implicacion productivos en explataciones alpaqueras del Depto de Puno. Alpaka 1(2):11–35.

5. Christensen, N. O. 1969. Some aspects of congenital defects and neonatal diseases in zoo animals. Acta Zool. Pathol. Antwerpen 48:275.

6. Dagg, A. I. 1974. The locomotion of the camelid. J. Zool. (Lond.) 174:67–73.

7. Dennis, S. M., and Leipold, H. W. 1979. Ovine congenital defects. Vet. Bull. 49:23–39.

8. Elsas, L. J., and Priest, J. H. 1979. Medical genetics. In W. A. Sodeman, Jr., and T. M. Sodeman. Pathologic Physiology, 6th ed. Philadelphia: W. B. Saunders, pp. 49–109.

9. Emery, A. E. H., and Rimoin, D. L., eds. 1983. Principles and Practice of Medical Genetics, vols. 1, 2. Edinburgh: Churchill Livingstone.

10. Erickson, F., Saperstein, G., McKinley, J., and Leipold, H. W. 1977. Congenital defects of dogs. Canine Pract. (Aug):45–61; (Oct):52–61; (Dec):4–53.

11. Fenwick, B. W., Fowler, M. E., and Kock, M. 1982. Complete choanal atresia in a llama. J. Am. Vet. Med. Assoc. 181:1409–10.

12. Fowler, M. E. 1982. Angular limb deformities in young llamas. J. Am. Vet. Med. Assoc. 181:1338–42.

13. ______. 1984. Congenital and hereditary diseases of llamas. Proc. 26th Int. Symp. Erkr. Zootiere 26:153–57.

14. ______. 1985a. It is hereditary. 3L Llama (26):23–25.

15. ______. 1985b. Umbilical hernias (llama care question). Llamas 30 (Nov.-Dec.):11–12.

16. ______. 1986. Form, function, conformation, and soundness. Llamas 35 (Nov.-Dec.):45–53.

17. ______. 1987. Blood typing and parentage verification in llamas. Llamas 1(4):81–84.

18. Gandarillas, H. 1971. (Preliminary identification of the genes involved in heredity of color of llamas and alpacas) Identificaciones preliminar de los genes involucrados en la herencia del color de los llamas y alpacas. Bol. Exp. 49. Durna de investigaciones agricolas, LaPaz, Bolivia, pp. 4–28.

19. Gentz, E. J., and Yates, T. L. 1986. Genetic identification of hybrid camelids. Zoo Biol. 5:349–54.

20. Graham, D. 1986. The hidden llama—Color coat inheritance in llamas. Llamas (34):38–46.

21. Griner, L. A. 1983. Pathology of zoo animals. Zool. Soc. San Diego, p. 505.

22. Hamori, D. 1983. Constitutional Disorders and Hereditary Diseases in Domestic Animals. Amsterdam: Elsevier.

23. Huston, R., Saperstein, G., and Leipold, H. W. 1977. Congenital defects in foals. J. Equine Med. Surg. 1:146–61.

24. Huston, R., Saperstein, G., Schoneweis, D., and Leipold, H. W. 1978. Congenital defects in pigs. Vet. Bull. 48:645–75.

25. Ingram, K. A., and Sigler, R. L. 1983. Cataract removal in a young llama. Proc. Am. Assoc. Zoo Vet., Tampa, Fla., pp. 95–97.

26. Keeler, R. F. 1978. Reducing incidence of plant-caused congenital deformities in livestock by grazing management. J. Range Manage. 31:355–60.

27. ______. 1984. Teratogens in plants. J. Anim. Sci. 58:1029–39.

28. Kolaczkowski, J., and Soboncinski, M. 1971. (A case of persistent arterial trunk in a guanaco) Przypadek Przetrwalego Pnia Tentiniczego u Lamy Givanako, Folia Morphol. (Warsz.) 30:233. (Polish)

29. Larramendy, M. L., Vidal R., L., Bianchi, M., and Bianchi, N. 1984. (Genetic studies in South American camelids) Camelidos Sudamericanos: Estudios geneticos. Bol. Lima 6(35):92–96.

30. Lasley, J. F. 1978. Genetics of Livestock Improvement, 3rd ed. Englewood Cliffs, N.J.: Prentice Hall.

31. Leipold, H. W. 1980. Congenital defects in zoo and wild mammals. In R. J. Montali and G. Migaki, eds. Comparative Pathology of Zoo Animals. Washington, D.C.: Smithsonian Institute Press, pp. 457–70.

32. Leipold, H. W., and Dennis, S. M. 1984. Congenital defects of domestic and feral animals. Issues and Reviews in Teratology, vol. 2. New York: Plenum, pp. 91–155.

33. Leipold, H. W., Huston, K., and Dennis, S. M. 1983. Bovine congenital defects. Adv. Vet. Sci. Comp. Med. 27:197–269.

34. McDonald, L. E. 1980. Veterinary Endocrinology and Reproduction, 3rd ed. Philadelphia: Lea & Febiger.

35. McKusick, V. A. 1986. Mendelian Inheritance in Man, 7th ed. Baltimore: Johns Hopkins Univ. Press.

36. Mayr, B., Auer, H., Schleger, W., Czaker, R., and Burger, H. 1985. Nucleolus organizer regions in the chromosomes of the llama. J. Hered. 76:222–23.

37. Miller, P. J., Hollander, P. J., and Franklin, W. L. 1985. Blood typing South American camelids. J. Hered. 76:369–71.

38. Nicholas, F. W. 1987. Veterinary Genetics. New York: Clarendon Press; Oxford Univ. Press.

39. Noden, D. M., and de Lahunta, A. 1985. The Embryology of Domestic Animals. Baltimore: Williams & Wilkins.

40. Penedo, M. C. T., Fowler, M. E., Bowling, A., Anderson, D. L., and Gordon, L. 1988. Genetic variation in the blood of llamas, *Lama glama,* and alpacas, *Lama pacos.* Anim. Genet. In press.

41. Ralls, K., Brugger, K., and Glick, A. 1980. Deleterious effects of inbreeding on a herd of captive Dorcas gazelle. In P. J. S. Olney, ed. International Zoo Yearbook 20. London: Zoological Society, pp. 137–46.

42. Saperstein, G., Leipold, H. W., and Dennis, S. M. 1975. Congenital defects of sheep. J. Am. Vet. Med. Assoc. 167:314–22.

43. Saperstein, G., Harris, S., and Leipold, H. W. 1976. Congenital defects in domestic cats. Feline Pract. 6:18–44.

44. Sumar, K. J. 1968. (Shortened maxillary bone in alpacas or mandibular prognathism) Maxilares deprimidos en alpacas or prognatismo mandibular. Bol. Extraordinario 3:50–53.

45. ______. 1983. Studies on reproductive pathology in alpacas. Dep. Obstet. Gynaecol. Fac. Vet. Med. (Uppsala, Sweden), pp. 1–90.

46. Tachdjian, M. O. 1972. Pediatric Orthopedics, vol. 2. Philadelphia: W. B. Saunders, pp. 1359–72.

47. Taibel, A. M., and Grilletto, R. 1966. (Actavic polydactyla in the fore-limb of a llama *Lama glama*). Zool. Gart. 33:174–81. German

48. Taylor, K. M., Hungerford, D. A., Snyder, R. L., and Ulmer, F. A., Jr. 1968. Uniformity of karyotypes in the camelidae. Cytogenetics 7:8–15.

49. Tillman, J. 1983a. Coat color inheritance in llamas and alpacas. I. Llama World 1(3):4–9.

50. ______. 1983b. Coat color inheritance in llamas and alpacas. II. Llama World 1(4):18–22.

51. Wallach, J. D., and Boever, W. J. 1983. Diseases of Exotic Animals: Medical and Surgical Management. Philadelphia: W. B. Saunders, p. 327.

52. Webb, S. D. 1972. Locomotor evolution in camels (and llamas). Form. Funct. 5:99–112.

23 Toxicology

ONLY A FEW INSTANCES of poisoning have been reported in lamoids, yet it is likely that they are susceptible to many of the noxious substances that affect other domestic and wild animals (4). Numerous texts deal with the effects of poisonous substances in humans and domestic animals (1, 3, 7–14). The reader is directed to these sources for details of the diagnosis and treatment of specific toxicants.

Although examples of toxicities will be given and tables presented to list known toxic substances that might affect lamoids, the primary focus will be enumeration of basic concepts. Understanding these may make it possible to advise clients on how to avoid poisoning by altering potentially dangerous situations.

Lamoids outside the Andes have been removed from their native habitat, wherein they may be resistant to the substances encountered over millennia. Toxicity is often thought to be a wholly artificial phenomenon, which humans have complete power to cause or prevent. This is a naive belief, because toxicants are as much a part of any environment as are substances that nourish an animal. Adaptation to the ingestion of poisonous substances is a basic part of evolution. Just as a certain animal population may develop resistance to a microorganism, so do many animals develop tolerance to a given toxicant. The problem is that nothing is known about the resistance of lamoids to toxicants.

ADAPTATION TO TOXICANTS

Animals cope with toxicants through one or more of the following strategies: avoidance, dilution, degradation, or detoxification (4). Should these strategies fail, the animal will be adversely affected and may ultimately die.

Avoidance is a crucial skill that must be learned early in life. It would be natural for lamoids in their native habitat to avoid unpalatable (potentially toxic) plants unless driven by extreme hunger. Lamoids in North America have been transported to a wide variety of new habitats and have had no opportunity to learn appropriate avoidance skills. Fortunately, lamoids are fastidious in food selection, so they may be partially protected.

Few irrigated and managed pastures are totally free of poisonous plants. As many as 40% of the plants growing on native rangelands may contain secondary plant compounds (poisonous substances). Harvested hays and prepared feeds may contain harmful weeds.

An animal with a choice of plants may *dilute* a toxicant by ingesting only small quantities that fail to reach the threshold level for production of toxicity. Lamoids are highly adapted to eating small quantities of a variety of plants, if given a choice.

A toxicant ingested by a lamoid may be *degraded* within the digestive tract. The multicompartmented stomach of camelids and their close relatives, the ruminants, is well designed to degrade toxic compounds, but the animal must depend on crucial gastrointestinal (GI) microorganisms to assist in rendering the toxicant harmless.

Once the toxic agent is absorbed from the GI tract, the body must either excrete it unchanged, sequester it in a nonactive storage site, *detoxify* it by molecular rearrangement, or suffer the ill-effects caused by the toxicant. All vertebrates have general detoxification pathways that can deal with many different substances. Some have specialized mechanisms, unique to a given species. Specific mechanisms are unknown in lamoids. Much detoxification is carried out by hepatic microsomal enzyme activity. Enzyme systems require priming and periodic reactivation by exposure to nonlethal quantities of toxicants. The intensively managed lamoid may never be given an opportunity to stimulate these systems and may be at a great risk if suddenly exposed.

DIAGNOSIS OF POISONING

The clinical signs caused by most potential toxicants in lamoids are unknown. Rarely will a diagnosis of poisoning be evident on initial examination. No pathognomonic signs of poisoning have been identified, and a limited number of pathognomonic lesions have been reported.

Diagnosis of poisoning depends upon analyzing a detailed history, evaluation of clinical signs, utilizing special laboratory diagnostic procedures, and, in some cases, necropsy and chemical analyses of tissue. Other possible disease conditions must be eliminated simultaneously by a thorough examination and medical workup.

Poisoning cases frequently result in litigation. It is imperative that detailed records be kept. It is unwise for the veterinarian to casually intimate, "It looks like a poison." A diagnosis of poisoning is not valid if based solely on the premise that no other disease entity or cause could be determined.

TREATMENT OF POISONING

The basic principles of treating a suspected case of poisoning include removal of the source and removal of the toxicant from the animal. If the toxicant has been applied externally, the animal must be bathed. This is difficult with lamoids, but copious amounts of water should be used to attempt to penetrate the coat and rinse the toxicant from the surface of the skin.

Emetics are inappropriate for use in lamoids. The volume of ingesta in compartment one (C-1) of the stomach precludes effective gavage. Catharsis may be produced by using magnesium oxide (10–20 g), magnesium sulfate (0.2 g/kg), or mineral oil (10 ml/kg). Activated charcoal may adsorb toxicants and may be administered via gastric intubation (100–200 g in 2 L water, 1–3 g/kg).

A limited number of general and specific antidotes are available. General antidotes include 20% calcium gluconate, 10% glucose, and 10–20% sodium thiosulfate. Specific antidotes include calcium versenate against lead, sodium thiosulfate and sodium nitrite against cyanide, and atropine against anticholinesterase compounds used as insecticides or parasiticides.

Early in the course of most poisonings, symptomatic and supportive therapy should be instituted, which will be of benefit in infectious or metabolic disease as well. Maintaining hydration with fluids, supporting respiration with oxygen and circulation with steroids and cardioactive drugs, and controlling central nervous system (CNS) stimulation with diazepam are indicated.

PREVENTION OF POISONING

Three basic concepts are important in the prevention of poisoning in lamoids. The most important is elimination of exposure to the toxicant. Purchased hay should be carefully inspected for quality and the presence of weeds or foreign material. Processed feeds must be of the highest quality. Since it is impossible to inspect certain types of processed feeds for poor or toxic ingredients, the integrity of the processor is of primary importance. Pastures should be walked periodically and unknown plants identified.

The second concept is avoidance of stress that enhances toxic effects. The third concept is provision of sufficient quantity and quality of nutrients in the diet to sustain healthy populations of GI microflora and microfauna.

CLASSES OF POISONS

Poisons that may be encountered in lamoids include insecticides, rodenticides, disinfectants, cleansing agents, paints, antifreeze, plant toxins, mycotoxins, drugs, and animal venoms. Tables 23.1 and 23.2 provide a short list of potential poisons in lamoids. Specific examples follow.

Insecticides

Lamoids are probably as susceptible to insecticides as other livestock species. A case of suspected organic phosphate insecticide poisoning has been reported (12). The clinical signs observed were typical of organic phosphate poisoning (depression, salivation, miosis, and diarrhea), but there was no muscle fasciculation.

Three llamas were given therapeutic doses of a drug used for treating lice infestations, chlorpyrifos (25 mg/kg body weight), followed by plasma levels of pseudocholinesterase. Plasma pseudocholinesterase activity decreased to as low as 38% of baseline by 5 days and returned to 90% baseline in approximately 36 days. None of the three exhibited overt signs of toxicity. Twenty-one healthy llamas were used to establish a baseline level of plasma pseudocholinesterase activity. The mean was 209 ± 29.16 IU/L (range = 150–252) (12).

Administration of atropine sulfate is the standard therapy for organic phosphate and carbamate insecticide poisoning. Poisoned animals are resistant to the effects of atropine, so the initial dose should be 0.2 – 0.4 mg/kg rather than the usual mammalian dose of 0.04 mg/kg. If possible, half the dose should be given intravenously and the rest subcutaneously. Pralidoxime (2-PAM) is effective against organic phosphate poisoning, but it is not recommended for carbamate poisoning. The dose is 20 mg/kg. Activated charcoal should be administered orally at 1–3 g/kg if the organic phosphate was taken orally.

Table 23.1. Miscellaneous toxicants with similar effects on all species

Toxicant	Source for llamas	Clinical signs	Special diagnostic procedures	Pathology	Management
Iodine	Therapeutic overdose	Dermal hyperemia and scaling, lacrimation	History and signs	Dermatitis	Removal
Fluoride	Rodenticides "1080", NaF	Hyperirritability, cardiac arrhythmias, trembling, colic, convulsions, death within 15–30 min	History and signs, chemical analysis of stomach, liver, and kidney	Biochemical lesion	Nonspecific, diazepam, anesthesia, calcium gluconate
Insecticides					
Organophosphates	Parasiticides	Salivation, colic, diarrhea, vomiting, dyspnea, miosis, muscle twitching, tetany, depression	History and signs, analysis of cholinesterase activity	No lesions	Removal of substances, atropine (0.4 mg/kg) 2-PAM (20 mg/kg)
Organochlorides	Insecticides	Hypersensitivity, muscle fasciculation, tonic/clonic convulsions, depression	History and signs, chemical analysis of liver, kidney, and stomach contents	No lesions	Removal, symptomatic, anesthesia
Rodenticides					
Strychine	Rodent bait	Tenseness, tetany, convulsions following stimulation, mydriasis	Chemical analysis of stomach contents	No lesions	Removal, sedation and anesthesia
Anticoagulants	Rodent bait	Hemorrhages at trauma sites	Clincal pathology, prolonged clotting time, bleeding time and clot retraction	Hemorrhages	Blood transfusion (20 ml/kg), vitamin K (20–30 mg)

Table 23.2. Heavy metal poisoning in lamoids

Metal	Source for llamas	Clinical signs	Diagnosis	Pathology	Management
Lead (Pb)	Contaminated forage, paint	Depression[a], anorexia, stomach atony, colic, diarrhea, ataxia, circling, blindness	Blood, liver, and kidney analysis	Encephalopathy, gastroenteritis	Calcium EDTA (110 mg/kg) for 5 days
Arsenic (As)	Contaminated forage, pesticides, herbicides	Colic[a], weakness, salivation, trembling, diarrhea, depression dehydration, shock	Chemical analysis of liver, kidney, and stomach contents	Gastroenteritis	Removal, symptomatic, fluids, prevent secondary infection
Selenium (Se)	Plants containing high Se, therapeutic overdose	See Nutrition, Chapter 2	Chemical analysis of liver and kidney	Pansystemic, hepatic necrosis, renal necrosis	Removal, symptomatic
Copper (Cu)	Water contamination, insecticides, food supplements	See Nutrition, Chapter 2	Chemical analysis	Hemolytic anemia, hepatic necrosis	Nothing for acute toxicity, add molybdenum
Molybdenum (Mo)	Plants high in Mo and low in Cu	See Nutrition, Chapter 2. Diarrhea, coat depigmentation, decreased fertility, emaciation, anemia	Response to Cu supplementation	Microcytic, hypochromic anemia, hemosiderosis, emaciation	Cu supplementation, Cu injection

Note: Signs listed are a composite.
[a]Clinical syndrome has not been described in lamoids. Signs are variable in livestock.

Rodenticides

No cases of rodenticide poisoning in lamoids have been reported, but these agents affect a broad host range, and lamoids are likely to be susceptible if exposed. Owners should be cautioned about the use of rat and mouse bait in impregnated grain that may be placed where lamoids can gain access.

Heavy Metals

Lead, arsenic, mercury, copper, and molybdenum are used in agricultural products and paints. It should be assumed that lamoids are susceptible. Clinical signs and lesions are presumed to be similar to those of poisoned cattle and sheep.

Plants

The only reports of plant poisoning in lamoids in North America involve oleander, *Nerium oleander,* and various species of the family Ericaceae (6). No plant poisonings have been reported from South America. Llamas browse a wide variety of plants and may be affected, in certain circumstances, by the plants listed in Tables 23.3 and 23.4 (Figs. 23.1–23.18). Alpacas are primarily grazers and hence are less likely to consume shrubbery. Other plants may also affect lamoids, but little benefit may be gained by listing every poisonous plant that has ever been suspected of causing poisoning in any species of animal. It is better for the veterinarian and the llama owner to become knowledgeable about a few key, likely plants than to bother with hundreds of less likely plants

Table 23.3. Poisonous plants that may affect llamas on trek

Common name	Scientific name	Habitat	Poisonous principle	Signs of poisoning	Therapy
Arrowgrass	*Triglochin maritina*	Meadows at low to moderate elevations	Cyanogenic glycoside	Muscle twitching, convulsions, dyspnea, bright red blood	Methylene blue, sodium thiosulfate
False hellebore, corn lily (Fig. 23.1)	*Veratrum californicum*	High mountain meadows	Alkaloids	Vomiting, salivation, convulsions, fast irregular heart beat	S
Death camas, sandcorn (Fig. 23.2)	*Zigadenus* sp.	Hillsides, fields, meadows in spring of year	Alkaloids	Foaming at mouth, convulsions, ataxia, vomiting, fast weak pulse	S
Nightshade (Fig. 23.3)	*Solanum* sp.	Ubiquitous	Alkaloid-glycoside solanine	Vomiting, weakness, groaning	S
Jimsonweed, thornapple (Fig. 23.4)	*Datura metaloides*	Waste places	Alkaloid-atropine	Dry mucous membranes, dilated pupil, mania	Parasympathomimetics
Chokecherry, wild cherry (Fig. 23.5)	*Prunus virginiana*	Streamsides	Cyanogenic glycoside	Dyspnea, convulsions, rapid death, bright red blood	Sodium nitrite and sodium thiosulfate
Western sneezeweed (Fig. 23.6)	*Helenium hoopesii*	High mountain meadows	Glycoside	Vomiting, depression, frothing at mouth, coughing, weak irregular pulse	S
Laborador tea (Fig. 23.7)	*Ledum glandulosum*	Around lakes, meadows, streams	Andromedotoxin (diterpene), arbutin	Vomiting, colic, paresis, anorexia, muscle twitches	S
Black laurel, Mt. laurel (Fig. 23.8)	*Leucothoe davisiae*	Around lakes, meadows, streams	Andromedotoxin (diterpene), arbutin	Vomiting, colic, paresis, anorexia, muscle twitches	S
Western azalea (Fig. 23.10)	*Rhododendron occidentale*	Around lakes, meadows, streams	Andromedotoxin (diterpene), arbutin	Vomiting, colic, paresis, anorexia, muscle twitches	S
Rhododendron (Figs. 23.9, 23.10)	*Rhododendron* sp.	Around lakes, meadows, streams	Andromedotoxin (diterpene), arbutin	Vomiting, colic, paresis, anorexia, muscle twitches	S
Oleander (Fig. 23.19)	*Nerium oleander*	Ornamental	Cardioactive glycoside	Diarrhea, colic, cardiac irregularities, cyanosis	S, gastrotomy
Castorbean (Fig. 23.11)	*Ricinus communis*	Ornamental, may escape	Ricin, water-soluble albumitoxin	Anaphylactic shock, diarrhea	Treat for shock, fluids
Tobacco, tree tobacco (Fig. 23.12)	*Nicotiana* sp.	Waste places	Alkaloid, nicotine	Stimulation of CNS, then depression; sweating, muscle twitches, convulsions	S

Note: S = Symptomatic. In most cases of poisoning from ingestion of poisonous plants, there is no specific antidote; rather, it is necessary to treat symptomatically.

Table 23.4. Additional plants that may poison lamoids

Common name	Scientific name	Poisonous principle	Habitat	Signs of poisoning	Therapy
Black locust (Fig. 23.13)	*Robinia pseudoacacia*	Alkaloids	Around homes and public buildings, in parks and farmyards	Diarrhea, collapse, shock	S
Purple fox glove (Fig. 23.14)	*Digitalis purpurea*	Digitalis	In gardens, cool shaded places, coastal areas of northern California	Diarrhea, colic, cardiac irregularities, cyanosis	S, gastrotomy and emptying contents
Yew (Fig. 23.15)	*Taxus baccatta*	Alkaloid	In gardens and parks, as trees or hedges, similar species found wild in California	Sudden death, dyspnea, collapse, diarrhea	S
Lantana (Fig. 23.16)	*Lantana camara*	Hepatotoxins	Ground cover, shrubs in gardens and parks, escapes into waste areas	Photosensitization, icterus, other signs of hepatic insufficiency	S
Water hemlock (Fig. 23.17)	*Cicuta douglasii*	Resinoids	In marshes or swamps with water present for majority of the year	Convulsions, trembling, death in 15–30 min	None, S
Milk weed (Fig. 23.18)	*Asclepias* sp.	Alkaloidal glycosides	Along roadsides, edges of cultivated fields, waste places, woodlots	Depression, weakness, convulsions, intestinal stasis early, diarrhea late	S

Note: S = Symptomatic. In most cases of poisoning from ingestion of poisonous plants, there is no specific antidote; rather, it is necessary to treat symptomatically.

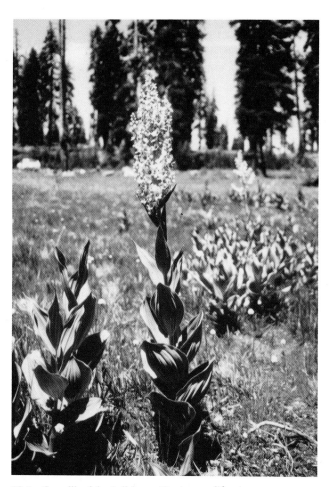

23.1 Corn lily, false hellebore, *Veratrum californicum*.

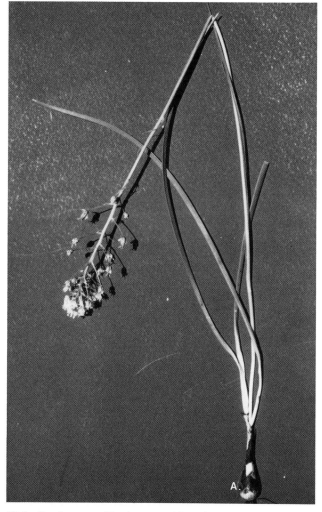

23.2 Death camus, *Zigadenus* sp.: **(A)** underground corm.

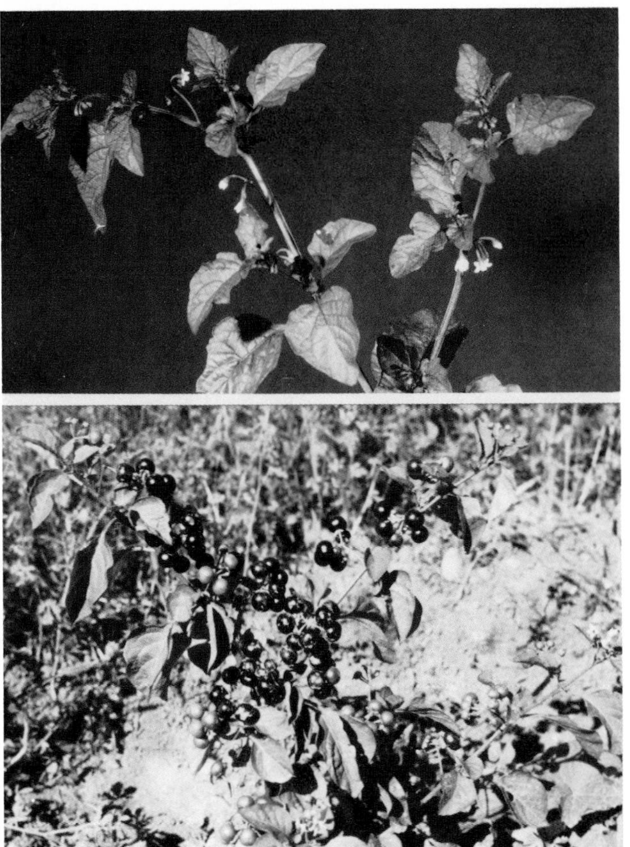

23.3 Night shade: (top) *Solanum sarrachoides,* (bottom) *S. nigrum.*

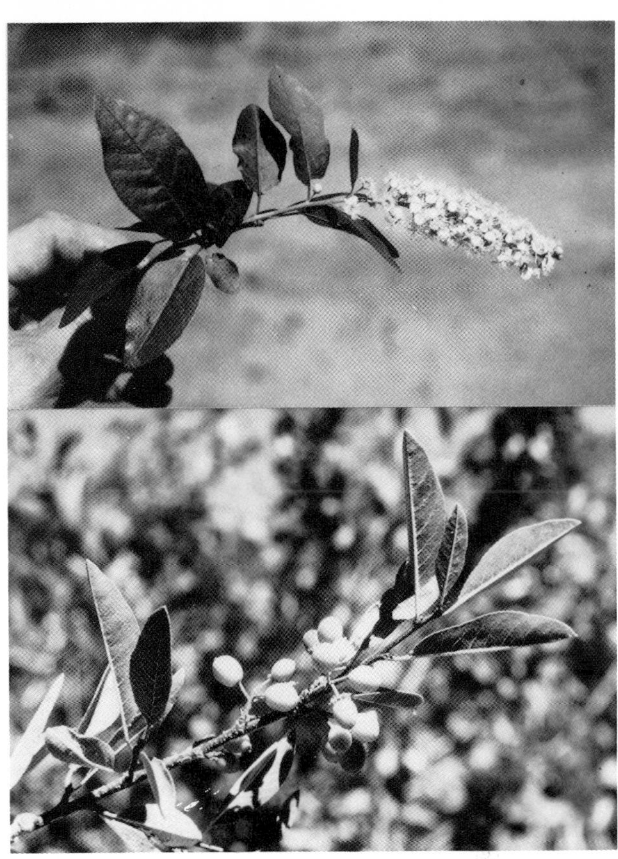

23.5 Chokecherry: (top) *Prunus demissa,* (bottom) *P. emarginata.*

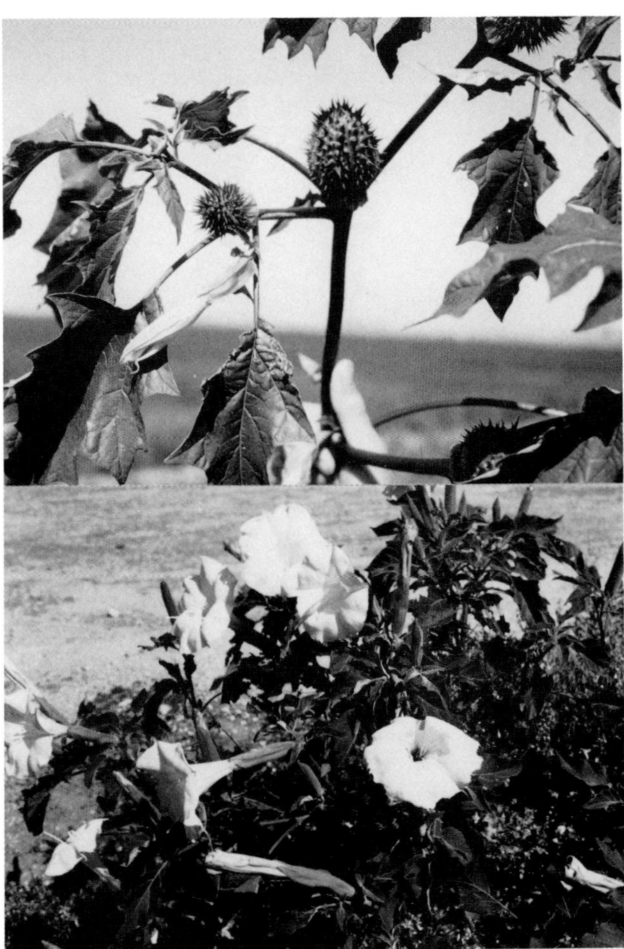

23.4 Datura: (top) jimson weed, *Datura stramonium,* (bottom) tolguacha, *D. metaloides.*

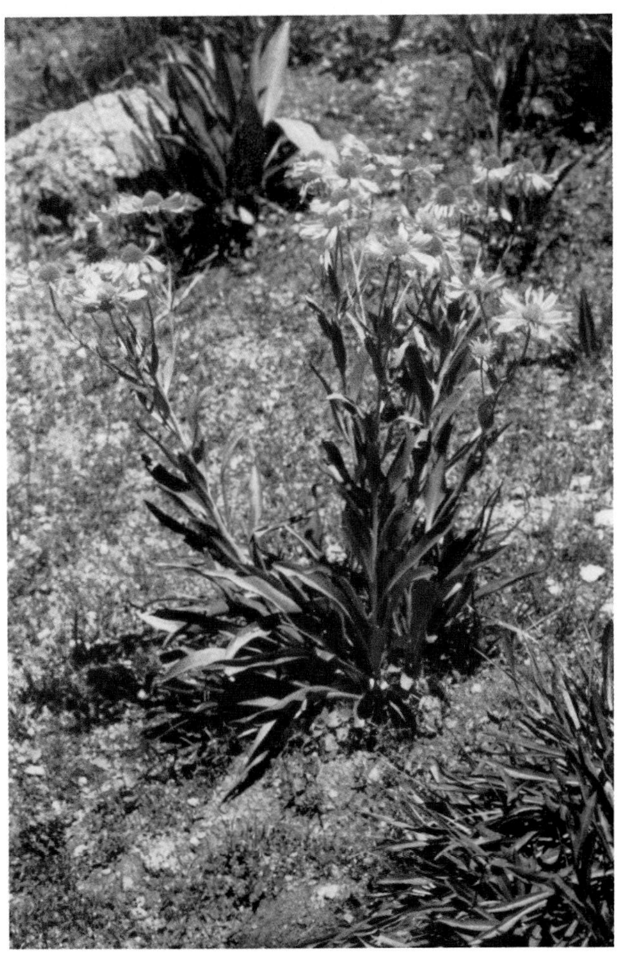

23.6 Western sneezeweed, *Helenium hoopesii.*

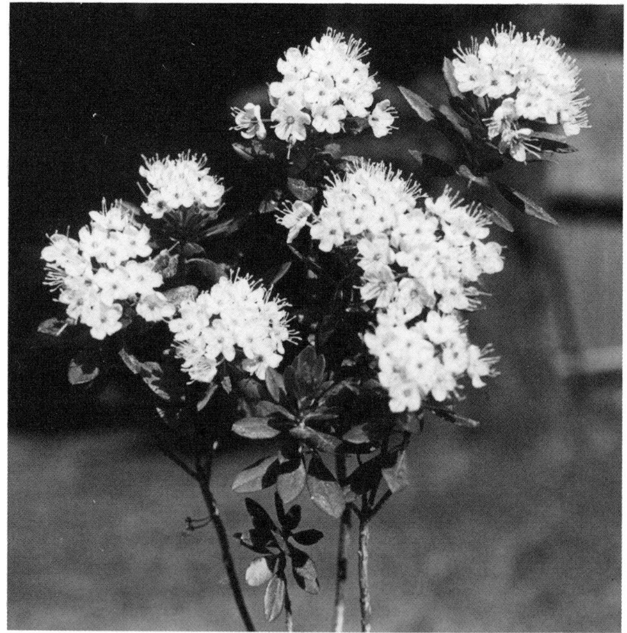

23.7 Labrador tea, *Ledum glandulosum*.

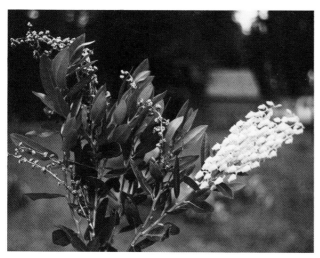

23.8 Black laurel, Mt. laurel, *Leucothoe davisiae*.

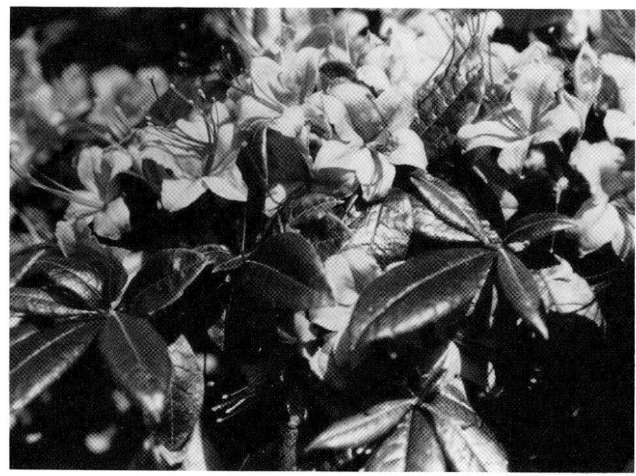

23.9 Azalea, *Rhododendron* sp.

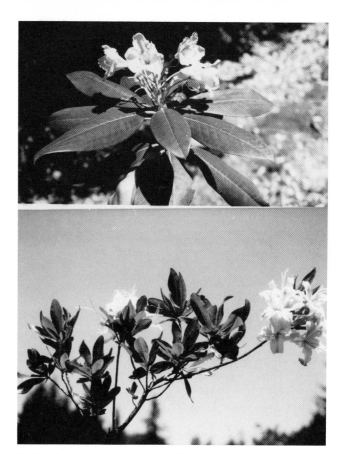

23.10 California rosebay, (top) *Rhododendron macrophyllum,* (bottom) western azalea, *R. occidentale*.

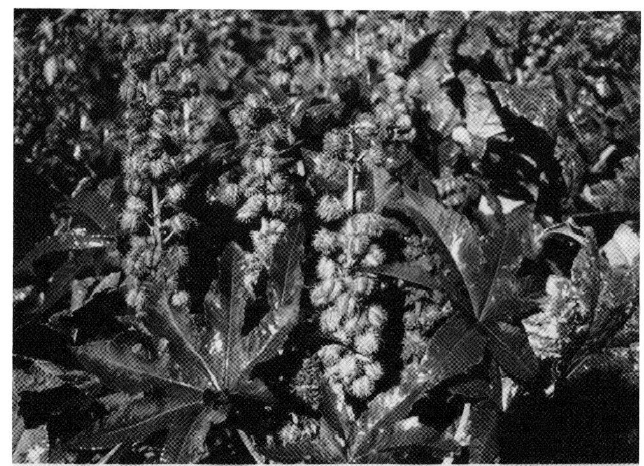

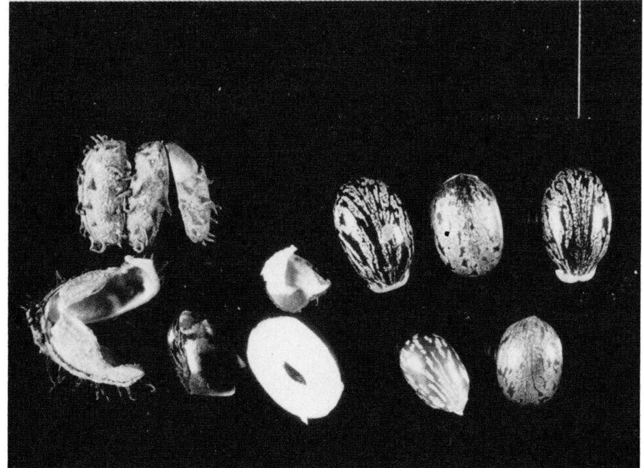

23.11 Castorbean, *Ricinus communis*.

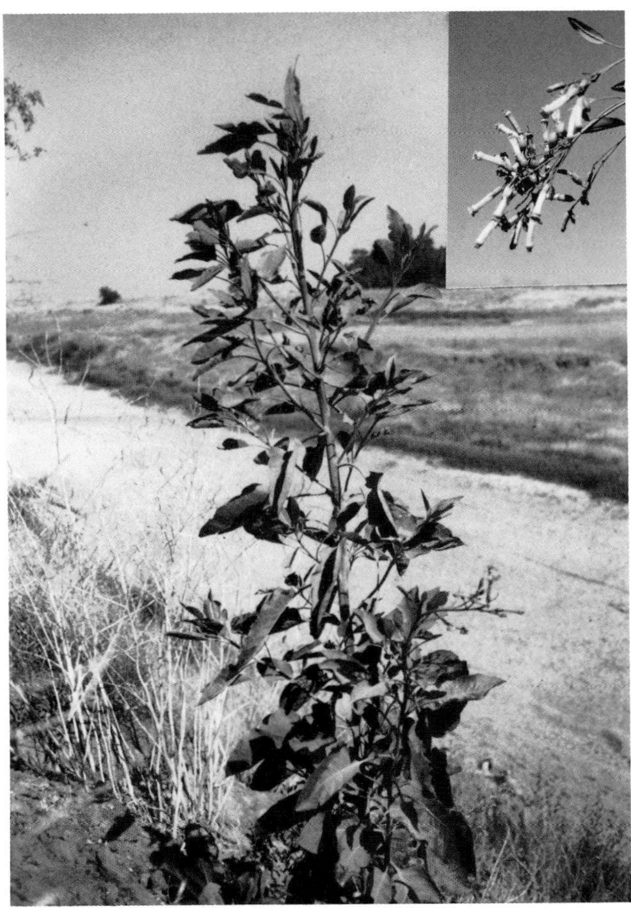

23.12 Tree tobacco, *Nicotiana glauca.*

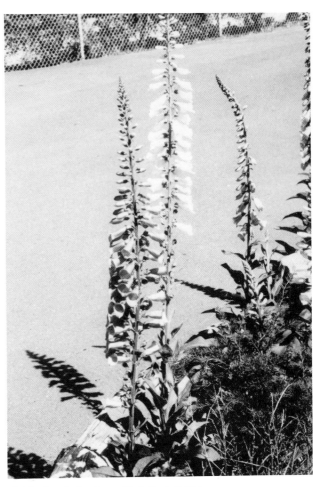

23.14 Purple foxglove, *Digitalis purpurea.*

23.13 Black locust, false acacia, *Robinia pseudoacacia.*

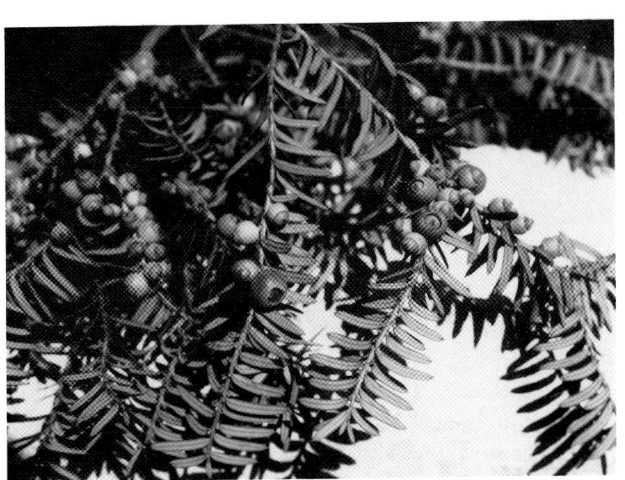

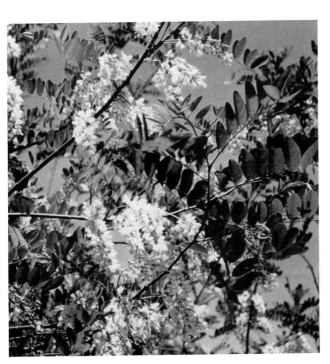

23.15 Yew, *Taxus* sp.

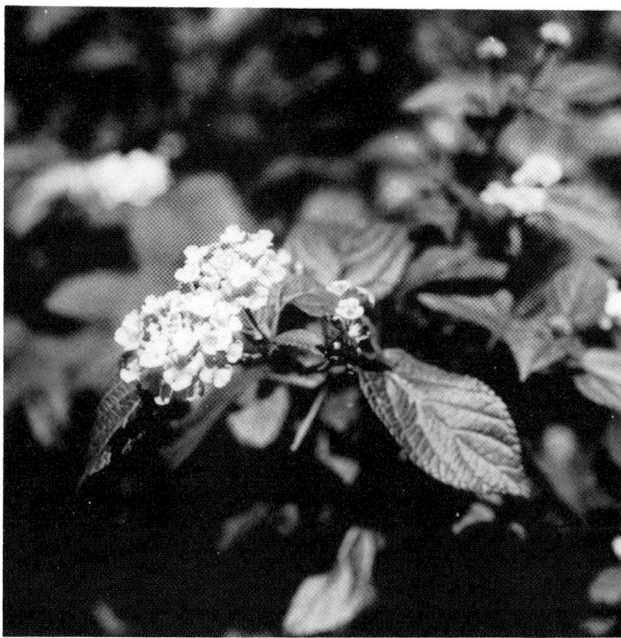

23.16 Lantana, *Lantana camara.*

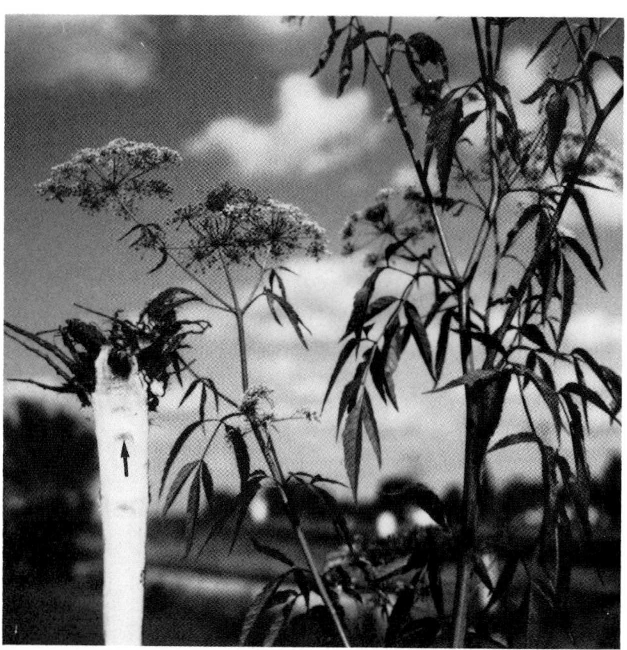

23.17 Water hemlock, *Cicuta douglasii.*

(Tables 23.3, 23.4). References are listed, if greater detail is desired.

Ornamental plants are a special hazard for llamas. Unfortunately, such plants may not be listed in poisonous plant lists and booklets of the region, since many ornamentals are not native.

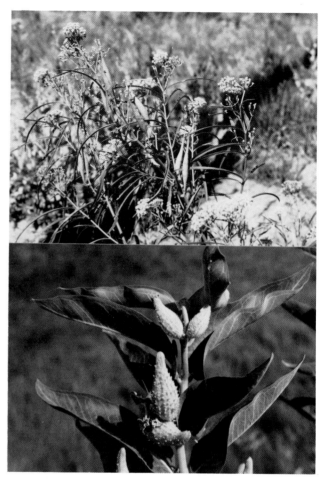

23.18 Milkweeds: (top) Mexican whorled milkweed, *Asclepias fasicularis,* (bottom) showy milkweed, *A. speciosa.*

RHODODENDRON POISONING. A number of genera and species within the plant family Ericaceae contain a resin called andromedotoxin and a glycoside, arbutin, which produce an identical syndrome in a broad host range. A description of the history and clinical signs of two llamas poisoned with Sierra laurel, *Leucothoe davisiae,* follows (5).

Two pack llamas were tied to some shrubs near a grassy area at the edge of a small lake during a lunch stop. The first clinical sign was noted 1.5 hours later when one llama began to cough and appeared to be choking. Within an hour, he was recumbent and refused to rise. The second llama began foaming (shaving cream consistency) from the mouth. He, too, began coughing and choking. Both llamas ultimately began projectile vomiting between episodes of rolling, retching, and groaning. Depression, anorexia, vomiting, groaning, and symptoms of colic persisted for 2 days. On the third day the animals had recovered sufficiently to slowly move out of the mountain to a trailhead.

The signs observed in these llamas are similar to those seen by the author in cases of rhododendron poisoning in both llamas and domestic livestock. The composite of the clinical signs includes anorexia, repeated swallowing, salivation, depression, vomiting, bloat, colic (straining, rolling, groaning, grinding of the teeth), weakness, ataxia, prostration, dyspnea (aspiration pneumonia), bradycardia, and hypotension. Hepatopathy may be a sequel.

Treatment of rhododendron poisoning is nonspecific. Administration of a cathartic such as magnesium oxide (10–20 g) is appropriate. Activated charcoal (100–200 g) is a general antidote and may be administered by stomach tube. A drench consisting of a slurry of activated charcoal in water may be given, but such therapy is dangerous in a vomiting animal. Atropine (0.04 mg/kg) may be used to alleviate bradycardia. Other symptomatic treatment is indicated.

OLEANDER POISONING. Oleander, *Nerium oleander,* is one of the most toxic shrubs to which a lamoid or any other mammal may be exposed. The lethal oral dose of either green or dried leaves is 225 mg/kg. For a 150 kg (330 lb) llama, this would mean less than 35 g of leaves (15 medium-sized leaves or 1 leaf/10 kg body weight). The poisonous principle is a cardioactive glycoside, similar in action to digitalis.

Oleander is a beautiful ornamental shrub, grown extensively throughout California and along the southern tier of the United States (Fig. 23.19). As a potted shrub that can be moved inside during the winter, it may be found almost anywhere. Llamas may obtain oleander leaves in a variety of ways. Rarely will they ingest leaves directly from the living shrub. However, if cuttings or lawn clippings containing leaves are placed where llamas can get at them, there is great risk. A sprig of oleander that had been chewed on was found in the manger of an 8-month-old llama that died with signs of oleander toxicity.

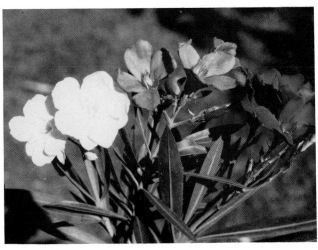

23.19 Oleander, *Nerium oleander.*

In another instance, oleander leaves and branches were included with other tree cuttings and run through a shredder. The mulch was then spread along a path next to a llama pasture. Some of the dried mulch blew into the pasture. Within 24 hours, one of three llamas was sick and died 4 days later. Another llama became ill but recovered.

The clinical signs of oleander poisoning are similar in all species of mammals. Llamas become anorectic, depressed, and lie down unless forced to rise. The major observable sign is frequent, projectile, catarrhal to hemorrhagic diarrhea. Colicky signs may accompany the diarrhea. If the ingested dose is high, the animal may die of cardiac complications before diarrhea develops.

The cardioactive glycoside has a direct effect on the cardiac musculature. Various conduction abnormalities may be heard on auscultation over a period of a few minutes because of the rate and rhythm change. There may be bradycardia, tachycardia, drop beats, and partial and complete blocks. Impaired circulation may result in cyanosis, muscle tremors, patchy perspiration, and dyspnea. Terminally, tachycardia progresses to ventricular fibrillation and agonal struggling.

Clinical signs in ruminants may develop 5–24 hours after ingestion. Lamoids may develop clinical signs sooner because C-1 of the stomach has an absorptive mucosa (see Chap. 13). Death may occur within 10 hours or after 3–4 days. The severity of clinical signs is not directly correlated with possible mortality.

At necropsy, lesions are limited to enteritis plus petechial or ecchymotic hemorrhages of the GI serosa or of the epicardium, endocardium, or pericardium. Stomach contents of all three compartments should be carefully examined for the presence of leaf segments. Oleander leaves have a unique vein pattern, with a single midrib and parallel secondary ribs (Fig. 23.20). Finding even a small segment of a leaf in the stomach contents would justify a diagnosis of oleander poisoning.

Treatment of oleander poisoning is difficult. The regimen for treating an overdose of digitalis in humans is not satisfactory for lamoids (lowering serum calcium by titration with sodium versenate, administration of potassium glutamate). The use of various drugs to counter arrhythmias has not been worked out. If a definitive diagnosis is made, the logical recourse is to remove the remaining oleander material from the digestive tract. This means that a gastrotomy must be performed (see Chap. 6). All of the contents of C-1 must be removed and the lumen washed out. Small leaf segments left in the

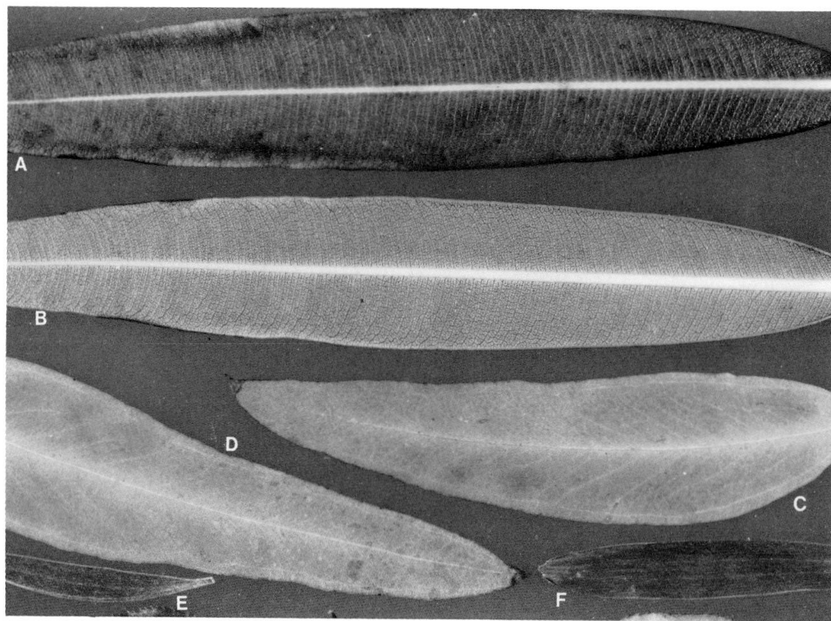

23.20 Veination of leaves that may be confused with oleander: **(A)** oleander, top view, **(B)** oleander, bottom view, **(C)** eucalyptus, *Eucalyptus* sp., top view, **(D)** eucalyptus, bottom view, **(E)** acacia, *Acacia* sp., top view, **(F)** acacia bottom view.

stomach may be lethal. The microorganisms from C-1 must be replaced by a transplant from another llama or a cow.

Unfortunately, patients with circulatory deficiencies are not good surgical anesthetic risks. Gastrotomy may be performed in the standing llama under local anesthesia, but it will be more difficult.

Animals in a herd are not all equally curious and all may not consume leaves in their enclosure. However, all exposed animals should be examined for cardiac irregularities. A cathartic may be administered to hasten emptying of the GI tract. Oleander is so toxic, it is dangerous to wait for symptoms to appear.

PYRROLIZIDINE ALKALOID POISONING (2). Dozens of pyrrolizidine alkaloids are found in plants broadly distributed throughout the world. These alkaloids vary in toxicity from no effect to pronounced effect on the liver of the host. Many animals have some innate resistance to pyrrolizidine alkaloids. The alkaloid must be metabolically altered to an active metabolite before toxicity occurs, and certain species such as sheep degrade the alkaloid, avoiding production of the active metabolite. Of the domestic animals studied, horses are the most susceptible, next are cattle, then swine. Humans seem to be as susceptible as the horse. It is not known just where lamoids fit on the scale, but poisoning has been diagnosed.

Pyrrolizidine alkaloid poisoning is a regional problem in California and other Pacific Northwest areas where alkaloid-containing plants thrive. Following is a short discussion of some of the major plants involved in toxicity of livestock and, potentially, of lamoids.

Fiddleneck, *Amsinckia intermedia* (Fig. 23.21), is in the family Boraginaceae. It is a common weed of abused native pastures and often contaminates oat hay and first-cutting alfalfa hay. Poisoning is most likely to occur when lamoids are fed hay or processed feeds containing the weed. The alkaloid is concentrated in the tiny (2–3 mm) nutlike seeds.

The genus *Senecio* contains over 500 species and is

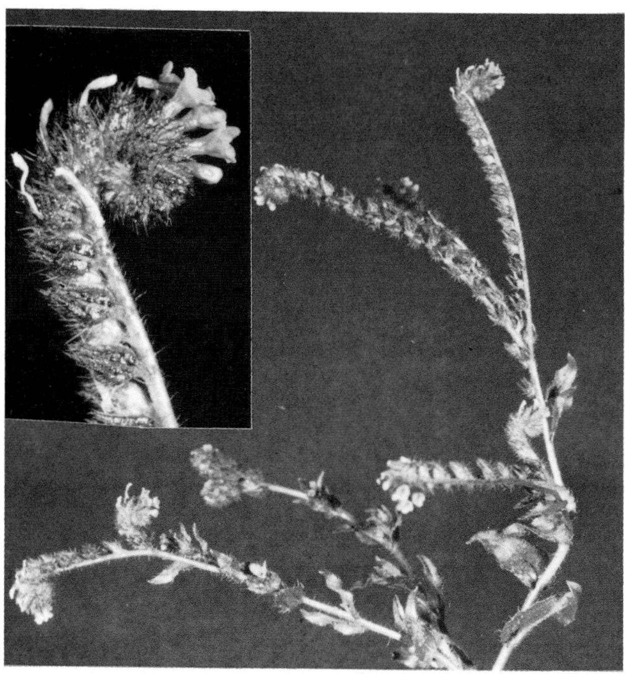

23.21 Fiddleneck, *Amsinckia intermedia:* (inset) enlarged floral head.

distributed worldwide. Only a few species have harmful levels of toxic alkaloids, but all members of the genus should be suspect until proven otherwise. Two particularly troublesome species found in North America are common groundsel, *Senecio vulgaris* (Fig. 23.22), and tansy ragwort, *Senecio jacobea* (Fig. 23.23). Groundsel is a common weed of waste places and a frequent contaminant of first-cutting alfalfa hay in California. Tansy ragwort is a biennial and a widespread weed of pastures in the Pacific Northwest.

Poisoning from pyrrolizidine alkaloids may occur from a single large ingestion or be accumulative over a period of days or weeks. The alkaloid acts directly on the hepatocyte, but expression of that damage may not occur for as long as 6 months after ingestion. This is an important factor when dealing with llamas having liver malfunction, where pyrrolizidine alkaloid poisoning may be suspected. Young growing animals are more susceptible than adults. The fetus may be affected in utero, and the alkaloid is found in the milk of cattle, goats, and women.

The clinical signs of pyrrolizidine alkaloid poisoning are those of hepatic insufficiency, indistinguishable from signs caused by other hepatotoxic agents and infectious diseases. The syndrome in lamoids has not been described but is likely to be similar to the syndrome in cattle. Icterus is common but not always present. Affected animals are anorectic and depressed. Various degrees of hepatic coma produce aimless wandering, incoordination, head pressing, pushing through or over obstacles in the path, apparent blindness, recumbency, and forced running activities while recumbent. Horses bite at fences, other animals, and humans, but this has not been seen in cattle. *For operator safety, in rabies-endemic areas, any animal exhibiting the foregoing signs should be handled as though it may be rabid.*

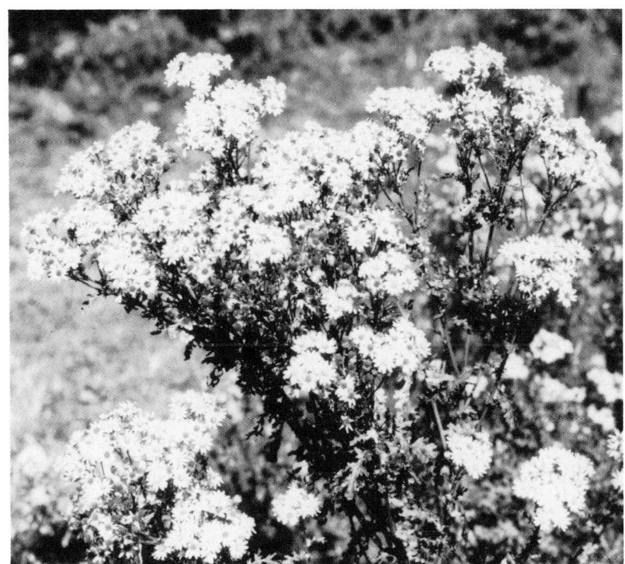

23.23 Tansy ragwort, *Senecio jacobea.*

Hemoglobinuria may be seen, and photosensitization develops on nonpigmented areas of the skin not covered by thick wool or otherwise protected from exposure to ultraviolet (sun) light. Body temperature may be normal or elevated. Secondary infection of the damaged liver is frequent. A neutrophilia and left shift is common on the hemogram.

A tentative diagnosis may be made on the basis of clinical signs and the hemogram. Serum enzymes may be normal, but liver function tests such as bromosulfo-

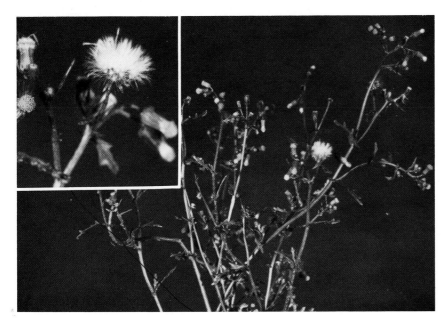

23.22 Groundsel, *Senecio vulgaris:* (inset) enlarged flowering head.

phthalein are markedly altered. A definitive diagnosis is based on histologic examination of liver samples collected by liver biopsy (see Chap. 4). Cardinal lesions are megalocytosis and karyomegaly of the hepatocytes, hepatic fibrosis, and bile duct hyperplasia.

On gross necropsy, the liver may be small, swollen, roughened, and have variable color. The consistency of the liver is firm, and it may be cut only with difficulty. Icterus may be prominent. Gross lesions are not pathognomonic, but microscopic lesions are.

No treatment is effective for pyrrolizidine alkaloid poisoning. Once the liver has been damaged to the extent that clinical signs appear, the damage to the liver is irreversible, and the animal will die. It may be desirable to examine other lamoids that may also have been exposed. A definitive prognosis may be provided by a combination of liver function tests and liver biopsy.

MECHANICALLY INJURIOUS PLANTS. Many plants and grasses have fruits or seeds that contain barbs or hooks, which aid in their distribution within the environment. Grass awns, clover burs, and other plant parts catch on the fiber coat and work their way deeply into the coat, much to the chagrin of lamoid groomers. Of greater concern are grass awns or plant foreign bodies that lodge in the conjunctival sac, ear, nostril, or mouth.

Foxtails, *Hordeum* sp. (Fig. 23.24), are a special problem in the western United States. These grasses are widespread weeds of pastures and hayfields. If weedy hay is fed to llamas, the awns may lodge alongside the tongue and in the buccal cavity. The tongue of the llama is not highly mobile and rarely protrudes from the mouth. The immobility of the tongue may inhibit the clearing of foxtails from the mouth.

Foxtails have also been extracted from the conjunctival sac and the external ear canal, producing signs of head shaking, head tilt, exudation from the ear canal, lacrimation, photophobia, blepharospasm, and depression. In one case, the foxtail had penetrated the tympanic membrane, entered the middle ear, worked its way through the inner ear and the temporal bone, and finally became lodged in the contiguous brain stem, producing an abscess and subsequent death of the llama. See Chapter 19 for a discussion of ear disorders.

Another mechanically injurious plant is yellow bristle grass, *Setaria lutescens* (Fig. 23.25). The grass causes no problem in a pasture; in fact, it is probably good forage. The problem arises with dried grass in hay. The dried brittle awns of the seed head become tiny needles. Yellow bristle grass is a common weed of irrigated alfalfa hay. If the grass constitutes more than 25% of the hay, there is a risk of mechanical injury to animals that consume the hay.

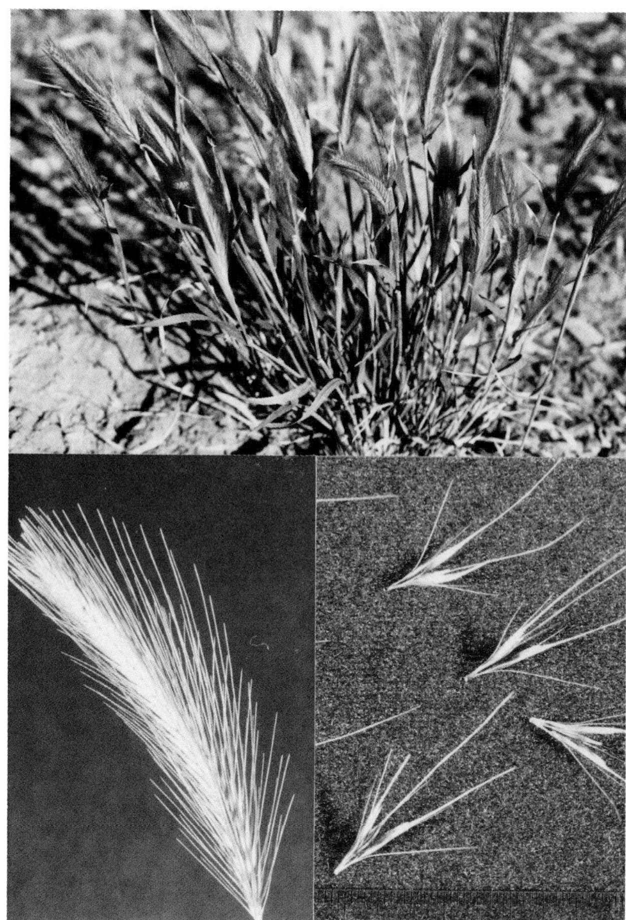

23.24 Foxtail, *Hordeum jubatum.*

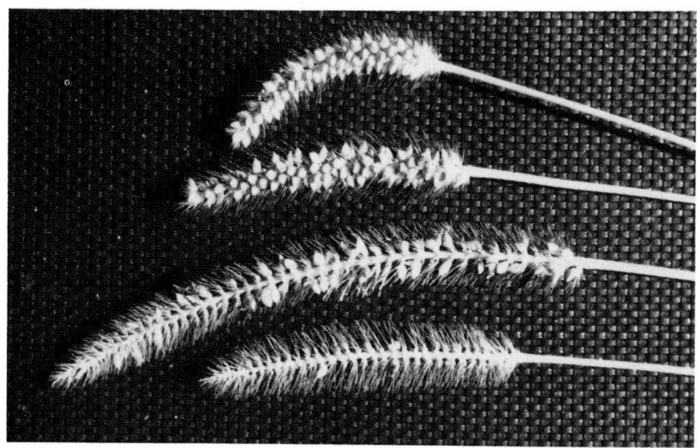

23.25 Yellow bristle grass, *Setaria lutescens.*

Clinical Signs. The awns penetrate the mucous membranes of the tongue, lips, gingiva, and buccal cavity. Ulcers varying in size from 1 to 3 cm in diameter are characterized by the protrusion of dozens of awn segments. The lips may be swollen. Salivation is common, and prehension and mastication are inhibited.

Treatment. The awn segments must be curetted from the surface of each ulcer. The application of disinfectants or other medication to the ulcers is superfluous. The weedy hay must be eliminated from the diet.

Tarweed, *Hemizonia* sp., exudes a dark resin onto the leaves and stems that may stick to the fiber and skin of grazing animals (Fig. 23.26).

MISCELLANEOUS PLANT POISONINGS. Mycotoxicosis has not yet been reported in lamoids but should be considered. Aflatoxicosis has a broad host range, as does ergotism.

Cyanide and nitrate poisoning have not yet been reported, but lamoids have a stomach capable of hydrolyzing cyanogenic glycosides to free cyanide and reducing nitrates to nitrites to produce methemoglobinemia. The syndrome and recommendation for management of these toxicities would be the same as for cattle. Figures 23.1–23.18 illustrate other potential plants that may cause poisoning in lamoids (see also Tables 23.3, 23.4).

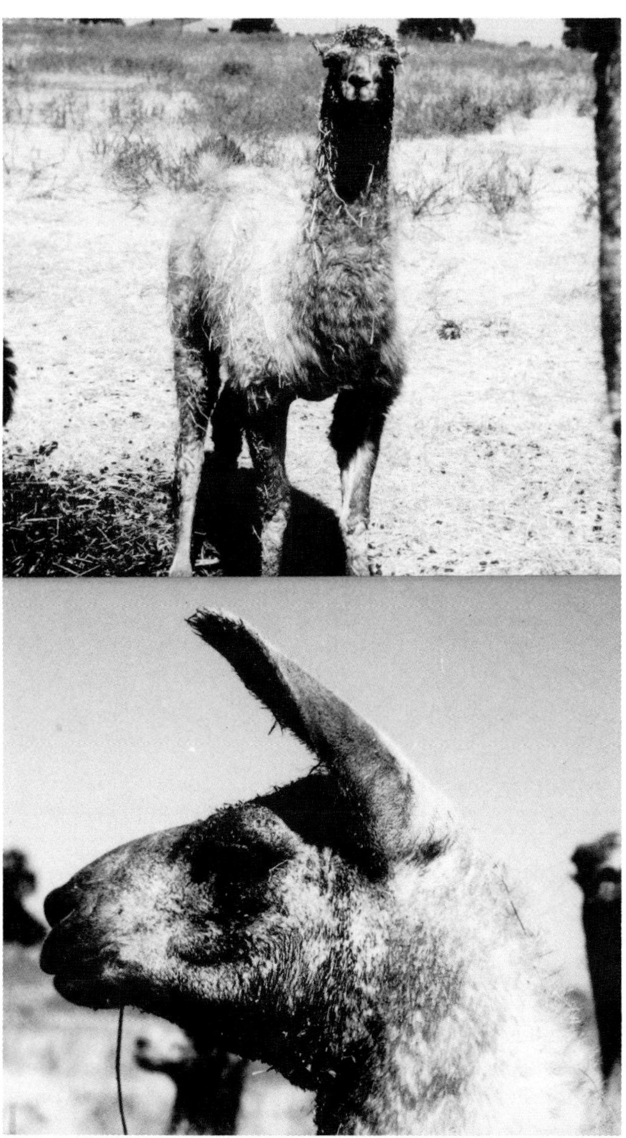

23.26 Plant resins on face, neck, and limbs from grazing in tarweed, *Hemazonia kelloggii.*

Snake Envenomation

Four types of venomous snakes are found in the United States: rattlesnake, *Crotalus* sp.; copperhead, *Agkistrodon contortrix;* water moccasin (cottonmouth), *Agkistrodon piscivorus;* and coral snake, *Micrurus sp.*

Copperheads are found in eastern North America, but their venom has low toxicity and serious envenomation is unlikely to occur in lamoids. Water moccasins are found in the swampy, marshy areas of southeastern North America, and lamoids are unlikely to encounter them. Coral snakes are small, inoffensive, secretive snakes of Florida, Texas, and Arizona and pose little threat to lamoids. Only the larger species of rattlesnake, genus *Crotalus,* are likely to be a hazard to lamoids. The author has dealt with three rattlesnake bites in llamas, one of them being fatal.

Llamas, especially juveniles, are curious and may be bitten on the nose while investigating the strange animal. Nose bites are especially hazardous to lamoids, because local swelling may occlude the nostrils. Since lamoids are primarily obligate nasal breathers, dyspnea and suffocation may ensue.

Clinical signs of rattlesnake bite include local tissue swelling at the bite site that spreads proximally and may involve any tissue or organ. Figure 23.27 is of a llama 4 hours after a bite, Figure 23.28, 24 hours after the bite, Figure 23.29, 48 hours after the bite, and Figure 23.30, 72 hours after the bite. Although not yet observed in bites of llamas, the swelling may progress to necrosis and sloughing of the skin in other species. Bites on the limb show unilateral edema of the limb proximal to the bite.

Systemic manifestations of envenomation are absent or minimal in large animals such as lamoids. However, the bite from a large eastern diamond back rattlesnake, *Crotalus adamanteus,* could produce effects on the kidney and cardiovascular system (hypotension) as well as the local necrotizing effects.

The diagnosis may not always be clear if the bite was not observed, since trauma may produce similar signs. Supportive and symptomatic therapy may be instituted while monitoring the progress of the swelling.

The principal therapeutic measure in lamoids is to maintain air flow via a tracheostomy (see Chap. 6). The tracheostomy tube must be maintained until the animal can breathe properly with the orifice of the tube oc-

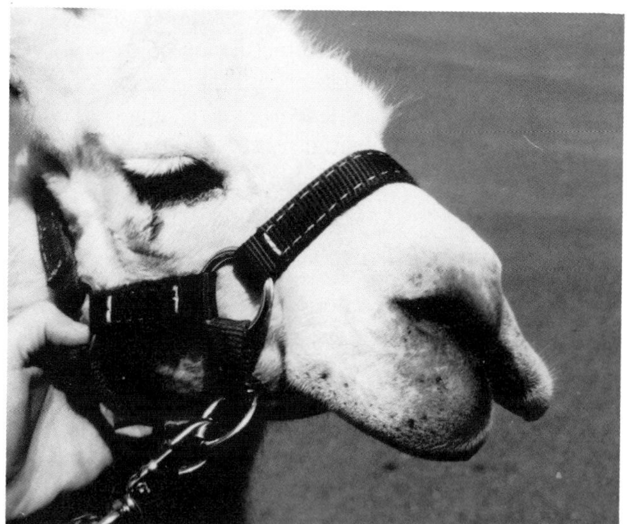

23.27 Rattlesnake bite on muzzle 4 hours after bite.

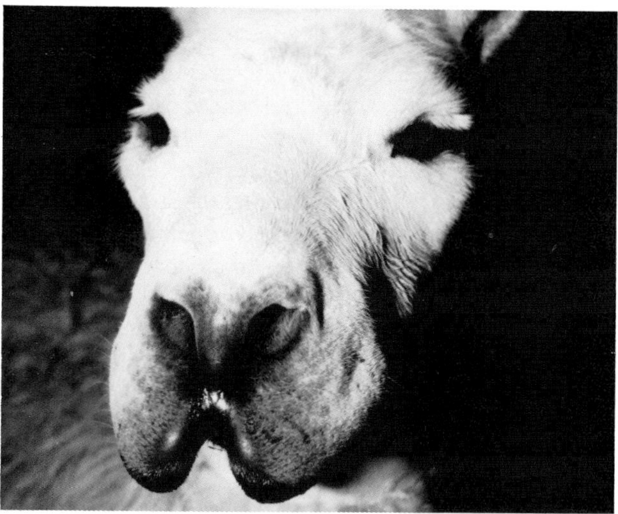

23.28 Rattlesnake bite 24 hours after bite.

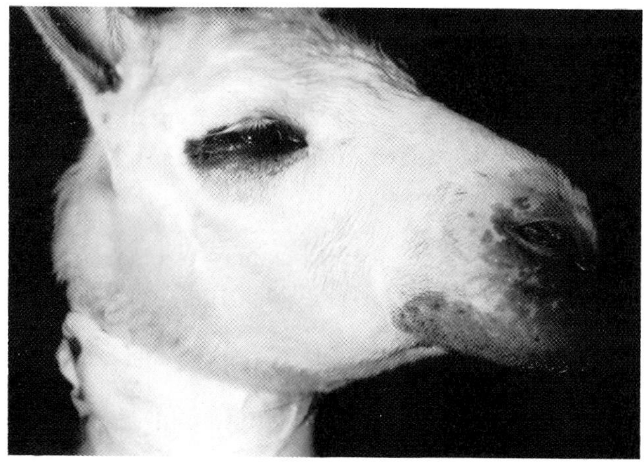

23.29 Rattlesnake bite 48 hours after bite.

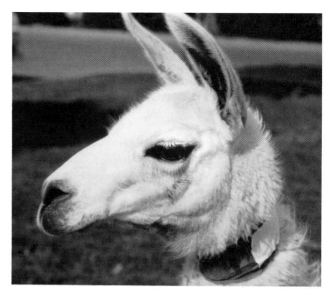

23.30 Rattlesnake bite 72 hours after bite.

cluded, usually 2–3 days. The use of specific antivenin in rattlesnake bites of large animals is controversial. Antivenin does not necessarily counter the local tissue necrosis effects, and since systemic effects are minimal, the use of antivenin is questionable. Antivenin is prepared from horse serum and may sensitize the llama to future use of any equine-prepared serum product.

Early in the course of a bite, cold water packs or spraying with water from a garden hose will tend to restrict spread of the edematous process. After 24 hours, the use of warm water packs and spray are indicated to enhance circulation and drainage of accumulated fluid and tissue breakdown products. Corticosteroids have been administered but are of questionable value. Antihistamines are contraindicated because of their potential hypotensive action, which may be additive to the hypotensive action of the venom.

Miscellaneous Animal Bites and Stings

Occasionally, all animals are stung or bitten by insects or arachnids (wasps, bees, ants, mosquitos, and spiders). Reactions vary but are unlikely to produce serious illness. The local inflammatory response produced by venom injection cannot easily be differentiated from contusions or foreign body penetration (slivers). Multiple bee or wasp stings may produce systemic manifestations, and horses and cattle subjected to a swarm attack from a disturbed hive of bees or wasps have died from the envenomation. Fire ants, found in the southeastern United States, have produced serious injury and even death to livestock that are tied near an ant hill and unable to flee.

There have been no reports of scorpion envenomation in lamoids, but it is likely that stings have occurred or will occur if lamoids are exposed to these arachnids. Likewise, envenomation from the black widow spider, *Latrodectus mactans,* or the brown recluse spider (violin spider), *Loxosceles reclusa,* has not been reported. Both of these spiders are poisonous to humans but are unlikely to inflict other than transiently painful bites to animals. The bite of the brown recluse spider causes a slow-healing ulcerous wound in humans, while the black widow spider causes muscle spasms and CNS depression.

DRUG TOXICITY

No drugs have been cleared for use in lamoids by the Federal Drug Administration in the United States, and none have been tested for efficacy or safety in lamoids. Nonetheless, it is necessary to use these drugs in order to practice good medicine and surgery. That some risk may be involved in such use must be recognized. On balance, thousands of experiences indicate that lamoids tolerate the use of drugs as do other livestock species. Empirical dosages are given, usually based on size and consideration of doses between those for cattle and sheep. No unique drug idiosyncrasies have been reported in lamoids, but drug toxicities have been seen.

Suspected toxicity of chlorpyrifos was described previously. Lidocaine toxicity was described in Chapter 5. Aminoglycoside antibiotics may be nephrotoxic. Gentamicin has produced renal tubular degeneration in a llama, but the animal died from a brain abscess before assessment of the renal lesion could be completed.

Prostaglandin Toxicity

Prostaglandins are used extensively in veterinary medical practice. Numerous commercial products result in different pharmacologic effects, depending on the form of prostaglandin employed. One such, $PGF_{2\alpha}$, is prescribed as a smooth muscle activator or for its luteolytic action. The effects of $PGF_{2\alpha}$ are vasoconstriction, bronchiolar constriction, intestinal muscle contraction, uterine muscle contraction, and luteolysis if a corpus luteum is present.

Tromethamine is an aqueous solution, with benzyl alcohol as a preservative. Generally, $PGF_{2\alpha}$ is considered to be nontoxic. However, there are species differences as to effective doses. The toxic dose for lamoids is unknown, but three llama females died shortly after administration of $PGF_{2\alpha}$, used to produce luteolysis. In all cases the llamas were determined to have retained corpora lutea.

CONDITIONS OF TOXICITY. Case one was a 16-year-old female llama with a cria at side. Dinoprost tromethamine (15 mg total dose) was administered intramuscularly at 3:00 P.M. The llama was found dead the next morning. Excessive fluid was found in the lungs at necropsy.

Case two was a 7-year-old female. Dinoprost tromethamine (20 mg total dose) was administered intramuscularly at 7:00 P.M. She was found dead 1 hour later. Pulmonary edema and intestinal hyperemia were noted at necropsy.

Case three was a mature female. Miscommunication resulted in an overdose (50 mg) of dinoprost tromethamine administered intramuscularly. She was returned to the owner's ranch but died within an hour from what was described as anaphylactic shock. Although the response was immediate, it is unlikely that this was an anaphylactic response but rather a direct toxic effect of $PGF_{2\alpha}$.

Three other females have exhibited dramatic, but temporary, clinical responses to therapeutic doses of tromethamine.

CLINICAL SIGNS. The three llamas that died were not observed prior to death. The presence of pulmonary edema would indicate that they were dyspneic. The three females that developed transient signs reacted within 5 minutes. Two females rolled on the ground and foamed from the mouth. The client described periodic abdominal spasms, somewhat like hiccups.

The pharmacologic effect of producing constriction of the intestinal musculature is likely to produce spasmodic colic and the signs of colic as described. One llama was observed to become extremely dyspneic, with open- mouth breathing and marked salivation within 5 minutes of a therapeutic dose (Fig. 23.31). The three dead animals had pulmonary edema, and if they had been observed would have exhibited dyspnea and terminal signs of suffocation. Since none of the animals were examined by veterinarians, it is not known whether the heart rate was altered or if blood pressure was elevated. Prostaglandins are often used to produce abortion or initiate parturition of a term fetus. This action requires 48–72 hours.

Based on limited observations and evaluations, it would appear that colic is the primary and immediate clinical sign to be observed. Bronchiolar constriction and pulmonary edema produce dyspnea and are probably causes of death.

THERAPY. Unfortunately, no antiprostaglandins are available that can be given intravenously to counter the toxic effects of $PGF_{2\alpha}$. Signs develop rapidly and culminate within an hour by recovery or death. Unless

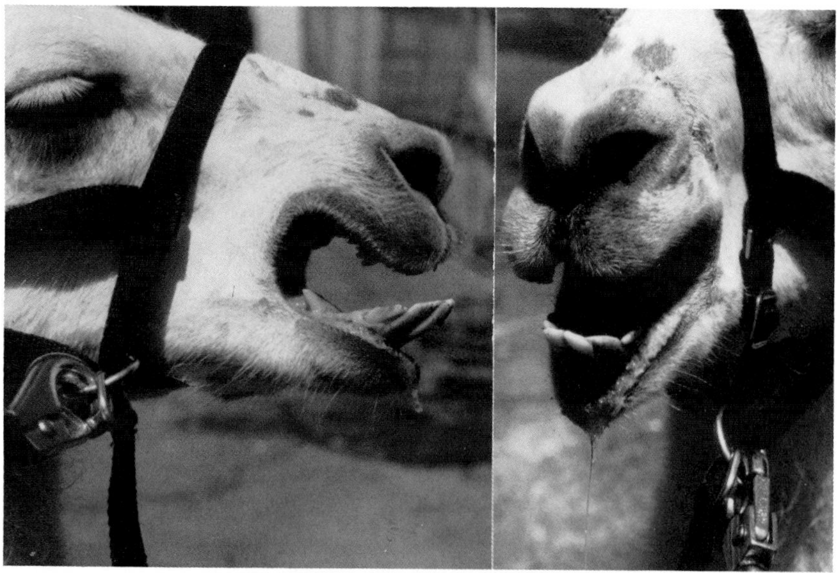

23.31 Prostaglandin $F_{2\alpha}$ toxicity.

the veterinarian had remained for an hour after administration of the drug, the animal would be dead before it could be reached.

Oxygen insufflation, via a face mask, may aid the llama with mild pulmonary edema or bronchiolar constriction. If pulmonary edema is severe, the only effective treatment is administration of oxygen under positive pressure. This requires anesthesia and tracheal intubation and is not likely to be available in the field.

COMMENTS. Prostaglandins are valuable therapeutic agents for dealing with infertility, but their use is not without risk. The animal should be kept under observation for at least an hour following administration of $PGF_{2\alpha}$. An apparatus for administration of oxygen ought to be available in the event of a reaction.

REFERENCES

1. Buck, W. B., Osweiler, G. D., and Van Gelder, G. A. 1976. Clinical and Diagnostic Veterinary Toxicology, 2nd ed. Dubuque, Iowa: Kendall/Hunt.

2. Fowler, M. E. 1968. Pyrrolizidine alkaloid poisoning in calves. J. Am. Vet. Med. Assoc. 152:1131–37.

3. ______. 1980. Plant Poisoning in Companion Animals. St Louis: Ralston Purina Co.

4. ______. 1983. Plant poisoning in freeliving wildlife: A review. J. Wildl. Dis. 19:34–43.

5. ______. 1985a. Plant poisoning in two pack llamas. Calif. Vet. 39:17–20.

6. ______. 1985b. Plant poisoning in llamas. 3L Llama 25 (Jan/Feb):23–24.

7. Fowler, M. E., Craigmill, A. L., Norman, B. B., and Michelsen, P. 1982. Livestock Poisoning Plants of California. Univ. Calif. (Berkeley) Div. Agric. Sci. Leafl. 21268.

8. Fuller, T., and McClintock, E. 1987. Poisonous Plants of California. Berkeley: Univ. of California Press.

9. Keeler, R. F., Van Kampen, K. R., and James, L. F., eds. 1978. Effects of Poisonous Plants on Livestock. New York: Academic Press.

10. Kingsbury, J. M. 1964. Poisonous Plants of the United States and Canada. Englewood Cliffs, N.J.: Prentice-Hall.

11. Lewis, W. H. 1977. Medical Botany. New York: John Wiley and Sons.

12. Pearson, E. G., Craig, A. M., and Lassen, E. D. 1986. Suspected chlorpyrifos toxicosis in a llama, and plasma pseudocholinesterase activity in llamas given chlorpyrifos. J. Am. Vet. Med. Assoc. 189:1062–64.

13. Schmitz, E. M., Freeman, B. N., and Reed, R. E. 1968. Livestock Poisoning Plants of Arizona. Tucson: Univ. of Arizona Press.

14. Youngken, H. W. 1951. Pharmaceutical Botany, 7th ed. Philadelphia: Blakiston.

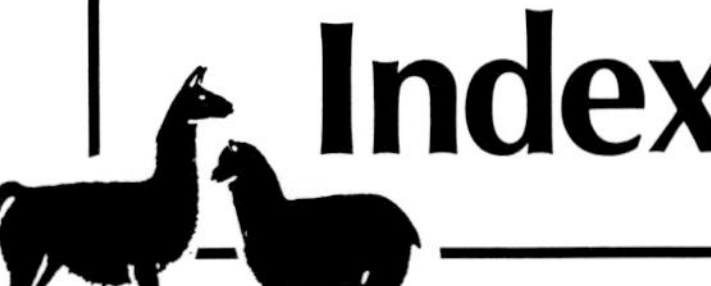

Index

Page numbers followed by f refer only to figures; page numbers followed by t refer to information found in tables.